WENNER-GREN CENTER
INTERNATIONAL SYMPOSIUM SERIES

VOLUME 22

DYNAMICS OF DEGENERATION AND GROWTH IN NEURONS

Already published in this series:

OLFACTION AND TASTE *Edited by* Y. Zotterman, 1963.

LIGHTING PROBLEMS IN HIGHWAY TRAFFIC *Edited by* E. Ingelstam, 1963.

THE STRUCTURE AND METABOLISM OF THE PANCREATIC ISLETS *Edited by* S. E. Brolin, B. Hellman and H. Knutson, 1964.

TOBACCO ALKALOIDS AND RELATED COMPOUNDS *Edited by* U. S. von Euler, 1965.

MECHANISMS OF RELEASE OF BIOGENIC AMINES *Edited by* U. S. von Euler, S. Rosell and B. Uvnäs, 1966.

COMPARATIVE LEUKAEMIA RESEARCH *Edited by* G. Winqvist, 1966.

THE FUNCTIONAL ORGANIZATION OF THE COMPOUND EYE *Edited by* C. G. Bernhard, 1966.

OLFACTION AND TASTE II *Edited by* T. Hayashi, 1967.

MAGNETIC RESONANCE IN BIOLOGICAL SYSTEMS *Edited by* A. Ehrenberg, B. G. Malmström and T. Vanngard, 1967.

STRUCTURE AND FUNCTION OF INHIBITORY NEURONAL MECHANISMS *Edited by* C. von Euler, S. Skoglund and U. Söderberg, 1967.

GROUND WATER PROBLEMS *Edited by* E. Eriksson, Y. Gustafsson and K. Nilsson, 1968.

PHYSIOLOGY AND PATHOPHYSIOLOGY OF PLASMA PROTEIN META-BOLISM *Edited by* G. Birke, R. Norberg and L.-O. Plantin, 1969.

THE POSSIBILITIES OF CHARTING MODERN LIFE, *Edited by* S. Erixon and Assisted by G. Ardwidsson and H. Hvarfner, 1970.

EVALUATION OF NOVEL PROTEIN PRODUCTS *Edited by* A. E. Bender, R. Kihlberg, B. Lofqvist and L. Munck, 1970.

VESTIBULAR FUNCTION ON EARTH AND IN SPACE *Edited by* J. Stahle, 1970.

THE STRUCTURE OF METABOLISM OF THE PANCREATIC ISLETS *Edited by* S. Falkner, B. Hellman, and I. B. Taljedal, 1970.

HUMAN ANTI-HUMAN GAMMAGLOBULINS *Edited by* R. Grubb and G. Samuelsson, 1971.

CIRCUMPOLAR PROBLEMS *Edited by* G. Berg, 1973.

International Symposium

on

Dynamics of Degeneration and Growth in Neurons
held in Wenner-Gren Center, Stockholm, May 16–18, 1973

Sponsored by

The Swedish Medical Research Council

The Wenner-Gren Center Foundation

The Committee for Cooperation between the Swedish Research Councils and the Wenner-Gren Center Foundation

Karolinska Institutet

Astra Pharmaceuticals AB

AB Bofors Nobel-Pharma

AB Ferrosan

Roche-Produkter AB

Burroughs Wellcome & Co

Sandoz AB

Squibb AB

DYNAMICS OF DEGENERATION AND GROWTH IN NEURONS

PROCEEDINGS OF THE INTERNATIONAL SYMPOSIUM
HELD IN WENNER-GREN CENTER, STOCKHOLM,
MAY 1973

Edited by

Kjell Fuxe, Lars Olson, and Yngve Zotterman

PERGAMON PRESS

Oxford · New York · Toronto
Sydney

Pergamon Press Ltd., Headington Hill Hall, Oxford

Pergamon Press Inc., Maxwell House, Fairview Park, Elmsford, New York 10523

Pergamon of Canada Ltd., 207 Queen's Quay West, Toronto 1

Pergamon Press (Aust.) Pty. Ltd., 19a Boundary Street, Rushcutters Bay, N.S.W. 2011, Australia

First edition 1974

Library of Congress Cataloging in Publication Data

International Symposium on Dynamics of Degeneration and
Growth in Neurons, Stockholm, 1973.
Dynamics of Degeneration and growth in neurons.

(Wenner-Gren Center international symposium series, v. 22)
Sponsored by the Swedish Medical Research Council and others.
1. Nervous system—Degeneration and regeneration—
Congresses. 2. Neurons—growth—Congresses. I. Fuxe,
Kjell, 1938–   ed. II. Olson, Lars, ed.
III. Zotterman, Yngve, ed. IV. Sweden. Medicinal-
styrelsen. Vetenskapliga rad. V. Title. VI. Series.
QP363.I534 1973   599'.01'88   74–7251

Printed in Great Britain by A. Wheaton & Co., Exeter
ISBN 0 08 017917 7

CONTENTS

Opening Address—Y. ZOTTERMAN   1

DEGENERATION PROCESSES IN PERIPHERAL AND CENTRAL
    NEURONS

Session I

Chairman: H. THOENEN   3

The Light and Electron Microscopical Appearance of Anterograde and Retro-
    grade Neuronal Degeneration—G. GRANT and F. WALBERG   5
The Degeneration Pattern of the Nigro-neostriatal Dopamine System after
    Electrothermic or 6-Hydroxy-Dopamine Lesions—T. HÖKFELT and U. UNGER-
    STEDT   19
Structure–Activity Correlations in Trihydroxyphenethylamines and Dihydroxy-
    tryptamines. Relationship to Cytotoxicity in Adrenergic and Serotonergic
    Neurons—J. DALY, J. LUNDSTRÖM, and C. R. CREVELING   29
Neurotoxic Action of 6-Hydroxy-Dopa on Central Catecholamine Neurons—
    CH. SACHS   43
Microfluorimetric and Neurochemical Studies on Degenerating and Regenerating
    Adrenergic Nerves—G. JONSSON   61
Late and Early Biochemical Changes in Central Catecholamine Neurons after
    Axotomy—N.-E. ANDÉN, T. MAGNUSSON, and G. STOCK   77
Biochemical and Morphological Changes after Mechanical or Chemical De-
    generation of the Dopaminergic Nigro-neostriatal Pathway—F. JAVOY, Y.
    AGID, J. GLOWINSKI, and C. SOTELO   85
Changes in Catecholamine Synthesizing Enzyme Activities during Neuronal Growth
    and Degeneration—M. GOLDSTEIN, B. ANAGNOSTE, L. S. FREEDMAN, M.
    ROFFMAN, and K. P. LELE   99
Some Aspects of the Reaction of Central and Peripheral Noradrenergic Neurons
    to Injury—D. J. REIS, R. A. ROSS, and T. H. JOH   109
Effects of Bretylium, Related Quaternary Ammonium Compounds, and Mitosis
    Inhibitors on the Degeneration Activity in the Sympathetically Innervated
    Periorbital Smooth Muscle in the Conscious Rat—D. LUNDBERG   127

v

Noradrenaline Nerve Terminals in the Rat Cerebral Cortex following Lesion of the Dorsal Noradrenaline Pathway: A Study on the Time Course of their Disappearance—P. LIDBRINK   141

Session II

Chairman: O. ERÄNKÖ   151

Studies on the Neurotoxic Properties of Hydroxylated Tryptamines—H. G. BAUMGARTEN, A. BJÖRKLUND, A. S. HORN, and H. G. SCHLOSSBERGER   153

Studies on Central 5-Hydroxytryptamine Neurons using Dihydroxytryptamines: Evidence for Regeneration of Bulbospinal 5-Hydroxytryptamine Axons and Terminals—K. FUXE, G. JONSSON, L.-G. NYGREN, and L. OLSON   169

Effects of Drugs on Sympathetic Nerve Cells and Small Intensely Fluorescent (SIF) Cells—O. ERÄNKÖ and L. ERÄNKÖ   181

The Effect of Industrial Solvents on Adrenergic Transmitter Mechanisms— B. HOLMBERG and T. MALMFORS   191

AXOPLASMIC TRANSPORT AS A MECHANISM FOR AXONAL SUPPORT AND GROWTH

Session I

Chairman: O. ERÄNKÖ   201

Dynamics and Mechanics of Neuroplasmic Flow—P. A. WEISS   203

Effects of Degeneration and Axoplasmic Transport Blockade on Synaptic Ultrastructure, Function, and Protein Composition—M. CUÉNOD, P. MARKO, E. NIEDERER, C. SANDRI, and K. AKERT   215

Axonal Transport of Proteins in Growing and Regenerating Neurons—J. SJÖSTRAND and M. FRIZELL   225

The Role of Axoplasmic Flow in Trophism of Skeletal Muscle—S. THESLEFF   237

Session II

Chairman: U. S. VON EULER   243

Differential Accumulation of Enzymes in Constricted Nerves According to their Subcellular Localization—P. LADURON   245

Importance of Axoplasmic Transport for Transmitter Levels in Nerve Terminals— J. HÄGGENDAL, A. DAHLSTRÖM, S. BAREGGI, and P.-A. LARSSON   257

Intra-axonal Transport Mechanisms in the Noradrenergic Neuron—P. BANKS and D. MAYOR   269

Proximodistal Transport of Acetylcholine in Peripheral Cholinergic Neurons— A. DAHLSTRÖM, J. HÄGGENDAL, E. HEILBRONN, P.-O. HEIWALL, and N. R. SAUNDERS   275

Axonal Transport of Dopamine-β-hydroxylase by Abnormal Human Sural Nerves—S. BRIMIJOIN and P. J. DYCK   291

GROWTH

Session I

Chairman: U. S. VON EULER   295

Control Mechanisms of the Adrenergic Neuron—R. LEVI-MONTALCINI   297

Regulation of Enzyme Synthesis by Neuronal Activity and by Nerve Growth Factor—H. THOENEN, I. A. HENDRY, K. STÖCKEL, U. PARAVICINI, and F. OESCH   315

Assay of Nerve Growth Factor (NGF) in Mouse Tissue and the Role of NGF and Depolarizing Stimuli in the Long-term Regulation of Tyrosine Hydroxylase Activity in Adrenergic Neurons—L. L. IVERSEN, I. A. HENDRY, and A. V. P. MACKAY   329

The Nerve Growth Factor Receptor: Demonstration of Specific Binding in Sympathetic Ganglia—S. H. SNYDER, S. P. BANERJEE, P. CUATRECASAS, and L. A. GREENE   347

DNA Synthesis and Cell Division in Differentiating Avian Adrenergic Neuroblasts—A. M. COHEN   359

Session II

Chairman: K. FUXE   371

Collateral Reinnervation in the Central Nervous System—G. RAISMAN   373

Growth of Adrenergic Neurons in the Adult Mammalian Nervous System—R. Y. MOORE   379

Has Nerve Growth Factor a Role in the Regeneration of Central and Peripheral Catecholamine Neurons?—A. BJÖRKLUND, B. BJERRE, and U. STENEVI   389

Session III

Chairman: K. FUXE   411

The Noradrenergic Innervation of Cerebellar Purkinje Cells: Localization, Function, Synaptogenesis and Axonal Sprouting of Locus Coeruleus—F. E. BLOOM, H. KREBS, J. NICHOLSON, and V. PICKEL   413

Biochemical Aspects of the Catecholaminergic Neurons in the Brain of the Fetal and Neonatal Rat—J. T. COYLE   425

Ontogenesis of Central and Peripheral Adrenergic Neurons in the Rat following Neonatal Treatment with 6-Hydroxydopamine—J. DE CHAMPLAIN and B. SINGH   435

Session IV

Chairman: G. BURNSTOCK   447

Agglutinins of Formalinized Erythrocytes: Changes in Activity with Development of *Dictyostelium discoideum* and Embryonic Chick Brain—S. H. BARONDES, S. D. ROSEN, D. L. SIMPSON, and J. A. KAFKA   449

Growth and Development of Cholinergic and Adrenergic Neurons in a Sympathetic Ganglion: Reciprocal Regulation at the Synapse—I. B. BLACK   455

Heterogenous Reinnervation of Sympathetic Lumbar Ganglia with Sympathetic Postganglionic Nerves—A. SURIA and S. H. KOSLOW   469

Ontogenesis of Central Noradrenaline Neurons after 6-Hydroxydopamine Treatment at Birth—CH. SACHS, C. PYCOCK, and G. JONSSON   479

Effects of Vinblastine on Peripheral Autonomic Nerves: Degeneration and Formation of New Nerve Fibers—I. HANBAUER, I. J. KOPIN, and D. M. JACOBOWITZ   485

Nerve Growth Specificity and Regulation as Revealed by Intraocular Brain Tissue Transplants—L. OLSON and Å. SEIGER   499

Degeneration and Oriented Growth of Autonomic Nerves in Relation to Smooth Muscle in Joint Tissue Cultures and Anterior Eye Chamber Transplants— G. BURNSTOCK   509

Electrophysiological and Histochemical Properties of Fetal Human Spinal Cord in Tissue Culture—L. HÖSLI, E. HÖSLI, and P. F. ANDRÈS   521

RECEPTOR CHANGES IN RELATION TO DEGENERATION AND DEVELOPMENT OF NEURONS AND DRUG TREATMENT

Session I

Chairman: S. THESLEFF   533

Autonomic Neuro-receptor Mechanisms in Brain Vessels—CH. OWMAN, L. EDVINSSON, and K. C. NIELSEN   535

Pharmacological Approaches to Monoamine Receptors during Brain Development —P. LUNDBORG and C. KELLOGG   561

Brain and Peripheral Monoamines: Possible Role in the Ontogenesis of Normal and Drug-induced Responses in the Immature Mammal—L. D. LYTLE and F. C. KEIL   575

Enhanced Accumulations of Cyclic AMP in Brain Slices Elicited by Norepinephrine after Intraventricular Pretreatment of Rats with 6-Hydroxydopamine— M. HUANG and J. W. DALY   593

Enhanced Sensitivity to the Noradrenaline Receptor Stimulating Agent, Clonidine, following Degeneration of Noradrenaline Pathways: Studies on Arterial Pressure, Heart Rate, and Respiration—P. BOLME, K. FUXE, L.-G. NYGREN, L. OLSON, and CH. SACHS   597

Learning Deficits in Offspring of the Nursing Mothers given Penfluridol— J. ENGEL, S. AHLENIUS, R. BROWN, and P. LUNDBORG   603

Effects of Pre- and Postnatal Injection of 6-Hydroxydopamine on Sleep and Biogenic Amines of Adult Rat—J. L. VALATX and J. F. PUJOL   607

OPENING ADDRESS

Yngve Zotterman

Ever since the days of Bell and Magendic the interneuronal transport of matter has been a constant source of speculation. When in 1926 I was working on the heat production of the nerve fibre with A. V. Hill in London he gave a series of lectures before a "juvenile auditory" at the Royal Institution and I have never forgotten the way he dealt with this problem saying:

"What the influence of the nerve cells is upon the fibre we have no notion. Why a nerve which may be yards long in a large animal should remain alive for many years provided it is in connection with its nerve cell, yet dies at once if the nerve cell is cut away from it, we do not know. As Sir William Hardy once pointed out in a lecture to the Chemical Society it would take almost geological time for any actual substance to be transmitted by transfusion along such a nerve fibre from the cell to which it belongs; and anything diffusing down would certainly get lost before it reached the bottom. It must presumably be something different from that, something (for want of a better name) I have called an 'influence'. Either the passage of nerve messages along a fibre is necessary for its continued health, or else there is some organization of its molecules, something analogous to the structure of a crystalline liquid transmitted from molecule to molecule along the nerve, which collapses as soon as the fibre is cut off from the influence of a similar organization in the parts lying near to it. Anyhow, the fact of this influence of the nerve cell on the nerve fibre remains and it is one of the most entrancing mysteries in biology."

The first proper advance came in the 1940s when my dear friend Paul Weiss got the crazy idea of putting *Schnürrings* on nerve stems and found that the axoplasma piled up and distended the axons centrally to the *Schnürring*. In those years the fundamental discoveries of catecholamines were being made by U. S. von Euler and others. One of Euler's assistants, C. G. Schmiterlöw, working in my laboratory at the Veterinary College, determined the content of noradrenalin in different parts of the neuron. The results gave him the idea of suggesting in his doctoral thesis in 1948 that catecholamines were synthesized in the pericaryon and transported down the axon to the terminals where they accumulated and were liberated at the arrival of the nerve impulses.

1

This transport of catecholamine was investigated in the 1960s by Annika Dahlström with the aid of the fluorescence method developed by the late Dr. Åke Hillarp. She and Jan Häggendal were the first to determine the rate of the transport of catecholamine granulas in the nerve fibre and they arrived at values of about 5–10 mm/h.

These unexpectedly high speeds raise a lot of questions which importunately insist upon solution. And with this I leave it to you ladies and gentlemen to give us in these three days your views and your deep understanding of the problems encountered in your own research concerning the dynamics of degeneration and growth of neurons.

DEGENERATION PROCESSES IN PERIPHERAL AND CENTRAL NEURONS

SESSION I

Chairman: H. THOENEN

THE LIGHT AND ELECTRON MICROSCOPICAL APPEARANCE OF ANTEROGRADE AND RETROGRADE NEURONAL DEGENERATION

GUNNAR GRANT AND FRED WALBERG

Department of Anatomy, Karolinska Institutet, Stockholm, Sweden, and Anatomical Institute, University of Oslo, Oslo, Norway

SUMMARY

A review is given of the light and electron microscopical appearance of anterograde and retrograde neuronal degeneration as this appears in neurons of the central nervous system and in ganglion cells. The three main types of anterograde degeneration are described, and details of the retrograde degeneration as this occurs in young animals are presented. The aim of the presentation is to give students interested in the tracing of neuronal connections a description of the neuronal changes that can safely be relied upon in experimental studies.

INTRODUCTION

The transection of axons in vertebrates leads to marked morphological changes, peripheral as well as central to the lesion. The changes are very characteristic and are usually more pronounced in newborn animals. In the present report a review is given of the light and electron microscopical appearance of anterograde and retrograde degenerative changes as these occur in neurons within the central nervous system and in ganglion cells that send their axons to the spinal cord and brain stem. The review will mainly be based on findings in the cat, but reference will be made to other mammals and to submammalian species. Transneuronal changes will not be included in this report. Neither will the glial reactions related to degenerative changes in the neurons be considered in detail. Students interested in the problems reviewed here will benefit from the comprehensive report by Raisman and Matthews (1972). Valuable information is also found in the monograph edited by Nauta and Ebbesson (1970).

ANTEROGRADE NEURONAL DEGENERATION

1. THE LIGHT MICROSCOPICAL APPEARANCE OF ANTEROGRADE DEGENERATION

Although the Marchi method in the hands of experienced neuroanatomists has given valuable information as to the origin and termination of degenerating fiber tracts (see especially Smith, 1951, 1956a, b; Smith *et al.*, 1956), it is clear that this method is no longer used routinely in neurobiological laboratories. One reason for this is obviously that only degenerating myelin and not the axoplasm itself is stained when this method is used. Degenerating unmyelinated fiber tracts can therefore not be studied with the Marchi method, and myelinated fiber systems can only be followed to the region where myelin terminates. Ultrastructural studies from the last two decades have, however, shown that afferent fibers to many nuclei and regions especially within the spinal cord and brain stem are covered with myelin almost to the region where the boutons emerge. The Marchi method can therefore in such regions be used since fibers down to about 0.5μ are impregnated. The Marchi "dust" is in these areas showing the terminal field of the afferent fibers. In spite of this fact the Marchi method has, however, not regained its earlier popularity, and it remains to be seen whether the method will be able to compete with all the currently applied silver methods.

Some of the silver impregnation methods used today visualize normal as well as degenerating neurons. Others are modifications which allow silver percipitate to occur mostly (only) on degenerating structures. The early methods, such as the Bielschowsky, the Reumont Lhermitte, and the Glees techniques, belong to the first group, the so-called "nonsuppressive" stains. Although in some laboratories valuable information has been collected with nonsuppressive stains, it was only after the introduction of the Nauta modifications (the Nauta–Gygax and Nauta–Laidlaw techniques; see Nauta, 1957) that the silver methods became popular. The Nauta–Gygax and Nauta–Laidlaw modifications are in many laboratories today standard methods.

Successfully impregnated Nauta–Gygax or Nauta–Laidlaw sections permit the student to trace in great detail degenerating fibers from a damaged area to the field of termination of the fibers. The degenerating fibers are easily seen, and stand out clearly against a yellowish or brown background, where in optimal sections the staining of normal fibers is negligible.

The light microscopical appearance of fiber degeneration in Nauta sections is very characteristic. The degenerating coarse axons appear as black fragmented fibers. The argyrophilic particles are often lying in a row so that the course of the fibers can be followed. The argyrophilic particles are irregularly outlined, beaded, and tortous.

The light microscopical picture has a somewhat different appearance in areas where the fibers terminate. The thin fragmented degenerating fibers present in a terminal region have a very beaded appearance. Furthermore, the smallest particles observed in the light microscope are irregular, oval, or round. They can lie close to perikarya or be more freely dispersed in the neuropil.†

Although it is quite clear that the Nauta–Gygax and Nauta–Laidlaw modifications give a good indication of the field of termination for a fiber tract, considerable difficulties are involved when the student tries to interpret the nature of the argyrophilic particles present in the sections. The coarser particles are, of course, local deposit of silver in thick degenerating fibers, but it is virtually impossible from light microscopical sections alone to reveal whether the smallest argyrophilic particles in a section partly (or only) are degenerating terminal fibers, or also (only) degenerating boutons. We had no possibility to make statement on this important point until the electron microscope was introduced into neuro-

---

† Pericellular aborization of such small argyrophilic particles is very characteristic, and was earlier considered to be a sign of axosomatic distribution of afferent fibers. Electron microscopy has shown that these particles in many regions to a great extent are fragments of terminal myelinated fibers.

biological research. At the time when the electron microscope became available, evidence had, however, emerged which quite clearly showed that the Nauta modifications were not optimal for the demonstration of degenerating boutons (Heimer, 1967). Heimer had thus been able to convincingly demonstrate that the modified silver impregnation method introduced by Fink and himself (1967) permitted degenerating boutons to be visualized in areas where the Nauta method failed to show degeneration (see also Heimer and Wall, 1968). Electron microscopy of silver-stained Nauta and Fink–Heimer stained sections have substantiated the information obtained in the light microscope (Heimer, 1970; Heimer and Peters, 1968; Walberg, 1971, 1972).

The Fink–Heimer method should be used when information is wanted concerning the distribution of afferent fibers as well as their boutons in the area of termination for these fibers. Of great importance is, however, that the fine dust, i.e. the degenerating boutons and fine terminal axonal ramifications, only occurs at certain critical survival times. The reason for this is that the degenerating terminal structures in many places are removed by glial cells shortly after the onset of degeneration. Since, thus, the fine dust in Fink–Heimer sections obviously demonstrates degenerating boutons and fine terminal axonal ramifications, it is advantageous for the student to have a detailed knowledge of the glial activity and of the speed with which degenerating terminal structures are removed in a nucleus. This requires electron microscopy of the area. Good results may, however, also be obtained without concomitant electron microscopical investigations. A sequence of series where the interval between the survival times is very short, can give the student the necessary information.

2. THE ELECTRON MICROSCOPICAL APPEARANCE OF ANTEROGRADE DEGENERATION

The experimental electron microscopical studies made in the last decade have shown that there are three types of morphological changes that can be observed when fiber tracts are damaged in the central nervous system. They are observed in mammals as well as in sub-mammalian species. However, the same fiber system can in different species react differently (the optic tract is a particularly good example, see below). The reason for this is at present unclear. Histochemical and biochemical studies may clarify whether there is a relation between the morphological appearance of the degeneration and the chemical reactions leading to disintegration of the neuron.

Some students have given evidence for the existence of types of degeneration diverging from those to be described here. Since these descriptions are based on observations made only in a few places, unexperienced students should not use these criteria alone for a safe identification of degenerating axons and boutons. These changes are briefly considered at the end of this chapter.

The Dark Type of Degeneration

The dark type of degeneration is conspicuous and easily diagnosed. The reaction was first described by Colonnier and Gray (1962). The most striking feature is the darkening of the degenerating boutons. This is largely due to the appearance of a finely granular background substance of the matrix in which the vesicles and mitochondria are included. The darkening is probably also caused by a shrinkage of the bouton. The degenerating bouton therefore often develops an indented outline which contrasts sharply with the normal shape.

Most mitochondria become dark. Their inner architecture changes, and this leads to a disrupture of the organelle or to a shrinkage. Other degenerating mitochondria appear initially to swell. The darkening of the bouton leads ultimately to a disappearance of vesicles and mitochondria, so that it virtually may be impossible to identify any organelles in the matrix.

The experimental observations made in the early 1960s appeared to indicate that there was a relation between the morphology of the degenerating bouton and the survival time. Such observations were taken as an indication that it could be possible to map the relative distribution of two afferent pathways ending within the same area if an operated animal after a certain survival time was reoperated and allowed to survive for a few more days. The evidence later gathered showed that this assumption was wrong. Double operations can therefore not be used in this way in experimental electron microscopy. (The technique can, however, be used if two fiber systems ending in the same area react differently on a lesion; see Walberg and Mugnaini, 1969.)

Degenerating terminal myelinated and unmyelinated fibers show matrix changes similar to those observed in the boutons. The myelinated thin fibers (about 0.5 μ in diameter) shrink and swell, and this leads to the light microscopically well-known beading and fragmentation of the terminal fibers seen in silver sections. Thick myelinated degenerating fibers are also easily identified in electron micrographs since their degenerating axoplasm shows the same dark reaction as does that of the terminal myelinated fibers. Concomitant degenerative changes of the myelin sheath are, however, difficult to recognize. Such changes appear to occur only after very long survival times.

The Filamentous Type of Degeneration

Degenerating boutons of the filamentous type are very characteristic. The boutons show a conspicuous swelling, and their main constituent is a filamentous material arranged in bundles or groups running in different directions. The synaptic vesicles are in such boutons easily recognized, and are grouped in the center of the swelling bouton together with the mitochondria, or are located close to the plasmalemma. Crowding of synaptic vesicles at the synaptic specialization of the membrane may be observed. The number of vesicles appears to be reduced, but this may be deceptive on account of the degenerating boutons being much larger than the normal ones.

The mitochondria, like the synaptic vesicles, are located either in the center or peripherally in the degenerating boutons. They are mostly normal, a finding that conspicuously contrasts to what is observed in degenerating boutons of the dark type. However, changed mitochondrial profiles may be encountered. Such mitochondria have cristae with unusual patterns (Mugnaini and Walberg, 1967). Furthermore, some boutons can show tubular or saccular smooth-surfaced profiles, which lie close to mitochondria or to the plasmalemma. All structural components mentioned here: filaments, synaptic vesicles, mitochondria, and smooth-surfaced profiles, lie dispersed in an electron lucid matrix.

Degenerating myelinated fibers, terminal and larger, are also characterized by an unusual amount of filaments in the axoplasm. The fibers are very characteristic, and swollen and constricted portions give them a beaded appearance. The smooth endoplasmic reticulum can be hypertrophic, but microtubules are scarce or absent in the swellings. Myelin changes are not observed. Boutons *en passant* can be connected to other boutons by constricted unmyelinated fibers.

The filamentous type of degeneration was first described by Gray and Hamlyn (1962) in the optic tectum of the chick. Later studies have shown that the filamentous reaction occurs in certain fiber systems in the central nervous system in various animal species. However, the same fiber system does not always show the same reaction. Thus, whereas the retino-geniculate fibers primarily react with a neurofilamentous degeneration in the cat (Szentá-gothai et al., 1966) and monkey (see especially Colonnier and Guillery, 1964; Glees et al., 1966, Guillery, 1965), the same pathway shows an electron dense reaction in the rat (McMahon, 1967). The causes for this difference are poorly understood. Jones and Rockel (1973) have recently, based on findings in the inferior colliculus, postulated that an ac-cumulation of shell fragments from complex vesicles is a necessary prerequisite for a neuro-filamentous reaction, and that the protein of the shells is reorganized into neurofilaments.

Although such postulates are interesting, it is only from chemical studies that decisive information can be obtained. The pilot study by Cuénod et al. (1973) is a valuable first effort to verify the type of protein that disappears during the filamentous type of degenera-tion. After removal of the retina in the pigeon the authors observed that one component of the protein (the pt band) decreased or disappeared within a few days.† Comparative biochemical studies could reveal interesting differences between optic tract fibers of various vertebrate species. Another fiber system to compare is the cerebellar Purkinje cell axons and boutons which so far have been studied with the electron microscope in operated rats and cats (Sotelo, 1968; Mugnaini and Walberg, 1967).

Light microscopists who want to study degenerating filamentous fiber systems while these exclusively show the filamentous type of degeneration should not rely upon the Nauta–Laidlaw or the Fink–Heimer techniques. The Eager method should be tried. This has been demonstrated in a recent electron microscopical study (Walberg, 1972). Since only the three mentioned methods were examined in the study, it is not clear whether any silver modifica-tions other than the Eager technique can be used.

The Pale (Electron-lucent) Type of Degeneration

Experimental studies from the last years have given evidence that there is also a third type of initial reaction of degenerating axons and boutons in the central nervous system. This type of reaction was first described in detail by Anderson and Westrum (1972), who made their observations in the olfactory tubercle of the rat. Their observations extend information given in reports from previous students who have mentioned an electron-lucent type of degeneration (for reference, see O'Neal and Westrum, 1973).

The operated animals show initially a reduction in the number of synaptic vesicles with a tendency for the remaining ones to gather into one or more clusters in the boutons. No alteration in vesicle morphology is observed. The cytoplasmic matrix is electron-lucent, and the degenerating boutons become distended with swollen mitochondria. Similar

---

† We are, however, here dealing with a very complex process, since filamentous degenerating fibers and boutons after a certain survival time in some species are transformed to dark structures. Transformation of filamentous degenerating fibers and boutons was first described in the cat by Mugnaini and Walberg (1967). The same sequence is observed in the pigeon (Cuénod et al., 1970). A similar process was not considered to occur in the monkey (see Colonnier and Guillery, 1964; Glees et al., 1966; Pecci-Saavedra et al., 1969; Levay, 1971). Recent studies have, however, clearly demonstrated that filamentous degenerating fibers and boutons also in the monkey at later survival stages show an increased electron density (Wong-Riley, 1972a). McMahon's (1967) detailed study in the rat has, however, failed to show an initial filamentous reaction of the degenerating optic fibers and terminals of this animal. He studied rats from 1 day after enucleation to 300 days after operation.

alterations are found in degenerating terminal axons which, because of their electron-lucent matrix and swollen mitochondria, can easily be distinguished from normal fibers. O'Neal and Westrum (1973) recently observed the same changes in the lateral cuneate nucleus of the cat, in which they have been able to demonstrate that degenerating fibers and boutons showing this type of reaction are gradually transformed to degenerating structures of the electron-dense type. The transformation to the electron-dense type occurs, however, very rapidly, and the electron-lucent type of degeneration may therefore escape recognition if the survival times of the animals are not appropriately selected. O'Neal and Westrum (1973) have given a clear documentation of this important point. Grofová and Rinvik (in prep.) have recently described the same type of changes in the nucleus ventralis lateralis thalami, following lesions of the entopeduncular nucleus in the cat.

Other Types of Degenerative Reactions

Several students have described changes in neuronal organelles as signs to be used for an identification of the earliest stages of axonal and bouton degeneration. Such changes are, however, not consistently found, and are not always easy to detect. Some of them may also be characteristic only of some fiber systems and certain species.

Vesicle flattening as a result of degeneration has been noted by several students (see, e.g., Holländer *et al.*, 1969), and initial swelling or shrinkage resulting in electron density of mitochondria has also been reported, as has also hypertrophy of the smooth endoplasmic reticulum. In addition, swollen synaptic vesicles have been reported to be an early sign of bouton degeneration (Pinching, 1969; Akert *et al.*, 1971; Cuénod *et al.*, 1970). Accumulation of glycogen in degenerating boutons has also been described. We will, however, warn unexperienced students against an acceptance of *such criteria alone* as sufficient in operated animals for a classification of boutons and axons as being in a state of degeneration. Sotelo and Palay (1971) have shown convincingly that an increase in the density of the cytoplasmic matrix, hyperplasia of the cisternae of the smooth endoplasmic reticulum, formation of concentric laminar arrays, assemblies of closely packed parallel tubules, giant mitochondria, decreased number of synaptic vesicles, and an increased number of lysosomes, not infrequently are observed in unoperated rats. Some of these apparently "degenerative" changes, which according to Sotelo and Palay (1971) probably reflect a continuing re-modelling of synaptic connections in unoperated animals, have also been observed in unoperated cats (see, e.g., Walberg, 1966). Such observations make it imperative to make a detailed ultrastructural analysis of so-called normal animals before any operations are performed. We would because of this highly *recommend that only the three above-mentioned types of degeneration are used by unexperienced students in electron microscopical studies of fiber projections.* The "pale" type of reaction should, furthermore, only be relied upon if a transformation from this to the dark type of reaction is observed.

RETROGRADE NEURONAL DEGENERATION

In the adult central nervous system the retrograde cellular reaction after a peripheral nerve lesion is usually followed by a restitution of the neuron. In some instances, however, the retrograde reaction is followed by a degeneration and disappearance of the neuron. This degeneration, which can be demonstrated with the suppressive silver techniques, starts with the perikaryon and the dendrites and is followed by a degeneration of the axon (and the myelin sheath) proceeding distalward from the cell body. The same type of degeneration may also occur in neurons of nuclei in the central nervous system which do not send their axons out of it.

Although this retrograde neuronal degeneration may occur in the adult nervous system, it is more easily provoked in the immature nervous system (Grant, 1970). This is most probably due to the fact that the retrograde reaction after axonal lesions seems to be much more intense in immature neurons than in adult ones (see, e.g., Brodal, 1940; La Velle and La Velle, 1958b). With this fact in mind the retrograde neuronal degeneration has been studied in the immature nervous system during the last years both at the light microscopical level, with the aid of suppressive silver technique, and at the electron microscopical level (see Grant, 1970). It has then turned out that retrograde neuronal degeneration has been possible to provoke in all neuronal populations examined so far.

1. LIGHT AND ELECTRON MICROSCOPICAL APPEARANCE OF RETROGRADE NEURONAL DEGENERATION

Cells

The retrograde cellular *reaction* after an axonal lesion can be demonstrated with the aid of ordinary Nissl stains. These have, therefore, been used extensively in studies where lesions have been made with the aim to localize cells of origin of various peripheral nerves and nerve fiber tracts. The modified Gudden method of Brodal (1939, 1940), which makes use of the fact that nerve cells of very young animals seem to be more susceptible to axon damage than nerve cells of adult animals, has proved especially valuable for such studies. Several, sometimes all, of the morphologically changed Nissl stained nerve cells shown with that method have been in a state of degeneration or on the way to degenerate, since prolonged postoperative survival periods were demonstrated to result in a loss of nerve cells (see, e.g., Brodal, 1939). However, specific techniques for demonstrating degenerating neurons were not available until the introduction of the suppressive silver techniques.

In silver-impregnated material from immature animals, the characteristic cells undergoing a retrograde neuronal degeneration have an appearance which very much resembles Golgi impregnated nerve cells but with the exception that the nuclei of the cells do not seem to be completely impregnated (Grant and Aldskogius, 1967; Grant, 1968). The impregnation of the cell nucleus seems to be restricted to one or a few small globules. These might be degenerating nucleolar material (cf. La Velle and La Velle, 1958a). By embedding ordinary silver-impregnated sections containing impregnated cells in Araldite and preparing semithin sections from this material, it has been possible to study the impregnation of the cells more in detail (Grant and Holländer; in preparation). These studies have shown that the cell nucleus escapes impregnation except for the type of globules mentioned. In addition they have demonstrated the occurrence of vacuoles in such globules, a finding which may be of interest when considering the observations of vacuolation of nucleoli in connection with the chromatolytic reaction after axonal lesions (see, e.g., Lieberman, 1971).

Strongly argyrophilic cells with an appearance very similar to that described for the cells in the immature animals have been reported also in material from adult animals. Campos-Ortega *et al.* (1970) found such cells in the lateral geniculate and the inferior and lateral pulvinar nuclei of young adult macaque monkeys following visual cortical lesions.† Heimer

† See footnote on p. 12.

(1968) demonstrated similar cells in the prepyriform cortex of rats following olfactory bulb lesions. He used both young and adult rats for his experiments. Although it does not appear from his description in which type of animals the cells were encountered, they were found in both young and adult rats (Heimer, personal communication).

In some instances in adult animals only a faint impregnation of cells may occur. Guillery (1959), Cragg (1962), and Powell and Cowan (1964) described fine, diffuse, granular deposits of silver in Nauta-impregnated preparations from thalamic nuclei of cats and rabbits following cortical lesions. This deposit, which they interpreted as caused by an impregnation of remnants of perikarya (and dendrites) in a state of retrograde degeneration, was clearly visible only under high power view.

In a study on retrograde neuronal degeneration in the lateral cervical nucleus of the kitten, Grant and Westman (1969) shortly described the electron microscopical appearance of a few structures which they interpreted as nerve cells in a state of retrograde cellular degeneration. Recently, however, Torvik published an investigation of the facial nucleus of newborn rabbits, part of which was devoted to the question of the electron microscopical appearance of retrograde cellular degeneration and in which more detailed observations were made (Torvik, 1972). He compared the appearance of retrograde cellular degeneration with that of retrograde cellular regeneration of the same neuronal system, which was also examined (Torvik and Söreide, 1972). The two types of reactions were achieved by nerve section and crush lesion of the nerve, respectively. After an initial period of retrograde changes, which were identical in the two different situations, the nerve cells developed the changes interpreted as characteristic of degeneration and regeneration, respectively. The degenerative changes comprised a rapid disappearance of the cisterns of the granular endoplasmic reticulum and a disaggregation of the ribosomal clusters and membrane bound ribosomes into free single elements (Torvik, 1972). These latter changes were considered as "true degenerative phenomena". That polyribosomal disaggregation would necessarily be a degenerative phenomenon has been questioned, however (Barron et al., 1973). The degenerative process was also reported to comprise a rapid depletion of most of the other cytoplasmic and nuclear organelles. The regenerative changes described will not be commented upon here.

Ultrastructural observations on retrograde nerve cell degeneration in adult animals have been made in some recent studies (e.g. Torvik and Skjörten, 1971; Wong-Riley, 1972;[†] Barron et al., 1973[†]). An increased electron density and densely packed mitochondria seem to be two common characteristic features of the degenerative nerve cells most often encountered.

Dendrites

With suppressive silver techniques, retrograde degeneration of dendrites is characteristically visualized as beaded strands of fibers emerging from an impregnated perikaryon. Usually these can be traced only a few cell diameters away from the cell body in the same section. The reason for this is probably not poor impregnation of degenerating dendrites, but that the impregnated sections are usually not thicker than about 20 μ. Occasionally, ramifications into dendritic branches of higher orders can be seen.

† The findings were made in thalamic nuclei after cortical lesions. Because of the reciprocal connections which exist between thalamic nuclei and the cerebral cortex, a transneuronal effect can therefore not be ruled out. That such an effect would be the single cause of the degeneration does not seem probable, however. Deafferentation of a nucleus may, however, probably add to the retrograde effect caused by transection of axons from that nucleus so as to result in degeneration (cf. Glees et al., 1951).

Dendrites of this type were first described in material from immature animals (Grant, 1965; see also Grant, 1970). Campos-Ortega *et al.* (1970) have, however, demonstrated the occurrence of an obviously identical type of dendrite in continuity with impregnated perikarya in the pulvinar and the lateral geniculate nucleus of young adult macaque monkeys (cf. above). As was mentioned above, some investigators (Guillery, 1959; Cragg, 1962; Powell and Cowan, 1964) have described a fine, diffuse, granular deposit of silver in Nauta-impregnated sections from thalamic nuclei of adult cats and rabbits following cortical lesions. This deposit, which was clearly visible only under high power view, was interpreted as impregnation of remnants of dendrites (and perikarya) in a state of retrograde degeneration.

In studies on retrograde neuronal degeneration in the lateral cervical nucleus of kittens, Grant and Westman (1968, 1969) described the electron microscopical appearance of retrograde degeneration of dendrites. The dendritic profiles were characterized by an increased electron density, which was very similar to that found during the dark type of anterograde fiber degeneration. They contained large mitochondria, which were sometimes fragmented. Occasionally these electron-dense dendrites showed bundles of filaments and small dense granules. After short postoperative survival periods the dendrites were found to be beset with apparently normal synaptic contacts. In animals with longer survival times a larger part of the dendritic surface appeared to be covered with astroglial cell processes. Even in these cases, however, the boutons showed a normal appearance.

Although the electron-dense type of degenerating dendrites described above were found in immature animals, later observations on electron microscopical material have demonstrated their occurrence also in adult animals (see, e.g., Wong-Riley, 1972b).

Axons—Myelin Sheaths

Fiber degeneration in association with retrograde neuronal degeneration was described in Marchi studies already around the turn of this century (e.g. Bregman, 1892; van Gehuchten, 1903; see also review by Beresford, 1965). van Gehuchten (1903, 1906) seems to have made the most informative and most extensive study of this type of fiber degeneration. He produced the degeneration by pulling various nerves in adult rabbits. Among other things he deduced from his experiments that rapid atrophy followed by cell death was the phenomenon on which the degeneration was based. In these early studies on Marchi-impregnated material it was also demonstrated that the degeneration, which closely resembled Wallerian degeneration, had a proximo-distal progression starting close to the cell body and proceeding in a distal direction. This progression of the degeneration has later been confirmed in material impregnated with silver according to the Nauta techniques (Cowan *et al.*, 1961). Furthermore, it was shown that the degeneration appeared later than the Wallerian degeneration affecting the fiber peripheral to the lesion. This is compatible with the mechanism that the degeneration of the fiber is caused indirectly via an effect on the cell perikaryon following the lesion of the fiber. van Gehuchten proposed the term "indirect Wallerian degeneration" for this special type of fiber degeneration. He suggested that this term should replace the currently used expressions "retrograde fiber degeneration" and "ascending degeneration". We do indeed agree in this suggestion, since it also helps to prevent confusion with the true retrograde changes occurring close to a lesion.†

† Originally Grant and collaborators included in this term also the retrograde changes affecting the cell body and the dendrites. Later they found it more appropriate to reserve the term indirect Wallerian degeneration solely for the changes affecting the axon with the surrounding myelin sheath (see p. 185 in Grant, 1970).

With suppressive silver techniques, indirect Wallerian fiber degeneration may appear as ordinary "direct" Wallerian degeneration with pictures suggesting axon fragmentation and vacuolation. A much more striking feature, however, which has been found in studies on young animals is a granulation along the course of the fibers (Grant and Aldskogius, 1967; Grant and Westman, 1969). Whether this is due to a very rapid breakdown of the fibers in the young animals or to other factors, is at present not known.

Whereas the electron microscopical appearance of retrograde cellular and dendritic degeneration is fairly well known, it was not until recently that the ultrastructural fiber changes were described. In a short abstract, Aldskogius (1973) reported on indirect Wallerian fiber degeneration in kitten hypoglossal neurons. About one week after the operation he found degenerative changes in the intramedullary root fibers on the side of the operation. The axoplasm had a dark appearance and was in many fibers disintegrated. The myelin sheaths were extensively split and disrupted, and often formed myelin bodies. In addition to these degenerative fiber changes, glial cell changes and signs of phagocytosis were reported. After longer postoperative survival periods the number of nerve fibers seemed to be reduced.

CONCLUDING REMARKS AS REGARDS RETROGRADE AND ANTEROGRADE NEURONAL DEGENERATION USED AS "MARKING" TECHNIQUES

Whereas anterograde degeneration has been a well known phenomenon widely used for tracing neuronal connections, retrograde degeneration has attracted very little attention. This is most probably due to the fact that this type of degeneration has been observed only exceptionally in the adult nervous system. Most frequently it seems to have been observed in thalamic nuclei after cortical lesions.† van Gehuchten (1903, 1906), who has made the most extensive investigation on indirect Wallerian degeneration in adult animals, was successful in provoking such degeneration in various peripheral rabbit motor nerves. He produced the degeneration by pulling the nerves and made it visible with the aid of the Marchi technique. He used this approach for tracing the intramedullary course of the motor nerves.

In the immature nervous system, cell loss or a heavy retrograde cellular reaction in response to axonal transection have been well known phenomena which have been used for localizing the cellular origin of various nerve fiber tracts (Gudden, 1870;‡ Brodal, 1940). It is not until recently, however, that retrograde neuronal degeneration has been investigated in detail in immature animals (see above). It has by these experiments turned out that this type of degeneration can be provoked in all neuronal populations examined so far. Furthermore, it has been shown to be possible to visualize the degeneration both by light and electron microscopical techniques. From a practical point of view it seems, therefore, that retrograde neuronal degeneration applied to the immature nervous system could be used as a basis for an additional neuroanatomical tracing or "marking" technique. This should then make possible the selective identification of the whole neuron proximal to an axon transection. It seems that this might be especially valuable at the electron microscopical level, where the problems of identifying specific populations of neurons, including dendritic

† See footnote on p. 12.

‡ As commented upon by Brodal (1940), Gudden originally did not realize that the cellular changes which he observed were of a retrograde nature.

and axonal arborizations, are great. Since the boutons contacting neurons in a state of retrograde degeneration can retain their normal ultrastructural appearance (see above), it should be possible, for the purpose of tracing neuronal connections, to combine the retrograde technique with selective transection of various afferent fiber systems terminating on the "marked" neurons. The anterograde degenerating boutons contacting the retrograde changed cells could after such double operations be identified electron microscopically.

The fact that the technique described above is based upon the use of very young animals, where morphological maturational changes can still be expected, is naturally a limiting factor. This has been commented upon earlier (see Grant, 1970). It is therefore of importance that retrograde neuronal degeneration may be brought about also in older animals, although their neurons are more resistant to axonal damage. A detailed knowledge of the various factors known to be of importance for causing the retrograde cellular response is therefore necessary for the strategy to be used for provoking retrograde degeneration in adult neurons.†

Another way to use retrograde neuronal degeneration for a tracing of neuronal connections has been described by Grant et al. (1970). They transected peripheral branches of the vestibular nerve in very young rabbits and found degeneration centrally within regions of the vestibular nuclei known to receive primary vestibular fibers. Electron microscopy confirmed that the degeneration was terminal (i.e. included degenerating boutons). The central‡ degeneration was interpreted as secondary to a "retrograde" degeneration of the ganglion cells following transection of their peripheral branches. This was found permissible since the time course indicated that the central degeneration had not been caused by a primary affection of the ganglion cells.

Recently, Grant and Arvidsson have found a corresponding type of degeneration in the trigeminal nuclei of kittens following transection of the mandibular or the ophthalmic branches of the Vth nerve (unpublished observations). In this instance a primary affection of the ganglion cells could definitely be excluded since the nerves were cut very peripherally and precautions were taken not to cause traction of the nerves at the operations.

These last described findings indicate that it is possible to make selective mapping in the central nervous system of centrally directed fibers of ganglion cells subjected to lesions of their peripheral branches. Thereby the obstacle presented by the sensory ganglia may be overcome. Future experiments will show whether also adult animals can be used for such studies.

REFERENCES

AKERT, K., CUÉNOD, M., and MOOR, H. (1971) Further observations on the enlargement of synaptic vesicles in degenerating optic nerve terminals of the avian tectum. *Brain Res.* **25**, 255–263.

ALDSKOGIUS, H. (1973) Indirect Wallerian degeneration in the hypoglossal nerve of the kitten. An electron microscopical study. *J. Ultrastruct. Res.* **42**, 409 (Abstract).

ANDERSON, C. A., and WESTRUM, L. E. (1972) An electron microscopic study of the normal synaptic relationships and early degenerative changes in the rat olfactory tubercle. *Z. Zellforsch.* **127**, 462–482.

BARRON, K. D., MEANS, E. D., and LARSEN, E. (1973) Ultrastructure of retrograde degeneration in thalamus of rat. I. Neuronal somata and dendrites. *J. Neuropathol. Expl. Neurol.* **32**, 218–244.

BERESFORD, W. A. (1965) A discussion on retrograde changes in nerve fibres. In *Progress in Brain Research*, vol. 14: *Degeneration Patterns in the Nervous System* (M. Singer and J. P. Schadé, eds.), pp. 33–56, Elsevier, Amsterdam.

---

† It is also possible that a deafferentation of a nerve cell group may facilitate the retrograde response to an axonal transection (see also footnote on p. 12).

‡ The term central is here used for the ganglion cell axon entering the brain stem.

BREGMAN, E. (1892) Über experimentelle aufsteigende Degeneration motorischer und sensibler Hirnnerven. *Arb. neurol. Inst. Univ. Wien* **1**, 73–97.

BRODAL, A. (1939) Experimentelle Untersuchungen über retrograde Zellveränderungen in der unteren Olive nach Läsionen des Kleinhirns. *Z. ges. Neurol. Psychiat.* **166**, 646–704.

BRODAL, A. (1940) Modification of Gudden method for study of cerebral localization. *Archs. Neurol.* **43**, 46–58.

CAMPOS-ORTEGA, J. A., HAYHOW, W. R., and CLÜVER, P. F. DE V. (1970) The descending projections from the cortical visual fields of Macaca Mulatta with particular reference to the question of a cortico-lateral geniculate-pathway. *Brain Behav. Evol.* **3**, 368–414.

COLONNIER, M., and GRAY, E. G. (1962) Degeneration in the cerebral cortex. In *Electron Microscopy*, Fifth International Congress for Electron Microscopy, vol. 1, p. U-3 (S. S. Breese Jr., ed.), Academic Press, New York and London.

COLONNIER, M., and GUILLERY, R. W. (1964) Synaptic organization in the lateral geniculate nucleus of the monkey. *Z. Zellforsch.* **62**, 333–355.

COWAN, W. M., ADAMSON, L., and POWELL, T. P. S. (1961) An experimental study of the avian visual system. *J. Anat. Lond.* **95**, 545–563.

CRAGG, B. G. (1962) Centrifugal fibers to the retina and olfactory bulb, and composition of the supraoptic commissures in the rabbit. *Expl. Neurol.* **5**, 406–427.

CUÉNOD, M., SANDRI, C., and AKERT, K. (1970) Enlarged synaptic vesicles as an early sign of secondary degeneration in the optic nerve terminals of the pigeon. *J. Cell Sci.* **6**, 605–613.

CUÉNOD, M., MARKO, P., and NIEDERER, E. (1973) Disappearance of particulate tectal protein during optic nerve degeneration in the pigeon. *Brain Res.* **49**, 422–426.

FINK, R. P., and HEIMER, L. (1967) Two methods for selective silver impregnation of degenerating axons and their synaptic endings in the central nervous system. *Brain Res.* **4**, 369–374.

GLEES, P., SOLER, J., and BAILEY, R. A. (1951) Retrograde axonal changes of the de-afferentated nucleus gracilis following mid-brain tractotomy. *J. Neurol. Neurosurg. Psychiat.* **14**, 281–286.

GLEES, P., MELLER, K., and ESCHNER, J. (1966) Terminal degeneration in the lateral geniculate body of the monkey; an electron-microscope study. *Z. Zellforsch.* **71**, 29–40.

GRANT, G. (1965) Degenerative changes in dendrites following axonal transection. *Experientia* **21**, 722.

GRANT, G. (1968) Silver impregnation of degenerating dendrites, cells and axons central to axonal transection: II, A Nauta study on spinal motor neurones in kittens. *Expl. Brain Res.* **6**, 284–293.

GRANT, G. (1970) Neuronal changes central to the site of axon transection: A method for the identification of retrograde changes in perikarya, dendrites and axons by silver impregnation. In *Contemporary Research Methods in Neuroanatomy* (W. J. H. Nauta and S. O. E. Ebbesson, eds.), pp. 173–185, Springer, Berlin, Heidelberg, and New York.

GRANT, G., and ALDSKOGIUS, H. (1967) Silver impregnation of degenerating dendrites, cells and axons central to axonal transection: I, A Nauta study on the hypoglossal nerve in kittens. *Expl. Brain Res.* **3**, 150–162.

GRANT, G., and WESTMAN, J. (1968) Degenerative changes in dendrites central to axonal transection: electron microscopical observations. *Experientia* **24**, 169–170.

GRANT, G., and WESTMAN, J. (1969) The lateral cervical nucleus in the cat: IV, A light and electron microscopical study after midbrain lesions with demonstration of indirect Wallerian degeneration at the ultrastructural level. *Expl. Brain Res.* **7**, 51–67.

GRANT, G., EKVALL, L., and WESTMAN, J. (1970) Transganglionic degeneration in the vestibular nerve. In *Vestibular Function on Earth and in Space* (J. Stahle, ed.), pp. 301–305, Pergamon Press, Oxford and New York.

GRAY, E. G., and HAMLYN, L. H. (1962) Electron microscopy of experimental degeneration in the avian optic tectum. *J. Anat. Lond.* **96**, 309–316.

GUDDEN, B. (1870) Experimentaluntersuchungen über das peripherische und centrale Nervensystem. *Arch. Psychiat. Nervenkr.* **2**, 693–723.

GUILLERY, R. W. (1959) Afferent fibres to the dorso-medial thalamic nucleus in the cat. *J. Anat. Lond.* **93**, 403–419.

GUILLERY, R. W. (1965) Some electron microscopical observations of degenerative changes in central nervous synapses. In *Degeneration Patterns in the Nervous System, Progress in Brain Research*, vol. 14 (M. Singer and J. P. Schadé, eds.), pp. 57–76, Elsevier, Amsterdam.

HEIMER, L. (1967) Silver impregnation of terminal degeneration in some forebrain fiber systems: a comparative evaluation of current methods. *Brain Res.* **5**, 86–108.

HEIMER, L. (1968) Synaptic distribution of centripetal and centrifugal nerve fibres in the olfactory system of the rat: an experimental anatomical study. *J. Anat. Lond.* **103**, 413–432.

HEIMER, L. (1970) Bridging the gap between light and electron microscopy in the experimental tracing of fiber connections. In *Contemporary Research Methods in Neuroanatomy* (W. J. H. Nauta and S. O. E. Ebbesson, eds.), pp. 162–172, Springer, Berlin, Heidelberg, and New York.

HEIMER, L., and PETERS, A. (1968) An electron microscope study of a silver stain for degenerating boutons. *Brain Res.* **8**, 337–346.

HEIMER, L., and WALL, P. D. (1968) The dorsal root distribution to the substantia gelatinosa of the rat with a note on the distribution in the cat. *Expl. Brain Res.* **6**, 89–99.

HOLLÄNDER, H., BRODAL, A., and WALBERG, F. (1969) Electronmicroscopic observations on the structure of the pontine nuclei and the mode of termination of the cortipontine fibres: an experimental study in the cat. *Expl. Brain Res.* **7**, 95–110.

JONES, E. G., and ROCKEL, A. J. (1973) Observations on complex vesicles, neurofilamentous hyperplasia and increased electron density during terminal degeneration in the inferior colliculus. *J. Comp. Neurol.* **147**, 93–118.

LA VELLE, A. and LA VELLE, F. W. (1958a) The nucleolar apparatus and neuronal reactivity to injury during development. *J. Exp. Zool.* **137**, 285–315.

LA VELLE, A., and LA VELLE, F. W. (1958b) Neuronal swelling and chromatolysis as influenced by the state of cell development. *Am. J. Anat.* **102**, 219–241.

LEVAY, S. (1971) On the neurons and synapses of the lateral geniculate nucleus of the monkey and the effects of eye enucleation. *Z. Zellforsch.* **113**, 396–419.

LIEBERMAN, A. R. (1971) The axon reaction: a review of the principal features of perikaryal responses to axon injury. In *International Review of Neurobiology*, vol. 14 (C. C. Pfeiffer and J. R. Smythies, eds.), pp. 49–124, Academic Press, New York and London.

McMAHON, U. J. (1967) Fine structure of synapses in the dorsal nucleus of the lateral geniculate body of normal blinded rats. *Z. Zellforsch.* **76**, 136–146.

MUGNAINI, E., and WALBERG, F. (1967) An experimental electron microscopical study on the mode of termination of cerebellar corticovestibular fibres in the cat lateral vestibular nucleus (Deiters' nucleus). *Expl. Brain Res.* **4**, 212–236.

NAUTA, W. J. H. (1957) Silver impregnation of degenerating axons. In *New Research Techniques of Neuroanatomy* (W. F. Windle, ed.), pp. 17–26, Thomas, Springfield, Ill.

NAUTA, W. J. H., and EBBESSON, S. O. E. (1970) *Contemporary Research Methods in Neuroanatomy*, Springer, Berlin, Heidelberg, and New York.

O'NEAL, J. T., and WESTRUM, L. E. (1973) The fine structural synaptic organization of the lateral cuneate nucleus: a study of sequential alterations in degeneration. *Brain Res.* **51**, 97–124.

PECCI-SAAVEDRA, J., MASCITTI, T. A., VACCAREZZA, O. L., and READER, T. A. (1969) Non-synaptic ring images in silver-impregnated lateral geniculate nucleus. *Brain Res.* **14**, 733–738.

PINCHING, A. J. (1969) Persistence of postsynaptic membrane thickenings after degeneration of olfactory nerves. *Brain Res.* **16**, 277–281.

POWELL, T. P. S., and COWAN, W. M. (1964) A note on retrograde fibre degeneration. *J. Anat. Lond.* **98**, 579–585.

RAISMAN, G., and MATTHEWS, M. R. (1972) Degeneration and regeneration of synapses. In *The Structure and Function of Nervous Tissue*, vol. IV (G. H. Bourne, ed.), pp. 61–104. Academic Press, New York and London.

SMITH, M. C. (1951) The use of Marchi staining in the later stages of human tract degeneration. *J. Neurol. Neurosurg. Psychiat.* **14**, 222–225.

SMITH, M. C. (1956a) Observations on the extended use of the Marchi method. *J. Neurol. Neurosurg. Psychiat.* **19**, 67–73.

SMITH, M. C. (1956b) The recognition and prevention of artifacts of the Marchi method. *J. Neurol. Neurosurg. Psychiat.* **19**, 74–83.

SMITH, M. C., STRICK, S. J., and SHARP, P. (1956) The value of the Marchi method for staining tissues stored in formalin for prolonged periods. *J. Neurol. Neurosurg. Psychiat.* **19**, 62–64.

SOTELO, C. (1968) Axon terminals in the lateral vestibular nucleus of the rat: an electron microscopic and experimental study. *Electr. Micr.* 539–540.

SOTELO, C., and PALAY, S. L. (1971) Altered axons and axon terminals in the lateral vestibular nucleus of the rat: possible example of axonal remodeling. *Lab. Invest.* **6**, 653–671.

SZENTÁGOTHAI, J., HÁMORI, J., and TÖMBÖL, T. (1966) Degeneration and electron microscope analysis of the synaptic glomeruli in the lateral geniculate body. *Expl. Brain Res.* **2**, 283–301.

TORVIK, A. (1972) Phagocytosis of nerve cells during retrograde degeneration. An electron microscopic study. *J. Neuropathol. Expl. Neurol.* **31**, 132–146.

TORVIK, A., and SKJÖRTEN, F. (1971) Electron microscopic observations on nerve cell regeneration and degeneration after axon lesions: I, Changes in the nerve cell cytoplasm. *Acta neuropath. Berlin* **17**, 248–264.

TORVIK, A., and SÖREIDE, A. J. (1972) Nerve cell regeneration after axon lesions in newborn rabbits. Light and electron microscopical study. *J. Neuropathol. Expl. Neurol.* **31**, 683–695.

VAN GEHUCHTEN, A. (1903) La dégénérescence dite rétrograde ou dégénérescence Wallérienne indirecte. *Le Névraxe* **5**, 3–107.

VAN GEHUCHTEN, A. (1906) *Anatomie du système nerveux de l'homme*, ed. 4, Louvain.

WALBERG, F. (1966) The fine structure of the cuneate nucleus in normal cats and following interruption of afferent fibres: an electron microscopical study with particular reference to findings made in Glees and Nauta sections. *Expl. Brain Res.* **2**, 107–128.

WALBERG, F. (1971) Does silver impregnate normal and degenerating boutons? A study based on light and electron microscopical observations of the inferior olive. *Brain Res.* **31**, 47–65.

WALBERG, F. (1972) Further studies on silver impregnation of normal and degenerating boutons: a light and electron microscopical investigation of a filamentous degenerating system. *Brain Res.* **36**, 353–369.

WALBERG, F., and MUGNAINI, E. (1969) Distinction of degenerating fibres and boutons of cerebellar and peripheral origin in the Deiters' nucleus of the same animal. *Brain Res.* **14**, 67–75.

WONG-RILEY, M. T. T. (1972a) Terminal degeneration and glial reactions in the lateral geniculate nucleus of the squirrel monkey after eye removal. *J. Comp. Neurol.* **144**, 61–92.

WONG-RILEY, M. T. T. (1972b) Changes in the dorsal lateral geniculate nucleus of the squirrel monkey after unilateral ablation of the visual cortex. *J. Comp. Neurol.* **146**, 519–548.

THE DEGENERATION PATTERN OF THE NIGRO-NEOSTRIATAL DOPAMINE SYSTEM AFTER ELECTROTHERMIC OR 6-HYDROXY-DOPAMINE LESIONS

Tomas Hökfelt and Urban Ungerstedt

Department of Histology, Karolinska Institute, Stockholm, Sweden

INTRODUCTION

The degeneration of neurons in the central nervous system has been studied with different techniques at the light and the electron microscopic level (for reference, see Nauta, 1957; Alksne *et al.*, 1966; Grant, 1970; Guillery, 1970; Heimer, 1970a, b), and the results from such studies form the basis for our knowledge of the connections between various brain areas. Recent histochemical methods to identify central neurons on the basis of their transmitter content (Carlsson *et al.*, 1962; Falck *et al.*, 1962; Fuxe *et al.*, 1970) opens up possibilities to map and to study the degeneration patterns of such "chemically homogeneous" systems. In the present paper we will briefly summarize some light and electron microscopic studies on the nigro-neostriatal dopamine (DA) system after electrothermic and chemical lesions (see Hökfelt and Ungerstedt, 1969, 1973).

LESIONS ON THE NIGRO-NEOSTRIATAL DA PATHWAY

The nigro-neostriatal DA pathway has been thoroughly mapped out with the formaldehyde fluorescence technique (Andén *et al.*, 1964, 1965, 1966; Dahlström and Fuxe, 1964; Fuxe, 1965; Ungerstedt, 1971a) and recently also with immunohistochemistry using antibodies to dopadecarboxylase (Hökfelt *et al.*, 1973). Unilateral lesions (spherical in shape with a diameter of about 1 mm) on this system were made by electrocoagulations placed at the level of the rostral end of the decussatio supramamillaris involving most of the median forebrain bundle and parts of the Forel's fields. In a second set of experiments 6-hydroxy-DA (6-OH-DA), a DA analog assumed to cause degeneration of catecholamine (CA) neurons (Tranzer and Thoenen, 1967a, 1968; Ungerstedt, 1968, 1971b; Bloom *et al.*, 1969; Iversen and Uretsky, 1970) was injected close to the substantia nigra (for details, see Hökfelt and Ungerstedt, 1969, 1973).

Two types of experiments were carried out. A detailed description of the material studied and the principles for the quantitative evaluations have been described elsewhere (Hökfelt and Ungerstedt, 1969, 1973).

Firstly, the anterograde degeneration of nerve terminals in the striatum was studied. At varying time intervals after both types of lesions slices of the striatum incubated with α-methyl-noradrenaline (NA) (Hökfelt, 1968) or 5-hydroxydopamine (5-OH-DA) (Tranzer and Thoenen, 1967a, b) and fixed with potassium permanganate ($KMnO_4$) (Richardson, 1966) were analyzed quantitatively in the electron microscope. With this procedure the nerve endings (boutons) of monoamine neurons can be identified at the ultrastructural level on the basis of their content of small granular vesicles (SGV) (Hökfelt, 1968). The occurrence of dense degenerating boutons in the striatum was determined in glutaraldehyde-OsO_4 fixed material at varying time intervals after 6-OH-DA injections.

Secondly, the site of injection and the substantia nigra were examined in glutaraldehyde-OsO_4 fixed material at various time intervals after 6-OH-DA lesions, mainly with the aim to study to what extent 6-OH-DA causes unspecific brain damage in addition to the postulated degeneration of DA cell bodies.

EFFECTS ON THE STRIATAL MONOAMINE BOUTONS

In the striatum of unoperated rats, of shamoperated rats or of the control side the percentage of boutons with SGV (Figs. 1 and 2) has been calculated to 10–15% (Hökfelt, 1968; Hökfelt and Ungerstedt, 1969, 1973). The figure 15% was obtained in the early study, but since mainly the frontal part of the head of the striatum was studied and since the material was limited in this study, the figures 10–11% as calculated in the two subsequent, more extensive studies, may be more representative for the head of the striatum.

After both types of lesions decreases in the percentage of boutons with SGV were observed (Figs. 4A, B). After the 6-OH-DA injections a marked decrease was observed at 18 h (to 6.5%) and the lowest figure was reached at 48 h (0.5%). During all following time intervals studied (up to 2 months) the percentage of boutons with SGV remained below 2% indicating a long-lasting, irreversible degeneration. Since no effect was observed at 12 h, the degeneration seems to start somewhere between 12 and 18 h after the lesion. Although after electrocoagulation a similar curve was obtained, the onset of degeneration seemed to be slightly postponed since no certain effects were observed at 24 h, whereas at 48 h the percentage of SGV was very low (1%).

Parallel to the decrease in percentage of boutons with SGV typical dense, degenerating boutons, mostly surrounded by glial elements (Fig. 3), appeared in the striatum (Fig. 4c). In the 6-OH-DA material the highest percentage was found 48 h (2.3%) and 72 h (1.5%) after the injection, whereas low figures were observed at 24, 96, 120, and 144 h.

The present findings demonstrate that after either an electrothermic or a chemical, uni-lateral lesion of the ascending nigro-neostriatal DA pathway there is a marked fall in the percentage of boutons with SGV (from 11% to below 1%) indicating a rapid anterograde degeneration of the DA nerve terminals in the striatum. The degeneration starts between 12 and 18 h and the initial phase, i.e. the loss of the uptake and/or storage mechanism seems to be complete within 48 h. The appearance of dense boutons occurs, subsequently reaching a maximum at 48 h. Since only few dense boutons are seen at the 96 h interval, there is obviously a rapid glial engulfment and removal of the dense boutons. The fact that we never observed a higher percentage of dense boutons than 2.2% as compared to 11% of boutons with SGV in the control side, further underlines the asynchronous degeneration course.

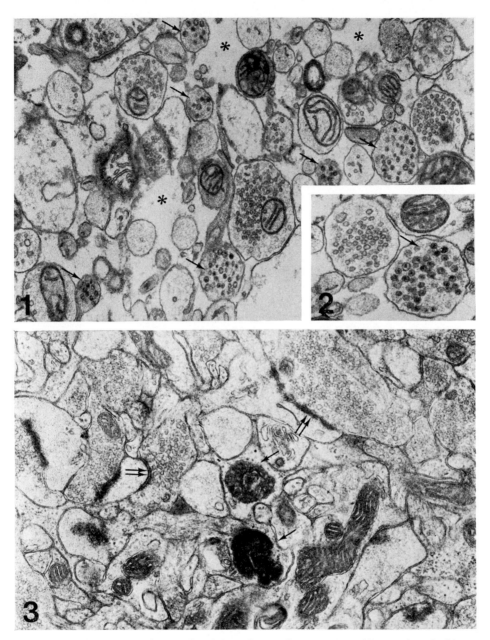

FIGS. 1 and 2. Electron micrographs of the striatum of untreated rat. Slice incubated with α-methyl-noradrenaline (10 μg/ml) and fixed with potassium permanganate. Several boutons (arrows) contain small granular vesicles but the majority contain only agranular (synaptic) vesicles. Note extracellular swelling (asterisks) due to incubation procedure. Magnification ×25,000 and ×35,000 respectively. (From Hökfelt, 1968).

FIG. 3. Electron micrographs of the striatum of rat after an injection of 6-OH-DA close to the substantia nigra. Fixation with glutaraldehyde perfusion followed by osmium tetroxide. Two dense degenerating boutons (arrows) are seen. The surrounding neuropil has a seemingly normal fine structure. Note synaptic complexes (double arrows). Magnification × 30,000.

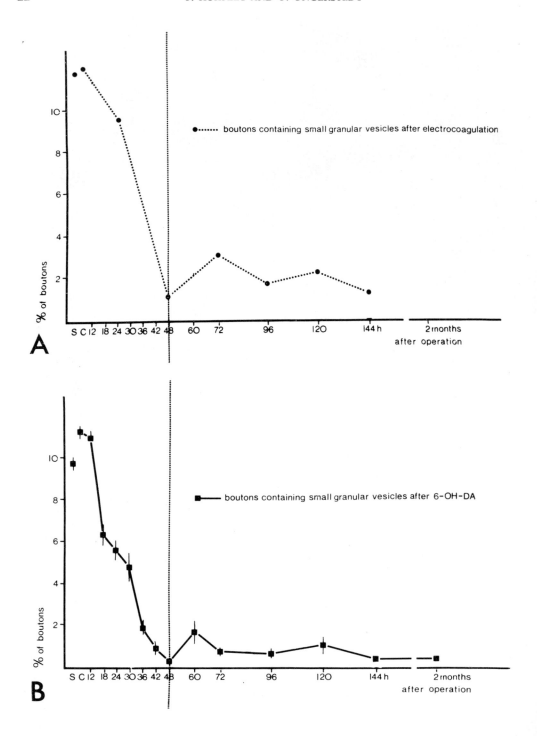

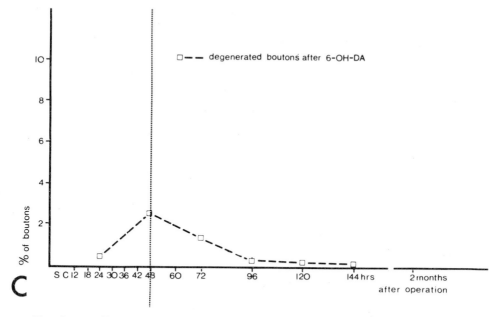

FIG. 4A–C. Effects of electrothermic lesions (A) or 6-OH-DA injection (B, C) close to the substantia nigra on striatal boutons. The percentage of boutons with SGV in striatal slices incubated with α-methyl-NA or 5-OH-DA and fixed with $KMnO_4$ was calculated after both types of lesions (A and B, respectively). The percentage of dense degenerating boutons in glutaraldehyde-OsO_4 fixed striatal tissue (C). The percentage of boutons with SGV falls from 11% in the controls to below 1% 48 h after both types of lesions and remains low during all following time intervals. The percentage of dense boutons reaches a maximum of about 2% 48 h after the lesion. (From Hökfelt and Ungerstedt, 1969, 1973).

It seems justified to draw two conclusions from these experiments which may be valid for ultrastructural degeneration studies based only on dense degenerating boutons. Firstly, due to the asynchronous degeneration it is not possible to obtain a correct figure of the number of the boutons of a special system by counting at a given time the number of degenerating dense boutons after lesions of this system, since this will in all probability give a much too low number. Secondly, dense degenerating boutons are present in a relative high number only during a relative short time period. This period may vary considerably for different systems: NA axons seem to degenerate at a considerably slower rate (Heller and Moore, 1968; Reis et al., this symposium) than the DA axons. Thus, studies of degenerating neuron systems must include a number of time intervals to guarantee detection of dense boutons.

EFFECTS ON THE NIGRAL DA CELL BODIES

The substantia nigra was studied after injections of 6-OH-DA close to the nigral DA cell bodies. The aim of this part of the study was to evaluate the selectivity of the intracerebral 6-OH-DA injections, i.e. whether this lesion technique causes a selective destruction of DA neurons or whether, in addition, unspecific brain damage occurs. It has previously been demonstrated that in the peripheral nervous system where the 6-OH-DA can be administered intravenously, there seems to be a selective destruction of the NA nerve terminals (Tranzer and Thoenen, 1967a, 1968). In the central nervous system, however, in addition to destruction of CA neuron systems (Ungerstedt, 1968, 1971b; Bloom *et al.*, 1969; Iversen and Uretsky, 1970) there seems to occur varying degrees of unselective brain tissue damage (Ungerstedt, 1971b; Poirier *et al.*, 1972; Hökfelt and Ungerstedt, 1973; Javoy *et al.*, this symposium).

After intracerebral injections of 8 μg 6-OH-DA dissolved in 4 μl 0.9% NaCl during 4 min, the following structural changes could be observed at the injection site and in the substantia nigra 24 h or 48 h after the injection.

(1) Unspecific destruction of brain tissue was seen along the track of the injection cannula (Figs. 5 and 7).

(2) A zone of unspecific damage was observed extending from the injection cannula mainly in the direction of the infusion. The size of this zone varied markedly within individual series of experiments and also during the course of the last 4 years. Mostly the zone was very small, confined to the immediate neighborhood of the injection site but occasionally a necrotic zone with a diameter of about 1 mm (Fig. 6), and in very rare instances even an empty hole with a diameter of 1–2 mm could be observed. During our last series, 2 out of 17 rats had a marked unspecifically damaged zone (Fig. 6). We have so far not been able to determine which factor(s) are responsible for this variation in the specificity of the lesion.

(3) In the substantia nigra a specific cell population with a localization closely resembling the distribution of DA cell bodies as seen in the fluorescence microscope with the Falck–Hillarp technique showed marked changes in the light and electron microscope (Figs. 5, 7, and 8). In our glutaraldehyde-OsO$_4$ fixed material, markedly swollen cell bodies and dendrites were observed intermingled with neurons of an apparently normal fine structure. It could be established that at least two neuron populations are present in the control substantia nigra, the first characterized by a sparse and irregular rough endoplasmic reticulum, a light cytoplasm and a richly indented nucleus, and the second by a dense, regular rough endoplasmic reticulum, a dense cytoplasm and a smooth nuclear envelope. The latter cell type was markedly affected by 6-OH-DA, whereas the first one mostly remained seemingly unchanged after the lesions. It may therefore be concluded that the second type of neurons represent DA neurons. Autoradiographic evidence for this view has recently been obtained (Gulley and Wood, 1972).

The present results thus suggest that 6-OH-DA administered intracerebrally in comparatively low doses and concentrations causes a comparatively specific lesion of the DA cell bodies of the substantia nigra and therefore represents a useful tool in elucidation of the functional role of this system. However, since in a varying but mostly low percentage of animals there occurs a comparatively large, unspecific lesion, it is necessary to evaluate with histological and histochemical (e.g. Falck–Hillarp) techniques the extent of the unspecific damage as also pointed out by Poirier *et al.* (1972).

CONCLUSIONS

The nigro-neostriatal DA system of rats undergoes a rapid anterograde degeneration after electrothermic or 6-OH-DA induced lesions. The degeneration process starts 12–18 h after the lesion and the degenerating dense boutons are to a large extent removed by glial elements within 96 h. The percentage of monoamine boutons of total striatal boutons falls from about 11% to below 1%, and remains low, indicating an irreversible process. With the 6-OH-DA injection technique when used under proper conditions, comparatively specific lesions of central catecholamine systems can be obtained although in a small number of animals extensive unspecific damage may occur.

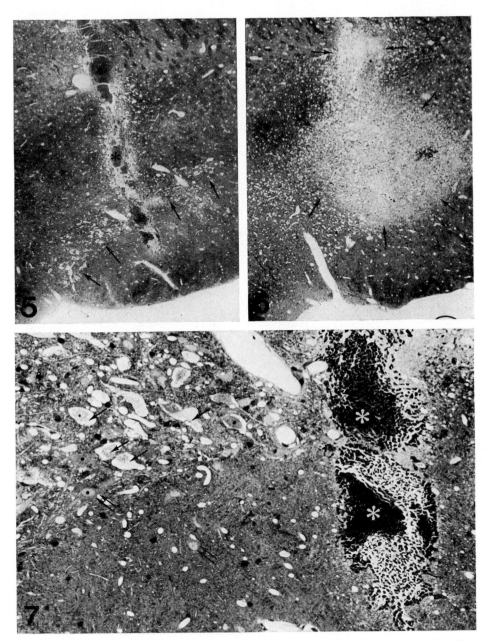

FIGS. 5–7. Light micrographs of the substantia nigra after 6-OH-DA injections close to this area. In Figs. 5 and 7 a successful injection is shown with only little unspecific damage. The track of the injection needle is shown at the asterisks. Arrows in Fig. 5 show the zone containing swollen, degenerating cell bodies, and processes. In Fig. 7 the track made by the tip of the injection needle and the degenerating cells (arrows) are seen at a higher magnification. Note apparently normal cell bodies (double arrows) intermingled with the affected cells. In Fig. 6 a large zone of unspecific damage is seen. Magnifications $\times 50$ (Figs. 5 and 6) and $\times 400$ (Fig. 7). (From Hökfelt and Ungerstedt, 1973).

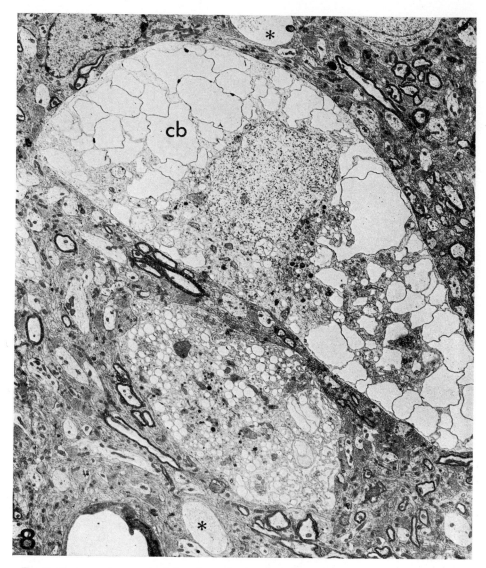

Fig. 8. Electron micrograph of the substantia nigra 24 h after a 6-OH-DA injection. One big, markedly affected cell body (cb) with a vacuolated cytoplasm and a nucleus is seen. Below a large dendrite or the periphery of a cell body is shown. Two small swollen dendrites (asterisks) are seen. Note that the surrounding neuropil appears unaffected. Magnification ×40,000. (From Hökfelt and Ungerstedt, 1973).

ACKNOWLEDGEMENTS

This work was supported by grants from the Swedish Medical Research Council (B73-O4X-2887-O4C, B73-14P-3262-O3C, B73-O4X,3574-O2A) and by grants from Karolinska Institutets Forskningsfonder, Ollie och Elof Ericssons Stiftelse, Margarethahemmet, and from Magn. Bergvalls Stiftelse. The skilful technical assistance of Miss E. Henriksson and Mrs. W. Hiort is gratefully acknowledged.

REFERENCES

ALKSNE, J. F., BLACKSTAD, T. W., WALBERG, F., and WHITE, L. E., Jr. (1966) Electron microscopy of axon degeneration: a valuable tool in experimental neuroanatomy. *Ergebn. Anat. EntwGesch.* **39**, 1–32.

ANDÉN, N.-E., CARLSSON, A., DAHLSTRÖM, A., FUXE, K., HILLARP, N.-Å., and LARSSON, K. (1964) Demonstration and mapping out of nigro-neostriatal dopamine neurons. *Life Sci.* **3**, 523–530.

ANDÉN, N.-E., DAHLSTRÖM, A., FUXE, K., and LARSSON, K. (1965) Further evidence for the presence of nigro-neostriatal dopamine neurons in the rat. *Am. J. Anat.* **116**, 329–334.

ANDÉN, N.-E., DAHLSTRÖM, A., FUXE, K., LARSSON, K., OLSON, L., and UNGERSTEDT, U. (1966) Ascending monoamine neurons to the telencephalon and diencephalon. *Acta physiol. scand.* **67**, 313–326.

BLOOM, F. E., ALGERI, S., GROPPETTI, A., REVUELTA, A., and COSTA, E. (1969) Lesions of central norepinephrine terminals with 6-OH-dopamine: biochemistry and fine structure. *Science* **166**, 1284–1286.

CARLSSON, A., FALCK, B., and HILLARP, N.-Å. (1962) Cellular localization of brain monoamines. *Acta physiol. scand.* **56**, 1–27.

DAHLSTRÖM, A. and FUXE, K. (1964) Evidence for the existence of monoamine-containing neurons in the central nervous system: I, Demonstration of monoamines in the cell bodies of brain stem neurons. *Acta physiol. scand.* **62**, Suppl. 232, 1–55.

FALCK, B., HILLARP, N.-Å., THIEME, G., and TORP. A. (1962) Fluorescence of catecholamines and related compounds condensed with formaldehyde. *J. Histochem. Cytochem.* **10**, 348–354.

FUXE, K. (1965) Evidence for the existence of monoamine neurons in the central nervous system: III. The monoamine nerve terminal. *Z. Zellforsch.* **65**, 573–596.

FUXE, K., HÖKFELT, T., JONSSON, G., and UNGERSTEDT, U. (1970) Fluorescence microscopy in neuroanatomy. In *Contemporary Research in Neuroanatomy*, pp. 275–314. (Ebbesson *et al.*, eds.), Springer, New York.

GRANT, G. (1970) Neuronal changes central to the site of axon transection: a method for the identification of retrograde changes in perikarya, dendrites and axons by silver impregnation. In *Contemporary Research Methods in Neuroanatomy*, pp. 173–183 (Nauta *et al.*, eds.), Springer, New York, Heidelberg, and Berlin.

GUILLERY, R. W. (1970) Light- and electron-microscopical studies of normal and degenerating axons. In *Contemporary Research Methods in Neuroanatomy*, pp. 77–104 (Nauta *et al.*, eds.), Springer, New York, Heidelberg, and Berlin.

GULLEY, R. L., and WOOD, R. L. (1972) The fine structure of the neurons in the rat substantia nigra. *Tissue & Cell* **3**, 675–690.

HEIMER, L. (1970a) Selective silver impregnation of degenerating axoplasm. In *Contemporary Research Methods in Neuroanatomy*, pp. 106–129. (Nauta *et al.*, eds.), Springer, New York, Heidelberg and Berlin.

HEIMER, L. (1970b) Bridging the gap between light and electron microscopy in the experiments tracing of fiber connections. In *Contemporary Research Methods in Neuroanatomy*, pp. 162–172 (Nauta *et al.*, eds.), Springer, New York, Heidelberg, and Berlin.

HELLER, A., and MOORE, R. Y. (1968) Control of brain serotonin and norepinephrine by specific neural systems. *Adv. Pharmac.* **6A**, 191–206.

HÖKFELT, T. (1968) *In vitro* studies on central and peripheral monoamine neurons at the ultrastructural level. *Z. Zellforsch.* **91**, 1–74.

HÖKFELT, T., and UNGERSTEDT, U. (1969) Electron and fluorescence microscopical studies on the nucleus caudatus putamen of the rat after unilateral lesions of ascending nigro-neostriatal dopamine neurons. *Acta physiol. scand.* **76**, 415–426.

HÖKFELT, T., and UNGERSTEDT, U. (1973) Specificity of 6-hydroxydopamine induced degeneration of central monoamine neurones: An electron and fluorescence microscopic study with special reference to intracerebral injection on the nigro-striatal dopamine system. *Brain Res.* **60**, 269–297.

HÖKFELT, T., FUXE, K., and GOLDSTEIN, M. (1973) Immunohistochemical studies on monoamine containing cell systems. *Brain Res.* **62**, 461–469.

IVERSEN, L. L., and URETSKY, N. J. (1970) Regional effects of 6-hydroxy-dopamine on catecholamine containing neurones in rat brain and spinal cord. *Brain Res.* **24**, 364–367.

NAUTA, W. J. H. (1957) Silver impregnation of degenerating axons. In *New Research Techniques of Neuroanatomy*, pp. 17–26. (W. F. Windle, ed.), Thomas, Springfield, Illinois.

POIRIER, L. J., LANGELIER, P., ROBERGE, A., BOUCHER, R. and KITSIKIS, A. (1972) Non-specific histopathological changes induced by the intracerebral injection of 6-hydroxy-dopamine (6-OH-DA). *J. Neurol. Sci.* **16**, 401–416.

RICHARDSON, K. C. (1966) Electron microscopical identification of autonomic nerve endings. *Nature, Lond.* **210**, 756.

TRANZER, J. P., and THOENEN, H. (1967a) Ultramorphologische Veränderungen der sympathischen Nervenendigungen der Katze nach Vorbehandlung mit 5- und 6-Hydroxy-Dopamin. *Arch. exp. Path. Pharmak.* **257**, 343.

TRANZER, J. P., and THOENEN, H. (1967b) Electron-microscopic localization of 5-hydroxydopamine (3,4,5-trihydroxy-phenylethylamine), a new "false" sympathetic transmitter. *Experientia* **23**, 743.

TRANZER, J. P., and THOENEN, H. (1968) An electron-microscopic study of selective, acute degeneration of sympathetic nerve terminals after administration of 6-hydroxydopamine. *Experientia* **24**, 155–156.

UNGERSTEDT, U. (1968) 6-Hydroxydopamine induced degeneration of central monoamine neurons. *Europ. J. Pharmacol.* **5**, 107–110.

UNGERSTEDT, U. (1971a) Stereotaxic mapping of the monoamine pathways in the rat brain. *Acta physiol. scand.* **82**, Suppl. 367, 1–48.

UNGERSTEDT, U. (1971b) Histochemical studies on the effects of intracerebral and intraventricular injections of 6-hydroxydopamine on monoamine neurons in the rat brain. In *6-Hydroxydopamine and Catecholamine Neurons*, pp. 101–127 (Malmfors *et al.*, eds.), North-Holland, Amsterdam.

STRUCTURE–ACTIVITY CORRELATIONS IN TRIHYDROXYPHENETHYLAMINES AND DIHYDROXYTRYPTAMINES

RELATIONSHIP TO CYTOTOXICITY IN ADRENERGIC AND SEROTONERGIC NEURONS

J. Daly, J. Lundström† and C. R. Creveling

National Institutes of Health, Bethesda, Maryland 20014

SUMMARY

With trihydroxyphenethylamines, the neurodegenerative activity towards noradrenergic structures is clearly dependent upon an active uptake and concentration of the amine into the axoplasm of the neuronal terminal, followed by a rapid cyclical oxidation, reduction, and reoxidation to a *para* quinone with concomitant formation of hydrogen peroxide during oxidation. The *para*-quinones can react with macromolecular nucleophiles and can undergo cyclization and "isomerization" to di-hydroxyindoles. The exact nature of the biochemical alteration or alterations which lead to "degeneration" of the terminal is as yet unknown and may be related to the rapid formation of reactive quinones and/or hydrogen peroxide from trihydroxyphenethylamines. In the case of dihydroxytryptamines, sufficient data is not yet available to delineate the nature of their cytotoxic activity towards serotonergic structures. The compounds do have high affinities for serotonin-transport systems in nerve terminals. Effects on noradrenergic structures have, however, been reported for 5,6-, 5,7-, and 6,7-dihydroxytryptamines. It is surprising that dihydroxytryptamines, which are autoxidized at very slow rates compared to 6-hydroxydopamine, would be quite efficacious in eliciting neurodegeneration, especially if this occurs via a similar mechanism involving intracellular oxidation to aminochrome-like compounds (quinone-amines) and hydrogen peroxide. The blockade of the long-term effects of the dihydroxytryptamines on cardiac noradrenergic mechanisms by inhibition of monoamine oxidase is unexpected and suggestive of monoamine oxidase-catalyzed formation of a toxic metabolite.

INTRODUCTION

2,4,5-Trihydroxyphenethylamine (6-hydroxydopamine) has become in the last 6 years a valuable pharmacological tool for the selective degeneration of noradrenergic nerve terminals (see Malmfors and Thoenen, 1971) in both peripheral organs such as heart, iris,

---

†Visiting Fellow, Public Health Service, 1970–1971. Present address: Socialstyrelsen, Läkemedels Avdelningen, Fack 10401 Stockholm, Sweden.

and vas deferens, and in the central nervous system (Hedreen and Chalmers, 1972) where after intracerebral, ventricular, or cisternal injection it interacts primarily with structures containing norepinephrine and to a lesser extent with those containing dopamine (Breese and Traylor, 1970; Simmonds and Uretsky, 1970; Uretsky and Iversen, 1970). The neurodegenerative actions of 6-hydroxydopamine appear dependent upon a selective concentration of the amine into the axoplasm of neuronal structures by specific amine transport systems. In agreement with this hypothesis, the effects of 6-hydroxydopamine on noradrenergic terminals in both peripheral and central neurons are effectively blocked by effective inhibitors of norepinephrine uptake, such as desmethylimipramine (Malmfors and Sachs, 1968; Corrodi *et al.*, 1971b; Bennett *et al.*, 1970; Stone *et al.*, 1964a; Jonsson and Sachs, 1970). Conversely, tricyclic compounds of the latter type do not effectively block either the effect of 6-hydroxydopamine on dopaminergic terminals or the uptake of dopamine by the amine transport system of such terminals (Taylor and Laverty, 1972; Evetts and Iversen, 1970). The lack of effect of 6-hydroxydopamine on cell bodies as in the sympathetic ganglia or in the adrenal gland (Thoenen and Tranzer, 1968) is in all likelihood due to the lower activity of the amine transport systems in the plasma membranes of such cells. Uptake of 6-hydroxydopamine into noradrenergic storage granules, with a concomitant release of norepinephrine, is not necessary for manifestation of neurodegenerative effects, since prior treatment with reserpine, an agent which blocks uptake–storage of amines into such granules, is without marked effect on the neurodegenerative activity of 6-hydroxydopamine (Malmfors and Sachs, 1968; Corrodi *et al.*, 1971b; Bennett *et al.*, 1970). The neurodegenerative activity of 6-hydroxydopamine does not appear due to formation of a metabolite by the action of either monoamine oxidase or catechol-*O*-methyltransferase, since inhibition of these enzymes either has no effect or potentiates the degenerative effect of 6-hydroxydopamine (Malmfors and Sachs, 1968; Corrodi *et al.*, 1971b). In addition, α-methyl-6-hydroxydopamine, a compound which is not substrate for monoamine oxidase, is as active or more active as a neurodegenerative agent than 6-hydroxydopamine itself (Stone *et al.*, 1964b; Tranzer and Thoenen, 1973). The monoamine oxidase inhibitor, pargyline, has been shown to greatly potentiate the 6-hydroxydopamine-elicited long-term depletion of dopamine, but not that of norepinephrine in the central nervous system (Breese and Traylor, 1971).

BIOLOGICAL EFFECTS OF 6-HYDROXYDOPAMINE

The effects of 6-hydroxydopamine and related compounds on neuronal structures may be assessed in a number of ways. Release of radio-labeled tissue stores of norepinephrine provides an index related to uptake of 6-hydroxydopamine at both plasma and granule membranes and to the efficacy of 6-hydroxydopamine as an amine-releasing agent. Low concentrations of 6-hydroxydopamine have been shown to displace endogenous norepinephrine without eliciting long-term effects on the nerve terminal (Thoenen and Tranzer, 1968). Long-term effects have been assessed (i) by measurement of endogenous levels of the catecholamines, norepinephrine and dopamine, in the tissue, (ii) with fluorescent histochemistry as a measure of levels and localization of catecholamines *in situ*, and (iii) by direct electron microscopic examination of tissue slices for evidence of neurodegeneration of noradrenergic neuronal structures. Lack of uptake of radioactive norepinephrine or other amines in the tissue, lack of binding of radioactive reserpine (Manara *et al.*, 1972), or loss of tyrosine hydroxylase, dopa decarboxylase or dopamine-β-hydroxylase activity provides further evidence for the destruction of presynaptic noradrenergic terminals. The levels of other enzymes such as monoamine oxidase and catechol-O-methyltransferase, that are not present primarily in such nerve terminals, are not decreased by treatment with 6-hydroxydopamine (Breese and Traylor, 1970; Uretsky and Iversen, 1970; Lowe and Horita, 1970). Compensatory increases in enzymes such as tyrosine hydroxylase in "neuronal" cell bodies of sympathetic ganglia and adrenal gland or phenethanolamine N-methyltransferase in adrenal gland have, however, been reported as a result of "chemical sympathectomy" by 6-hydroxydopamine (Thoenen *et al.*, 1970; Mueller *et al.*, 1969; Thoenen *et al.*, 1969; Brimijoin and Molinoff, 1971).

Assessment of neurodegenerative effects by indirect biochemical techniques has afforded results which are *in toto* quite compatible with direct histological and histochemical evidence for neurodegeneration. However, long-term depletion of norepinephrine in brain tissue without observable ultrastructural damage has been reported (Bartholini *et al.*, 1970a, b) and classical histochemical techniques have been purported to give evidence for generalized tissue damage in response to intracerebral injection of 6-hydroxydopamine (Poirier *et al.*, 1972).

The degenerative effects elicited by 6-hydroxydopamine are accompanied by long-term retention of radioactive 6-hydroxydopamine in neuronal structures as a part of macromolecules, i.e. 6-hydroxydopamine or a transformation product has reacted in an essentially irreversible manner with macromolecular neuronal constituents (Porter *et al.*, 1965; Thoenen and Tranzer, 1968). Evidence for reaction of oxidation products of 6-hydroxydopamine with nucleophilic moieties in macromolecules has been obtained (Saner and Thoenen, 1971).

After administration of 6-hydroxydopamine, the time course for the appearance of effects of the drug on noradrenergic terminals has been investigated (Bennett *et al.*, 1970; Haeusler, 1971). The rate of appearance of these effects will, of course, be dose dependent, but certain generalizations may be made. Release of norepinephrine due to displacement by 6-hydroxydopamine appears to be complete within 15–20 min. Uptake of radioactive norepinephrine is found to be blocked within 1–3 h. In heart and nictitating membrane, nerve transmission appears to be blocked approximately 1 h after the drug (Haeusler, 1971). The appearance of morphological changes occurs more slowly over a period of 3–4 h. Rupture of axon membranes, dispersal and subsequent coagulation of vesicles, and appearance of necrotic abnormal mitochondria precedes the ultimate disappearance of the morphologically identifiable neuronal structures within Schwann cell sheaths. Effects of 6-hydroxydopamine treatment on neurotubules of axons have been reported (Cheah *et al.*, 1971). In addition, high doses have been reported to cause a long-lasting blockade of α-adrenergic receptors which was proposed to be due to site-directed reaction of the drug with the α-receptor (Haeusler, 1971). The rate of subsequent regeneration of neuronal structures after destruction with 6-hydroxydopamine depends on the tissue with fairly rapid recovery in peripheral structures (Haeusler *et al.*, 1969; de Champlain, 1971; Goldman and Jacobowitz, 1971) and with virtually no recovery in the central nervous system.

The recent introduction of 2,4,5-trihydroxyphenylalanine (6-hydroxydopa) as a research tool (Ong *et al.*, 1969) has allowed the study of the effects of a compound which passes the blood brain barrier. The results obtained with this amino acid precursor of 6-hydroxydopamine are compatible with the proposal that the compound must be decarboxylated to 6-hydroxydopamine in order to elicit demonstrable effects on noradrenergic neurons. The effects elicited by 6-hydroxydopa have been similar to those evoked with lower doses of

6-hydroxydopamine (Clarke et al., 1972; Thoa et al., 1972; Kostrzewa and Jacobowitz, 1972, 1973; Jacobowitz and Kostrzewa, 1971; Sachs and Jonsson, 1972a, b; Corrodi et al., 1971a) except in the adrenal gland, where the high doses of 6-hydroxydopa do cause a significant depletion of catecholamines (Berkowitz et al., 1970).

Few in vitro studies on the effects of 6-hydroxydopamine have been published. Such studies would be invaluable for a determination of the exact locus or loci of the degenerative action of this compound. In vitro incubation of atria, irides, vas deferens, and superior cervical ganglia with 6-hydroxydopamine resulted in gradual displacement of norepinephrine as shown by fluorescent histochemistry (Jonsson and Sachs, 1970, 1972). 6-Hydroxydopamine uncoupled oxidative phosphorylation, but did not inhibit monoamine oxidase activity in mitochondria present in liver homogenates (Wagner and Trendelenburg, 1971). 6-Hydroxydopamine inhibits the growth of neuroblastoma cells (Prasad, 1970).

CHEMISTRY OF 6-HYDROXYDOPAMINE

6-Hydroxydopamine, because of its low oxidation-reduction potential is subject to rapid autoxidation in aqueous solution to the para-quinone anion (Fig. 1). This para-quinone was initially assumed based on ultraviolet spectral data to have undergone a rapid intramolecular 1,4-cyclization to 4,6,7-trihydroxyindoline (Senoh and Witkop, 1959). This is not the

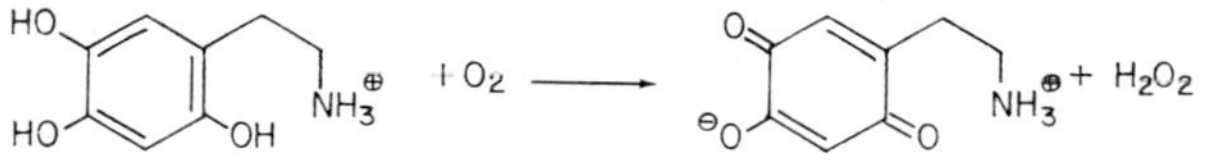

FIG. 1. Probable major route for autoxidation of 6-hydroxydopamine at physiological pH.

case, and the initial autoxidation product of 6-hydroxydopamine has now been shown to be quite stable with spectral properties compatible with its formulation as the red-colored para-quinone (Adams et al., 1972; Powell and Heacock, 1973; Wehrli et al., 1972). At pH values below approximately 5, the compound exists as a yellow-colored uncharged hydroxyquinone (Wehrli et al., 1972) (Fig. 2). A slow cyclization of para-quinone anions of this type to hydroxyindoles in basic media has been demonstrated (Blank et al., 1972; Wehrli et al., 1972; Harley-Mason, 1953; Powell and Heacock, 1973). The slow rate of reaction of the para-quinone of 6-hydroxydopamine with the nucleophilic nitrogen of the side chain strongly suggests that it will also react slowly with amine nucleophiles in macromolecules. Thus the reaction of "oxidized 6-hydroxydopamine" with bovine serum album (Saner and Thoenen, 1971) may well involve nucleophilic sulfhydryl rather than amine groups on the protein (cf. Fig. 3). 5,6-Dihydroxyindole can undergo autoxidation to an aminochrome followed by nucleophilic attack or formation of polymeric melanins (Fig. 3). It is important to note that the rate of formation of 5,6-dihydroxyindole is quite slow in comparison to the initial rapid autoxidative formation of the para-quinone from 6-hydroxydopamine.

Autoxidation of 6-hydroxydopamine produces, in addition to the para-quinone, another reactive product, hydrogen peroxide, and it has been suggested that hydrogen peroxide generated within the noradrenergic terminal may indeed be the active agent in the elicitation of neurodegenerative changes (Heikkila and Cohen, 1971, 1972a, b). Since 6-hydroxydopamine and the para-quinone exist in a reversible oxidation-reduction system, a cyclic mechanism can pertain in vivo with ascorbate (Heikkila and Cohen, 1972a) and other reducing agents such as reduced pyridine nucleotides or perhaps even glutathione supplying

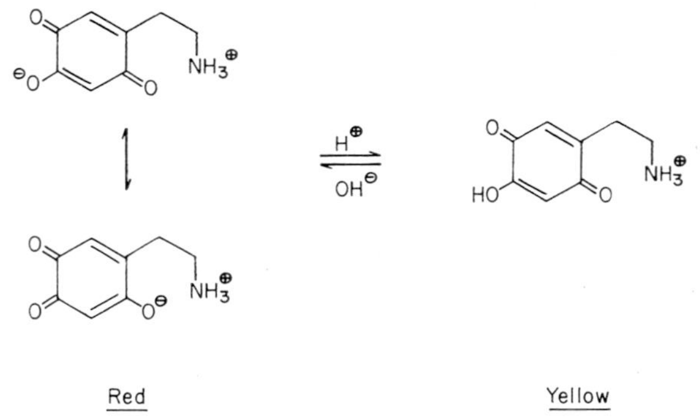

FIG. 2. Formulation of *para*-quinone oxidation product of 6-hydroxydopamine. The two anionic structures to the right represent canonical forms of the same compound. Colors are as designated. (Wehrli *et al.*, 1972.)

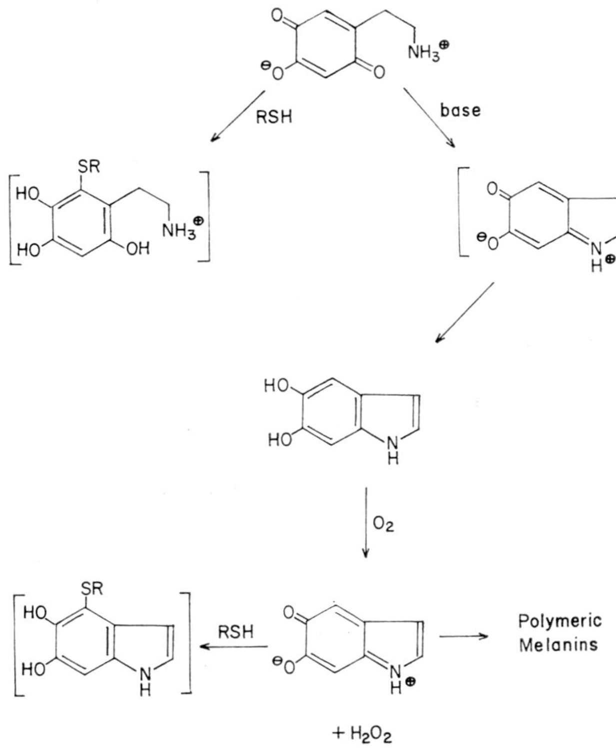

FIG. 3. Further reactions of the intermediate *para*-quinone oxidation product from 6-hydroxy-dopamine. The reactions with sulfhydryl groups are tentative formulations based on analogous reactions and the resultant compounds would then undergo further autoxidation.

the requisite reducing equivalents (Fig. 4). Recent results showing that *in vivo* administration of the *para*-quinone of 6-hydroxydopamine (Heikkila *et al.*, 1973) elicits neurodegeneration similar to that elicited by 6-hydroxydopamine is strong evidence for the rapid and quantitative reduction of the quinone *in vivo*, since the *para*-quinone itself would *not* be expected to have a high affinity for the norepinephrine-transport system. Heikkila and Cohen (1973b) have recently demonstrated that superoxide dismutase retards oxygen uptake during autoxidation of 6-hydroxydopamine.

The original demonstration of 6-hydroxydopamine, as an autoxidation product of dopamine (Senoh *et al.*, 1959a, b) has thus led to an ever-expanding literature on the chemistry and pharmacology of this substance. Recently, Stein and Wise (1971) have even proposed that overproduction of this compound in human brain may be implicated in the

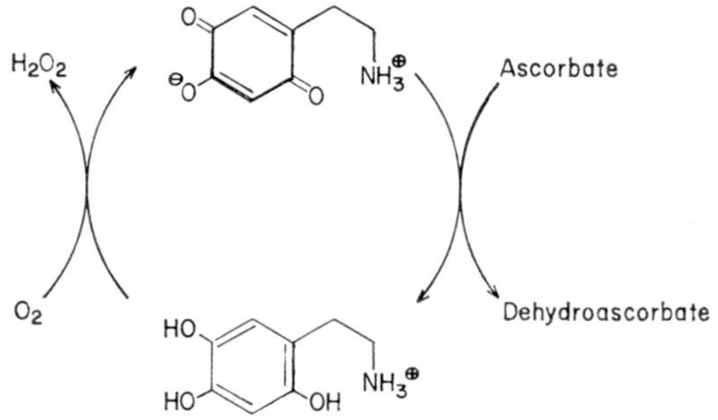

FIG. 4. Proposed sequence of cyclic generation of H_2O_2 from 6-hydroxydopamine. (Heikkila and Cohen, 1972.)

etiology of schizophrenia. This proposal has renewed interest in the mechanism of formation of 6-hydroxydopamine from dopamine *in vivo*. Adams (1972) has drawn attention to the fact that in the absence of ascorbate and with one molecule of dopamine serving as electron donor, dopamine-β-hydroxylase will form the necessary intermediate, dopamine-ortho-quinone (Levin and Kaufman, 1961). The intermediate can then add water to form 6-hydroxydopamine, cyclize and oxidize to aminochromes, or react by 1,4-addition with other nucleophiles such as amino acids (Adams, 1972) (Fig. 5).

STRUCTURE ACTIVITY CORRELATIONS IN TRIHYDROXYPHENETHYLAMINES

Recent studies (Siggins *et al.*, 1973; Tranzer and Thoenen, 1973) have confirmed the early data (Stone *et al.*, 1964b) that indicated that 6-aminodopamine and α-methyl-6-hydroxydopamine would cause a neurodegeneration of noradrenergic nerve terminals similar to that elicited by 6-hydroxydopamine. These results are not surprising since these compounds should have high affinity for amine transport systems and should, like 6-hydroxydopamine, undergo rapid autoxidation to afford hydrogen peroxide and, respectively, a *para*-quinone-amine and a *para*-quinone. The facile oxidation of 6-aminodopamine and the subsequent cyclization to 5,6-dihydroxyindole has now been demonstrated by Blank *et al.* (1972). It is surprising the 6-hydroxynorepinephrine, which is rapidly autoxidized and which has been reported to cause release of cardiac norepinephrine (Daly *et al.*, 1966), has no apparent neurodegenerative activity (Sachs, 1972). Release of cardiac norepinephrine by 6-hydroxynorepinephrine could, however, not be confirmed (A. Rotman, J. Daly and C. R. Creveling, unpublished results).

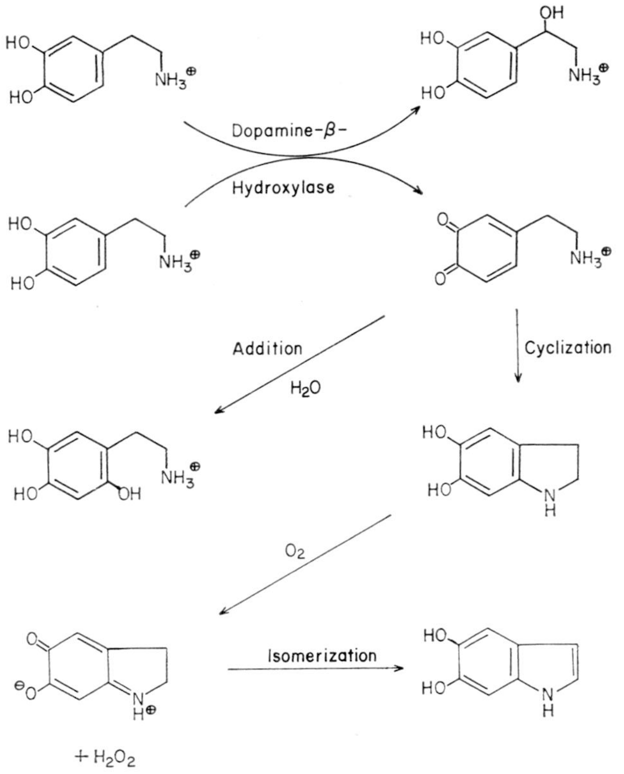

FIG. 5. Scheme for the enzymatic formation of 6-hydroxydopamine and aminochromes from dopamine. (Adopted from Adams, 1972.)

A variety of trihydroxyphenethylamines have now been investigated with respect to (i) uptake into neurons as measured by both inhibition of uptake of ^{3}H-norepinephrine into heart and displacement of ^{3}H-norepinephrine from prelabeled cardiac stores, (ii) rate of autoxidation of the amine as measured by oxygen uptake at pH 7, and (iii) long-term "neurodegenerative effects" on cardiac adrenergic neurons as measured by percent inhibition of ^{3}H-norepinephrine uptake into heart 5 days after administration at the amine (Lundstrom *et al.*, 1973a, b) (Table 1). The results indicate that only compounds which have a high affinity for noradrenergic uptake mechanisms and which are, in addition, rapidly autoxidized to *para*-quinones elicit long-term "neurodegeneration". It is noteworthy that the *para*-quinone of 2,3,5-trihydroxyphenethylamine should yield 5,7-dihydroxyindole on cyclization rather than the 5,6-dihydroxyindole that results from cyclization of the oxidation products derived from 6-hydroxy- and 6-aminodopamine. Certain tetrahydroxyphenethyl-amines also elicited neurodegeneration and were even more readily autoxidized than the effective trihydroxy-compounds (Lundstrom *et al.*, 1973a, b).

In an independent study of structure activity relationships, α-methyl-6-hydroxydopamine, 2,3,5-trihydroxyphenethylamine, 6-aminodopamine, 2,5-dihydroxy-4-aminophenethyl-amine, and 2,4-dihydroxy-5-aminophenethylamine, but not the corresponding dihydroxy-nitrophenethylamines, were found to cause both long-term depletion of norepinephrine and neurodegeneration in peripheral adrenergic organs (Tranzer and Thoenen, 1973). All of

TABLE 1. TRIHYDROXYPHENETHYLAMINES: RELATIVE ACTIVITIES RELATED TO THEIR EFFECT ON NEURONAL STRUCTURES[a]

$R = CH_2CH_2-NH_2$	A Rate autoxidation	B ED_{50} for inhibition of uptake norepinephrine	C ED_{50} for release of norepinephrine	D Long-term inhibition of uptake of norepinephrine
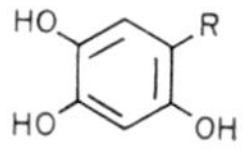 (structure)	276	0.7	7	++
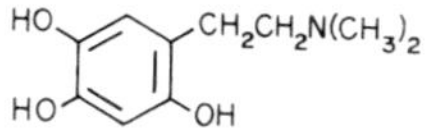 (structure, $CH_2CH_2N(CH_3)_2$)	269	n.i.	—	n.i.
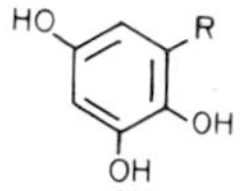 (structure)	288	1.2	63	+
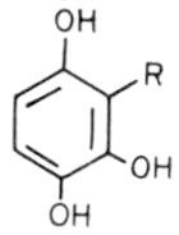 (structure)	287	2.2	>1000	n.i.
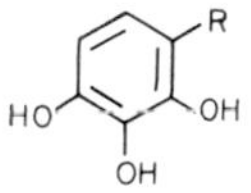 (structure)	22	0.6	74	n.i.
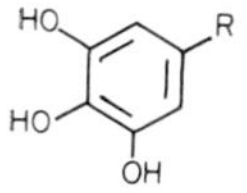 (structure)	20	0.05	10	n.i.
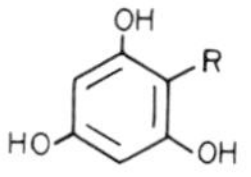 (structure)	<2	n.i.	>400	n.i.

[a]A, oxygen consumption (nmole/min) of 0.5 M solution. B, ED_{50} (μmoles/kg) for inhibition of uptake of ^{3}H-norepinephrine into mouse heart *in vivo* on coadministration (intravenous) with ^{3}H-norepinephrine. n.i. = no inhibition. C, ED_{50} (μmoles/kg) for release of ^{3}H-norepinephrine from mouse heart *in vivo* when administered subcutaneously 1 h after ^{3}H-norepinephrine. D, relative activity with regard to long-term inhibitory effects on uptake of ^{3}H-norepinephrine into mouse heart *in vivo* measured with the ^{3}H-norepinephrine administered 5 days after the test compound. ED_{50} <50 μmoles/kg, ++; ED_{50} 50–150 μmoles/kg, +; marginal effects, ±; and no inhibition, n.i. (Lundstrom *et al.*, 1973b and unpublished results).

the active compounds are again those which will readily autoxidize to *para*-quinones. The quinones from two of the amino compounds (Fig. 6, I and III) should cyclize to yield 5(6)-hydroxy-6(5)-aminoindoles.

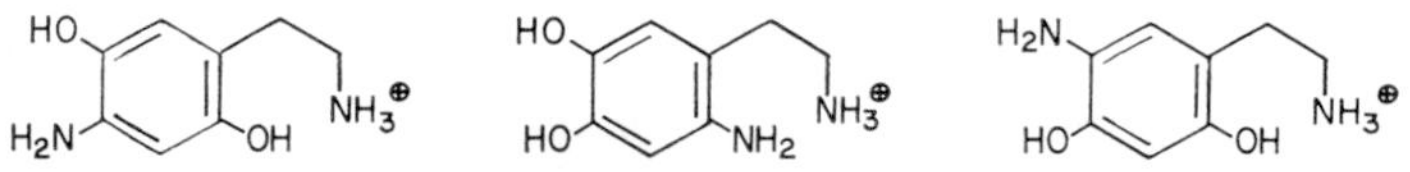

I   II   III

FIG. 6. Dihydroxyaminophenethylamines that are active as neurodegenerative agents towards noradrenergic terminals. The nitro compounds that correspond to compounds I and III were inactive. (Tranzer and Thoenen, 1973.)

DIHYDROXYTRYPTAMINES

The successful development of 6-hydroxydopamine as a tool for the selective degeneration of catecholamine containing neurons, led to the search for an agent with similar effects on serotonergic neurons. 5,6-Dihydroxytryptamine has now been demonstrated as such a compound (Baumgarten et al., 1971). Intraventricular injection of this compound rather specifically depletes brain of serotonin particularly in brain stem, causes disappearance of serotonin-containing nerve terminals and a long-term loss of uptake of radioactive serotonin in slices prepared from hypothalamus and spinal cord (Baumgarten and Lachenmayer, 1972a; Baumgarten et al., 1972a–e, 1973a; Costa et al., 1972; Daly et al., 1972, 1973). Intracerebral injection of 5,6-dihydroxytryptamine proximate to serotonin tracts provides a method for analysis of morphology and function of central serotonin neurons (Daly et al., 1972, 1973). A certain degree of nonspecificity of effects of 5,6-dihydroxytryptamine on neuronal structures was evident in both the degeneration of tissue elicited by proximal intracerebral injection of the amine (Daly et al., 1973) and in the reduction of brain catecholamine and tyrosine hydroxylase levels after intraventricular administration of large doses of the amine (Baumgarten et al., 1972c). 5,6-Dihydroxytryptamine has been shown to have high affinity for the serotonin-transport system of brain slices and low affinity for the dopamine-transport system (Heikkila and Cohen, 1973a). Peripherally, 5,6-dihydroxytryptamine causes release of norepinephrine (Daly et al., 1966) and an acute pressor effect apparently mediated by direct interaction with serotonin receptors (Baumgarten et al., 1972d). A mild degree of peripheral noradrenergic neurodegeneration has been reported after large doses of 5,6-dihydroxytryptamine (Baumgarten et al., 1972b). Unfortunately, 5,6-dihydroxytryptamine is quite toxic both by peripheral and intraventricular administration.

5,7-Dihydroxytryptamine is perhaps a more satisfactory agent for the selective neurodegeneration of central serotonin neurons since it is less toxic and somewhat more active with regard to effects on serotonin neurons (Baumgarten and Lachenmayer, 1972b, Fuxe, personal communication). Like the 5,6-isomer, 5,7-dihydroxytryptamine has, however, effects on both serotonin and catecholamine neurons. Both compounds have recently been shown to decrease brain tryptophan hydroxylase levels (Victor et al., 1973; Baumgarten et al., 1973b).

Structure activity correlations with respect to effects on central catecholamine and serotonin neurons are under investigation for the dihydroxytryptamines (Fuxe et al., unpublished results). The effects of these compounds on certain other systems have also been measured (Lundstrom et al., 1973a): (i) rate of autoxidation, (ii) inhibition of ^{3}H-norepinephrine uptake into heart, (iii) efficacy as releasing agents towards cardiac stores of ^{3}H-norepinephrine, and (iv) long-term effects on uptake of ^{3}H-norepinephrine into cardiac tissue (Table 2). It is apparent that all of the compounds auto-oxidize at extremely low rates compared to 6-hydroxydopamine, and that the 5,6- and 5,7-dihydroxytryptamine have low but significant affinity for the norepinephrine-transport system of heart. In spite of their low rate of autoxidation, two of the three dihydroxytryptamines do elicit long-term reductions in uptake of ^{3}H-norepinephrine into cardiac stores, evidence suggestive of degenerations of noradrenergic terminals and all three dihydroxytryptamines apparently can cause neurodegeneration of central serotonergic and noradrenergic terminals (Fuxe, personal communication).

The effects of trihydroxyphenethylamines in regard to long-term neurodegeneration are

TABLE 2. DIHYDROXYTRYPTAMINES: RELATIVE ACTIVITIES RELATED TO THEIR EFFECT ON NEURONAL STRUCTURES[a]

R = CH_2—CH_2—NH_{22}	A Rate autoxidation	B ED_{50} for inhibition of uptake of norepinephrine	C ED_{50} for release of norepinephrine	D Long-term inhibition of uptake of norepinephrine
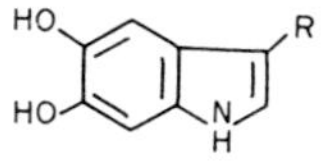 *(structure)*	2	10	41	±
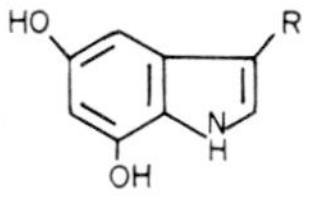 *(structure)*	3	10	109	+
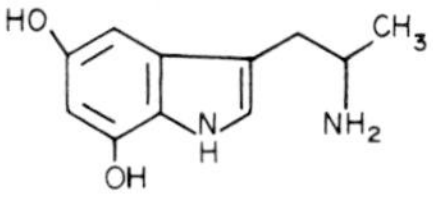 *(structure)*	—	—	10	n.i.
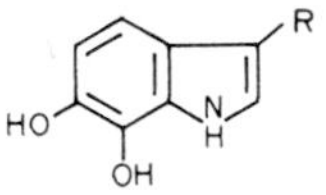 *(structure)*	—	n.i.	—	+

[a]For significance of columns A–D, see notes to Table 1.

slightly potentiated by inhibition of monoamine oxidase (see above). Surprisingly, the long-term effects of 5,7-dihydroxytryptamine on cardiac uptake of ^{3}H-norepinephrine are *blocked* by inhibition of monoamine oxidase and are absent in the α-methyl analog of 5,7-dihydroxytryptamine (Fig. 7). α-Methyl-5,7-dihydroxytryptamine is, however, much more

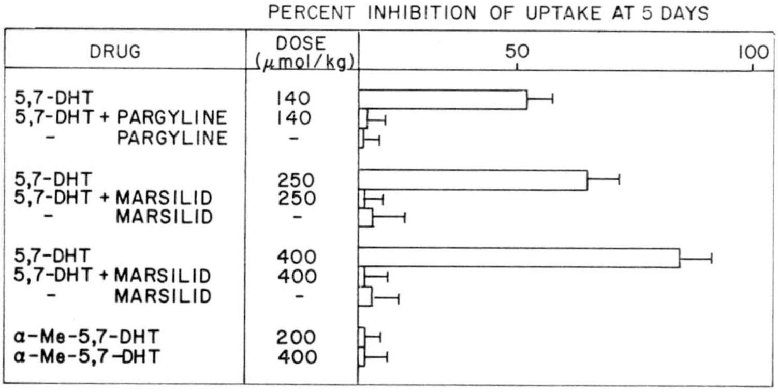

PERCENT INHIBITION OF UPTAKE AT 5 DAYS

DRUG	DOSE (μmol/kg)	
5,7-DHT	140	
5,7-DHT + PARGYLINE	140	
- PARGYLINE	-	
5,7-DHT	250	
5,7-DHT + MARSILID	250	
- MARSILID	-	
5,7-DHT	400	
5,7-DHT + MARSILID	400	
- MARSILID	-	
α-Me-5,7-DHT	200	
α-Me-5,7-DHT	400	

FIG. 7. Long-term effects of 5,7-dihydroxytryptamine (5,7-DHT) and α-methyl-5,7-dihydroxytryptamine (α-Me-5,7-DHT) on the *in vivo* uptake of ^{3}H-norepinephrine in mouse heart: blockade by inhibition of monoamine oxidase. (Lundstrom, J., Creveling, C. R., McNeal, E., and Daly, J. W., unpublished results.) Pargyline (50 mg/kg s.c.) or marsilid (150 mg/kg, s.c.) was administered 18 h prior to administration of the 5,7-DHT. ^{3}H-Norepinephrine was administered intravenously to mice 5 days after subcutaneous administration of the dihydroxytryptamine and levels of radioactivity in heart were measured 15 min later. (Cf. Lundstrom *et al.*, 1973b.)

active than the parent compound as a releasing agent for ^{3}H-norepinephrine (Table 2) and inhibition of monoamine oxidase slightly potentiates the norepinephrine releasing activity of 5,7-dihydroxtryptamine. A tentative explanation is that the action of monoamine oxidase converts 5,7-dihydroxytryptamine into a highly active cytotoxic agent within the noradrenergic nerve terminal. Further studies are in progress on this and other aspects of the action of dihydroxytryptamines.

REFERENCES

ADAMS, R. N. (1972) Stein and Wise theory of schizophrenia: a possible mechanism for 6-hydroxydopamine formation *in vivo*. *Behavioral Biology* **7**, 861–866.

ADAMS, R. N., MURRILL, E., McCREERY, R., BLANK, L., and KAROLCZAK, M. (1972) 6-Hydroxydopamine, a new oxidation mechanism. *Eur. J. Pharmac*. **17**, 287–292.

BARTHOLINI, G., PLETSCHER, A., and RICHARDS, J. (1970a) 6-Hydroxydopamine-induced inhibition of brain catecholamine synthesis without ultra-structural damage. *Experientia* **26**, 598–600.

BARTHOLINI, G., RICHARDS, J., and PLETSCHER, A. (1970b) Dissociation between biochemical and ultra-structural effects of 6-hydroxydopamine in rat brain. *Experientia* **26**, 142–144.

BAUMGARTEN, H. G., and LACHENMAYER, L. (1972a) Chemically induced degeneration of indoleamine-containing nerve terminals in rat brain. *Brain Res*. **38**, 228–232.

BAUMGARTEN, H. G., and LACHENMAYER, L. (1972b) 5,7-Dihydroxytryptamine: Improvement in chemical lesioning of indoleamine neurons in the mammalian brain. *Z. Zellforsch*. **135**, 399–414.

BAUMGARTEN, H. G., BJÖRKLUND, A., LACHENMAYER, L., NOBIN, A., and STENEVI, U. (1971) Long lasting selective depletion of brain serotonin by 5,6-dihydroxytryptamine. *Acta physiol. scand*., *Suppl*. 373.

BAUMGARTEN, H. G., BJÖRKLUND, A., LACHENMAYER, L., and NOBIN, A. (1972a) Chemical degeneration of indolamine axons in rat brain by 5,6-dihydroxytryptamine. *Z. Zellforsch*. **129**, 256–271.

BAUMGARTEN, H. G., BOTHERT, M., HOLSTEIN, A. F., and SCHLOSSBERGER, H. G. (1972b) Chemical sympathectomy induced by 5,6-dihydroxytryptamine. *Z. Zellforsch*. **128**, 115–134.

BAUMGARTEN, H. G., EVETTS, K. D., HOLMAN, R. B., IVERSEN, L. L., VOGT, M., and WIJSON, G. (1972c) Effects of 5,6-dihydroxytryptamine on monoaminergic neurones in the central nervous system of the rat. *J. Neurochem*. **19**, 1587–1597.

BAUMGARTEN, H. G., GOTHERT, M., SCHLOSSBERGER, H. G., and TUCHINDA, P. (1972d) Mechanism of pressor effect of 5,6-dihydroxytryptamine in pithed rats. *Naunyn-Schmiedeberg's Arch. exp. Path. Pharmak*. **274**, 375–384.

BAUMGARTEN, H. G., LACHENMAYER, L., and SCHLOSSBERGER, H. G. (1972e) Evidence for a degeneration of indolamine containing nerve terminals in rat brain, induced by 5,6-dihydroxytryptamine. *Z. Zellforsch*. **125**, 553–569.

BAUMGARTEN, H. G., LACHENMAYER, L., BJORKLUND, A., NOBIN, A., and ROSENGREN, E. (1973a) Long-term recovery of serotonin concentrations in the rat CNS following 5,6-dihydroxytryptamine. *Life Sci*., Part I, 12, 357–364.

BAUMGARTEN, H. G., VICTOR, S. J., and LOVENBERG, W. (1973b) Effect of intraventricular injection of 5,7-dihydroxytryptamine on regional tryptophan hydroxylase of rat brain. *J. Neurochem*. **21**, 251–253.

BENNETT, T., BURNSTOCK, G., COBB, J. L. S., and MALMFORS, T. (1970) An ultrastructural and histochemical study of the short-term effects of 6-hydroxydopamine on adrenergic nerves in the domestic fowl. *J. Pharmac*. **38**, 802–809.

BERKOWITZ, B. A., SPECTOR, S., BROSSI, A., FOCELLA, A. and TEITEL, S. (1970) Preparation and biological properties of (−) and (+)-6-hydroxydopa. *Experientia* **26**, 982–983.

BLANK, C. L., KISSINGER, P. T., and ADAMS, R. N. (1972) 5,6-Dihydroxyindole formation from oxidized 6-hydroxydopamine. *Eur. J. Pharmac*. **19**, 391–394.

BREESE, G. R., and TRAYLOR, T. D. (1970) Effect of 6-hydroxydopamine on brain norepinephrine and dopamine: evidence for selective degeneration of catecholamine neurons. *J. Pharmac. Exp. Ther*. **174**, 413–420.

BREESE, G. R., and TRAYLOR, T. D. (1971) Depletion of brain noradrenaline and dopamine by 6-hydroxydopamine. *Br. J. Pharmac*. **42**, 88–99.

BRIMIJOIN, S., and MOLINOFF, P. B. (1971) Effects of 6-hydroxydopamine on the activity of tyrosine hydroxylase and dopamine-β-hydroxylase in sympathetic ganglia of the rat. *J. Pharmac. Exp. Ther*. **178**, 417–424.

CHEAH, T. B., GEFFEN, L. B., JARROTT, B., and OSTBERG, A. (1971) Action of 6-hydroxydopamine on lamb sympathetic ganglia, vas deferens and adrenal medulla: a combined histochemical, ultrastructural and biochemical comparison with the effects of reserpine. *Br. J. Pharmac*. **42**, 543–557.

CLARKE, D. E., SMOOKLER, H. H., HADINATA, J., CHI, C., and BARRY, H., III (1972) Acute effects of 6-hydroxydopa and its interaction with dopa on brain amine levels. *Life Sci.* **11**, 97–102.

CORRODI, H., CLARK, W. G., and MASUOKA, D. I. (1971a) The synthesis and effects of DL-6-hydroxydopa. In *6-Hydroxydopamine and Catecholamine Neurons* (eds. Malmfors, T. and Thoenen, N.), North-Holland, Amsterdam, pp. 187–192.

CORRODI, H., MASUOKA, D. T., and CLARK, W. G. (1971b) Effect of 6-hydroxydopamine on rat heart noradrenaline. *Eur. J. Pharmac.* **15**, 160–163.

COSTA, E., LEFEVRE, H., MEEK, J., REVUELTA, A., SPANO, F., STRADA, S., and DALY, J. (1972) Serotonin and catecholamine concentrations in brain of rats injected intracerebrally with 5,6-dihydroxytryptamine. *Brain Res.* **44**, 304–308.

DALY, J. W., CREVELING, C. R., and WITKOP, B. (1966) The chemorelease of norepinephrine from mouse hearts: structure-activity relationships: I, Sympathomimetic and related amines, *J. Med. Chem.* **9**, 273–280.

DALY, J. W., FUXE, K., and JONSSON, G. (1972) 5,6-Dihydroxytryptamine: a new tool in mapping out central 5-HT neurons, Abstr., *4th Int. Congr. Histochem. and Cytochem.*, *Kyoto*, pp. 487–488.

DALY, J. W., FUXE, K., and JONSSON, G. (1973) Effects of intracerebral injections of 5,6-dihydroxytryptamine on central monoamine neurons: evidence for selective degeneration of central 5-hydroxytryptamine neurons. *Brain Res.* **49**, 476–382.

DE CHAMPLAIN, J. (1971) Degeneration and regrowth of adrenergic nerve fibers in the rat peripheral tissues after 6-hydroxydopamine. *J. Physiol. Pharmac.* **49**, 345–355.

EVETTS, K. D., and IVERSEN, L. L. (1970) Effects of protriptyline on the depletion of catecholamines induced by 6-hydroxydopamine in the brain of the rat. *J. Pharm. Pharmac.* **22**, 540–543.

GOLDMAN, H., and JACOBOWITZ, D. (1971) Correlation of norepinephrine content with observations of adrenergic nerves after a single dose of 6-hydroxydopamine in the rat. *J. Pharmac. Exp. Ther.* **176**, 119–133.

HAEUSLER, G. (1971) Early pre- and postjunctional effects of 6-hydroxydopamine. *J. Pharmac. Exp. Ther.* **178**, 49–62.

HAEUSLER, G., HAEFELY, W., and THOENEN, H. (1969) Chemical sympathectomy of the cat with 6-hydroxydopamine. *J. Pharmac. Exp. Ther.* **170**, 50–61.

HARLEY-MASON, J. (1953) Melanin and its precursors: IV, Further syntheses of 5,6-dihydroxyindole and its derivatives. *J. Chem. Soc.* 200–203.

HEDREEN, J. C., and CHALMERS, J. P. (1972) Neuronal degeneration in rat brain induced by 6-hydroxydopamine: a histological and biochemical study. *Brain Res.* **47**, 1–36.

HEIKKILA, R., and COHEN, G. (1971) Inhibition of biogenic amine uptake by hydrogen peroxide: a mechanism for toxic effects of 6-hydroxydopamine. *Science* **172**, 1257–1258.

HEIKKILA, R., and COHEN, G. (1972a) Further studies on the generation of hydrogen peroxide by 6-hydroxydopamine. *Molec. Pharmac.* **8**, 241–248.

HEIKKILA, R. E., and COHEN, G. (1972b) *In vivo* generation of hydrogen peroxide from 6-hydroxydopamine. *Experientia* **28**, 1197.

HEIKKILA, R. E., and COHEN, G. (1973a) The inhibition of H-biogenic amine uptake by 5,6-dihydroxytryptamine: a comparison with the effects of 6-hydroxydopamine. *Eur. J. Pharmac.* **21**, 66–69.

HEIKKILA, R., and COHEN, G. (1973b) 6-Hydroxydopamine: Evidence for superoxide radical as an oxidative intermediate. *Science* **181**, 456–457.

HEIKKILA, R. E., MYTILINEOU C., COTE, L., and COHEN, G. (1973) Evidence for degeneration of sympathetic nerve terminals caused by the *ortho*- and *para*- quinones of 6-hydroxydopamine. *J. Neurochem.* **20**, 1345–1350.

JACOBOWITZ, D., and KOSTRZEWA, R. (1971) Selective action of 6-hydroxydopa on noradrenergic terminals: mapping of preterminal axons of the brain. *Life Sci.* **10**, 1329–1342.

JONSSON, G., and SACHS, C. (1970) Effects of 6-hydroxydopamine on the uptake and storage of noreadrenaline in sympathetic adrenergic neurons. *Eur. J. Pharmac.* **9**, 141–155.

JONSSON, G., and SACHS, C. (1972) Degenerative and nondegenerative effects of 6-hydroxydopamine on adrenergic nerves. *J. Pharmac. Exp. Ther.* **180**, 625–635.

KOSTRZEWA, R., and JACOBOWITZ, D. (1972) The effect of 6-hydroxydopa on peripheral adrenergic neurons. *J, Pharmac. Exp. Ther.* **183**, 284–297.

KOSTRZEWA, R., and JACOBOWITZ, D. (1973) Acute effects of 6-hydroxydopa on central monoaminergic neurons. *Eur. J. Pharmac.* **21**, 70–80.

LEVIN, E. Y., and KAUFMAN, S. (1961) Studies on the enzyme catalyzing the conversion of 3,4-dihydroxyphenethylamine to norepinephrine. *J. Biol. Chem.* **236**, 2043–2049.

LOWE, M. C., and HORITA, A. (1970) Stability of cardiac monoamine oxidase activity after chemical sympathectomy with 6-hydroxydopamine. *Nature* **228**, 175–176.

LUNDSTROM, J., MCNEAL, E. T., DALY, J. W., and CREVELING, C. R. (1973a) Acute and chronic effects of trihydroxyphenethylamines and dihydroxytryptamines on adrenergic mechanisms in the murine heart. *Fed. Proc.* **32**, 769 Abs.

LUNDSTROM, J., ONG, H., DALY, J. W., and CREVELING, C. R. (1973b) Isomers of 2,4,5-trihydroxyphenethyl-amine (6-hydroxydopamine): long term effects on the *in vivo* accumulation of H-norepinephrine in mouse heart. *Molec. Pharmac.* **9**, 505–513.

MALMFORS, T., and SACHS, C. (1968) Degeneration of adrenergic nerves produced by 6-hydroxydopamine. *Eur. J. Pharmac.* **3**, 89–92.

MALMFORS, T., and THOENEN, H. (eds.) (1971) 6-*Hydroxydopamine and catecholamine neurons*, North-Holland, Amsterdam.

MANARA, L., MENNINI, T., and CARMINATI, P. (1972) Reduced binding of ^{3}H-reserpine to hearts of 6-hydro-xydopamine-pretreated rats. *Eur. J. Pharmac.* **17**, 183–185.

MUELLER, R. A., THOENEN, H., and AXELROD, J. (1969) Adrenal tyrosine hydroxylase: compensatory increase in activity after chemical sympathectomy. *Science* **163**, 468–469.

ONG, H. H., CREVELING, C. R., and DALY, J. W. (1969) The synthesis of 2,4,5-trihydroxyphenylalanine (6-hydroxydopa). A centrally active norepinephrine-depleting agent. *J. Med. Chem.* **12**, 458–461.

POIRIER, L. J., LANGELIER, P., ROBERGE, A., BOUCHER, R., and KITSIKIS, A. (1972) Non-specific histo-pathological changes induced by the intracerebral injection of 6-hydroxydopamine (6-OH-DA). *J. Neurol. Sci.* **16**, 401–416.

PORTER, C. C., TOTARO, J. A., and BURCIN, A. (1965) The relationship between radioactivity and nore-pinephrine concentrations in the brains and hearts of mice following administration of labeled methyl-dopa or 6-hydroxydopamine. *J. Pharmac. Exp. Ther.* **150**, 17–22.

POWELL, W. S., and HEACOCK, R. A. (1973) The oxidation of 6-hydroxydopamine. *J. Pharm. Pharmac.* **25**, 193–200.

PRASAD, K. N. (1970) Effect of dopamine and 6-hydroxydopamine on the growth of mouse neuroblastoma cells *in vitro*. *J. Cell Biol.* **41**, 160a.

SACHS, C. (1972) Failure of 6-hydroxynoradrenaline to produce degeneration of catecholamine neurons. *Eur. J. Pharmac.* **20**, 149–155.

SACHS, C., and JONSSON, G. (1972a) Selective 6-hydroxy-DOPA induced degeneration of central and peri-pheral noradrenaline neurons. *Brain Res.* **40**, 563–568.

SACHS, C. and JONSSON, G. (1972b) Degeneration of central and peripheral noradrenaline neurons produced by 6-hydroxy-dopa. *J. Neurochem.* **19**, 1561–1575.

SANER, A., and THOENEN, H. (1971) Model experiments on molecular mechanism of action of 6-hydro-xydoparnine. *Molec. Pharmac.* **7**, 147–154.

SENOH, S., and WITKOP, B. (1959) Formation and rearrangements of aminochromes from a new metabolite of dopamine and some of its derivatives. *J. Am. Chem. Soc.* **81**, 6231–6235.

SENOH, S., CREVELING, C. R., UDENFRIEND, S., and WITKOP, B. (1959a) Chemical, enzymatic and metabolic studies on the mechanism of oxidation of dopamine. *J. Am. Chem. Soc.* **81**, 6236–6240.

SENOH, S., WITKOP, B., CREVELING, C. R. and UDENFRIEND, S. (1959b) 2,4,5-Trihydroxyphenylamine, a new metabolite of 3,4-dihydroxyphenethylamine. *J. Am. Chem. Soc.* **81**, 1768.

SIGGINS, G. R., FORMAN, D. S., BLOOM, F. E., SIMS, K. L., and ADAMS, R. N. (1973) Destruction of peripheral and central adrenergic nerves by 6-aminodopamine. *Fed. Proc.* **32**, 692A.

SIMMONDS, M. A., and URETSKY, N. J. (1970) Central effects of 6-hydroxydopamine on the body temperature of the rat. *Br. J. Pharmac.* **40**, 630–638.

STEIN, L., and WISE, C. D. (1971) Possible etiology of schizophrenia: Progressive damage to the noradren-ergic reward system by 6-hydroxydopamine. *Science* **171**, 1032–1036.

STONE, C. A., PORTER, C. C., STAVORSKI, J. M., LUDDEN, C. T., and TOTARO, J. A. (1964a) Antagonism of certain effects of catecholamine depleting agents by antidepressant and related drugs. *J. Pharmac. Exp. Ther.* **144**, 196–204.

STONE, C. A., STAVORSKI, J. M., LUDDEN, C. T., WENGER, H. C., ROSS, C. A., TOTARO, J. A., and PORTER, C. C. (1964b) Comparison of some pharmacologic effects of certain 6-substituted dopamine derivatives with reserpine, guanethidine and metaraminol. *J. Pharmac. Exp. Ther.* **142**, 147–156.

TAYLOR, K. M., and LAVERTY, R. (1972) The effects of drugs on the behavioural and biochemical actions of intraventricular 6-hydroxydopamine. *Eur. J. Pharmac.* **17**, 16–24.

THOA, N. B., EICHELMAN, B., RICHARDSON, J. S., and JACOBOWITZ, D. (1972) 6-Hydroxydopa depletion of brain norepinephrine and facilitation of aggressive behavior. *Science* **178**, 75–77.

THOENEN, H., and TRANZER, J. P. (1968) Chemical sympathectomy by selective destruction of adrenergic nerve endings with 6-hydroxydopamine. *Naunyn-Schmiedebergs' Arch. exp. Path. Pharmak.* **261**, 271–288.

THOENEN, H., MUELLER, R. A., and AXELROD, J. (1969) Increased tyrosine hydroxylase activity after drug-induced alteration of sympathetic transmission. *Nature* **221**, 1264.

THOENEN, H., MUELLER, R. A. and AXELROD, J. (1970) Neuronally dependent induction of adrenal phenyl-ethanolamine-*N*-methyltransferase by 6-hydroxydopamine. *Biochem. Pharmac.* **19**, 669–673.

TRANZER, J. P., and THOENEN, H. (1973) Selective destruction of adrenergic nerve terminals by chemical analogues of 6-hydroxydopamine. *Experientia* **29**, 314–316.

URETSKY, N. J. and IVERSEN, L. L. (1970) Effects of 6-hydroxydopamine on catecholamine containing neurones in the rat brain. *J. Neurochem.* **17,** 269–278.

VICTOR, S. J., BAUMGARTEN, H. G., and LOVENBERG, W. (1973) Effect of intraventricular administration of 5,6- and 5,7-dihydroxytryptamine on regional tryptophan hydroxylase activity in rat brain. *Fed. Proc.* **32,** 564 Abs.

WAGNER, K., and TRENDELENBURG, U. (1971) Effect of 6-hydroxydopamine on oxidative phosphorylation and on monoamine oxidase activity. *Naunyn-Schmiedeberg's Arch. exp. Path. Pharmak.* **269,** 112–116.

WEHRLI, P. A., PIGOTT, F., FISCHER, U., and KAISER, A. (1972) Oxydations Produkte von 6-Hydroxydopamin. *Helv. chim. Acta* **55,** 3057–3061.

NEUROTOXIC ACTION OF 6-HYDROXY-DOPA ON CENTRAL CATECHOLAMINE NEURONS

Charlotte Sachs

Department of Histology, Karolinska Institutet, Stockholm

SUMMARY

The neurotoxic effects of 6-hydroxy-DOPA (6-OH-DOPA)† in combination with MAO-inhibition is studied on central catecholamine neurons in the mouse. 6-OH-DOPA administration led to a rapid and long-lasting decrease in ^{3}H-amine uptake in NA neurons which paralleled a similar decrease in endogenous NA concentration. The NA terminals in the cerebral cortex were quantitatively more affected than those in the hypothalamus. The effect of 6-OH-DOPA (100 mg/kg i.p.) was selective on NA neurons, while DA and 5-HT neurons were left intact. However, there was no absolute selectivity, since after higher doses, also DA neurons were attacked. In long-term experiments there were signs of regeneration of NA nerve fibers, mostly pronounced in the hypothalamus.

Fluorescence histochemical examinations also showed a selective effect by 6-OH-DOPA on NA neurons, with a disappearance of terminals in many brain regions. The most conspicuous fluorescence histochemical observation was strongly fluorescent accumulations of NA in the preterminal axons, making it possible to trace NA axons for long distances in the same animal. The NA cell bodies appeared intact. Certain NA neuron systems were preferentially attacked by 6-OH-DOPA, i.e. mainly the NA fibers emanating from cell bodies in the locus coeruleus area. 6-OH-DOPA has, due to its selectively destroying NA terminals and building up accumulations in NA tracts, become a valuable tool in the mapping of NA pathways in the brain. 6-OH-DOPA may also be of value for functional studies of central NA neurons.

INTRODUCTION

6-Hydroxydopamine (6-OH-DA) can produce a selective degeneration of catecholamine nerve terminals in the central and peripheral nervous system (see symposium volume edited by Malmfors and Thoenen, 1971). This unique property of 6-OH-DA has led to its extensive use as a denervation tool for the elucidation of various aspects of catecholamine transmitter mechanisms. However, in order to markedly affect the central catecholamine neurons, 6-OH-DA has to be injected locally into the brain since the compound does not

†Abbreviations used: 6-OH-DOPA = 2,4,5-trihydroxyphenylalanine, 6-OH-DA = 6-hydroxydopamine, NA = noradrenaline, MA = metaraminol, MAO = monoamine oxidase, COMT = catechol-*O*-methyl transferase DA = dopamine, 5-HT = 5-hydroxytryptamine, DMI = desipramine.

readily pass the blood–brain barrier (Ungerstedt, 1968, 1971a; Bloom *et al.*, 1969; Uretsky and Iversen, 1969).

The 6-OH-DA precursor, 6-OH-DOPA, may pass from the blood circulation into the brain and induce marked decrease in brain NA concentration (Ong *et al.*, 1969; Berkowitz *et al.*, 1970; Corrodi *et al.*, 1971a), which is related to selective destruction and degeneration of NA nerve terminals (Jacobowitz and Kostrzewa, 1971; Sachs and Jonsson, 1972a, b). In order to obtain a degenerative effect by 6-OH-DOPA, it must be decarboxylated to 6-OH-DA (Fig. 1), which is responsible for the neurotoxic action (Sachs and Jonsson, 1972b). The purpose of the present paper is to review some recent work on 6-OH-DOPA from our laboratory, dealing with effects of 6-OH-DOPA on central catecholamine neurons, i.e. changes in NA uptake–storage mechanisms and the use of 6-OH-DOPA as a tool in neuroanatomical studies by fluorescence histochemistry.

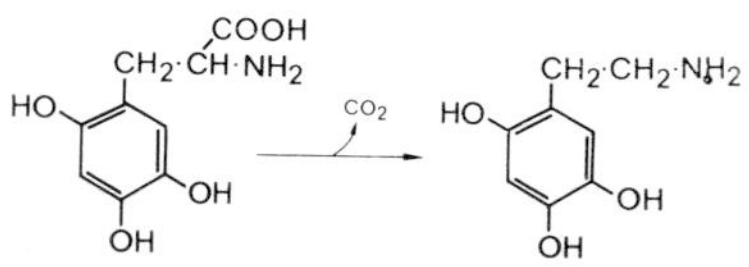

FIG. 1.

6-OH-DOPA-INDUCED NA DEPLETION AND REDUCTION OF ^{3}H-AMINE UPTAKE

One limiting factor when working with 6-OH-DOPA is its severe general toxicity. The highest dose of 6-OH-DOPA (H88/61, AB Hässle) which was tolerated by mice for prolonged survival was 100 mg/kg i.p., a dose which could be repeated several times with 24 h intervals. One single dose (100 mg/kg i.p.) was found not to have any effect on the catecholamine nerve terminals of cortex cerebri, measured as *in vitro* uptake of ^{3}H-NA in cortical slices (Sachs and Jonsson, 1972b), but when repeated once there was an approximately 40% decrease of ^{3}H-NA uptake. When 6-OH-DOPA was given 6 times with 24 h intervals, there was a 55% reduction in ^{3}H-NA uptake. Kostrzewa and Jacobowitz (1973) have, however, showed marked effects of single 6-OH-DOPA injections (100 or 150 mg/kg) on the endogenous NA content of mouse brain especially after intravenous administrations. The reason for the differences between these and the present results is unclear, but may be related to differences in mouse strains and/or due to differences in the 6-OH-DOPA substances used. In the search for a drug to reinforce the effect of 6-OH-DOPA, it was found that pretreatment of mice with the MAO-inhibitor, nialamide (100 mg/kg i.p.) 2 h before 6-OH-DOPA (100 mg/kg i.p.), resulted in a pronounced potentiation of the reduction of ^{3}H-NA uptake, compared with 6-OH-DOPA given alone (Fig. 2).

Therefore, in most of the studies reported here the animals were treated with nialamide (100 mg/kg i.p., 2 h) before the 6-OH-DOPA administration.

Studying the short-term effects of 6-OH-DOPA (100 mg/kg i.p.) in nialamide pretreated mice, a rather rapid decrease of ^{3}H-NA uptake in cerebral cortex slices was found (Fig. 3). The decrease was maximal already 2 h after the 6-OH-DOPA injection, being about 40% of control value. The decrease in ^{3}H-NA uptake was less pronounced in hypothalamic

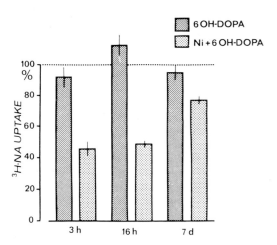

FIG. 2. Effect of nialamide + 6-OH-DOPA on the *in vitro* uptake of ^{3}H-NA (10^{-7} M, 10 min) in slices of cerebral cortex. The mice were treated with 6-OH-DOPA (100 mg/kg i.p., 3 h, 16 h, or 7 days) with or without pretreatment with nialamide (100 mg/kg i.p., 2 h). The values are expressed as percent of untreated control. Each value is the mean ± SEM of eight determinations. (Sachs and Jonsson, 1972b.)

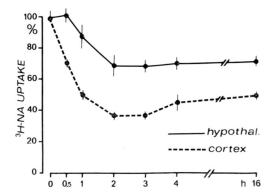

FIG. 3. Time-course of nialamide + 6-OH-DOPA-induced reduction of ^{3}H-NA (10^{-7} M, 10 min) uptake *in vitro* in slices of hypothalamus and cerebral cortex. The mice were treated with nialamide (100 mg/kg i.p.) 2 h before 6-OH-DOPA (100 mg/kg i.p.). The animals were killed at various periods of time after the 6-OH-DOPA injection. The values are expressed as percent of untreated control and each value represents the mean ± SEM of six to ten determinations.

slices and the onset of the 6-OH-DOPA effect seemed somewhat slower. It is possible that part of the ^{3}H-NA taken up in cerebral cortex after nialamide + 6-OH-DOPA treatment is localized in DA nerve terminals. This is supported by the finding that DMI causes a more effective inhibition of ^{3}H-NA uptake in slices of cerebral cortex from untreated mice than in slices from mice treated with nialamide + 6-OH-DOPA. It is known that DMI is an effective inhibitor of the membrane pump of NA neurons, but not of DA neurons (Carlsson *et al.*, 1966; Hamberger, 1967).

The long-term effects of nialamide + 6-OH-DOPA (3 × 100 mg/kg i.p., 24 h intervals) was studied on ^{3}H-amine uptake in slices from cerebral cortex, hypothalamus, nucl. caudatus putamen, and on endogenous NA concentration in whole brain (Fig. 4). There

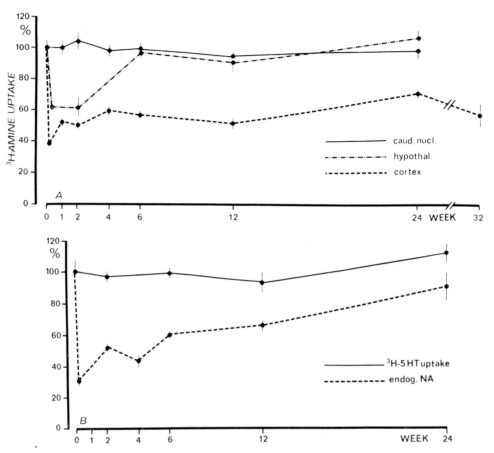

FIG. 4. Time-course of nialamide + 6-OH-DOPA induced effects on the *in vitro* uptake of
^{3}H-amine in slices from various parts of the brain and on the endogenous NA concentration
of whole brain. The mice were treated with nialamide (100 mg/kg i.p.) 2 h before 6-OH-DOPA
(3×100 mg/kg i.p., 24 h intervals). The mice were killed at various periods of time after the
last 6-OH-DOPA injection. The values are expressed as percent of untreated control and each
value represents the mean $\pm$ SEM of six to ten determinations. Endogenous NA was measured
according to Bertler *et al.* (1958) on five pooled mouse brains. The values are expressed as
percent of untreated control and each value represents the mean $\pm$ SEM of three determinations. Control brain contained 0.36 ± 0.02 μg/g.
A. ●——● ^{3}H-MA uptake (10^{-7} M, 10 min) in nucleus caudatus.
   ●–·–·–● ^{3}H-NA uptake (5×10^{-8} M, 10 min) in hypothalamus.
   ●– – –● ^{3}H-MA uptake (10^{-7} M, 10 min) in cerebral cortex.
B. ●——● ^{3}H-5-HT uptake (5×10^{-8} M, 10 min)in cerebral cortex.
   ●– – –● Endogenous NA concentration in whole brain.

was a pronounced reduction in ^{3}H-amine uptake at 16 h in slices from cerebral cortex and
hypothalamus and also of endogenous NA concentration of whole brain. The amine uptake
in slices of caudate nucleus was unchanged, indicating that the DA neurons were not
affected after this 6-OH-DOPA treatment. 6-OH-DOPA had also no apparent effect on
^{3}H-5-HT uptake in cerebral cortex (cf. Berkowitz *et al.*, 1970; Sachs and Jonsson, 1972b.
The present results show a selective effect of 6-OH-DOPA on NA neurons, which has also
been described by Jacobowitz and Kostrzewa (1971) and Kostrzewa and Jacobowitz (1973).

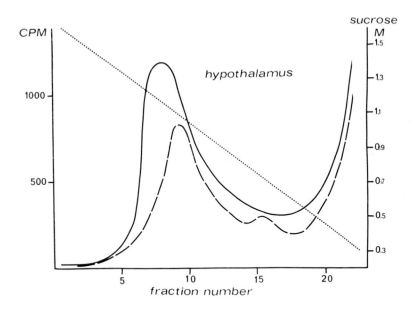

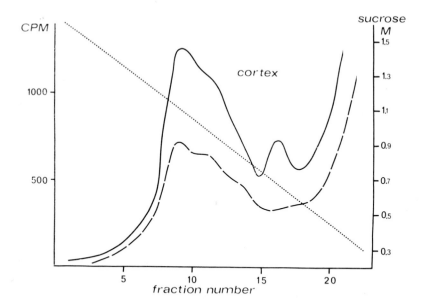

FIG. 5. Distribution of radioactivity of homogenates from mouse cerebral cortex and hypo-thalamus (incubated in ^{3}H-NA or ^{14}C-NA 5×10^{-8} M, 20 min) in a continuous sucrose density gradient, ranging from 0.3 to 1.6 M. The gradients were centrifuged at 75,000 g for 120 min, 4 drop-fractions were collected, and the radioactivity determined. The homogenates were made from untreated mice (———) and from mice treated with nialamide + 6-OH-DOPA (– – – –). Nial-amide (100 mg/kg i.p.) was injected 2 h before 6-OH-DOPA (100 mg/kg i.p.) and the mice killed 48 h later. (Pycock, unpublished results.)

The effects of 6-OH-DOPA were long-lasting, indicating a severe damage and degeneration of NA nerve fibers, which also is supported by the fluorescence histochemical observations (see below). Present results (Fig. 4) and results from Jacobowitz and Kostrzewa (1971) show an increase in endogenous NA levels with time, indicating a regeneration of the NA fibers. However, the NA recovery may also in part be related to a "collateral accumulation" of NA granules (see Andén et al., 1966). There was a recovery of ^{3}H-NA uptake in the hypothalamus up to control value in 6 weeks, while there was only a slight increase in ^{3}H-amine uptake in the cortex cerebri over the 32 weeks studied. Thus the nerve terminals of the cerebral cortex seem less capable of regenerating compared with the terminals of the hypothalamus, which may be related to a damage relatively closer to the cell bodies. Enzymatic determination according to Saelens et al. (1967) of the endogenous NA concentration of the cerebral cortex 24 weeks after 6-OH-DOPA treatment showed that it was lower (65 $\pm$ 5% of control value, $n = 4$) than the NA concentration of whole brain (see Fig. 4B), while the NA level in hypothalamus was up to control value, pointing to a regional difference in restitution of NA nerve terminals in the brain after 6-OH-DOPA (unpublished observations).

The radioactivity distribution of homogenates from cerebral cortex and hypothalamus incubated in ^{3}H-NA was studied in continuous sucrose density gradients ranging from 0.3 M to 1.6 M sucrose (Fig. 5). The mice were pretreated with nialamide (100 mg/kg i.p.) 2 h before 6-OH-DOPA (100 mg/kg i.p.) and killed 48 h later. Nerve-ending particles were prepared from the cerebral cortex and hypothalamus according to Green et al. (1969) and incubated in vitro in ^{3}H-NA (5 $\times$ 10^{-8} M, 20 min). The nerve-ending particles were thereafter run on continuous sucrose gradients (75,000 g, 120 min). In the hypothalamus of the 6-OH-DOPA-treated animals there was a shift in the radioactivity peak towards a less dense region of the gradient. The control peak was at 1.17 M sucrose ($n = 4$) and the peak of 6-OH-DOPA-treated mice was at 1.09 M sucrose ($n = 4$). There was no such shift in peaks in the cortical synaptosomes, but only a general reduction of the radioactivity (Pycock, unpublished results). These results may indicate that a certain population of nerve terminals in the hypothalamus are preferentially destroyed by 6-OH-DOPA, possibly NA nerve terminals emanating from the so called dorsal NA bundle and locus coeruleus cell bodies (Ungerstedt, 1971b).

In order to investigate the possibility of further increasing the neurotoxic effect of 6-OH-DOPA, newborn mice were treated with nialamide and 6-OH-DOPA (3 $\times$ 100 mg/kg i.p., 24 h intervals) (Sachs and Jonsson, 1972b). The animals were studied when adult by measuring ^{3}H-NA uptake in slices from cerebral cortex and nucl. caudatus. The nialamide + 6-OH-DOPA-induced decrease in ^{3}H-NA uptake in cerebral cortex was approximately the same as in mice treated as adults (cf. Fig. 4). However, it was observed that the ^{3}H-DA uptake in nucl. caudatus slices was decreased about 20%. Thus the 6-OH-DOPA effects seem to be somewhat less selective in the neonate mouse.

PHARMACOLOGICAL MODIFICATIONS OF 6-OH-DOPA EFFECTS

Investigations were made on the effect of drugs known to interfere in catecholamine transmitter mechanisms in modifying the action of 6-OH-DOPA. Three brain regions were studied—cerebral cortex, hypothalamus, and nucl. caudatus. As previously mentioned, the *MAO inhibitor*, nialamide, caused a marked potentiation of the decrease in ^{3}H-NA uptake compared with 6-OH-DOPA alone (Fig. 2). The decrease in uptake was more pronounced

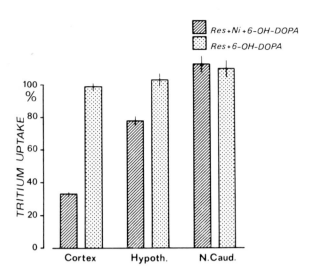

FIG. 6. Effect of reserpine (Res) on the 6-OH-DOPA-induced changes of *in vitro* uptake of ^{3}H-NA (10^{-7} M, 10 min) in slices from cerebral cortex and hypothalamus and uptake of H-DA (10^{-7} M, 10 min) in slices from nucl. caudatus. The mice were treated with reserpine (5 mg/kg i.p.) 6 h before nialamide (100 mg/kg i.p.), which was injected 2 h before 6-OH-DOPA (100 mg/kg i.p.), and were killed 48 h thereafter. The mice received in addition another dose of nialamide (100 mg/kg i.p.) 2 h before death, in order to obtain an efficient MAO inhibition when measuring the radioactivity uptake after reserpine. The values are expressed as percent of the respective control when 6-OH-DA was omitted. Each value represents the mean ± SEM of eight to ten determinations. (Jonsson and Sachs, 1973a.)

in the slices from cerebral cortex than from hypothalamus, indicating a greater sensitivity of the cortex NA terminals to the neurotoxic action of 6-OH-DA. There was no effect of nialamide + 6-OH-DOPA on ^{3}H-amine uptake in slices from the nucl. caudatus (Jonsson and Sachs, 1973a). The reason for the potentiating effect of MAO inhibition may be that the 6-OH-DA, formed from 6-OH-DOPA, is a substrate for this enzyme. Thus after MAO inhibition, increased tissue levels of formed, unchanged 6-OH-DA may be reached, and there will be a diminished intraneuronal breakdown of 6-OH-DA. In many nerve terminals the 6-OH-DA concentration will attain the critical level, required for producing neuronal degeneration (Thoenen and Tranzer, 1968; Jonsson and Sachs, 1970, 1971). Also the effect of 6-OH-DA is clearly augmented by MAO inhibition, especially when using low doses of 6-OH-DA (cf. Breese and Traylor, 1970; Jonsson *et al.*, 1972). There is also an increased uptake-accumulation of ^{3}H-6-OH-DA after nialamide pretreatment (Jonsson and Sachs, 1971).

Pretreating mice with *reserpine* (5 mg/kg i.p.) 6 h before 6-OH-DOPA did not result in any apparent change in ^{3}H-amine uptake (Fig. 6), compared with nialamide + 6-OH-DOPA treatment. However, a small protective effect of reserpine was found in the hypothalamus. Thus reserpine, which blocks the ATP-Mg^{2+} dependent uptake mechanism of the amine storage granules, did not markedly modify the neurotoxic action of 6-OH-DOPA. These results agree with findings in mouse heart and iris after 6-OH-DA (Jonsson and Sachs, 1970; Corrodi *et al.*, 1971b; Jonsson *et al.*, 1972), indicating that an intact granular uptake–storage mechanism is not a prerequisite for 6-OH-DA to produce neuronal degeneration, although intact amine granules may under certain conditions maintain the high intraneuronal 6-OH-DA levels, necessary for inducing degeneration (Jonsson *et al.*, 1972).

Treatment with the *"membrane pump" inhibitor*, DMI counteracted the nialamide + 6-OH-DOPA-induced reduction in uptake of ^{3}H-amine in cerebral cortex and hypothalamus (Fig. 7). These results indicate that uptake of 6-OH-DA formed extraneuronally from 6-OH-DOPA or reuptake of intraneuronally formed and released 6-OH-DA is important and necessary for the production of neuronal degeneration (cf. Kostrzewa and Jacobowitz, 1973).

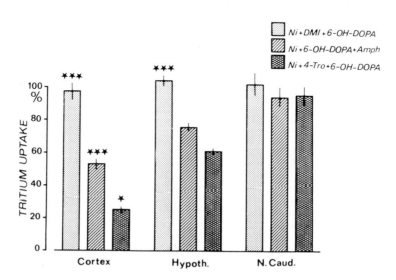

FIG. 7. Effect of DMI, amphetamine (amph), and 4-tropolone acetamide (4-tro) on the nialamide + 6-OH-DOPA-induced changes of *in vitro* uptake of ^{3}H-NA or ^{3}H-DA in brain slices (as in Fig. 6). Nialamide (100 mg/kg i.p.) was injected 2 h before 6-OH-DOPA (100 mg/kg i.p.) and the mice were killed 48 h thereafter. DMI (25 mg/kg i.p.) was injected 30 min before, and amphetamine (1 mg/kg i.v.) 15 min after the 6-OH-DOPA injection. 4-Tropolone acetamide (100 mg/kg i.p.) was given in two doses, 30 min before and 30 min after the 6-OH-DOPA injection. The values are expressed as percent of untreated control. Each value represents the mean ± SEM of six to ten determinations. The difference in experimental group and treatment with nialamide + 6-OH-DOPA was tested with Student's *t*-test. * $0.05 < p > 0.01$, *** $p < 0.001$. (Jonsson and Sachs, 1973a.)

Injection of *amphetamine* in a low dose (1 mg/kg i.v.) after the 6-OH-DOPA treatment resulted in a small counteraction of the 6-OH-DOPA-induced decrease in ^{3}H-amine uptake (Fig. 7). Amphetamine at this dose level is suggested to release mainly extragranular catecholamines from the axoplasm (Carlsson *et al.*, 1966) and may therefore release 6-OH-DA formed from 6-OH-DOPA, thereby decreasing the intraneuronal concentration of 6-OH-DA.

Inhibition of COMT, by 4-tropolone acetamide (100 mg/kg, 30 min before and 30 min after the 6-OH-DOPA injection) resulted in a small potentiation of the nialamide + 6-OH-DOPA induced decrease in ^{3}H-amine uptake (Fig. 7). COMT inhibition has been shown to increase the neurotoxic effects of 6-OH-DA also in sympathetic adrenergic nerves of the heart (Corrodi *et al.*, 1971b). Neither amphetamine nor 4-tropolone acetamide itself affected the uptake. 6-OH-DOPA may therefore, like L-DOPA to a certain extent be metabolized by COMT (Kuruma *et al.*, 1972).

Pretreatment with a *NA synthesis inhibitor*, H44/68 (α-methyl-*p*-tyrosine methylester) led to a counteraction of the nialamide + 6-OH-DOPA induced reduction in ^{3}H-NA uptake in cerebral cortex and hypothalamus (Fig. 8). This counteraction was most effective when H44/68 was given 16 h before 6-OH-DOPA, when the NA depletion is most pronounced. In the peripheral nervous system, on the other hand, H44/68 potentiated the effect of 6-OH-DOPA and 6-OH-DA (Jonsson and Sachs, 1973b). No sufficient explanation for this clear-cut difference of NA synthesis inhibition in the central and peripheral nervous system has been presented so far. It has been proposed that the critical intraneuronal concentration of 6-OH-DA needed for degeneration, may be related mainly to the extragranular concentration (Bennett *et al.*, 1970). If this is the case, the granules may play a

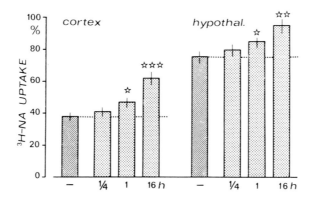

FIG. 8. Effect of H44/68 (α-methyl-*p*-tyrosine methylester) on the nialamide + 6-OH-DOPA-induced changes in the *in vitro* uptake of ^{3}H-NA (10^{-7} M, 10 min) in slices from cerebral cortex and hypothalamus. The mice were pretreated with nialamide (100 mg/kg i.p.) 2 h before 6-OH-DOPA (100 mg/kg i.p.) and killed 4 h later. H44/68 (500 mg/kg i.p.) was given 15 min, 1 h, or 16 h before the 6-OH-DOPA injection. The values are expressed as percent of the ^{3}H-NA uptake in *untreated control*. The striped columns represent nialamide + 6-OH-DOPA controls. Each column represents the mean ± SEM of eight to twelve determinations. Difference in values between the nialamide ± 6-OH-DOPA treatment and the additional H44/68 treatment was tested with Student's *t*-test. * $p < 0.05$, ** $p < 0.01$, *** $p < 0.001$. (Jonsson and Sachs, 1973b.)

protective role by binding 6-OH-DA; 6-OH-DA can be taken up in amine storage granules (Jonsson and Sachs, 1970; Bennett *et al.*, 1970). If 6-OH-DOPA is decarboxylated at a rather slow rate and the formed 6-OH-DA could be incorporated more efficiently in the amine granules after the depletion of the NA stores by H44/68, the result would be a protective effect. After H44/68 pretreatment the granules may more efficiently take up and retain 6-OH-DA than in the untreated control (cf. Jonsson *et al.*, 1969; Sachs, 1970). The results obtained by using reserpine or H44/68 are difficult to fully explain, but show that the granular uptake–storage mechanism may modulate the neurotoxic action of 6-OH-DA.

There may be differences in the rate of introduction of 6-OH-DA from 6-OH-DOPA into the neuron or in the granular uptake–storage mechanisms *per se* in central and peripheral NA neurons. The present results on pharmacological modification of the 6-OH-DOPA effect are relatively complicated, and it is impossible to draw any definite conclusions which may be related to a complex action of the neurotoxic compound 6-OH-DA.

FLUORESCENCE HISTOCHEMICAL STUDIES AFTER 6-OH-DOPA

Fluorescence histochemical studies according to the method of Falck and Hillarp (Falck *et al.*, 1962; Falck, 1962) revealed that after nialamide + 6-OH-DOPA treatment there was a marked decrease of fluorescing NA nerve terminals in many brain regions, e.g. in cerebral and cerebellar cortex and in periventricular areas of hypothalamus (Sachs and Jonsson, 1972a, b; cf. Jacobowitz and Kostrzewa, 1971). The NA cell bodies, e.g. in the locus coeruleus, appeared unaffected. The DA cell bodies in substantia nigra and its nerve terminals in the nucleus caudatus and the DA nerve terminals in the external layer of the median eminence also appeared unaffected by the nialamide + 6-OH-DOPA treatment (3 × 100 mg/kg i.p., 24 h intervals, and studied 16 h to 3 weeks after last dose). No notable effect was obtained by 6-OH-DOPA alone, without nialamide. When very high doses of 6-OH-DOPA (400 mg/kg) were used, there was also an effect on the DA neurons (Sachs *et al.*, 1973). The nigro-neostriatal DA axons became strongly fluorescent in the same way as the NA tracts, but the cell bodies located in the substantia nigra were unaffected. However, the DA cell bodies of the nucl. arcuatus (Fig. 9) developed a yellowish fluorescence with an emission spectrum, which differed from the formaldehyde-induced catecholamine fluorescence. It is not known if this is due to any oxidized forms of 6-OH-DA or to a degenerative reaction of these DA neurons.

The 5-HT cell bodies in the raphe nuclei and the 5-HT nerve terminals in, e.g., nucleus suprachiasmaticus, were unaffected with the ordinary nialamide + 6-OH-DOPA treatment (3 × 100 mg/kg i.p., 24 h intervals). However, after a very high 6-OH-DOPA dose (400 mg/kg i.p., 4–6 h), *single* 5-HT fibers became more strongly yellow fluorescent, indicating that they could also be affected by 6-OH-DOPA (Sachs *et al.*, 1973). No yellow fluorescent accumulations were observed, supporting previous chemical-analytical results, that 5-HT neurons are resistant to the neurotoxic effects of 6-OH-DOPA (Berkowitz *et al.*, 1970; Sachs and Jonsson, 1972b).

The most conspicuous finding by the fluorescence histochemical studies was the appearance of intensely fluorescent retrograde accumulations (Fig. 10) of transmitter in a large number of the ascending NA axons (Jacobowitz and Kostrzewa, 1971; Sachs and Jonsson, 1972a, b). The marked accumulations of NA may in part be related to a piling up of amine storage granules proximal to the lesioned terminals (cf. Dahlström, 1966), but the very *longish* NA accumulations observed after 6-OH-DOPA, indicate a more diffuse damage of the axoplasma transport mechanism, e.g. the neurotubules, along the axon (cf. Cheah *et al.*, 1971). It is believed that the occurrence of accumulations is a sign of neuronal degeneration and there seems to be a relation between the number of accumulations occurring and the degree of terminal degeneration (Sachs *et al.*, 1973).

In order to study the properties of the NA accumulations formed, in some detail, nialamide + 6-OH-DOPA (3 × 100 mg/kg i.p., 24 h intervals) pretreated mice were after 7 days injected with reserpine (10 mg/kg i.p., 16 h) or H44/68 (500 mg/kg i.p., 16 h) and the

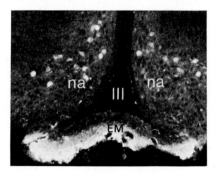

FIG. 9. Histochemical demonstration of catecholamines in the hypothalamus. Mice were injected with nialamide (100 mg/kg i.p.) 2 h before 6-OH-DOPA (400 mg/kg i.p.) and killed 6 h thereafter. The DA cell bodies in the nucl. arcuatus have become strongly yellowish fluorescent. III = third ventricle; na = nucl. arcuatus; EM = eminentia mediana. (×160).

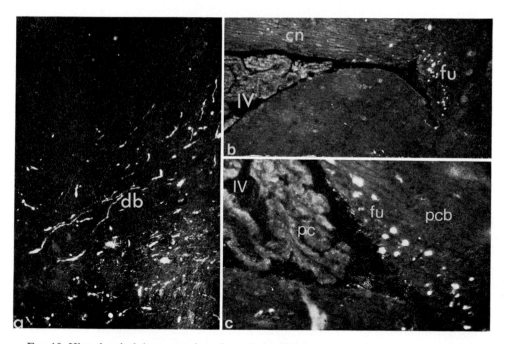

FIG. 10. Histochemical demonstration of catecholamines in mouse brain after treatment with nialamide (100 mg/kg i.p.) 2 h before 6-OH-DOPA (3 ×100 mg/kg i.p., 24 h intervals) and killed 16 h after the last injection. a, Horizontal section of mesencephalon showing extensive accumulations of transmitter in ascending NA axons. db = dorsal NA bundle. (×100). b, Sagittal section through rhombencephalon with overlying cerebellum. Transversally cut, strongly fluorescent NA fibers from the locus coeruleus are observed within the fasciculus uncinatus. IV = fourth ventricle; cn = cerebellar nuclei; fu = fasciculus uncinatus. (×100). c, Higher magnification of the NA fibers in the fasciculus uncinatus. IV = fourth ventricle; pc = plexus choroideus; fu = fasciculus uncinatus; pcb = pedunculus cerebelli. (×400.)
(Sachs *et al.*, 1973.)

fluorescence histochemistry of the dorsal NA bundle in the mesencephalon was studied. The NA accumulations were efficiently depleted by reserpine, which may indicate a granular localization of the accumulated NA. After H44/68 there was a slight reduction of fluorescence of the accumulations, suggesting at least some nerve-impulse-dependent release of accumulated NA. To study any possible replenishment of fluorescence in the depleted axonal "accumulations", mice were treated with nialamide (100 mg/kg i.p.) 2 h before L-DOPA (100 mg/kg i.p.) and killed 1 h later. There was a slight increase in fluorescence in the H44/68 pretreated mice and a stronger increase in the reserpinized mice, indicating that at least some of the axons in the dorsal NA bundle may have an intact uptake mechanism.

MAPPING OF CENTRAL NA TRACTS WITH 6-OH-DOPA

6-OH-DOPA has proven to be a valuable tool in the mapping of central NA pathways using the fluorescence method of Falck and Hillarp (Jacobowitz and Kostrzewa, 1971; Sachs and Jonsson, 1972a, b; Sachs *et al.*, 1973). NA tracts which are ordinarily not visible due to low NA levels, become conspicuous because of strongly fluorescent accumulations of endogenous NA along the axon after nialamide + 6-OH-DOPA treatment. In the dose level of 100 mg/kg 6-OH-DOPA, a dose which can be repeated with 24 h intervals, only NA neurons appear affected, while DA and 5-HT neurons are left intact. The main advantage of using 6-OH-DOPA compared with intracerebral administration of 6-OH-DA is that a differentiation of DA from NA pathways is possible by the selectivity of 6-OH-DOPA and also that the brain is not directly interfered with, which facilitates the microscopical investigations. A limitation using 6-OH-DOPA in the mapping of central NA tracts is that not all pathways are demonstrable by this method (Sachs *et al.*, 1973).

Fluorescence of NA axons was mainly observed in parts of the brain close to the NA cell bodies in the pons and medulla oblongata, and only few axons were observed either in the telencephalon or in the spinal cord. An exception was the axons of the dorsal NA bundle (Ungerstedt, 1971b), where accumulations were found at quite a long distance from the cell bodies in the locus coeruleus. The NA axons of the ventral bundle were not demonstrable after 6-OH-DOPA (100 mg/kg) which agrees with the finding that the terminals of the cerebral cortex are degenerated to a higher extent than the terminals of the hypothalamus (cf. Sachs and Jonsson, 1972c; Jonsson and Sachs, 1973a). The dorsal NA bundle innervates mainly the cortex cerebri and the ventral NA bundle mainly the hypothalamus and subcortical parts of the limbic system (Ungerstedt, 1971b; Olson and Fuxe, 1971, 1972).

By the nialamide + 6-OH-DOPA technique the NA accumulations were mainly found in fibers originating from the locus coeruleus, indicating that these are the most sensitive to the neurotoxic action of formed 6-OH-DA (Fig. 10). It was found that the dorsal NA bundle is subdivided into two bundles in the subthalamic area—a medial and a lateral one. Before the subdivision of the dorsal NA bundle, fibers are given off to the geniculate body and parts of the thalamus. The medial bundle becomes scattered in the lateral hypothalamus and the lateral bundle joins the inner surface of the capsula interna (Jacobowitz and Kostrzewa, 1971; Sachs *et al.*, 1973). *The medial NA fibers* reach the cerebral cortex mainly by looping back in the cingulum and the stria terminalis after having bypassed the septal area. The majority of the *lateral NA fibers* seem to reach the cerebral cortex by passing through the neostriatum, and only a minor part seemed to enter the stria terminalis (Fig.

11). Furthermore, NA fibers, arriving from cell bodies in the locus coeruleus, could be observed to reach cerebellum via the fasciculus uncinatus (Fig. 10b, c). The descending NA bundle from the "subcoeruleus area" could be traced into the dorso-medial reticular formation of the pons and medulla oblongata, down to the level of nucleus tractus solitarii.

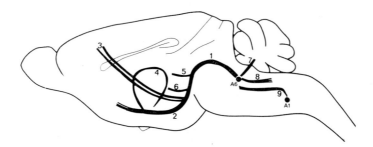

Fig. 11. Schematic diagram of NA bundles, projected on a midsagittal section of the mouse brain, made visible by nialamide + 6-OH-DOPA treatment. 1, Dorsal NA bundle. 2, NA bundle in lateral hypothalamic area. 3, NA bundle in capsula interna. 4, NA bundle in stria terminalis. 5, NA bundle to geniculate body. 6, NA bundle to the thalamus. 7, NA bundle in fasciculus uncinatus. 8, Descending medial reticular NA bundle. 9, Ascending lateral reticular NA bundle. (Sachs *et al.*, 1973.)

It is apparent that by the use of 6-OH-DOPA, mainly the projections from the NA cell bodies in the locus coeruleus area will be demonstrated (Fig. 11). The results confirm earlier reports on the wide spread of the axons and terminals from this nucleus (Loizou, 1969; Olson and Fuxe, 1971, 1972).

ON THE MODE OF ACTION OF 6-OH-DOPA

6-OH-DOPA itself has no apparent effect on NA neurons, but has to be decarboxylated to 6-OH-DA which causes the neuronal destruction. This statement is based on the findings that pretreatment of mice with a peripheral decarboxylase inhibitor, MK485 (100 mg/kg i.p.) could partially prevent the nialamide + 6-OH-DOPA induced decrease in ^{3}H-NA uptake in the peripheral nervous system, while there was no change in the cerebral cortex (Fig. 12). When using Ro4-4602 in a dose that inhibits aromatic L-amino acid decarboxylase both in the peripheral and central nervous system (Burkard *et al.*, 1964; Lotti and Porter, 1970), a complete counteraction was obtained of the decrease in ^{3}H-NA uptake produced by nialamide + 6-OH-DOPA, both in peripheral and central tissues (Sachs and Jonsson, 1972b). Although nothing is known about tissue toxicity or neurotoxicity of 6-OH-DOPA itself, it is very likely that the decarboxylation of 6-OH-DOPA to 6-OH-DA represents an accumulation process of the latter compound within the nerves, both when the decarboxylation takes place extraneuronally and intraneuronally. The decarboxylation of 6-OH-DOPA may occur both intra- and extraneuronally, since aromatic L-amino acid decarboxylase is not restricted to monoamine neurons (Andén *et al.*, 1965). When this process is intraneuronal, it will lead to a relatively slower increase in the intraneuronal 6-OH-DA concentration. Extraneuronally formed 6-OH-DA will be taken up by the efficient "membrane pump" of the nerves. The inhibition of the 6-OH-DOPA effects by the membrane pump inhibitor, DMI, may favor this view for the introduction of 6-OH-DA in the neuron, since

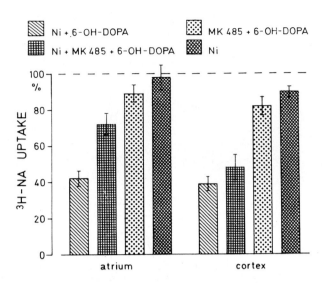

FIG. 12. Effect of a peripheral decarboxylase inhibition on nialamide + 6-OH-DOPA-induced changes in ³H-NA (10^{-7} M, 10 min) uptake in mouse atrium and cerebral cortex slices. The mice were treated with nialamide (100 kg/kg i.p., 18 h) or nialamide + 6-OH-DOPA (100 mg/kg i.p., 16 h), nialamide + MK 485 (100 mg/kg i.p., 16.5 h) + 6-OH-DOPA or MK 485 + 6-OH-DOPA. The values are expressed as percent of untreated control value. Each value represents the mean ± SEM of eight determinations. (Sachs and Jonsson, 1972b.)

the entrance of 6-OH-DA is inhibited, but not that of 6-OH-DOPA (cf. Carlsson *et al.*, 1966). In the peripheral nervous system this route may be of importance, leading to a relatively more rapid introduction of 6-OH-DA into the neuron. The neurotoxic effect of 6-OH-DOPA begins earlier in the peripheral than in the central nervous system (Sachs and Jonsson, 1972b).

Certain NA neuron systems were affected more than others, i.e. mainly those emanating from the locus coeruleus cell bodies. Histochemical and uptake studies, as well as results from gradient centrifugation of synaptosomes, pointed to a more pronounced destruction of cortical than of hypothalamic NA terminals. The reason for this is not clear, but factors explaining the difference observed, could be, e.g. differences in 6-OH-DOPA distribution, in uptake efficiency and intraneuronal uptake-storage and metabolism of the formed 6-OH-DA. In addition, there could also be a difference in surface/volume relationships of the nerve terminals of the different neuron systems. The hypothalamus and subcortical part of the limbic system contain two populations of nerve terminals, fine and thicker ones. The former may be derived from those fibers in the dorso-lateral hypothalamic areas which originate from the dorsal NA bundle assuming that the nerve terminals from the locus coeruleus are of the similar fine type in all parts of the brain. If surface/volume relationships are of importance for the production of neuronal degeneration, this is consistent with the view that mainly the fine terminals of the locus coeruleus are affected.

Great efforts have been devoted to the elucidation of the mode of action of 6-OH-DA, but it is not completely understood. It has been suggested that the neuronal degeneration results from covalent binding of oxidation products of 6-OH-DA to nucleophilic groups of proteins and other macromolecules of vital importance for the neuron, leading to destruction of the neuron (Saner and Thoenen, 1971). The selectivity of this reaction would be directed by the 6-OH-DA being selectively taken up and concentrated by the "membrane pump" of the catecholamine nerves, and a critical concentration of 6-OH-DA must be reached intraneuronally in order to induce neuronal degeneration (Thoenen and Tranzer, 1968; Jonsson and Sachs, 1970, 1972). Hydrogen peroxide, formed from 6-OH-DA, has been suggested as the agent responsible for the degenerative effects (Heikkila and Cohen, 1971, 1972). Furthermore, 6-OH-DA has been shown *in vitro* to uncouple oxidative phosphorylation, which may be associated with the early impairment of the "membrane pump" seen after 6-OH-DA and 6-OH-DOPA (Wagner, 1971).

ACKNOWLEDGEMENTS

These investigations have been supported by the Swedish Medical Research Council (04X-3881 and 04X-2295), Karolinska Institutet, C.-B. Nathorsts, and M. Bergvalls Stiftelser and Svenska Livförsäkrings-bolagen. The following companies are acknowledged for generous supplies of drugs: Swedish Pfizer (Niamid), Ciba (Serpasil), Geigy (Pertofran), and AB Hässle (DL 6-OH-DOPA, 6-OH-DA, 4-tropolone acetamide) through Dr. H. Corrodi. The skilful technical assistance of Ulla-Britt Finnman, Bodil Flock, and Eva Lindqvist is gratefully acknowledged.

REFERENCES

ANDÉN, N.-E., FUXE, K., and LARSSON, K. (1966) Effect of large mesencephalic-diencephalic lesions on the NA, DA and 5-HT neurons of the central nervous system. *Experientia* 22, 842–847.

ANDÉN, N.-E., MAGNUSSON, T., and ROSENGREN, E. (1965) Occurrence of dihydroxyphenylalanine decarboxylase in nerves of the spinal cord and sympathetically innervated organs. *Acta physiol. scand.* 66, 127–135.

BENNETT, T., BURNSTOCK, G., COBB, J. L. S., and MALMFORS, T. (1970) An ultrastructural and histochemical study of the short-term effects of 6-hydroxydopamine on adrenergic nerves in the domestic fowl. *Br. J. Pharmac.* 38, 802–809.

BERKOWITZ, B. A., SPECTOR, S., BROSSI, A., FOCELLA, A., and TEITEL, S. (1970) Preparation and biological properties of (−)- and (+)-6-Hydroxy-dopa. *Experientia* 26, 982–983.

BERTLER, Å., CARLSSON, A., and ROSENGREN, E. (1958) A method for the fluorimetric determination of adrenaline and noradrenaline in tissues. *Acta physiol. scand.* 44, 273–292.

BLOOM, F. E., ALGERI, S., GROPPETTI, A., REVUELTA, A., and COSTA, E. (1969) Lesions of central norepinephrine terminals with 6-OH-dopamine: biochemistry and fine structure. *Science* 166, 1284–1286.

BREESE, G. R., and TRAYLOR, T. D. (1970) Effect of 6-hydroxydopamine on brain norepinephrine and dopamine: evidence for selective degeneration of catecholamine neurons. *J. Pharmac. Exp. Ther.* 174, 413–427.

BURKARD, W. P., GEY, K. F., and PLETSCHER, A. (1964) Inhibition of decarboxylase of aromatic amino acids by 2,3,4-trihydroxybenzylhydrazine and its seryl derivatives. *Archs. Biochem.* 107, 187–196.

CARLSSON, A., FUXE, K., HAMBERGER, B., and LINDQVIST, M. (1966) Biochemical and histochemical studies on effects of imipramine-like drugs and (+)-amphetamine on central and peripheral catecholamine neurons. *Acta physiol. scand.* 67, 481–497.

CHEAH, T. B., GEFFEN, L. B., JARROTT, B., and OSTBERG, A. (1971) Action of 6-hydroxydopamine on lamb sympathetic ganglia, vas deferens and adrenal medulla: a combined histochemical, ultrastructural and biochemical comparison with the effects of reserpine. *Br. J. Pharmac.* 42, 543–557.

CORRODI, H., CLARKE, W. G., and MASUOKA, D. I. (1971a) The synthesis and effects of DL-6-hydroxydopa. In: *6-Hydroxydopamine and Catecholamine Neurons* (eds. T. Malmfors and H. Thoenen), North-Holland, Amsterdam, pp. 187–192.

CORRODI, H., MASUOKA, D. T., and CLARK, W. G. (1971b) Effect of 6-hydroxy-dopamine on rat heart noradrenaline. *Eur. J. Pharmac.* 15, 160–163.

DAHLSTRÖM, A. (1966) The intraneuronal distribution of noradrenaline and the transport and life-span of amine storage granules in the sympathetic adrenergic neuron, M.D. thesis, Stockholm.

FALCK, B. (1962) Observations on the possibilities of the cellular localization of monoamines by a fluorescent method. *Acta physiol. scand.* 56, Suppl. 197.

FALCK, B., HILLARP, N.-Å., THIEME, G., and TORP, A. (1962) Fluorescence of catechol amines and related compounds condensed with formaldehyde. *J. Histochem. Cytochem.* 10, 348–354.

GREEN, A. I., SNYDER, S. H., and IVERSEN, L. L. (1969) Separation of catecholamine-storing synaptosomes in different regions of rat brain. *J. Pharmacol. Exp. Ther.* 168, 264–271.

HAMBERGER, B. (1967) Reserpine-resistant uptake of catecholamines in isolated tissues of the rat. *Acta physiol. scand.*, Suppl. 295.

HEIKKILA, R., and COHEN, G. (1971) Inhibition of biogenic amine uptake by hydrogen peroxide: a mechanism for toxic effects of 6-hydroxy-dopamine. *Science* 172, 1257–1258.

HEIKKILA, R., and COHEN, G. (1972) Further studies on the generation of hydrogen peroxide by 6-hydroxydopamine. *Molec. Pharmac.* 8, 241–248.

JACOBOWITZ, D., and KOSTRZEWA, R. (1971) Selective action of 6-hydroxy-dopa on noradrenergic terminals: mapping of preterminal axons of the brain. *Life Sci.* 10, 1329–1342.

JONSSON, G., and SACHS, CH. (1970) Effects of 6-hydroxydopamine on the uptake and storage of noradrenaline in sympathetic adrenergic neurons. *Eur. J. Pharmac.* 9, 141–155.

JONSSON, G., and SACHS, CH. (1971) Uptake and accumulation of ^{3}H-6-hydroxydopamine in adrenergic nerves. *Eur. J. Pharmac.* 16, 55–62.

JONSSON, G., and SACHS, CH. (1972) Degenerative and non-degenerative effects of 6-hydroxydopamine on adrenergic nerves. *J. Pharmac. Exp. Ther.* 180, 625–635.

JONSSON, G., and SACHS, CH. (1973a) Pharmacological modifications of the 6-hydroxy-DOPA induced degeneration of central noradrenaline neurons. *Biochem. Pharmac.* 22, 1709–1716.

JONSSON, G., and SACHS, CH. (1973b) Effect of tyrosine hydroxylase inhibition on the action of 6-hydroxydopamine. *Res. Communs. Chem. Path. Pharmac.* 5, 287–296.

JONSSON, G., HAMBERGER, B., MALMFORS, T., and SACHS, CH. (1969) Uptake and accumulation of ^{3}H-noradrenaline in adrenergic nerves of rat iris—effect of reserpine, monoamine oxidase and tyrosine hydroxylase inhibition. *Eur. J. Pharmac.* 8, 58–32.

JONSSON, G., MALMFORS, T., and SACHS, CH. (1972) Effects of drugs on the 6-hydroxydopamine induced degeneration of adrenergic nerves. *Res. Communs. Chem. Path. Pharmac.* 3, 543–556.

KOSTRZEWA, R., and JACOBOWITZ, D. (1973) Acute effects of 6-hydroxydopa on central monoaminergic neurons. *Eur. J. Pharmac.* 21, 70–80.

KURUMA, I., BARTHOLINI, G., and PLETSCHER, A. (1972) L-DOPA-induced accumulation of 3-*O*-methyldopa in brain and heart. *Eur. J. Pharmac.* 10, 189–192.

LOIZOU, L. A. (1969) Projections of the nucleus locus coeruleus in the albino rat. *Brain Res.* 15, 563–566.

LOTTI, V. J., and PORTER, C. C. (1970) Potentiation and inhibition of some central actions of L (−) DOPA by decarboxylase inhibitors. *J. Pharmac. Exp. Ther.* 172, 406–415.

MALMFORS, T., and THOENEN, H. (eds.) (1971) 6-*Hydroxydopamine and Catecholamine Neurons*, North-Holland, Amsterdam.

OLSON, L., and FUXE, K. (1971) On the projections from the locus coeruleus noradrenaline neurons: the cerebellar innervation. *Brain Res.* 28, 165–171.

OLSON, L., and FUXE, K. (1972) Further mapping out of central noradrenaline neuron systems: projections of the "subcoeruleus" area. *Brain Res.* 43, 289–295.

ONG, H. H., CREVELING, C. R., and DALY, J. (1969) The synthesis of 2,4,5-trihydroxyphenylalanine (6-hydroxydopa): centrally active norepinephrine-depleting agent. *J. Med. Chem.* 12, 458–461.

SACHS, CH. (1970) Noradrenaline uptake mechanisms in the mouse atrium. *Acta physiol. scand.* Suppl. 341.

SACHS, CH., and JONSSON, G. (1972a) Selective 6-hydroxy-DOPA induced degeneration of central and peripheral noradrenaline neurons. *Brain Res.* 40, 563–568.

SACHS, CH. and JONSSON, G. (1972b) Degeneration of central and peripheral noradrenaline neurons produced by 6-hydroxy-DOPA. *J. Neurochem.* 19, 1561–1575.

SACHS, CH., and JONSSON, G. (1972c) Degeneration of central noradrenaline neurons after 6-hydroxydopamine in newborn animals. *Res. Communs. Chem. Path. Pharmac.* 4, 203–220.

SACHS, CH., JONSSON, G., and FUXE, K. (1973) Mapping of central noradrenaline pathways with 6-hydroxy-DOPA. *Brain Res.* 63, 249–261.

SAELENS, J. K., SCHOEN, M. S., and KOVACSICS, G. B. (1967) An enzyme assay for norepinephrine in brain tissue. *Biochem. Pharmac.* 16, 1043.

SANER, A., and THOENEN, H. (1971) Contributions to the molecular mechanism of action of 6-hydroxydopamine. In: 6-*Hydroxydopamine and Catecholamine Neurons* (eds. T. Malmfors and H. Thoenen), North-Holland, Amsterdam, pp. 265–275.

THOENEN, H., and TRANZER, J. P. (1968) Chemical sympathectomy by selective destruction of adrenergic nerve endings with 6-hydroxydopamine. *Naunyn-Schmiedebergs Arch. exp. Path. Pharmak.* 261, 271–288.

UNGERSTEDT, U. (1968) 6-Hydroxy-dopamine induced degeneration of central monoamine neurons. *Eur. J. Pharmac.* 5, 107–110.

UNGERSTEDT, U. (1971a) Histochemical studies on the effect of intracerebral and intraventricular injections of 6-hydroxydopamine on monoamine neurons in the rat brain. In: 6-*Hydroxydopamine and Catecholamine Neurons* (eds. T. Malmfors and H. Thoenen), North-Holland, Amsterdam, pp. 101–127.

UNGERSTEDT, U. (1971b) Stereotaxic mapping of the monoamine pathways in the rat brain. *Acta physiol. scand.*, Suppl. 367, 1–48.

URETSKY, N. J., and IVERSEN, L. L. (1969) Effects of 6-hydroxydopamine on noradrenaline-containing neurones in the rat brain. *Nature* **221**, 557–559.

WAGNER, K. (1971) Uncoupling of oxidative phosphorylation by 6-hydroxy-dopamine. In: *6-Hydroxy-dopamine and Catecholamine Neurons* (eds. T. Malmfors and H. Thoenen), North-Holland, Amsterdam, pp. 277–278.

MICROFLUORIMETRIC AND NEUROCHEMICAL STUDIES ON DEGENERATING AND REGENERATING ADRENERGIC NERVES

Gösta Jonsson

Department of Histology, Karolinska Institutet, S-104 01 Stockholm 60, Sweden

SUMMARY

Noradrenaline uptake–storage mechanisms in de- and regenerating sympathetic adrenergic nerves have been studied using neurochemical techniques and the Falck–Hillarp fluorescence method in combination with quantitative scanning microfluorimetry. *Degenerating nerves* were studied in mouse and rat iris after axotomy produced by removal of the superior cervical ganglion. The results obtained support the view that the noradrenaline uptake–storage mechanisms are intact up to a certain time point after ganglionectomy after which these functions are very rapidly lost with a concomitant disappearance of the transmitter stores. After the onset of the axotomy induced changes, the deterioration of the uptake–storage mechanisms in the single nerve terminal is completed within about 1 h. The onset of these changes is somewhat varying for different nerve terminal systems. *Regenerating nerves* were investigated in mouse iris and atrium after a chemical sympathectomy produced by the neurotoxic compound 6-hydroxydopamine. The present results favor the view that regenerating adrenergic nerves directly develop the NA "membrane pump" uptake mechanism with similar kinetic properties as that of mature nerves. There is, however, a certain lag in the development of the NA storage capacity reflected by a lower endogenous NA concentration.

INTRODUCTION

The separation of the axon from its perikaryon will without any exception lead to degeneration of the separated part of the neuron. In the sympathetic adrenergic nerve terminals a number of changes of the neurotransmitter mechanisms will take place during the degeneration phase after axotomy, e.g. deterioration of the noradrenaline (NA) storage mechanism, loss of the ability to take up and retain exogenous NA, and ultimately a disappearance of the nerves as seen at the ultrastructural level (von Euler and Purkhold, 1951; Kirpekar *et al.*, 1962; Benmiloud and von Euler, 1963; Trendelenburg, 1963; Malmfors and Sachs, 1965; Roth and Richardson, 1969; van Orden *et al.*, 1967). The neurons of the peripheral nervous system possess the property of regenerating their peripherally directed axons after injury, and in most cases with a re-establishment of functional connections with the periphery. In this respect, the neurotoxic compound 6-hydroxydopamine (6-OH-DA) provides a very useful tool for studying regenerating sympathetic adrenergic nerves under fairly controlled conditions from the quantitative point of view (Jonsson and Sachs, 1972, 1974). This compound has been shown to cause an acute and selective degeneration of the terminal parts of the adrenergic neuron leaving their perikarya more or less intact (see symposium volume edited by Malmfors and Thoenen, 1971). Thus the adrenergic nerves can regenerate and reinnervate a tissue or an organ after a sympathectomy produced by 6-OH-DA (Haeusler et al., 1969; Jonsson and Sachs, 1970, 1972; de Champlain, 1971).

The present paper deals with recently performed studies in our laboratory aimed to elucidate the dynamics of the changes that take place in de- and regenerating adrenergic nerves. Special interest has been focused on changes in NA uptake–storage and synthesis mechanisms using neurochemical techniques and fluorescence histochemistry in combination with quantitative microfluorimetry. These studies have mainly been performed on adrenergic nerves in rat and mouse *iris*. *Degeneration* was studied after axotomy produced by removal of the superior cervical ganglion, while *regeneration* was followed after a chemical sympathectomy produced by 6-OH-DA.

DEGENERATION

FLUORESCENCE HISTOCHEMISTRY

The formaldehyde fluorescence technique of Falck and Hillarp (Falck et al., 1962; Corrodi and Jonsson, 1967; Fuxe et al., 1970) has been used for the histochemical demonstration of NA in the adrenergic nerves of the iris, prepared as a stretch-preparation (Malmfors, 1965). As seen in Fig. 1A, the mouse iris is very richly innervated by sympathetic adrenergic nerves forming a dense, evenly distributed network of varicose fibers which have their perikarya in the superior cervical ganglion. Removal of this ganglion leads to very small changes in the fluorescence morphology of the terminals up to about 10 h after ganglionectomy. Between 10 and 16 h there was a dramatic reduction of detectable nerve terminals, and after 16 h only very few nerves, most of them weakly fluorescent, could be observed. Practically no nerves could be seen 24 and 48 h after ganglionectomy. Twelve hours after ganglionectomy, approximately 50% of the fluorescent nerves could be detected, and the vast majority of these remaining nerve terminals displayed an unchanged appearance (Fig. 1B). However, the presence of a relatively small number of weakly fluorescent nerves could also be seen, with single weakly fluorescent varicosities (Fig. 1B). It was also the subjective impression that between 10 and 16 h after ganglionectomy a small population of the demonstrable varicosities appeared larger than normally, displaying a more intense fluorescence intensity. In either of the time intervals studied after ganglionectomy was it possible to restitute the disappeared nerves by exogenous administration of α-methyl-NA *in vitro* (1 μM, 30 min) or *in vivo* (0.2 mg/kg i.v., 20 min before sacrifice). This compound is efficiently taken up by adrenergic nerves and has the same fluorescence yield as NA (Jonsson, 1971). Exogenous administration of α-methyl-NA thus makes it possible to detect adrenergic nerves that have lost their endogenous NA but still have an intact axonal "membrane pump" uptake mechanism. It therefore seems clear that the nerves that have lost their endogenous NA and are not detectable in the microscope must have lost their NA uptake–storage functions in view of the negative outcome with α-methyl-NA. This seems also to be the case with the weakly fluorescent nerves, at least with respect to "membrane pump" function, since they appeared unaffected after administration of α-methyl-NA.

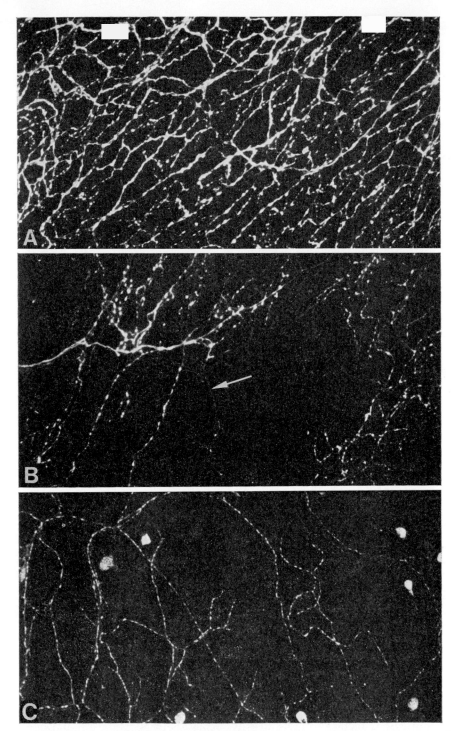

Fig. 1. Fluorescence histochemical demonstration of NA in sympathetic adrenergic nerves in mouse iris according to the technique of Falck and Hillarp. (×180.) A, *Untreated control.* A dense plexus of adrenergic nerves with characteristic varicosities can be seen. B, *Ganglionectomy, 12 h.* The density of the nerve plexus is considerably reduced and the majority of the remaining fibers show an unchanged fluorescence morphology. A few fibers (→) with a very weak fluorescence intensity can also be seen. C, *6-OH-DA* (2 × 50 mg/kg i.v., 4 weeks). The adrenergic nerve plexus is reduced in density compared with untreated, and the terminals exhibit a weaker fluorescence intensity.

SCANNING MICROFLUORIMETRY

A quantitative determination of the relative number of fluorescent adrenergic nerves (nerve density) remaining in the irides after ganglionectomy was carried out using scanning microfluorimetry (Fig. 2) (Sachs and Jonsson, 1973). With this technique the fluorescent nerve fibers are represented as spikes, and the number of spikes per unit scanning length is an index of the nerve density. Typical scans are shown in Fig. 3. Although there exist a concentration-dependent quenching of the NA fluorescence in the nerve terminals (Jonsson, 1969), this phenomenon does not affect the nerve density estimations. The reason for this is that this type of quantization is solely dependent on the sensitivity of the formaldehyde fluorescence method and the resolution of the microfluorimetric scanning procedure. The resolution of the present scanning technique is in fact very good, as has been shown by comparing the fluorescence microphotographs of irides with the corresponding recorder charts (Sachs and Jonsson, 1973). The fluorescent nerve terminals are distinctly represented.

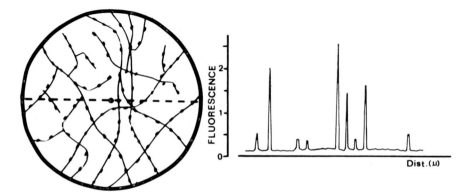

FIG. 2. Schematic representation of the scanning microfluorimetry. The view-field in the microscope with nerve fibers is to the left. The broken line indicates where the measuring field passes. As the specimen moves across the microscope stage, spikes are recorded (to the right) corresponding to fluorescent adrenergic nerve fibers passing the circular measuring field (diameter 1.5 μ, an area of approximately the same size as a varicosity). The number of spikes per unit length of the scanning is an index of nerve density, whereas the peak height is related to the fluorescence intensity of the recorded nerve terminal.

Moreover, the formaldehyde fluorescence method is very sensitive, since less than 10% of the endogenous NA level is needed for the fluorescence microscopical demonstration of the adrenergic nerve terminals in iris (Jonsson, 1969). Therefore the microfluorimetric scanning procedure used must be regarded as a rather precise technique for the evaluation of nerve density.

The number of nerve terminals was unchanged in mouse iris 6 h after ganglionectomy, whereas a small reduction (about 10%) was found after 10 h (Fig. 4). Between 10 and 16 h there was a drastic reduction in nerve density, being about 50% at 12 h and only 5% of control 16 h after removal of the ganglion.

NEUROCHEMISTRY

No significant changes of the endogenous NA content of mouse iris determined by using a radiometric enzyme–assay procedure (Saelens et al., 1967) was observed up to 10 h

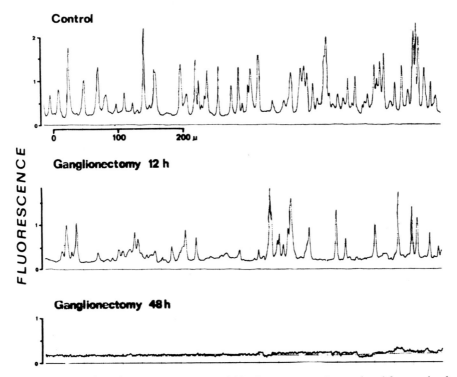

FIG. 3. Microfluorimetric scans across mouse irides from *untreated* control and from animals where the superior ganglion had been removed 12 or 48 h before sacrifice. (Sachs and Jonsson, 1973.)

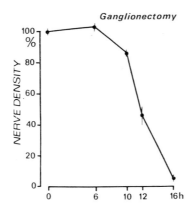

FIG. 4. Time-course changes in *nerve density* of mouse irides after ganglionectomy as estimated by scanning microfluorimetry. Each point represents the mean ± SEM of four determinations and are expressed as percentages of untreated control. (Sachs and Jonsson, 1973.)

after ganglionectomy. If anything, there was a tendency for an increased NA content at 10 h. Between 10 and 16 h the NA content was drastically reduced down to 20% of control which value was further reduced to 10% of control 48 h after ganglionectomy (Fig. 5). A similar time-course pattern was found when studying the *in vitro* uptake of ^{3}H-NA (0.1 μM, 10 min) or ^{3}H-metaraminol (^{3}H-MA; 0.1 μM, 10 min) in the irides various periods of time after ganglionectomy (Fig. 6). Also when following the ^{3}H-amine uptake–accumulation or retention, a similar pattern was observed (Fig. 7). When investigating the formation of ^{3}H-NA in control and denervated irides (12 h after ganglionectomy) after *in vitro* incubation in ^{3}H-DA (0.25 μM, 30 min), it was found that the ^{3}H-NA recovered from the irides was more reduced (about 25%) after ganglionectomy compared with control than was the reduction (about 50%) of recovered ^{3}H-DA (Fig. 8). The changes in formed ^{3}H-NA reflect deterioration of the intraneuronal storage granules whereas changes in ^{3}H-DA recovered from the irides will reflect effects on the "membrane uptake" mechanism.

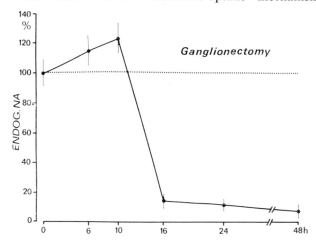

FIG. 5. Endogenous NA in mouse iris various periods of time after ganglionectomy. Each point represents the mean $\pm$ SEM (n = 6–10) and is expressed as percentages of untreated control. (Sachs and Jonsson, 1973.)

Since the above presented data on axotomy-induced changes of uptake–storage mechanisms were obtained from *in vitro* experiments, we wanted to use an *in vivo* approach to study these phenomena. For experimental–technical reasons this was made in rats. The experimental design was as follows: rat irides were unilaterally either sympathectomized (ganglionectomy) or decentralized (preganglionic cutting) immediately before intraocular injection of ^{3}H-NA (0.5 μCi in 5 μl) in both eyes, thereby labeling the storage pool of the adrenergic nerves in the iris. The unoperated side served as control. Various periods of time after the operation, the rats were sacrificed and ^{3}H-NA, taken up and retained in the irides, was determined. Immediately after the operation and up to a certain time point, the ganglionectomized and decentralized nerve terminals may be comparable, both preparations lacking nerve impulse flow. The time point when these two groups start to differ in ^{3}H-NA retention must be related to the onset of the axotomy-induced effects on the NA storage mechanisms. Thus, relating the ^{3}H-NA retention in irides after ganglionectomy to that after decentralization, it was observed that the ^{3}H-NA retention was unaffected up to 12 h after ganglionectomy (Fig. 9). Between 12 and 16 h there was, however, a very drastic reduction

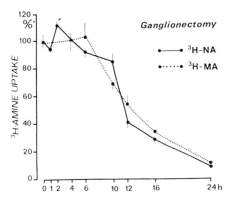

FIG. 6. *In vitro* uptake of ³H-NA and ³H-MA (0.1 μM, 10 min at $+37°$C) various periods of time after ganglionectomy. Each point represents the mean $\pm$ SEM ($n = 8$–22) and is expressed as percentages of untreated control. (Sachs and Jonsson, 1973.)

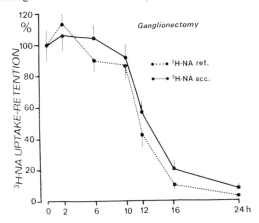

FIG. 7. *In vitro* accumulation and retention of ³H-NA in mouse irides various periods of time after ganglionectomy. The irides were first incubated in ³H-NA (0.1 μM, 20 min at $+37°$C) and thereafter either washed a few seconds in cold buffer (——) or reincubated for 30 min in fresh buffer $+37°$C (– – –). Each point represents the mean $\pm$ SEM ($n = 6$–8) and is expressed as percentages of untreated control. (Sachs and Jonsson, 1973.)

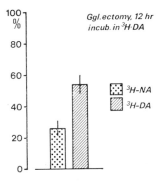

FIG. 8. Effect of ganglionectomy (12 h) on the formation of ³H-NA in mouse irides incubated *in vitro* in ³H-DA (0.25 μM, 30 min at $+37°$C). Each point represents the mean $\pm$ SEM ($n = 4$) and is expressed as percentages of untreated control. (Sachs and Jonsson, 1973.)

of retained ³H-NA, being about 10% of decentralized 16 h after ganglionectomy. An almost identical time-course pattern was found when measuring the *in vitro* uptake of ³H-NA (0.1 μM, 10 min) in irides following ganglionectomy.

COMMENTS AND CONCLUSIONS

Previous studies have shown that the disappearance of the endogenous NA from the sympathetic adrenergic nerves following axotomy is a rather rapid process (Malmfors and Sachs, 1965; van Orden *et al.*, 1967). The present results also underline this view of a rapid degeneration process in terms of deterioration and loss of the amine uptake–storage functions. The uptake–storage mechanisms in mouse iris are apparently unaffected up to a certain time point following axotomy, whereas between about 10 and 16 h the functions of these mechanisms are completely lost. In view of the close quantitative correlation between

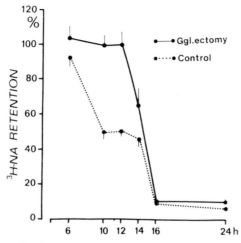

FIG. 9. Effect of decentralization or ganglionectomy on the retention of ³H-NA in rat iris after intraocular injection of ³H-NA. ³H-NA (0.5 μCi in 5 μl) was injected immediately after respective operation and the rats sacrificed 6–24 h later. Each point represents the mean ± SEM (*n* = 6–12) and is expressed as percentages of ³H-NA retained in decentralized irides for each time interval.

the time-course pattern of all the parameters measured (nerve density, uptake, and storage), it is conceivable to assume that the deterioration of the "membrane pump" uptake and the storage mechanisms occur approximately simultaneously, although the results from the studies on formation of ³H-NA from ³H-DA after ganglionectomy point to a somewhat earlier onset of the destruction of the storage function. Since the enzyme responsible for the conversion of DA to NA (DA-β-hydroxylase) is localized in the granules (Laduron and Belpaire, 1968), the more pronounced reduction of recovered ³H-NA than that of ³H-DA seen 12 h after ganglionectomy indicate that the deterioration of the storage capacity starts prior to that of the "membrane pump" function. This is consistent with the ultrastructural data reported by van Orden *et al.* (1967). Therefore the onset of the axotomy-induced changes in NA uptake and storage might initially start with a swelling of the terminals and a concomitant onset of the deterioration of the storage granules (Fig. 10). An observation in line with this view is the appearance of a small population of varicosities showing a

DEGENERATION COURSE

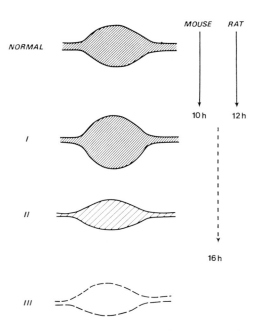

FIG. 10. Schematic representation of the time course of the axotomy-induced changes in NA uptake–storage mechanisms of sympathetic adrenergic nerves in the mouse and rat iris. After ganglionectomy these mechanisms are intact up to about 10 h for the mouse (about 12 h for the rat) after which they rapidly deteriorate (probably within less than 1 h for the single nerve terminal) and approximately at the same time. The onset of the degeneration is probably associated with an initial swelling (I) and concomitant start of the destruction of the storage capacity. In stage II most of the NA store has disappeared and the "membrane pump" uptake mechanism is lost. Soon thereafter the nerve terminals completely disappear (III).

larger size and increased fluorescence intensity during the degeneration phase. The destruction of the storage mechanism may initially be associated with a leakage of NA from granular storage sites into the extragranular space. This would lead to an increased fluorescence intensity in view of the existing concentration dependent quenching of the NA fluorescence in the terminals. The leakage of NA leads to a reduced average NA concentration in the nerve terminals, thereby reducing the quenching and increasing fluorescence intensity. However, the increase in fluorescence might also be related to the reduced NA release after axotomy and a continuation of the NA synthesis leading to increased NA levels. Thus, relating the endogenous NA levels to the nerve density, the present results (Fig. 4 and 5) show a significant increase ($p < 0.01$) in the endogenous NA content in the nerve terminals 10 h after ganglionectomy.

Although the destruction of the storage mechanism seems to start somewhat prior to that of the "membrane pump", the present data indicate a more rapid completion of this process for the "membrane pump." Thus a certain population of nerves during the degeneration phase displaying a very weak fluorescence and thus storing a certain amount of NA seemed to have lost their "membrane pump", since they were not able to take up and accumulate α-methyl-NA. Thus in the late phase there may be a certain storage capacity left, whereas the "membrane pump" function is completely destroyed. It should be under-lined, however, that these differences in onset and completion of axotomy-induced changes in NA uptake and storage are rather small, giving further support for the view of a sudden and rapid loss of the uptake–storage properties. This is further emphasized by the fact that there was a very good correlation between the quantitative changes in nerve density, ^{3}H-NA uptake and endogenous NA after axotomy, pointing to a very rapid destruction of these mechanisms which in the single neuron is in all probability completed within less than 1 h. A somewhat varying onset of these changes in different nerve terminal systems of the iris is certainly the explanation for the observations that it takes approximately 5 h for the complete disappearance of the NA uptake–storage functions of all the nerves in the iris.

The present results from *in vivo* studies on rat iris are very similar to the mouse iris data except that the onset of the changes in uptake–storage are delayed 2 h in rat. There is at present no clear explanation for this discrepancy, but might be related to differences in length of the axon (Emmelin, 1967; Lundberg, 1972; Sachs and Jonsson, 1973).

REGENERATION

FLUORESCENCE HISTOCHEMISTRY

The dose-schedule of 6-OH-DA (2×50 mg/kg i.v., 16 h interval) used produced a practically complete sympathetic denervation in the organs investigated, as evidenced by a practically complete disappearance of the fluorescent adrenergic nerves, of the ^{3}H-NA uptake and of the endogenous NA (Figs. 12 and 13; see also Jonsson and Sachs, 1970; Hökfelt *et al.*, 1972). The onset of the degeneration is very rapid (within 1 h) compared with surgical denervation, although both types of procedures show similar degenerative changes at the ultrastructural level, i.e. the dense type of degeneration. The difference in rate of onset is certainly related to 6-OH-DA acting directly on both axons and nerve terminals of the neuron.

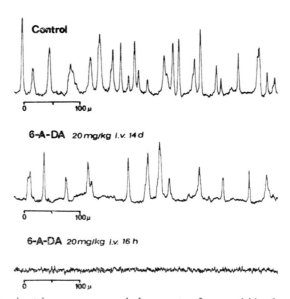

FIG. 11. Microfluorimetric scans across whole mounts of mouse irides from untreated and 6-A-DA (20 mg/kg i.v. 16 h or 14 days) treated mice. (Jonsson and Sachs, 1973.)

There is a reappearance with time of endogenous NA, ³H-NA uptake and fluorescent nerves after 6-OH-DA due to a growth and regeneration of adrenergic nerves. This regrowth starts very early and it takes about 2 months for a complete restitution of the nerve plexus (Haeusler *et al.*, 1969; Jonsson and Sachs, 1970; de Champlain, 1971). The morphology of the regenerating nerves is very similar to adult mature nerves, both as seen in the fluorescence microscope (Fig. 1c) and in the electron microscope (Hökfelt *et al.*, 1972). However, the regenerating nerve terminals display a weaker NA fluorescence intensity (Fig. 1c) while the nonterminal axons show a stronger fluorescence intensity and a more beaded appearance than do mature nerves. Microfluorimetric scanning of adrenergic nerves regenerated after 6-aminodopamine, a compound with similar neurotoxic actions as 6-OH-DA (Blank *et al.*, 1972; Jonsson and Sachs, 1973; Heikkila *et al.*, 1973), showed them to have a lower mean fluorescence intensity than mature nerve terminals (Fig. 11). These results thus indicate that the regenerating adrenergic nerves contain less endogenous transmitter compared with adult mature nerves. It was also observed that the fluorescence intensity of the regenerating adrenergic nerves could be increased after *in vitro* incubation in 1 μM NA for 30 min in contrast to nerves in irides from untreated mice. However, there was no observable increase in the number of nerve terminals.

NEUROCHEMISTRY

It has previously been reported that the recovery of ³H-NA uptake in mouse heart is more rapid than the endogenous NA after a 6-OH-DA-induced sympathectomy (Jonsson and Sachs, 1970). This discrepancy is maximal around 4 weeks after 6-OH-DA and is why a more detailed study of the NA uptake–storage and synthesis properties was studied at this time interval. It was thus observed that at 4 weeks after 6-OH-DA the ³H-NA uptake in mouse atrium was about 75%, whereas the endogenous NA level was about 40% of untreated control (Fig. 12). A similar discrepancy was observed in mouse iris, although less pronounced (Fig. 13). In the iris it was also found that the nerve density was well correlated with the ³H-NA uptake.

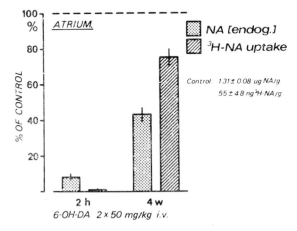

FIG. 12. Effect of 6-OH-DA (2 × 50 mg/kg i.v., 2 h or 4 weeks) on the endogenous NA concentration and the *in vitro* uptake of ³H-NA (0.1 μM, 10 min at +37°C) in mouse atrium. Each column represents the mean ± SEM (*n* = 4–8) and the values expressed as percentages of untreated control. (Jonsson and Sachs, 1972.)

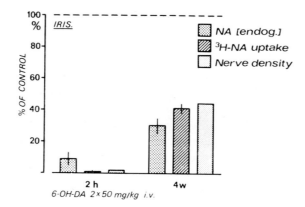

FIG. 13. Effect of 6-OH-DA (2 × 50 mg/kg i.v., 2 h and 4 weeks) on the endogenous NA, *in vitro* uptake of ³N-HA (0.1 μM, 10 min at +37°C) and nerve density in mouse iris. Each column represents the mean ± SEM (*n* = 4–8) and the values expressed as percentages of untreated control. (Jonsson and Sachs, 1972.)

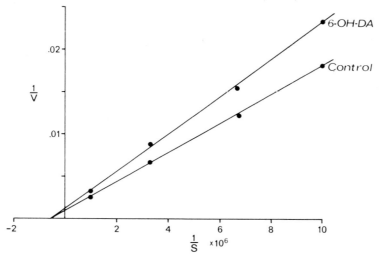

FIG. 14. Double reciprocal analysis of ³H-NA uptake (10 min at +37°C) *in vitro* in mouse atria from control (untreated) and 6-OH-DA (2 × 50 mg/kg i.v., 4 weeks) treated mice. Each point represents the mean of four determinations. Velocity (V) = ³H-NA uptake ng/g per 10 min. Substrate concentration (S) = M ³H-NA. (Jonsson and Sachs, 1972.)

Double reciprocal analysis of the ³H-NA uptake *in vitro* in atria from untreated and mice treated with 6-OH-DA (4 weeks) showed both groups to obey Michaelis–Menten kinetics having similar K_m values, whereas the V_{max} differed (Fig. 14).

Studies on the spontaneous release *in vitro* of ³H-NA previously taken up and accumulated *in vitro* (0.1 μM, 30 min) showed the regenerating nerves to have similar retention properties compared with mature nerves, although there was a tendency for a somewhat less efficient retention (Jonsson and Sachs, 1972).

The synthesis of ¹⁴C-catecholamines after *in vitro* incubation of atria in ¹⁴C-DOPA (10 μM, 60 min) was similarly reduced for both ¹⁴C-DA and ¹⁴C-NA after 6-OH-DA (4 weeks), being about 60% of control. Thus the catecholamine synthesis was somewhat less reduced compared with endogenous NA, but more reduced than ^{3}H-NA uptake after 6-OH-DA (4 weeks). Since the ^{3}H-NA uptake is an index of the relative number of nerve terminals, these data indicate that there is a small reduction in the formation of ^{14}C-catecholamines in the regenerating adrenergic nerves.

The subcellular distribution of ^{3}H-NA was investigated in mouse atria after intravenous injection of 20 μCi ^{3}H-NA (30 min). It was then found that the affinity of ^{3}H-NA to the microsomal fraction (P_2) was considerably lower in regenerating nerves. The ratio $\dfrac{P_2}{P_2 + S}$ $\times$ 100 (S = high speed supernatant) was 37 for untreated control, while 25 after 6-OH-DA (4 weeks). The microsomal fraction is believed to contain the amine storage granules.

COMMENTS AND CONCLUSIONS

The 6-OH-DA induced denervation of sympathetically innervated organs can be considered as a sympathectomy at the axonal level since the perikarya are not appreciably damaged after the 6-OH-DA treatment used. The regenerating adrenergic nerves show structural similarities both as revealed by fluorescence histochemistry and at the ultrastructural level (Jonsson and Sachs, 1972; Hökfelt et al., 1972). They also have very similar release properties as found by studying the field stimulation induced release of ^{3}H-NA from isolated atria (Farnebo et al., unpublished). However, the present microfluorimetric data clearly show that the regenerating nerves display a weaker NA fluorescence intensity, in all probability related to these nerves containing less endogenous NA than adult mature nerves. This is certainly also the explanation why the ^{3}H-NA uptake is higher than the endogenous NA in the recovery phase after 6-OH-DA. Similar results have been obtained on peripheral and central NA neurons during ontogenesis (Iversen et al., 1967; Coyle and Axelrod, 1971). The regenerating nerves have similar ^{3}H-NA uptake kinetics as adult mature nerves, since they showed identical K_m values. This is consistent with recently reported data on NA uptake in axonal sprouts from superior cervical ganglia in organ culture (Hanbauer et al., 1972). The different V_{max} values observed in all probability reflect differences in the total number of transport sites, and thus differences in the nerve density in view of the close correlation between ^{3}H-NA uptake and nerve density. Thus measurement of ^{3}H-NA uptake is a very good and simple method for the determination of the relative number of adrenergic nerve terminals.

During the regeneration phase after a 6-OH-DA-induced sympathectomy there is thus a more rapid recovery of ^{3}H-NA uptake than of the endogenous NA. This is certainly related to the regenerating nerves promptly developing the "membrane pump" uptake mechanism, whereas there is a certain lag in the development of the NA storage capacity as reflected by a lower endogenous NA content, less efficient ^{3}H-NA retention, less affinity for ^{3}H-NA to the microsomal fraction, and a reduced catecholamine synthesis. It is at present not known whether this lag is related to a "maturation" of the NA storage granules, changes in feedback mechanisms regulating NA synthesis, or dependent on a delay in synthesis and transport of amine storage granules.

ACKNOWLEDGEMENTS

The present study has been supported by research grants 04X-2295 and 04X-3881 from the Swedish Medical Research Council, M. Bergvalls and C-B. Nathorsts Stiftelser and Karolinska Institutet (Forskningsfonder).

The skilful technical assistance of Mrs. Ulla-Britt Finnman, Miss Bodil Flock, and Mrs. Eva Lindqvist is gratefully acknowledged. For generous supply of 6-OH-DA, the author is gratefully indebted to Dr. H. Corrodi.

REFERENCES

BENMILOUD, M., and VON EULER, U. S. (1963) Effects of bretylium, reserpine, guanethidine and sympathetic denervation on the noradrenaline content of rat submaxillary gland. *Acta physiol. scand.* **59**, 34–42.

BLANK, C. L., MURRILL, E., and ADAMS, R. N. (1972) Central nervous system effects of 6-aminodopamine and 6-hydroxydopamine. *Brain Res.* **45**, 635–637.

CORRODI, H., and JONSSON, G. (1967) The formaldehyde fluorescence method for the histochemical demonstration of biogenic monoamines: a review on the methodology. *J. Histochem. Cytochem.* **15**, 65–78.

COYLE, J. T., and AXELROD, J. (1971) Development of the uptake and storage of L-^{3}H-norepinephrine in the rat brain. *J. Neurochem.* **18**, 2061–2075.

DE CHAMPLAIN, J. (1971) Degeneration and regrowth of adrenergic nerve fibers in the rat peripheral tissues after 6-hydroxydopamine. *Can. J. Physiol. Pharmac.* **49**, 345–355.

EMMELIN, N. (1967) Parotid secretion after cutting the auriculotemporal nerve at different levels. *J. Physiol. Lond.* **188**, 44–45.

FALCK, B., HILLARP, N.-Å., THIEME, G., and TORP, A. (1962) Fluorescence of catechol amines and related compounds condensed with formaldehyde. *J. Histochem. Cytochem.* **10**, 348–354.

FUXE, K., HÖKFELT, T., JONSSON, G., and UNGERSTEDT, U. (1970) Fluorescence microscopy in neuroanatomy. In *Contemporary Research in Neuroanatomy* (S. Ebbesen and W. Nauta, eds.), Springer, Berlin, Heidelberg and New York.

HAEUSLER, G., HAEFLY, W., and THOENEN, H. (1969) Chemical sympathectomy of the cat with 6-hydroxydopamine. *J. Pharmac. Exp. Ther.* **170**, 50–61.

HANBAUER, I., JOHNSON, D. G., SILBERSTEIN, S. D., and KOPIN, I. J. (1972) Pharmacological and kinetic properties of uptake of ^{3}H-norepinephrine by superior cervical ganglion of rats in organ culture. *Neuropharmacology* **11**, 857–862.

HEIKKILA, R. E., MYTILINEOU, C., CÔTÉ, L. J., and COHEN, G. (1973) The biochemical and pharmacological properties of 6-aminodopamine: similarity with 6-hydroxydopamine. *J. Neurochem.* **21**, 111–116.

HÖKFELT, T., JONSSON, G., and SACHS, CH. (1972) Fine structure and fluorescence morphology of adrenergic nerves after 6-hydroxydopamine *in vivo* and *in vitro*. *Z. Zellforsch.* **131**, 529–543.

IVERSEN, L. L., DE CHAMPLAIN, J., GLOWINSKI, J., and AXELROD, J. (1967) Uptake, storage and metabolism of norepinephrine in tissues of the developing rat. *J. Pharmac. Exp. Ther.* **157**, 509–516.

JONSSON, G. (1969) Microfluorimetric studies on the formaldehyde-induced fluorescence of noradrenaline in adrenergic nerves of rat. *J. Histochem. Cytochem.* **17**, 714–723.

JONSSON, G. (1971) Quantitation of biogenic monoamines demonstrated with the formaldehyde fluorescence method. *Progr. Histochem. Cytochem.* **2**, 299–334.

JONSSON, G., and SACHS, CH. (1970) Effects of 6-hydroxydopamine on the uptake and storage of noradrenaline in sympathetic adrenergic neurones. *Eur. J. Pharmac.* **9**, 141–155.

JONSSON, G., and SACHS, CH. (1972) Neurochemical properties of adrenergic nerves regenerated after 6-hydroxydopamine. *J. Neurochem.* **19**, 2577–2585.

JONSSON, G., and SACHS, CH. (1973) 6-Aminodopamine induced degeneration of catecholamine neurons. *J. Neurochem.* **21**, 117–124.

JONSSON, G., and SACHS, CH. (1974) Histochemical and neurochemical studies on adrenergic nerves regenerated after chemical sympathectomy produced by 6-hydroxydopamine. In *Fluorescence Histochemistry of Biogenic Amines* (M. Fujiwara, ed.), Igaku-Shoin Ltd., Tokyo.

KIRPEKAR, S. M., CERVONI, P., and FURCHGOTT, R. F. (1962) Catecholamine content of the rat nictitating membrane following procedures sensitizing it to norepinephrine. *J. Pharmac. Exp. Ther.* **135**, 180–190.

LADURON, P., and BELPAIRE, F. (1968) Tissue fractionation and catecholamines: II, Intracellular distribution patterns of tyrosine hydroxylase, dopa decarboxylase, dopamine-β-hydroxylase, phenylethanolamine *N*-methyltransferase and monoamine oxidase in adrenal medulla. *Biochem. Pharmac.* **17**, 1127–1140.

LUNDBERG, D. (1972) Effects of colchicine, vinblastine and vincristine on degeneration transmitter release after sympathetic denervation studied in the conscious rat. *Acta physiol. scand.* **85**, 91–98.

MALMFORS, T. (1965) Studies on adrenergic nerves. *Acta physiol. scand.* **64**, Suppl. 248, 1–120.

MALMFORS, T., and SACHS, CH. (1965) Direct studies on the disappearance of the transmitter and changes in the uptake-storage mechanisms of degenerating adrenergic nerves. *Acta physiol. scand.* **64**, 211–223.

MALMFORS, T., and THOENEN, H. (eds.) (1971) 6-*Hydroxydopamine and Catecholamine Neurons*, North-Holland, Amsterdam.

ROTH, C. D., and RICHARDSON, K. C. (1969) Electron microscopical studies on axonal degeneration in the rat iris following ganglionectomy. *Am. J. Anat.* **124**, 341–359.

SACHS, CH., and JONSSON, G. (1973) Quantitative microfluorimetric and neurochemical studies on degenerating adrenergic nerves. *J. Histochem. Cytochem.* **21,** 902–911.

SAELENS, J. K., SCHOENEN, M. S., and KOVACSICS, G. B. (1967) An enzyme assay for norepinephrine in brain tissue. *Biochem. Pharmac.* **16,** 1043.

TRENDELENBURG, U. (1963) Time course of changes in sensitivity after denervation of the nictitating membrane of the spinal cat. *J. Pharmac. Exp. Ther.* **142,** 335–342.

VAN ORDEN, L. S., III, BENSCH, K. G., LANGER, S. Z., and TRENDELENBURG, U. (1967) Histochemical and fine structural aspects of the onset of denervation supersensitivity in the nictitating membrane of the spinal cat. *J. Pharmac. Exp. Ther.* **157,** 274–283.

VON EULER, U. S., and PURKHOLD, A. (1951) Effect of sympathetic denervation on the noradrenaline and adrenaline content of spleen, kidney and salivary glands in the sheep. *Acta physiol. scand.* **24,** 214–217.

LATE AND EARLY BIOCHEMICAL CHANGES IN CENTRAL CATECHOLAMINE NEURONS AFTER AXOTOMY

NILS-ERIK ANDÉN, TOR MAGNUSSON, AND GÜNTER STOCK†

Department of Pharmacology, University of Göteborg, Sweden

SUMMARY

A unilateral, transverse section in the caudal part of the rat forebrain (hemisection) induces a disappearance of both dopamine and noradrenaline frontal to the lesion on the operated side after 7 days, in all probability due to anterograde degeneration of the ascending catecholamine neurons. The dopamine, but not the noradrenaline, increases rapidly by about 60% after hemisection and remains elevated for 1 day. The increase is caused partly by a reduced release, but mainly by an increased synthesis of dopamine. Injections of 25% KCl, but not 20% NaCl, into the neostriatum eliminate the increase in dopamine both when given concomitantly with or after a hemisection, showing that the increase is caused by a blockade of the nerve impulse flow to the dopamine terminals. The increase in dopamine seen after hemisection may be partially mediated via a reduced dopamine receptor activity judging from experiments with receptor stimulating and blocking drugs.

INTRODUCTION

The dopamine (DA) and the noradrenaline (NA) in the forebrain (telencephalon plus diencephalon) are present in nerve terminals belonging to neurons whose cell bodies are localized in the lower brain stem (Andén *et al.*, 1966). The ascending pathways are rather scattered, and it is difficult to interrupt all of them by means of an electrolytic lesion. Therefore, the introduction of a complete, transverse section of the caudal part of the rat forebrain on one side (Hassler and Bak, 1969) has been of great value, particularly in biochemical experiments where a great number of samples is needed. The contents of DA and NA in the forebrain at different time intervals after such a hemisection are shown in Fig. 1 (Andén *et al.*, 1972). No significant changes are seen on the unoperated side. On the operated side, the DA is reduced to insignificant values after 7 days. The NA content is also markedly lowered at this time interval. These losses are in all probability caused by an anterograde degeneration of the ascending catecholamine neurons. The decline in percent

---

† Permanent address: Department of Physiology I, University of Heidelberg, D-6900 Heidelberg, Federal Republic of Germany.

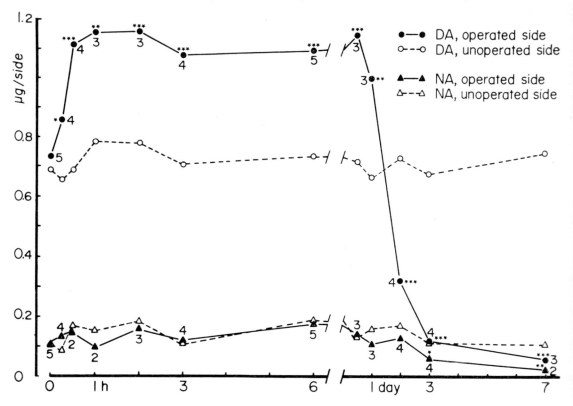

Fig. 1. Content of dopamine (DA) and noradrenaline (NA) in the rat forebrain at different intervals after a hemisection. Means, number of experiments, and statistical significances for the differences between the operated and unoperated side (***$p < 0.001$, **$p < 0.01$, *$p < 0.05$). (From Andén et al., 1972.)

of the original value is, however, smaller for the NA than for the DA. This difference between NA and DA may be due to the slower disappearance of the NA, but it may also be explained by a certain crossing of NA fibers from the opposite side (Magnusson, unpublished data). Anyhow, the reductions indicate that most of the ascending NA neurons and all of the ascending DA neurons are severed on the lesioned side.

EARLY INCREASE IN DOPAMINE AFTER AXOTOMY

Prior to the described lowerings of DA and NA, the forebrain DA on the operated side is markedly elevated (Andén et al., 1971; Andén et al., 1972). This increase in DA is seen already 15 min after the hemisection. The DA content reaches a plateau, about 160 % of the normal, after approximately 1 h. The DA remains at this elevated level for about 24 h and then the drop starts. In contrast to the DA, the NA is not increased on the operated side during the first postoperative day and, sometimes, the NA is even significantly reduced at the early intervals (Stock et al., 1973). Similarly to the NA, the 5-hydroxytryptamine in the forebrain does not show any marked increase after hemisection (Andén et al., 1972; Bédard et al., 1972). On the other hand, acetylcholine is increased to about the same degree as DA after axotomy (Pepeu and Mantegazzini, 1964; Kuhar et al., 1973).

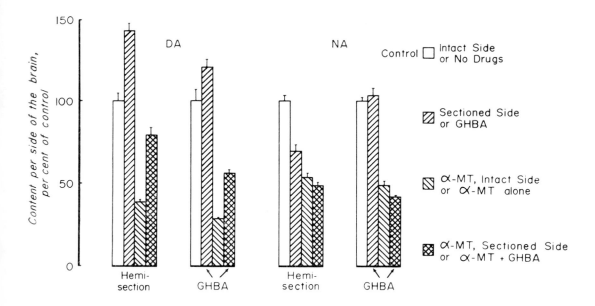

FIG. 2. Effect of hemisection and gammahydroxybutyric acid (GHBA, 1.5 + 1.0 g/kg i.p.) on the disappearance of dopamine (DA) and noradrenaline (NA) in the rat brain induced by α-methyltyrosine (α-MT, 250 mg/kg i.p. of its methylester H44/68 4 h before sacrifice). The α-MT was given immediately before the hemisection and the first injection of GHBA. Means ± SEM of 9–10 experiments. (From Stock *et al.*, 1973.)

Treatment with the tyrosine hydroxylase inhibitor α-methyltyrosine causes a marked reduction of DA when the neurons are intact but causes only a small loss when given immediately after an electrolytic lesion of the ascending DA axons, thus showing that the α-methyltyrosine-induced DA disappearance is highly dependent on the nerve impulse flow (Andén *et al.*, 1971). Since a hemisection produces an increase in brain DA, the effect of α-methyltyrosine has been investigated by giving it 10 min before the operation (Stock *et al.*, 1973). Under these circumstances, the DA in the forebrain is about twice as high on the operated as on the unoperated side when analyzed 4 h after the administration of α-methyltyrosine, in agreement with the findings after an electrolytic lesion (Fig. 2). In this context it is of interest to note that treatment with gammahydroxybutyric acid induces similar increases in DA and similar decelerations of the α-methyltyrosine-induced DA disappearance (Stock *et al.*, 1973) (Fig. 2) and that this compound has been shown to inhibit the firing of the DA cells in the substantia nigra (Walters *et al.*, 1972). A lack of nerve impulses, and a consequent blockade of release of DA, should cause an increase in DA if the synthesis continues. However, the loss of DA by the normal nerve impulse flow is probably rather slow to judge from the rate of disappearance of DA after treatment with α-methyltyrosine. Therefore a blockade of release can hardly be the only explanation for the rapid increase in DA seen after interruption of the nerve impulse flow. For that reason, it is likely that also the synthesis of DA is increased after axotomy. In fact, it has been observed that a hemisection causes a rapid and marked increase in the synthesis of the forebrain DA, analyzed by means of accumulation of DOPA after inhibition of the DOPA decarboxylase activity (Kehr *et al.*, 1972).

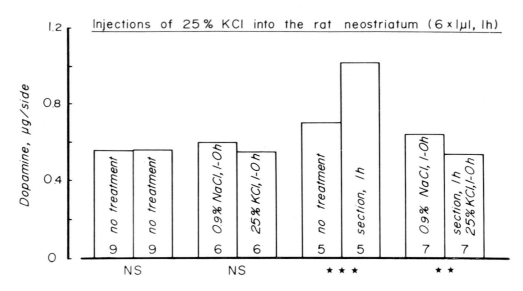

FIG. 3. Effect of 25% KCl, given into the neostriatum, on the increase in rat forebrain dopamine seen after hemisection. One side was used for the administration of 25% KCl and for hemisection. On the opposite side, 0.9% NaCl was given when 25% KCl was injected on the experimental side. The times denote the intervals in hours between the hemisection or injections and killing. The columns represent means. The figures show the number of right and left forebrain halves analyzed. Statistical significances for differences between the two sides (***p < 0.001, **p < 0.01).

POTASSIUM-INDUCED RELEASE OF DOPAMINE

After axotomy, the DA nerve terminals in the neostriatum are not depolarized by nerve impulses in the nigro-neostriatal DA neurons. In order to depolarize the DA nerve terminals in the neostriatum after hemisection, 25% KCl has been given locally into this nucleus (Stock et al., 1973). By means of stereotaxically implanted guide cannulae, the hyperosmotic KCl was given into the neostriatum of freely moving rats in a volume of 1 μl every 10 min. Such an administration of 25% KCl for 1 h into the neostriatum of rats with intact nigroneostriatal DA neurons does not change the normal DA content significantly (Fig. 3). However, this local treatment with 25% KCl completely prevents the increase in forebrain DA observed 1 h after hemisection. Actually, the DA is significantly lowered on the operated side after the treatment with KCl. Local injections of KCl are able to counteract the rise in DA also when they are given after the hemisection; thus, if KCl is administered into the neostriatum 1.5 to 2.5 h after a hemisection, the elevated DA is markedly reduced to values even lower than those seen without hemisection (Stock et al., 1973). In this latter case, the treatment with KCl releases in 1 h at least the amount of DA normally stored in the neostriatum. Since KCl does not induce any reduction of the DA in the intact nigroneostriatal DA neurons, it appears that the KCl has a special ability to release the newly synthesized DA. The DA accumulated after hemisection may, thus, be located in the granules in a fraction on which KCl or nerve impulses easily can act.

In order to study the duration of the effect of 25% KCl, this solution has been given into the neostriatum for 1 h, starting 1 h, 2 h, or 3 h before sacrifice, in combination with a hemisection performed 1 h before sacrifice (Stock et al., 1973). The effect of KCl is almost

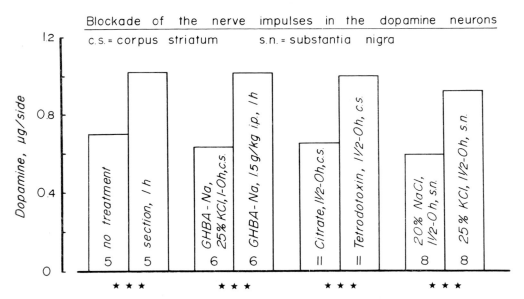

FIG. 4. Dopamine content in the rat brain after hemisection, intraperitoneal injection of gammahydroxybutyric acid (GHBA), injections of tetrodotoxin into the corpus striatum and injections of 25% KCl into the substantia nigra. For further details, see legend to Fig. 3.

completely eliminated when the treatment is discontinued 1 h before the hemisection, and it is partly eliminated when the KCl application is discontinued concomitantly with the hemisection.

Also a hyperosmotic solution of NaCl has been given into the neostriatum in a concentration of 20% which is equimolar to that of 25% KCl (Stock *et al.*, 1973). The increase in DA after a hemisection is not influenced by such a treatment, thus suggesting that the effect of KCl is not due to an unspecific effect. The experiments with 25% KCl and 20% NaCl indicate that the DA nerve terminals are in a good condition after hemisection since the DA is rapidly released in the former but not in the latter case. The reappearance of the effect of axotomy on the DA content after discontinuation of the KCl treatment strengthens this view.

It has been tried to block the nerve impulse flow to the DA nerve terminals in the neostriatum also by other means than axotomy (Fig. 4). Treatment with gammahydroxybutyric acid inhibits the firing of the DA cell bodies in the substantia nigra (Walters *et al.*, 1972), and it causes a rise in brain DA to about the same level and at about the same rate as seen after hemisection (Stock *et al.*, 1973). The fish poison tetrodotoxin blocks the nerve impulses by preventing the entry of sodium ions into the nerves. Administration of tetrodotoxin into the neostriatum of rats also elevates the DA to about the same degree as observed after hemisection (Stock *et al.*, 1973). Injections of 25% KCl, but not 20% NaCl, into the rat substantia nigra induce an increase in brain DA of about the same magnitude as the former treatments (Stock *et al.*, 1973). It can be speculated that the KCl persistently depolarizes the DA cell bodies in the substantia nigra or that it releases an inhibitory transmitter to these cells. Thus there is evidence from different kinds of experiments that a blockade of the nerve impulses to the DA nerve terminals in the neostriatum causes an increase in DA, indicating that these phenomena are related.

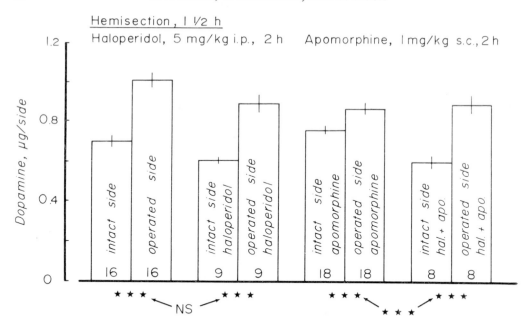

FIG. 5. Effect of apomorphine and haloperidol on the increases in rat forebrain dopamine
seen after hemisection. Means ± SEM. For further details, see legend to Fig. 3.

DOPAMINE RECEPTOR ACTIVITY

Drugs influencing monoamine receptors appear to change both the release and the synthesis of the corresponding monoamine via feedback (Andén *et al.*, 1969). Thus both the synthesis and release of DA are stimulated normally by the DA receptor blocking agent haloperidol and they are inhibited by the DA receptor stimulating agent apomorphine. Therefore these two drugs have been given in combination with a hemisection in order to investigate the influence of the DA receptor activity on the increase in DA (Andén *et al.*, 1973) (Fig. 5). After pretreatment with haloperidol, the DA on the operated side is significantly higher than on the unoperated side, and the difference between the two sides is not statistically significant from that seen after hemisection alone. After pretreatment with apomorphine, there is a small but significant decrease in DA on the operated side ($p < 0.001$) but not on the intact side ($p > 0.1$), causing a smaller difference between the two sides than after hemisection alone ($p < 0.001$). When haloperidol is given before apomorphine, about the same great difference in the DA content between the two sides is obtained as after pretreatment with haloperidol only.

The results with haloperidol and apomorphine indicate that DA receptors are involved in the elevation of DA seen after axotomy (cf. Kehr *et al.*, 1972). It is not clarified if such DA receptors are localized either on the effector cells or on the terminals or on both structures. After interruption of the nerve impulse flow, no DA will be released to the synaptic cleft and reach the receptors. The lack of receptor stimulation may, via feedback, increase the synthesis and content of DA. Hence, an additional blockade of these receptors by haloperidol should not lead to a further change in DA. On the other hand, restitution of the DA receptor stimulation by apomorphine should inhibit the effect of axotomy. The inhibition is, however, only partial, despite behavioral findings that the DA receptors are continuously overstimulated by the doses of apomorphine used. Since pretreatment with haloperidol counteracts the small effect of apomorphine, a reduced stimulation of DA receptors may be partially responsible for the increase in DA seen after interruption of the nerve impulse flow.

ACKNOWLEDGEMENT

This work was supported by the Swedish Medical Research Council (04X-502).

REFERENCES

ANDÉN, N.-E., DAHLSTRÖM, A., FUXE, K., LARSSON, K., OLSON, L., and UNGERSTEDT, U. (1966) Ascending monoamine neurons to the telencephalon and diencephalon. *Acta physiol. scand.* **67**, 313–326.

ANDÉN, N.-E., CARLSSON, A., and HÄGGENDAL, J. (1969) Adrenergic mechanisms. *A. Rev. Pharmac.* **9**, 119–134.

ANDÉN, N.-E., CORRODI, H., FUXE, K., and UNGERSTEDT, U. (1971) Importance of nervous impulse flow for the neuroleptic induced increase in amine turnover in central dopamine neurons. *Eur. J. Pharmac.* **15**, 193–199.

ANDÉN, N.-E., BÉDARD, P., FUXE, K., and UNGERSTEDT, U. (1972) Early and selective increase in brain dopamine levels after axotomy. *Experientia* **28**, 300–301.

ANDÉN, N.-E., MAGNUSSON, T., and STOCK, G. (1973) Effects of drugs influencing monoamine mechanisms on the increase in brain dopamine produced by axotomy or treatment with gammahydroxybutyric acid. *Naunyn-Schmiedeberg's Arch. Pharmac.* **278**, 363–372.

BÉDARD, P., CARLSSON, A., and LINDQVIST, M. (1972) Effect of a transverse cerebral hemisection on 5-hydroxytryptamine metabolism in the rat brain. *Naunyn-Schmiedeberg's Arch. Pharmac.* **272**, 1–15.

HASSLER, R., and BAK, I. J. (1969) Unbalanced ratios of striatal dopamine and serotonin after experimental interruption of strionigral connections in rat. In *Third Symposium on Parkinson's Disease* (F. J. Gillingham and I. M. L. Donaldson, eds.), Livingstone, Edinburgh and London, pp. 29–37.

KEHR, W., CARLSSON, A., LINDQVIST, M., MAGNUSSON, T., and ATACK, C. (1972) Evidence for a receptor-mediated feedback control of striatal tyrosine hydroxylase activity. *J. Pharm. Pharmac.* **24**, 744–747.

KUHAR, M. J., SETHY, V. H., ROTH, R. H., and AGHAJANIAN, G. K. (1973) Choline: selective accumulation by central cholinergic neurons. *J. Neurochem.* **20**, 581–593.

PEPEU, G., and MANTEGAZZINI, P. (1964) Midbrain hemisection: effect on cortical acetylcholine in the cat. *Science* **145**, 1069–1070.

STOCK, G., MAGNUSSON, T., and ANDÉN, N.-E. (1973) Increase in brain dopamine after axotomy or treatment with gammahydroxybutyric acid due to elimination of the nerve impulse flow. *Naunyn-Schmiedeberg's Arch. Pharmac.* **278**, 347–361.

WALTERS, J. R., AGHAJANIAN, G. K., and ROTH, R. H. (1972) Dopaminergic neurons: inhibition of firing by γ-hydroxybutyrate. In *Proc. Fifth Pharmacol. Congr.*, Abstract vol., San Francisco, p. 246.

BIOCHEMICAL AND MORPHOLOGICAL CHANGES AFTER MECHANICAL OR CHEMICAL DEGENERATION OF THE DOPAMINERGIC NIGRO-NEOSTRIATAL PATHWAY

F. Javoy, Y. Agid, J. Glowinski, and C. Sotelo†

Groupe NB (INSERM U.114) Laboratoire de Biologie Moléculaire Collège de France 11, place Marcelin Berthelot, Paris 5e

SUMMARY

The dopaminergic activity of dopamine (DA) containing nerve terminals was estimated in the neostriatum (NCP) immediately (30 min) or at a long time (30 days) after interruption of the DA nigro-neostriatal pathway. For this purpose, unilateral lesions of the substantia nigra (SN) were performed either by electrocoagulation or local injection of 6-hydroxy-dopamine (6-OH-DA).

An immediate rapid rise in DA levels was observed in NCP shortly after interruption of the nigro-neostriatal pathway. This increase reflects a diminished rate of DA utilization in nerve endings, probably induced by a decrease in the nerve impulse flow. Despite the high DA levels in the NCP, the amine synthesis was markedly enhanced. The present data support the concept of a receptor-mediated control of DA synthesis in neostriatal DA nerve endings. Morphological changes in the SN were studied 24 or 43 h after local 6-OH-DA administration. In zones far enough from the tip of the injection cannula, numerous dendritic profiles and neural perikarya exhibited an advance necrotic appearance. These selectively damaged neurons, probably the dopaminergic ones, were intermixed with normal neural perikarya and neuropil islands. The extension of the selective chemical lesion was shown to be directly dependent on the amount of 6-OH-DA injected. In the NCP of rats sacrificed 43 h after the nigral 6-OH-DA injection, some dark and shrunken degenerating axon terminals were observed. Some of them were still synapsing on dendritic profiles; however, the large majority of such degenerating terminals were already engulfed by astrocytic processes. The degenerating terminals have completely disappeared 30 days later, as indicated by the marked depletion of neostriatal DA.

When part of the DA nigro-neostriatal system had degenerated, a metabolic hyperactivity of the remaining intact DA neurons was observed as revealed by the increased rate of DA synthesis in the NCP.

INTRODUCTION

There is now good evidence for the existence of a monosynaptic dopaminergic nigro-neostriatal pathway (Andén *et al.*, 1964; Poirier and Sourkes, 1965; Faull and Laverty, 1969; Moore *et al.*, 1971; Hedreen and Chalmers, 1972) involved in extrapyramidal motor control (Hornykiewicz, 1972). The injection of 6-hydroxy-dopamine (6-OH-DA) into the

† Laboratoire de Neuromorphologie (INSERM U.106) Hôpital de Port Royal, Paris 75014.

substantia nigra (SN) (Ungerstedt, 1968; Sotelo *et al.*, 1973) or nigral electrothermal lesions (Andén *et al.*, 1964) induce degeneration of some fibers and axon terminals ending in the neostriatum (caudate nucleus + putamen) (NCP) of the rat. Both types of lesions lead to a depletion of striatal dopamine (DA) within a few days (Ungerstedt, 1968; Hökfelt and Ungerstedt, 1969; Agid *et al.*, 1973a). The importance of the DA decrease in the NCP, reflects the extent of the chemical lesion made into the SN. This lesion has been shown to be dependent on the dose of 6-OH-DA locally injected (Agid *et al.*, 1973a). The amount of DA still present in the NCP after incomplete nigral lesion may provide a good index of the number of intact remaining DA neurons in the SN since the drug very likely has, at a given dose, an all or nondestroying effect (Bennet *et al.*, 1970).

On the other hand, a rapid rise in neostriatal DA content has been observed immediately after the interruption of nerve impulses induced by nigral electrolytic lesions (Faull and Laverty, 1969). Furthermore, Ungerstedt (1971) has described an alteration of the retention of exogenous ^{3}H-DA in the NCP shortly after the injection of 6-OH-DA into the SN. However, at this early time no detectable morphological changes have yet appeared in DA nerve terminals (Hökfelt and Ungerstedt, 1969).

In the present study we have attempted to analyze DA metabolism in NCP (1) in the still undamaged nerve endings of DA neurons in the rat, immediately after interruption of the nigro-neostriatal pathway by electrolytic or 6-OH-DA induced lesions of the SN, and (2) in undamaged terminals several weeks after partial degeneration of DA nigral neurons induced by 6-OH-DA. These results will be discussed in regard to the morphological modifications occurring in the nigro-neostriatal system after partial chemical destruction of the SN.

MATERIAL AND METHODS

Experiments were performed on male Charles River rats (250 g) positioned in a stereotaxic apparatus. During the surgical procedure, the animals were anesthetized by circulating a mixture of halothane, oxygen, and nitrous oxide through a mask fitted over their nose.

Electrolytic lesions were performed unilaterally in the right SN, using a high frequency current generated through a Grass apparatus. 6-OH-DA was administered unilaterally into the rostromedial part of the zona compacta of the SN (Agid *et al.*, 1973a). 6-OH-DA (dihydrochloride, Hässle, Sweden) was dissolved at a concentration of 2 μg/μl in Merles solution containing ascorbic acid. Sham-operated animals received an injection of 6-OH-DA free Merles ascorbic acid solution.

Morphological observations were performed on animals sacrificed 24 and 43 h after 6-OH-DA administration (Sotelo *et al.*, 1973).

Three experimental approaches were utilized to estimate changes in neostriatal DA metabolism occurring 30 days (chronic animals) or 30 min (acute animals) after the operation. (1) ^{3}H-DA accumulated in the NCP was determined 10 min after an intravenous injection of L-3,5-^{3}H-tyrosine (49 c/mM, CEA, France). (2) ^{3}H-H$_2$O synthesized *in vivo* from L-3,5-^{3}H-tyrosine was estimated in NCP 3 min after intracerebral injections of the labeled amino acid (1 μl in 3 min) simultaneously made in both striata (Javoy *et al.*, 1974a). (3) The rate of striatal DA utilization was determined by blocking the amine synthesis with the help of a DOPA decarboxylase inhibitor, RO 4-4602. The drug was utilized at a dose (800 mg/kg i.p.) inhibiting both central and peripheral enzymes.

In all cases left and right striata were analyzed separately for their content in endogenous and labeled DA and tyrosine (Javoy *et al.*, 1972).

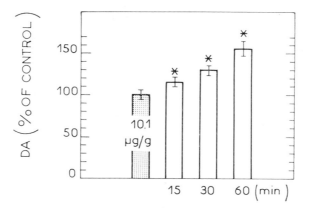

FIG. 1. Dopamine content in the rat right NCP at various time intervals after local injection of 6-OH-DA (8 μg) into the ipsilateral SN. Results are expressed as percentage of DA content found in the NCP of the sham-operated nigro-neostriatal system (Black bar). Differences between sham-operated and operated sides were estimated to be significant (*) for $p \leqslant 0.05$. Each estimation is the mean of data obtained on eight animals.

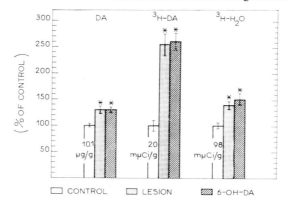

FIG. 2. Early effect of electrolytic lesions or 6-OH-DA injections into the SN on neostriatal DA metabolism. An electrolytic lesion, or an injection of 8 μg of 6-OH-DA, was performed unilaterally in the right SN. In all cases animals were sacrificed 30 min later for the analysis of DA metabolism in the right and left NCP. Accumulation of ^{3}H-DA was estimated 10 min after an intravenous injection of L-3,5-^{3}H-tyrosine (430 μC). ^{3}H-H$_2$O formation was determined 3 min after a local infusion of L-3,5-^{3}H-tyrosine (1.8 μCi) in both NCP simultaneously. All results are expressed as percentage of control values (control = NCP controlateral to the lesioned side). Differences were accepted as statistically significant for all p values $\leqslant 0.05$ (*). Experiments were made on groups of nine rats.

RESULTS AND DISCUSSION

1. EARLY CHANGES ON NEOSTRIATAL DA METABOLISM AFTER A 6-OH-DA INJECTION OR ELECTROLYTIC LESION INTO THE SN

The intracerebral injection of 8 μg of 6-OH-DA into the right SN induced a rapid rise in striatal DA levels (Fig. 1). As soon as 15 min after the drug administration, a detectable increase (15%) in DA content could be observed in DA terminals; it reached 150% of normal values after 60 min. As illustrated in Fig. 2, a similar effect was seen within the 30 min which followed the electrolytic destruction of DA cell bodies. Moreover, following intravenous injection of ^{3}H-tyrosine, a marked increase in the accumulation of newly synthesized ^{3}H-DA was observed when nigral cells had been injured by either procedures (Fig. 2). Tyrosine and ^{3}H-tyrosine levels in the NCP were unchanged when compared to the controlateral side. No increase in DA or ^{3}H-DA levels was observed in sham-lesioned animals.

The mechanism by which striatal DA metabolism was impaired has been examined. We attempted to determine which of DA synthesis or utilization was responsible for the disbalance in the DA and ^{3}H-DA levels observed as compared to the controlateral side.

Two observations are in favor of a decreased release of DA from the nerve terminals. Firstly, immediately after the unilateral injection of 6-OH-DA into the SN, as well as after the electrolytic nigral lesion, the rats developed an asymmetrical posture, rotating towards the operated side. This well known behavior has been observed previously by other workers after unilateral electrothermal lesions (Andén et al., 1966) as well as after 6-OH-DA (Ungerstedt and Arbuthnott, 1970) induced degeneration of the nigro-neostriatal DA neuronal system. It has been attributed to a decreased DA utilization in synapses. Secondly, there is biochemical evidence for a decreased DA utilization in the NCP when the SN has been destroyed by an electrolytic lesion. The initial rate of DA disappearance after inhibition of its synthesis was used as an index of the amine utilization. The inhibitor of DOPA-decarboxylase, RO 4-4602, which rapidly (Agid and Javoy, unpublished observations) induced a complete inhibition of DA synthesis, was used for this purpose. Therefore animals were treated with an intraperitoneal injection of either RO 4-4602 or saline (control rats) 30 min before death, immediately before performing an electrolytic lesion of the SN. As expected, DA levels in saline-treated animals were increased in the NCP ipsilateral to the damaged SN. A significant decrease in striatal DA could be seen on the intact nigro-neostriatal system of RO 4-4602-treated animals when compared to the concentrations of DA found in NCP of saline-treated rats (Fig. 3). DA concentrations were those of normal in the NCP of the lesioned system in RO 4-4602-treated animals. Since DA levels were not decreased in the NCP ipsilateral to the nigral lesion, these results suggest an immediate blockade of the transmitter utilization. A similar process seems to be induced shortly after a 6-OH-DA injection into the SN since the rate of utilization of exogenous ^{3}H-DA previously taken up in DA terminals was markedly reduced (Ungerstedt, 1971).

As it will be discussed later on, degenerative processes in the NCP appear much later after the operation. Metabolic changes observed in DA terminals are thus induced by events occurring at the level of nigral cell bodies. In this view, Ungerstedt (1971) has reported that DA cell bodies in the SN are affected already 5 min after the local injection of 6-OH-DA. On the other hand, the neurotransmitter utilization is known to be rapidly affected by interruption of nerve impulse activity (Andén et al., 1971). It has also been shown that transection of the nigro-neostriatal system in the cat immediately blocks the spontaneous release of newly synthesized ^{3}H-DA from DA terminals (Besson et al., 1973). In conclusion, the electrolytic destruction of the SN in the rat likely impairs neurotransmitter release by blocking normal nerve impulse flow. The similarity of the rapid biochemical changes observed in the NCP after electrolytic or 6-OH-DA-induced nigral lesions suggest that the latter procedure also affects nerve impulse activity as already proposed by Ungerstedt (1971).

Possible changes in DA metabolism occurring at the level of the first limiting step of the amine synthesis have been investigated. For this purpose a new method has been developed enabling the estimation of changes in the *in vivo* rate of tyrosine hydroxylation (Javoy et al.,

1974a). L-3,5-³H-tyrosine locally injected into the NCP is rapidly converted into ³H-DA (Javoy *et al.*, 1970). ³H-H₂O parallely formed during the hydroxylation of the labeled amine into ³H-DOPA provides a good index of the first step of the ³H-amine synthesis when its accumulation in tissues is estimated shortly after ³H-tyrosine injection. The complete blockade of ³H-H₂O formation after total degeneration of the DA nigro-neostriatal system or α-methyl-*p*-tyrosine treatment revealed the specificity of the method. Furthermore, the similarity of the results obtained in pharmacological studies with the ³H-H₂O technique and other methods used for the estimation of DA synthesis have demonstrated the validity of this approach (Javoy *et al.*, 1974a).

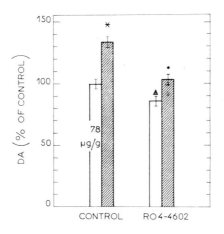

FIG. 3. Changes in striatal DA of normal or RO4-4602-treated animals after nigral lesion. An unilateral electrolytic lesion of the right SN was performed in normal or RO4-4602-treated animals. The drug was injected just before the destruction of the right SN. Results are expressed as percentage of control values (control = NCP of the unlesioned side of untreated animals). The open bars represent the normal side and the hatched bars, the lesioned side. Significant statistical difference ($p \leq 0.05$) (*) between the lesioned and unlesioned sides of control animals, (▲) between the unlesioned side of control or RO4-4602-treated animals, (●) between lesioned and unlesioned side of RO4-4602-treated animal. Results are the mean of groups of seven animals.

The *in vivo* initial accumulation (3 min) of ³H-H₂O formed from L-3,5-³H-tyrosine in the NCP was thus estimated 30 min after an injection of 6-OH-DA into the SN or a nigral electrolytic lesion. In both cases (Fig. 2) a 30% increase in ³H-H₂O formation was observed in the NCP corresponding to the lesioned side when compared with that of the contro-lateral NCP. These changes were not related to modifications of tyrosine specific activity in tissues, therefore they strongly suggest an activation of ³H-DA formation at the rate-limiting step of the amine synthesis. These results confirm and extend recent observations of Carlsson *et al.* (1972). These authors have reported that DA synthesis in the rat forebrain was stimulated rapidly after a cerebral hemisection.

This increase in DA synthesis is associated in time to the inhibition of the neurotransmitter release. Similarly we observed a rapid activation of DA synthesis shortly after the injection of γ-hydroxybutyrate (Javoy *et al.*, 1974b), a general anaesthetic which blocks DA release from DA terminals (Bustos and Roth, 1972). The lack of information at DA post- or presynaptic receptors sites may be, through a short feedback process, responsible for the activation of the neurotransmitter synthesis. Such a receptor-mediated control of striatal DA synthesis has already been suggested by Kehr *et al.* (1972). However, a direct relationship between cell bodies and nerve endings in regulatory processes of DA synthesis cannot be excluded. The impairment of DA metabolism in nerve terminals could result from their recent disconnection with cell bodies.

In a previous report we have demonstrated the existence of a regulation of DA synthesis by end-product inhibition at the tyrosine-hydroxylase step (Javoy *et al.*, 1972). In the present study, the increase in neostriatal DA levels seen after nigral lesions does not induce a slower rate of the amine synthesis. On the contrary, activation of synthesis is observed. Therefore, enhanced DA levels in the NCP result in an activation or an inhibition of the amine synthesis depending on the factor responsible for the changes in amine levels. After the interruption of nerve impulse flow by electrolytic lesion or 6-OH-DA intranigral injection, a rapid accumulation of DA occurs in DA nerve endings. The exceeding amine is likely mainly stored in vesicles, sites in which it is protected from enzymatic inactivation and not available for the regulation of its own synthesis. A different picture may be seen when DA levels in nerve endings have been increased after MAO inhibition or uptake of exogenous amine (Javoy *et al.*, 1972); the exceeding amine may be partly accumulated in extravesicular sites where it can act on DA synthesis regulation.

2. LONG TERM CHANGES ON NIGRAL DA NEURONS AND STRIATAL DA METABOLISM AFTER INJECTIONS OF 6-OH-DA INTO THE SUBSTANTIA NIGRA

Several papers have been already published (Ungerstedt, 1971; Frigyesi *et al.*, 1971; Poirier *et al.*, 1972; Sotelo *et al.*, 1973) on the morphological changes induced by injection of 6-OH-DA into the brain parenchyma, especially into the SN. In some of them it was claimed that 6-OH-DA mainly induces a catecholaminergic neuronal degeneration in addition to a small unspecific damage restricted to the tissue around the tip of the injection cannula (Ungerstedt, 1971; Frigyesi *et al.*, 1971). In others, for instance in the paper by Poirier *et al.* (1972), it was concluded that the intracerebral application of 6-OH-DA only produces unspecific lesions similar to those induced by electrolysis.

An explanation to this apparent discrepancy had been advanced in our recent study on the morphological changes induced by injection of 6-OH-DA into the SN (Sotelo *et al.*, 1973). It has been found in rats sacrificed 24 or 43 h after the drug administration that the nature of the lesion was directly dependent on the amount of 6-OH-DA injected. When this amount was from 0.5 to 4 μg, three types of cytopathological responses were obtained, each of them being characterized by a different morphological appearance, giving rise to three different zones: (1) a central zone, around the tip of the injection cannula, represented by an unselective necrotic lesion in which the edema was the most important feature: the extension of this edematous necrotic zone was directly related to the 6-OH-DA dose; (2) an intermediary zone composed of a narrow band of nervous parenchyma, concentrical to the central necrotic area. In this intermediary zone the extracellular edema was absent, but most of neuronal and glial elements exhibited clear unselective degenerative changes; (3) a peripheral zone in which only some neuronal elements exhibited degenerative changes. This latter area was considered as the zone of the selective action of 6-OH-DA on catecholaminergic neurons. In this zone altered neuronal perikarya, dendrites or axons could be encountered among normal nervous tissue. In the altered neurons the Nissl bodies were

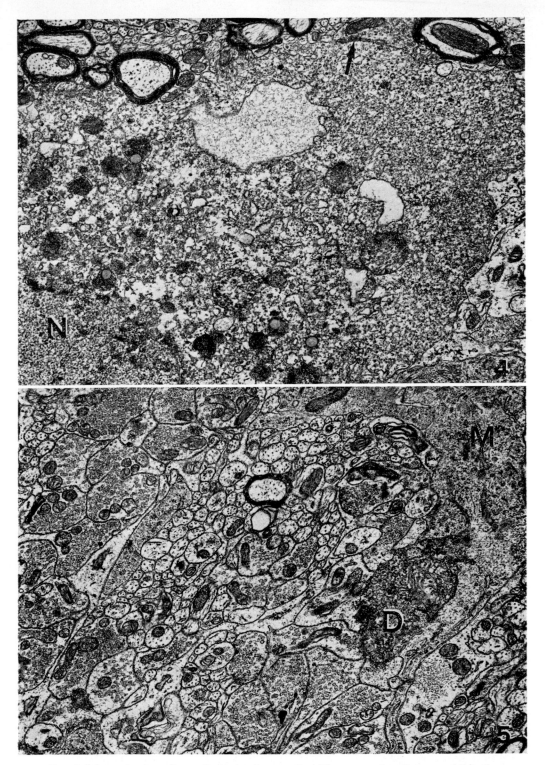

FIG. 4. Substantia nigra. Zone of selective degeneration. The neuronal perikaryon exhibits the features characterizing the early stage of degeneration: disaggregation of Nissl bodies; formation of micro sacs from the endoplasmic reticulum; alteration of mitochondria; and granular appearance of the cytoplasm. The picnosis of its nucleus (N) is evident. A normal axon terminal (arrow) is synapsing on the surface of the degenerating neuron. (×13,000.)

FIG. 5. Substantia nigra. Zone of selective degeneration. A dendritic profile (D), partially surrounded by microglial processes (M), exhibits a coagulated dark appearance, characteristic of its necrotic stage. In the neuropil, most of the neuronal elements appear normal. (×27,000.)

completely disaggregated (Fig. 4); their fragmentated endoplasmic reticular cisterns form small vesicular sacs which were floating in a granular hyaloplasmic matrix. At later stages of degeneration these neurons exhibited clear necrotic changes, explaining the neuronal loss observed in chronic animals. Necrotic changes were also evident in dendritic profiles (Fig. 5). Their cytoplasms had a coagulated dark appearance in which some altered mitochondria could still be recognized. Rare dark degenerating axon terminals and more frequent large axonal torpedos (Fig. 6) were present in the nigral neuropil. In conclusion, nigral dopaminergic neurons have the ability to take up 6-OH-DA throughout all their plasmamembranes (perikaryal, dendritic, or axonal), as such neurons do with tritiated exogenous catecholamines (Sotelo, 1971).

Concomitant studies in the ipsilateral NCP (Sotelo et al., 1973) have shown that 24 h after nigral administration of 6-OH-DA there is no detectable degenerative changes in axon terminals. However, in rats sacrificed 43 h after the drug administration, some rare dark and shrunken degenerating axon terminals were synapsing on dendritic profiles (Fig. 7). In most instances, and at this survival time, degenerating axon terminals had lost their synaptic attachments and were engulfed in astroglial processes (Fig. 8). Similar results have been obtained by Hökfelt and Ungerstedt (1969) in the neostriatum of rats killed 2 days after electrolytic lesions of nigro-neostriatal fibers.

Results obtained in the morphological study led us to analyze DA metabolism in remaining DA neurons in animals which had received various doses of 6-OH-DA (0.5, 4, 8 μg) in order to induce various degrees of degeneration of the DA nigro-neostriatal pathway. Animals were sacrificed 1 month after the operation. In agreement with our previous observations (Agid et al., 1973a), DA levels in the NCP ipsilateral to the lesion were decreased at a greater extent when larger doses of 6-OH-DA were injected into the SN (Fig. 9). No significant changes in striatal DA levels were observed between the two NCP of sham-operated animals which only received an injection of 4 μl of the Merles solution used to dissolve 6-OH-DA. It is interesting to note that no change in neostriatal tyrosine levels occurred after large lesions of the SN (Agid et al., 1973b). This is not surprising since DA nerve terminals represent only a small percentage of the overall cells and nerve endings populations of the NCP (Hökfelt, 1968).

When lesioned animals were injected intravenously with ^{3}H-tyrosine, the accumulation of newly synthesized ^{3}H-DA was decreased in the NCP ipsilateral to the lesion as compared to that found in the controlateral side (Fig. 9). Although no change in tyrosine specific activity (^{3}H-tyrosine/tyrosine) occurred in tissues, the initial accumulation of ^{3}H-DA was decreased to a lesser extent than the endogenous levels of DA (Fig. 9). In fact DA specific activity in the NCP ipsilateral to the lesion was greatly enhanced in all groups of lesioned animals. These data are in favor of an activation of DA turnover in remaining DA terminals. To confirm this hypothesis, ^{3}H-H$_2$O initial accumulation was estimated 3 min after the injection of L-3,5-^{3}H-tyrosine into the striatum in rats injected 1 month earlier with 0.5 μg of 6-OH-DA into the SN. ^{3}H-H$_2$O formation was not reduced in the NCP ipsilateral to the lesion when compared to the controlateral intact side (Fig. 10). The ^{3}H-H$_2$O/DA ratio was enhanced on the lesioned side (Fig. 10) indicating the existence of an activation of the first limiting step of DA synthesis.

As suggested in a previous study (Agid et al., 1973a), the dose dependent decrease in DA levels following intranigral injection of various doses of 6-OH-DA can be used as an index of the number of intact DA terminals still present in the NCP. However, endogenous levels of the amine give very little information about possible changes in the transmitter meta-

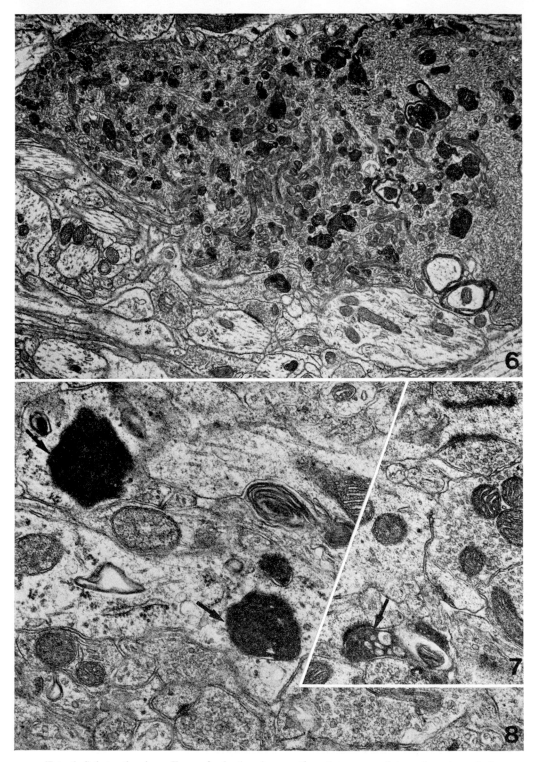

FIG. 6. Substantia nigra. Zone of selective degeneration. Large axonal torpedo surrounded by a normal looking neuropil. The axonal varicosity is filled with numerous mitochondria lysosome-like bodies, and tubular profiles of the smooth endoplasmic reticulum. (×12,000.)

FIG. 7. Ipsilateral neostriatum, 43 h after nigral 6-OH-DA administration. A dark degenerating axon terminal (arrow) is in synaptic contact with a small dendritic profile. (×29,000.)

FIG. 8. Some material as in Fig. 7. Two remnants of presynaptic terminals (arrows) are engulfed by astrocytic processes. (×33,000.)

bolism. Both the increased DA specific activity and the ^{3}H-H$_2$O/DA ratio observed in tissues when 25% of DA neurons were destroyed (Fig. 10) strongly suggest an acceleration of DA synthesis in remaining DA neurons of the lesioned side. It seems unlikely that the results obtained could be related to a greater delivery of ^{3}H-tyrosine in remaining DA neurons of the lesioned side since tyrosine content in DA terminals is negligible when compared to the amino-acid concentration in the NCP. The increased synthesis of DA observed in undamaged DA neurons very likely reflects changes in their activity. This may represent a compensatory mechanism. These results are in agreement with the observations made by Sharman *et al.* (1967) on lesioned monkeys, and by Berheimer and Hornykiewicz

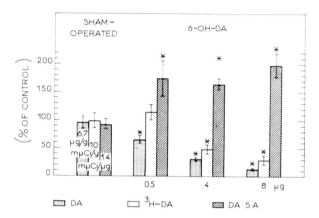

Fig. 9. Long term effect of 6-OH-DA-induced nigral lesions on striatal DA metabolism. Various doses (0.5, 4, and 8 μg) of 6-OH-DA were injected unilaterally in the right SN. Sham-operated animals received an injection of 6-OH-DA free Merles solution. Animals were killed 30 days later. Accumulation of ^{3}H-DA was estimated 10 min after an intravenous injection of ^{3}H-tyrosine (200 μCi). Left and right NCP were analyzed separately. DA, ^{3}H-DA, and DA specific activity (SA) are expressed as percentage of control values (control = NCP ipsilateral to the sham-operated side). The NCP ipsilateral to the sham-operated side is expressed as percentage of normal NCP. * represents significant statistical differences ($p \leqslant 0.05$) between lesioned and sham-operated sides. Data are the mean of groups of eight animals.

(1965) in Parkinsonian patients. The increase in the ratio of homovanillic acid to the DA content found in the caudate nucleus ipsilateral to the lesion when compared to the normal state also suggested an acceleration of DA turnover in remaining DA neurons.

CONCLUSION

Two mechanisms are involved in the rapid rise in DA levels and in the accumulation of newly synthesized ^{3}H-DA seen in the rat NCP shortly after the interruption of the nigro-neostriatal pathway by electrolytic or 6-OH-DA lesions made in the SN. As expected, the lack of nerve impulse flow is likely in both cases responsible for the blockade of transmitter release. Surprisingly, this effect is associated with an acceleration of DA synthesis. A rapid and local regulatory process linked to the modifications of the transmitter concentrations in the synaptic cleft seems to be involved in this effect. Presynaptic receptors have been recently shown to play an important role in release process in peripheral noradrenergic (Stjärne, 1973) and cholinergic neurons (Chang *et al.*, 1973). The existence of such receptors on DA terminals may contribute to the rapid triggering of DA synthesis seen after the interruption

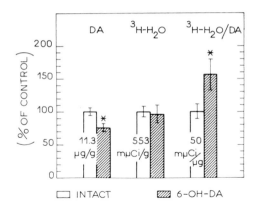

F<small>IG</small>. 10. *In vivo* estimation of the ^{3}H-H$_2$O formed from L-3,5-^{3}H-tyrosine in the intact remaining DA neurons of the NCP after incomplete destruction of the nigro-striatal pathway. 6-OH-DA (0.5 μg) was unilaterally injected in the right SN. Thirty days later, L-3,5-^{3}H-tyrosine (4 μCi) was locally infused in both NCP simultaneously. Animals were sacrificed 3 min later. Each NCP was analyzed separately for its ^{3}H-H$_2$O content. Results are expressed as percentage of control values (control = NCP controlateral to the lesioned side). * represents significant statistical difference ($p \leqslant 0.05$) between NCP of lesioned and unlesioned sides. Data are the mean of groups of eight rats.

of DA release. Further experiments are required to retain this hypothesis; postsynaptic receptors could be as well involved in this feedback mechanism.

As revealed by the present experiments the estimation of the initial accumulation of ^{3}H-DA formed from ^{3}H-tyrosine cannot provide alone information about changes in the transmitter synthesis. Complementary measurements of the *in vivo* rate of the first limiting step must be made. The new methodology developed, consisting in the *in vivo* estimation of ^{3}H-H$_2$O formation after the local injection of L-3,5-^{3}H-tyrosine, is and will be, a precious tool for further investigations on synthesis regulatory processes.

As illustrated by combined ultrastructural and biochemical studies, the gradual extent of degeneration of the nigro-striatal pathway which can be obtained by appropriate chemical lesions made with 6-OH-DA is particularly useful to study long-term compensatory mechanisms. The hyperactivity of remaining DA neurons revealed by the increased synthesis of striatal DA seen after partial degeneration of the nigro-striatal pathway should be taken into account to better understand the pathophysiology and the pharmacological therapeutics of Parkinson's disease. Investigations about the intraneuronal and interneuronal processes involved in the metabolic and eventual morphological changes occurring in remaining intact DA neurons should provide interesting information concerning the plasticity of central neuronal systems.

REFERENCES

A<small>GID</small>, Y., J<small>AVOY</small>, F., G<small>LOWINSKI</small>, J., B<small>OUVET</small>, D., and S<small>OTELO</small>, C. (1973a) Injection of 6-hydroxydopamine in the substantia nigra of the rat: II, Diffusion and specificity. *Brain Res.* **58**, 291–301.

A<small>GID</small>, Y., J<small>AVOY</small>, F., and G<small>LOWINSKI</small>, J. (1973b) Hyperactivity of the remaining dopaminergic neurons after partial destruction in the nigrostriatal dopaminergic system in the rat. *Nature*, **245**, 144, 150–151.

A<small>NDÉN</small>, N.-E., C<small>ARLSSON</small>, A., D<small>AHLSTRÖM</small>, A., F<small>UXE</small>, K., H<small>ILLARP</small>, N. A., and L<small>ARSSON</small>, K. (1964) Demonstration and mapping out of nigro-neostriatal dopamine neurons. *Life Sci.*, **3**, 523–530.

A<small>NDÉN</small>, N.-E., D<small>AHLSTRÖM</small>, A., F<small>UXE</small>, K., and L<small>ARSSON</small>, K. (1966) Functional role of the nigro-neostriatal dopamine neurons. *Acta pharmac. tox.* **24**, 263.

ANDÉN, N.-E., CORRODI, H., FUXE, K., and UNGERSTEDT, U. (1971) Importance of nervous impulse flow for the neuroleptic induced increase in amine turnover in central dopamine neurons. *Eur. J. Pharmac.* **15**, 193–199.

BENNET, T., BURNSTOCK, G., LOBB, J. L. S., and MALMFORS, T. (1970) An ultrastructural and histochemical study of the short term effects of 6-hydroxydopamine on adrenergic nerves in the domestic fowl. *Br. J. Pharmac.* **38**, 802–809.

BERHEIMER, H., and HORNYKIEWICZ, O. (1965) Herabgesetzte Koncentration der Homovanillinsaüre im gehirn von Parkinson Kranken Menschen als Ansdrück der Störung des zentralen Dopamin stoffwechsels. *Klin. Wschr.* **43**, 711–715.

BESSON, M. J., CHERAMY, A., GAUCHY, C., and GLOWINSKI, J. (1973) *In vivo* continuous estimation of ^{3}H-DA release and synthesis in the cat caudate nucleus: effect of α-methyl-*p*-tyrosine and of transection of the nigro-neostriatal pathway. *Arch. Pharm.* **278**, 101–105.

BUSTOS, G., and ROTH, R. H. (1972) Release of monoamines from the striatum and hypothalamus: effect of γ-hydroxybutyrate. *Br. J. Pharmac.* **46**, 101–115.

CARLSSON, A., KEHR, W., LINDQVIST, M., MAGNUSSON, T., and ATACK, C. T., (1972) Regulation of monoamine metabolism in the central nervous system. *Pharmac. Rev.* **24**, 371–384.

CHANG, C. C., CHEN, T. F., and LEE, C. Y. (1973) Studies of the presynaptic effect of β-burgarotoxin on neuromuscular transmission. *J. Pharmacol. Exp. Ther.* **184**, 339–345.

FAULL, R. L. M., and LAVERTY, R. (1969) Changes in dopamine levels in the corpus striatum following lesions in the substantia nigra. *Expl. Neurol.* **23**, 332–340.

FRIGYESI, T. L., IGE, A., IULO, A., and SCHWARTZ, R. (1971) Denigration and sensimotor disability induced by ventral tegmental injection of 6-hydroxydopamine in the cat. *Expl. Neurol* **33**, 78–87.

HEDREEN, J. C., and CHALMERS, J. P. (1972) Neuronal degeneration in the rat brain induced by 6-hydroxydopamine: a histological and biochemical study. *Brain Res.* **47**, 1–36.

HÖKFELT, T. (1968) *In vitro* studies on central and peripheral monoamines neurons at the ultrastructural level. *Z. Zellforsch.* **91**, 1–74.

HÖKFELT, T., and UNGERSTEDT, U. (1969) Electron and fluorescence microscopical studies on the nucleus caudatus putamen of the rat after unilateral lesions of ascending nigro-neostriatal dopamine neurons. *Acta physiol. scand.* **76**, 415.

HORNYKIEWICZ, O. (1972) Dopamine and extrapyramidal motor function and dysfunction. In *Neurotransmitters*, Res. Publ. ARNMD, **50**, 390–415.

JAVOY, F., HAMON, M., and GLOWINSKI, J. (1970) Disposition of newly synthesized amines in cell bodies and terminals of central catecholaminergic neurons: I, Effect of amphetamine and thioproperazine on the metabolism of CA in the caudate nucleus, the substantia nigra and the ventromedial nucleus of the hypothalamus. *Eur. J. Pharmac.* **10**, 178–188.

JAVOY, F., AGID, Y., BOUVET, D., and GLOWINSKI, J. (1972) Feedback control of DA synthesis in the dopaminergic terminals of the rat striatum. *J. Pharmac. Exp. Ther.* **182**, 454–463.

JAVOY, F., AGID, Y., and GLOWINSKI, J. (1974a) *In vivo* estimation of the first step of dopamine synthesis in the rat neostriatum *J. Pharm. Pharmac.* (in press).

JAVOY, F., AGID, Y., and GLOWINSKI, J. (1974b) Early effect of the interruption of the nigro-neostriatal pathway on the metabolism of dopamine in the caudate nucleus of the rat. *Brain Res.* (in press).

KEHR, W., CARLSSON, A., LINDQVIST, M., MAGNUSSON, T., and ATACK, C. (1972) Evidence for a receptor mediated feedback control of striatal tyrosine hydroxylase activity. *J. Pharm. Pharmac.* **24**, 744–747.

MOORE, R. Y., BHATNAGAR, R. K., and HELLER, A. (1971) Anatomical and chemical studies of a nigro-neostriatal projection in the cat. *Brain Res.* **30**, 119–135.

NYBACK, H. (1971) Effect of brain lesions and chlorpromazine on accumulation a disappearance of catecholamines formed *in vivo* from ^{14}C-tyrosine. *Acta physiol. scand.* **84**, 54–64.

POIRIER, L. J., and SOURKES, T. L. (1965) Influence of the substantia nigra on the catecholamine content of the striatum. *Brain Res.* **88**, 181–192.

POIRIER, L. J., SINGH, P., BOUCHER, R., BOUVIER, G., OLIVIER, A., and LAROCHELLE, P. (1967) Effect of brain lesions on the concentration of the striatal dopamine and serotonin in the cat. *Archs. Neurol.* **17**, 601–608.

POIRIER, L. J., LANGELIER, P., ROBERGE, A., BOUCHER, R., and KITSIKIS, A. (1972) Non-specific histopathological changes induced by intracerebral injection of 6-hydroxydopamine (6-OH-DA) *J. Neurol. Sci.* **16**, 401–416.

SHARMAN, D. F., POIRIER, L. J., MURPHY, G. F., and SOURKES, T. L. (1967) Homovanillic acid and dihydroxyphenylacetic acid in the striatum of monkeys with brain lesions. *Can. J. Physiol. Pharmac.* **45**, 57–62.

SOTELO, C. (1971) Two fine structural localization of norepinephrine-^{3}H in the substantia nigra and area postrema of the rat: an autoradiographic study. *J. Ultrastruct. Res.* **36**, 824–841.

SOTELO, C., JAVOY, F., AGID, Y., and GLOWINSKI, J. (1973) Injection of 6-hydroxydopamine in the substantia nigra of the rat: I, Morphological study. *Brain Res.* **58**, 269–290.

STJÄRNE, L. (1973) Alpha-adrenoceptor mediated feedback control of sympathetic neurotransmitter secretion in guinea pig vas deferens. *Nature* **241**, 190–191.

UNGERSTEDT, U. (1968) 6-hydroxydopamine induced degeneration of central monoamine neurons. *Eur. J. Pharmac.* **5**, 107–110.

UNGERSTEDT, U. (1971) Histochemical studies on the effect of intracerebral and intraventricular injections of 6-hydroxydopamine on monoamine neurons in the rat brain. In *6-Hydroxydopamine and Catecholamine Neurons* (T. Malmfors and H. Thoenen, eds.), North-Holland, Amsterdam, pp. 101–127.

UNGERSTEDT, U., and ARBUTHNOTT, G. (1970) Quantitative recording of rotational behavior in rats after 6-hydroxydopamine lesions of the nigro striatal dopamine system. *Brain Res.* **24**, 485–493.

CHANGES IN CATECHOLAMINE SYNTHESIZING ENZYME ACTIVITIES DURING NEURONAL GROWTH AND DEGENERATION

Menek Goldstein, Berta Anagnoste, Lewis S. Freedman, Mark Roffman, and Kusum P. Lele

Department of Psychiatry, Neurochemistry Laboratories and Department of Pharmacology, New York University Medical Center, New York, NY 10016

SUMMARY

Dopamine-β-hydroxylase activity was used as a marker for neuroblastoma tumor growth. The increase in enzyme activity in the tumor and in the serum of mice that bear the tumor is proportional to the increase in size of the tumor. The removal of the tumor causes a marked decline in serum DβH activity.

DβH activity in the cultured adrenergic cell line N-115-G of mouse neuroblastoma and in cultured cell line SK-N-SH of human neuroblastoma culture declines during early stages of growth while the total DβH activity increases. dB-cAMP causes a time-dependent increase in the specific activity of DβH. Changes in the specific DβH activity seem to be linked to changes in the cell morphology.

Pharmacological and immunochemical studies indicate that a single enzyme catalyzes the decarboxylation of L-Dopa and L-5HTP in the striatum.

The administration of 6-hydroxydopa causes a rise of DβH activity in the hypothalamus the first 2 days after treatment, and subsequently the enzyme activity falls below the control values. Two days after administration of 6-hydroxydopa, the enzyme activity in the brain stem decreases and remains below the control values on the eighth day posttreatment.

INTRODUCTION

Dopamine-β-hydroxylase (DβH)† is present in the norepinephrine containing vesicles and could serve as a marker for the localization of the noradrenergic nervous system. Mouse neuroblastoma C-1300 tumor cells synthesize acetylcholine and norepinephrine in culture and the micrographs of the tumor cells show clusters of dense-core vesicles in nerve terminals (Augusti-Tocco and Sato, 1969; Nelson *et al.*, 1969; Schubert *et al.*, 1969). Non-

† *Abbreviations.* DβH: Dopamine-β-hydroxylase (EC 1.14.2.1). AADC: Aromatic L-amino-acid decarboxylase (EC 4.1.1.28). BrdU: 5-Bromodeoxyuridine. Dopa: 3,4-Dihydroxyphenylalanine. 6-OH-DA: 6-Hydroxydopamine. 5-HTP: 5-Hydroxytryptophan. cyclic AMP: Adenosine 3'5'-monophosphate. dB-cAMP: N^6,O^2-Dibutyryl adenosine 3'5'-cyclic monophosphate.

dividing neuroblastoma cells are capable of neuronal differentiation, and it was reported that neural differentiation is associated with increased specific activity of acetylcholinesterase (Blume *et al.*, 1970), choline-*O*-acetyltransferase (Rosenberg *et al.*, 1971), and with an increased formation of acetylcholine receptors (Harris and Dennis, 1970) as well as with an increased development of axon-dendrites (Seeds *et al.*, 1970). The availability of adrenergic neuroblastoma clonal cell lines have made it possible to study the activities of catecholamine synthesizing enzymes. We will report on changes in DβH activities in neuroblastoma tumors and in neuroblastoma cultured cells during various phases of growth.

6-Hydroxydopamine (6-OH-DA) is known to produce a degeneration of the sympathetic nerve terminals (Tranzer and Thoenen, 1967). Several studies have shown that the 6-OH-DA-induced degeneration of the central neurons is associated with a depletion of catecholamine stores and with a reduction of catecholamine synthesizing enzyme activities (Anagnoste *et al.*, 1969; Uretsky and Iversen, 1969). More recently it was reported that

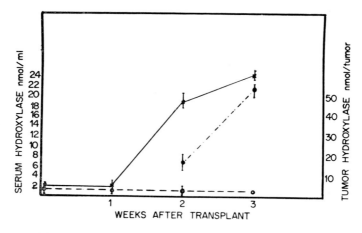

Fig. 1. DβH activity in mouse neuroblastoma and in sensor at different times after implantation. $\times$, activity of enzyme in serum C-1300 mice. $\bigcirc$, activity in serum of A/J mice; $\bullet$, activity in tumor tissue from C-1300 mice.

6-OH-Dopa causes a selective degeneration of central noradrenergic neurons (Ong *et al.*, 1969; Sachs and Jonsson, 1972). We have investigated the effects of 6-OH-Dopa on DβH activities in various regions of the brain. We have also studied the effects of 6-OH-DA-induced nigro-striatal degeneration on the AADC activity in the striatum.

DβH (EC 1.14.2.1) ACTIVITY IN C-1300 NEUROBLASTOMA TUMORS AND SERUM OF MICE

Figure 1 shows that tumors possess substantial DβH activity and that in growing tumors the amount of enzyme is proportional to their weight, the activity per gram of tumor being the same at day 14 as at day 21, although the size increased three to four times. DβH activity in the serum of mice that bear tumors is markedly increased over that of control mice 2 weeks after implantation of the tumor (Fig. 1). There was no difference 1 week after implantation when the tumors first became palpable. The increase in enzyme activity in the serum is proportional to the increase in size of the tumor, continuing from the fourteenth to the twenty-first day after implantation. We have investigated the decline of serum DβH activity following surgical removal of the tumors. The removal of the tumor causes a marked decline in serum DβH activity. The serum DβH activity approaches control values 24–48 h after removal of the tumor. A half-life of 3–4 h was calculated from the decline rate of the enzyme activity. This data demonstrates that the elevated levels of serum DβH are due to the secretion of the enzyme by the neural tumor (Anagnoste *et al.*, 1972).

THE EFFECTS OF 6-OH-DA OR OF BrdU ON TUMOR GROWTH AND ON DβH ACTIVITY

Administration of 6-OH-DA or of BrdU to neuroblastoma-bearing mice results in a noticeable slowing of tumor growth in the first 2 weeks after treatment. Subsequently tumor growth resumed, and concomitantly, the DβH activity increased in the tumor and serum of treated mice (Anagnoste *et al.*, 1970, 1972). The retardation of tumor growth induced by 6-OH-DA is most likely due to degeneration of catecholamine containing neurons in the tumor. Although the mechanism of the effects of BrdU on the growth of neuroblastoma is still obscure, it is conceivable that either the higher production of axon-like processes induced by BrdU (Schubert and Jacob, 1970) or the incorporation of the BrdU into DNA is responsible for its activity.

DβH AND AADC (EC 4.1.1.26) ACTIVITY IN TWO DIFFERENT CLONAL CELL LINES OF MOUSE C-1300 NEUROBLASTOMA TUMORS

The results in Table 1 show that DβH activity is ten times higher in the adrenergic clonal line N-115-G than in the nonadrenergic clonal line N-18-G. It is noteworthy that AADC activity was not detectable either in the N-115-G line or in the N-18-G line. It is conceivable that some inhibitors inactivate AADC activity or that the enzyme is rapidly released from the cells to the medium. Further studies are now in progress to determine the factors which are responsible for the absence of AADC activity in the cultured neuroblastoma cells.

TABLE 1. DβH ACTIVITY IN NEUROBLASTOMA TISSUE CULTURE

Cell line	DβH (nm/h/mg)	AADC
N-18-G	0.54 ± 0.08	ND
N-115-G	5.32 ± 0.15	ND

ND, not detectable.
Cultures assayed in stationary growth phase.
The activity is expressed as nm of *N*-methyl octopamine formed during 1 h of incubation per milligram of protein.
Results are the mean from five experiments ± SEM.

THE EFFECT OF dB-cAMP ON DβH ACTIVITY IN VARIOUS PHASES OF GROWTH

DβH activity in the adrenergic clonal cell line N-115-G was investigated in various phases of growth. The specific activity of DβH declines during the early stages of growth (Table 2) while the total DβH activity increases.

TABLE 2. EFFECT OF dB-cAMP ON DβH ACTIVITY IN
NEUROBLASTOMA CELL CULTURE (N-115-G)

Time (h)	DβH activity (nm/h/mg protein)		
	Control	dB-cAMP	% Control
48	2.06 ± 0.3	2.64 ± 0.4	128
72	1.48 ± 0.3	2.62 ± 0.3	177
96	0.84 ± 0.1	2.02 ± 0.3	240
120	1.04 ± 0.1	1.22 ± 0.1	117

N-115-G cells (5 × 10^5) cultured in 5 ml Dulbecco's modified Eagles medium supplemented with 10% calf serum in plastic T-flasks. dB-cAMP (1.0 mM) was administered in the media 24 h after plating. Cells were harvested after trypsinization (0.05% trypsin) and centrifugation. Cell pellets were washed free of media (3×); sonicated; and aliquots taken for enzyme and protein assay. Results are the mean from three experiments ± SEM.

In a previous study we have shown that cells of the line with a higher specific DβH activity have a greater tendency to produce axon-like processes than those with a line with lower specific activity (Anagnoste et al., 1972). We have therefore investigated the effects of dB-cAMP on the morphological differentiation and on DβH activity in the clonal cell line N-115-G. Gross observation of the living cells shows that dB-cAMP induces differentiation already 24 h after the addition of the nucleotide. The maximal effect was observed 3–4 days after the addition of dB-cAMP. These results are in agreement with the previously reported findings on dB-cAMP-induced differentiation in the nonclonal C-1300 neuroblastoma cells (Prasad and Hsie, 1971).

The histochemical studies of the N-115-G cell line show small nerve cells which exhibit fluorescence of very weak intensity unspecific for catecholamines (Fig. 2a). Forty-eight hours after addition of dB-cAMP the cells are much larger and the intensity of the specific fluorescence is much stronger (Fig. 2b) with a perinuclear location. Also some small catecholamine containing processes were observed. The maximal effects were observed 3–4 days after the addition of the cyclic nucleotide (Goldstein and Fuxe, unpublished data).

The results in Table 2 also show that dB-cAMP causes a time-dependent increase in the specific activity of DβH. The addition of dB-cAMP 1 day after replating the cells results in a significant increase in specific DβH activity 1–3 days later. Thus changes in the specific activity of DβH seem to be linked to changes in the cell morphology.

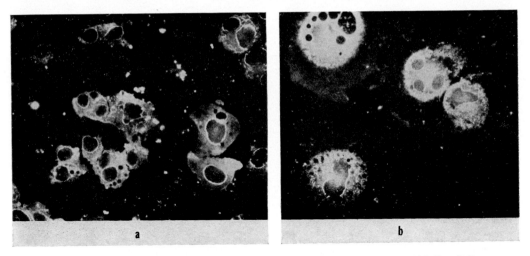

Fig. 2. Histochemical localization of catecholamine containing cells in N-115-G cell line.
(a) Cells without addition of dB-cAMP; (b) 72 h after addition of dB-cAMP.

DβH ACTIVITY IN CULTURED CELLS OF HUMAN NEUROBLASTOMA†
(Freedman *et al.*, 1973)

A cultured cell line SK-N-SH has been established *in vitro* and was maintained in culture for about 2 years. The gross observation of the living cells shows two types of cells; one type of cell (80%) of the total) consists of round neuroblastoma-like cells which tend to form dense clusters, and the second type consists of epithelioid cells. Figure 3 shows a parallel rise in the numbers of neuroblastoma cells and in the total protein content during the period of rapid growth. The specific activity of DβH declines during the early stages of growth and rises markedly during the stationary phase of growth. Thus, DβH, like other functional proteins, is synthesized at a low rate at a time period when structural proteins are preferentially synthesized, and at a high rate when functional proteins are preferentially synthesized.

THE EFFECTS OF INTRANIGRAL-STRIATAL ADMINISTRATION OF 6-OH-DA ON AADC ACTIVITY IN THE STRIATUM OF RATS‡

The question whether a single enzyme catalyzes the decarboxylation of L-Dopa and L-5-HTP in specific areas of the CNS is still unresolved (Christenson *et al.*, 1972; Sims *et al.*, 1973; Goldstein *et al.*, 1972). In order to investigate further this problem we have tested AADC activity in the striatum of rats with 6-OH-DA-induced lesions. Intranigro-striatal administration of 6-OH-DA causes a degeneration of the striatal dopamine terminals but does not affect the serotoninergic terminals. We have tested AADC activity on the lesion side and on the intact side of the striatum using both L-Dopa and L-5HTP as substrates.

---

† This study was carried out in collaboration with Dr. Helson and Dr. J. L. Biedler from Sloan Kettering Institute for Cancer Research, New York City.
‡ This study was carried out in collaboration with Dr. Urban Ungerstedt from Karolinska Institutet, Stockholm, Sweden.

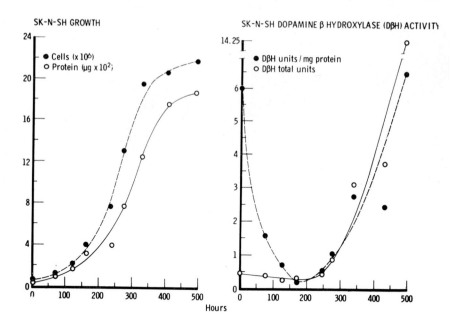

FIG. 3. DβH activity in cultured cells of human neuroblastoma during various phases of growth.

The results in Table 3 show that AADC activity is reduced on the lesion side of the striatum as compared with the corresponding intact side. The reduction in AADC activity is approximately the same when L-Dopa or L-5-HTP were used as substrates for the enzyme. These results suggest that a single enzyme catalyzes the decarboxylation of L-Dopa and L-5-HTP in the striatum.

TABLE 3. THE EFFECT OF INTRACEREBRAL INJECTION OF 6-OH-DA
ON AADC ACTIVITY IN THE STRIATUM OF RATS

Substrate	AADC Activity (cmp/g/tissue/10^3)		% Change
	Intact side	Lesion side	
DL-Dopa-1-C^{14}	280.0 ± 12.5	163.7 ± 3.1	41.5
DL-5-HTP-1-C^{14}	63.7 ± 3.1	32.0 ± 1.9	49.8

Results are the mean from four experiments $\pm$ SEM.

IMMUNOCHEMICAL STUDIES

We have also investigated the effects of a specific AADC antiserum on AADC activity using L-Dopa or L-5-HTP as substrates. The results in Table 4 show that AADC antiserum inhibits proportionately L-Dopa and L-HTP activity in various regions of the brain. Thus the Dopa decarboxylase and 5-HTP decarboxylase activities are indistinguishable immunochemically. It is noteworthy that the immunohistochemical studies corroborate

TABLE 4. SIMULTANEOUS IMMUNOLOGICAL TITRATION OF DOPA AND
5-HTP DECARBOXYLASE ACTIVITIES IN VARIOUS REGIONS OF THE
RAT BRAIN

Brain region	Antiserum (μl)	% Inhibition	
		Dopa	5-HTP
Striatum	10	40	35
	20	70	60
	40	90	90
Hypothalamus	10	30	25
	20	60	60
	40	90	90
Brain stem	10	40	40
	20	75	70
	40	95	90
Cerebellum	10	35	35
	20	60	55
	40	90	90

these findings (Hökfelt *et al.*, 1973). Although these results indicate that in various regions of the CNS a single enzyme catalyzes the decarboxylation of L-Dopa and L-5-HTP, it could be argued that a second enzyme exists which crossreacts with the antiserum. Thus our results cannot exclude the possibility that in some regions of the brain a specific L-5-HTP decarboxylase or an L-Dopa decarboxylase exists (Sims *et al.*, 1973).

THE EFFECT OF 6-HYDROXY-DOPA ON CENTRAL DβH ACTIVITY

Mice received a single injection of 6-OH-Dopa, 150 mg/kg i.v. and were sacrificed at various time intervals post-injection. The effect of 6-OH-Dopa on DβH activity was studied in two regions of the brain; hypothalamus, a region enriched in norepinephrine nerve terminals, and in the brain stem, a region enriched in norepinephrine cell bodies (Fig. 4). One day after the administration of 6-OH-Dopa the DβH activity in the hypothalamus rises significantly and remains elevated the second day after the administration of the drug. The third day the DβH activity falls below the control values and remains decreased on the eighth day after the administration of the drug. The administration of 6-OH-Dopa has no effect on the DβH activity in the brain stem on the first day after treatment, but falls on the second day and remains below the control values on the eighth day post-treatment.

Following 6-OH-Dopa-induced axonal degeneration, the nerve impulse dependent enzyme release from the nerve terminals might be impaired. The impairment in the enzyme release could be responsible for the initial rise in the DβH activity in the hypothalamus. The observed slight decrease in the DβH activity in the brain stem might be due to a 6-OH-Dopa-induced degeneration of nerve terminals within this region of the brain. Immunohistochemical studies are now in progress to determine the mechanisms involved in the 6-OH-Dopa-induced alterations in DβH activities in various regions of the CNS.

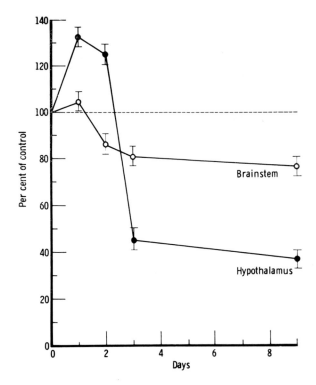

FIG. 4. The effect of 6-OH-Dopa administration on DβH activity in the hypothalamus and brain stem of mice.

ACKNOWLEDGEMENTS

The authors wish to thank Dr. Marshall W. Nirenberg from National Institutes of Health, Bethesda, Maryland, for providing us with the clonal cell line N-115-G.

This work was supported by USPHS Grant NS-06801 and NSF Grant GB 27603.

REFERENCES

ANAGNOSTE, B., BACKSTROM, T., and GOLDSTEIN, M. (1969) *Pharmacologist* **11**, 254.

ANAGNOSTE, B., GOLDSTEIN, M., and BROOME, J. (1970) *Pharmacologist* **12**, 269.

ANAGNOSTE, B., FREEDMAN, L. S., GOLDSTEIN, M., BROOME, J., and FUXE, K. (1972) *Proc. Natn. Acad. Sci. USA* **69**, 1883–1886.

AUGUSTI-TOCCO, B., and SATO, G. (1969) *Proc. Natn. Acad. Sci. USA* **64**, 311–316.

BLUME, A., GILBERT, F., WILSON, S., FARBER, J., ROSENBERG, R., and NIRENBERG, M. (1970) *Proc. Natn. Acad. Sci. USA* **67**, 786–791.

CHRISTENSON, J. G., DAIRMAN, W., and UDENFRIEND, S. (1972) *Proc. Natn. Acad. Sci. USA* **69**, (2) 343–347.

FREEDMAN, L. S., ROFFMAN, M., LELE, K. P., GOLDSTEIN, M., BIEDLER, J. L., SPENGLER, B. A., and HELSON, L. (1973) *Fed. Proc.* **32**, 708.

GOLDSTEIN, M., ANAGNOSTE, B., BATTISTA, A. F., NAKATANI, S., and OGAWA, M. (1972) *Neurotransmitters,* Res. Publ. ARNMD, **50**, 434–447.

HARRIS, A. J., and DENNIS, M. J. (1970) *Science* **167**, 1253–1255.

HÖKFELT, T., FUXE, K., and GOLDSTEIN, M. (1973) *Brain Res.* **53**, 175–180.

NELSON, P., RUFFNER, W., and NIRENBERG, M. (1969) *Proc. Natn. Acad. Sci. USA* **64**, 1004–1010.

ONG, H. H., CREVELING, C. R., and DALY, J. (1969) *J. Med. Chem.* **12**, 458–463.

PRASAD, K. N., and HSIE, A. W. (1971) *Nature New Biol.* **233**, 141–142.

ROSENBERG, R. N., VANDEVENTER, L., DE FRANCESCO, L., and FRIEDKIN, M. E. (1971) *Proc. Natn. Acad. Sci. USA* **68**, 1436–1440.

SACHS, C., and JONSSON, G. (1972) *J. Neurochem.* **19**, 1561–1575.

SCHUBERT, D., and JACOB, F. (1970) *Proc. Natn. Acad. Sci. USA* **67**, 247–254.

SCHUBERT, D., HUMPHREYS, S., BARONI, C., and COHN, M. (1969) *Proc. Natn. Acad. Sci. USA* **64**, 31–36.

SEEDS, N. W., GILMAN, A. G., AMANO, T., and NIRENBERG, M. (1970) *Proc. Natn. Acad. Sci. USA* **66**, 160–165.

SIMS, K. L., DAVIS, G. A., and BLOOM, F. E. (1973) *J. Neurochem.* **20**, 449–464.

TRANZER, J. P., and THOENEN, H. (1967) *Naunyn-Schmiedeberg's Arch. exp. Path. Pharmak.* **257**, 343–346.

URETSKY, N. J., and IVERSEN, L. L. (1969) *Nature, Lond.* **221**, 557–558.

SOME ASPECTS OF THE REACTION OF CENTRAL AND PERIPHERAL NORADRENERGIC NEURONS TO INJURY

Donald J. Reis, Robert A. Ross, and Tong H. Joh

Laboratory of Neurobiology, Department of Neurology, Cornell University Medical College, New York, NY

SUMMARY

Noradrenergic neurons of the central and peripheral nervous systems respond to axonal injury in qualitatively comparable ways. The *anterograde reaction* in the severed axons consists of a loss of the neurotransmitter norepinephrine (NE) and associated biosynthetic enzyme including tyrosine hydroxylase (TH), dopa-decarboxylase (DDC), and dopamine-β-hydroxylase (DBH). This results in a loss of the capacity of the terminals to synthesize, store, release, or inactivate by reuptake NE. In CNS the fall-off of NE and enzymes is retarded possibly as a consequence of survival of vesicular contents in glia.

The *retrograde reaction*, in neurons which recover, consists initially of an increase in NE content and a variable increase of TH and DBH activities over 1–2 days. This is followed by a second stage characterized by a rapid fall in the quantities of enzyme protein and a more gradual drop in NE. This stage persists for weeks and parallels the development of regenerative sprouts from the injured axons in brain and periphery. In peripheral ganglia the morphological characteristics of chromatolysis appear along with evidence of enhanced lysosomal activity, a possible mechanism for regulating intraneuronal quantities of the enzyme and transmitter. In brain NE neurons show biochemical changes and sprouting without evident chromatolysis. The biochemical events in the reactive cell body in central neurons are reflected in uninjured (sustaining) collaterals. After weeks the neurons may return to normal.

These findings lead to three general conclusions. Firstly, the reversible retrograde reaction of central noradrenergic neurons shares the biochemical and regenerative but not the morphological (chromatolytic) events with peripheral ganglion cells. This suggests, contrary to the widely held view, that intrinsic neurons of CNS may undergo the reversible biochemical events of the retrograde reaction, and these are intimately related to sprouting. Secondly that during the retrograde reaction the cell reorders priorities for protein biosynthesis favoring the production of proteins required for reconstitution of the cell surface at the expense of those required for function of the neuron as an excitable cell. Finally, the biochemical events triggered in a nerve cell by injury of axons in one area of brain may be signaled to other remote areas through sustaining collaterals. The significance of this remote transfer of neuronal activity might relate to the processes of transfer of functional activity from one brain area to another after injury leading thereby to physiological compensation.

I. INTRODUCTION

The nature of the response of neurons to axonal injury has long been a subject of intense interest to neurobiologists. Over the years, increasing knowledge of the morphological, biochemical, and functional consequences of neuronal damage has multiplied (Lieberman, 1971), but many fundamental problems still remain. These include the relationship of the reaction of the cell body (variously termed the retrograde response, the retrograde reaction or, when referring to the morphological concomitant, chromatolysis) to the process of regenerative sprouting, the role of sustaining collaterals in governing retrograde changes, the precise nature of the changes in protein biosynthesis and enzyme activities in the peri-karyon and their relationship to the functions of the reactive neuron as an excitable cell, and the nature of the signal to chromatolysis. One other problem of interest is whether intrinsic neurons of the CNS (i.e. neurons whose axons only make contact with other centrally situated neurons), demonstrate a retrograde response in the same manner as do axons whose cell bodies either lie outside of the CNS or whose axons project peripherally (e.g. hypoglossal neurons).

Over the past few years some new insights into the processes underlying the neural response to injury have come from analysis of the reactive processes in noradrenergic neurons. This group of specific neurons which synthesize, store, and release the neuro-transmitter norepinephrine (NE) has certain distinct advantages for studying the events elicited by axonal damage in both peripheral and central nervous systems. Firstly, the cell bodies of these systems are specifically located in peripheral ganglia and within identifiable nuclei within the brain (e.g. nucleus locus coeruleus [Ungerstedt, 1971]), lending themselves to morphological analysis at both the light and electron microscopic level. Secondly, the neurotransmitter produced by these cells is defined and easily measured. Thirdly, the enzymes involved in the biosynthesis of the transmitter are known, and their activities can be assayed in reasonably small quantities of tissue. More recently the availability of specific antibodies to most of these enzymes has permitted estimation of the amounts of specific enzyme protein. Fourthly, the cell body and processes of noradrenergic neurons can be visualized by specific histofluorescence (Dahlström and Fuxe, 1964) and more recently immuno-fluorescence techniques (Fuxe et al., 1971). Fifthly, these neurons have been shown to sprout within the central (Katzman et al., 1971) as in the peripheral (Matthews and Raisman, 1972) nervous system and hence can permit an analysis of the general problem of the rela-tionship of the retrograde reaction to regenerative sprouting.

Finally, the function of these neurons in the peripheral and, to an increasing extent, the central nervous systems, can be evaluated. Hence it is possible to relate the events of de-generation and regeneration to functional changes within the fields of innervation of these neurons.

In this paper we shall review in a selective fashion present knowledge of biochemical and morphological responses of peripheral and central noradrenergic neurons to injury. New information derived from analysis of this specific neuronal system, we believe, has shed new light onto some of the processes by which neurons, particularly in the CNS, respond to injury.

II. ANTEROGRADE AND RETROGRADE RESPONSES IN PERIPHERAL SYMPATHETIC NEURONS

A. ANTEROGRADE CHANGES

In peripheral postganglionic sympathetic neurons the severed axon rapidly degenerates losing its capacity, over days, to synthesize, store, release, or inactivate by specific re-uptake, the neurotransmitter NE (Potter et al., 1965; Malmfors and Sachs, 1965; Pilar and

Landmesser, 1972). Biochemically, the anterograde reaction is reflected, over 48 h, by a fall in the concentrations of NE in the terminals (Andén *et al.*, 1965). The activities of the enzymes required for the synthesis of the catecholamines, including tyrosine hydroxylase (TH), dopa-decarboxylase (DDC), and dopamine-β-hydroxylase (DBH), are reduced in parallel (Andén *et al.*, 1965; Sedvall and Kopin, 1967; Kopin and Silberstein, 1972).

Morphologically, the anterograde response is characterized by a gradual loss of specific histofluorescence for catecholamines, swelling of nerve endings, loss of vesicles, and incorporation of the cellular debris into Schwann cells (Hökfelt *et al.*, 1972). Degeneration of the terminal may be viewed as a consequence of the separation of the axon from the neuronal cell body which synthesizes the enzymes and organelles essential for transmitter biosynthesis which are then transported by axoplasmic flow into the terminals. It is in the axon terminals where the bulk of the neurotransmitter is synthesized and released (Geffen and Livett, 1971).

The peripheral sympathetic neuron has a considerable capacity for regeneration. Soon after a lesion, regenerating axons sprout from the ganglia and preterminal axons, grow, and ultimately establish normal physiological activities in target organs (Matthews and Raisman, 1972). Thus degeneration can be considered as prelude to regeneration.

B. RETROGRADE CHANGES

The retrograde response in the cell body of postganglionic noradrenergic neurons to axonal disruption is less well characterized. Within the first 48 h after injury inflicted by ligation or transection of postganglionic fibers, there is an increase in the amount of NE in the proximal axon and cell body (Jacobowitz and Woodward, 1968). This phase of augmentation, sometimes referred to as a "piling-up", is associated ultrastructurally with an increase of granular vesicles having a dense core in the axon and cell bodies (Kapeller and Mayor, 1969). This raises the possibility that soon after a lesion there is a brief flurry of increased biosynthesis of these organelles, enzymes, and possibly neurotransmitter itself. Following this brief and variable period of augmentation, a series of biochemical, histochemical, and morphological changes occur within the ganglion. It is this stage that coincides with the classically defined period of chromatolysis. It usually persists for several weeks.

Biochemically and histochemically, the "chromatolytic state" is characterized by a progressive decrease in the activities of several of the enzymes involved in transmitter biosynthesis, specifically TH and DBH (Kopin and Silberstein, 1972). While the concentrations of NE may remain elevated initially, it gradually declines, reflected in part by a reduction of the amounts transported distally by axoplasmic flow (Boyle and Gillespie, 1970). At this stage the activities of the enzymes and their capacities for induction by prolonged nerve impulse activity are reduced (Brimijoin and Molinoff, 1971). In addition the activities of monoamine oxidase (MAO) and cholinesterase, enzymes of importance in the metabolic inactivation of transmitters, fall (Härkönen, 1964; Huikuri, 1966).

The reduction of the activities of enzymes subserving transmitter and receptive functions, however, does not appear to be shared by other enzymes in the cell. During the chromatolytic phase there is a marked increase in the activity of acid phosphatase as determined histochemically (Huikuri, 1966), indicating activation of lysosomal systems in the cell. There is also a histochemically demonstrable increase in the activity of several oxidative enzymes suggesting an increased level of function of the metabolic systems required for energy production (Härkönen, 1964; Huikuri, 1966). In addition there is biochemical evidence of increased quantities of RNA in sympathetic ganglia (Causey and Strattman, 1956). Thus, as will be discussed below, it appears that during the retrograde reaction the sympathetic ganglia is reordering its priorities for protein biosynthesis to favor the production of those which are required for restitution of cell membranes at the expense of those subserving transmitter or receptor functions (Brattgård et al., 1957; Griffith and La Velle, 1971).

Morphologically, at the light microscopy level, the sympathetic ganglion undergoes the classical changes of chromatolysis including cell swelling, displacement, and indentation of the nucleus, and dispersion of the Nissl substance (Dixon, 1970; Matthews and Raisman, 1972). There is also central aggregation of dense bodies. Ultrastructurally, there is an interesting sequence of changes that has recently been detailed by Matthews and Raisman (1972). Three features may be noted. Firstly, from 3 to 14 days following postganglionic section there is a significant increase in the number of autophagic vacuoles and cytoplasmic dense bodies. This suggests an increase in lysosomal activity and correlates with the histo-chemical demonstration of increased acid phosphatase activity. Secondly, there is a decrease in the number of large and small dense core vesicles. This observation would correlate with the biochemically demonstrable decrease of NE and the vesicular enzyme DBH. Finally, there is evidence of sprouting from the soma and axons of these cell bodies, suggesting that at the time of involutional changes there is concomitantly a regenerative process going on within the cell. After many weeks the ganglion cells, if they survive, may regain a normal or near-normal appearance.

Thus the retrograde reaction in sympathetic ganglia may be viewed as a reversible sequence of changes probably correlating with the process of regeneration. During this phase there is evidence biochemically and morphologically that the neuron is functioning less as a unit specialized for neurotransmission and more as a cell working to establish contact with end organs. The physiological data would support this view since during chromatolysis in sympathetic and other neurons there is evidence of subsensitivity in the receptor and a reduction of activity within the neuron (Brown and Pascoe, 1954; Acheson and Remolina, 1955; Eccles et al., 1958; Kuno and Llinas, 1970).

III. ANTEROGRADE AND RETROGRADE RESPONSES TO AXONAL INJURY IN CENTRAL NORADRENERGIC NEURONS

A. NORADRENERGIC SYSTEMS IN THE BRAIN

1. *General Distribution*

The neuronal systems in the brain which synthesize, store, and release the neurotransmitter NE have been extensively mapped by histofluorescence techniques using the Falck–Hillarp method. The most recent and extensive contribution has been that of Ungerstedt (1971) who has clarified the trajectories of some of the noradrenergic pathways.

On the basis of lesions studies, Ungerstedt (1971) has defined two principal noredrenergic ascending systems in the lower brainstem: a ventral and dorsal NE pathway. The *ventral* ascending pathway arises from cell groups designated as A1, A2, A5, A7 (according to Dahlström and Fuxe, 1964) in the medulla oblongata and pons. In contrast the so-called dorsal noradrenergic pathway arises almost *in toto* from the nucleus of the locus coeruleus (A6), at least in rat.

2. *The Nucleus Locus Coeruleus*

The locus coeruleus of the rat is a brainstem nucleus comprising some 1400 medium-size nerve cells, mostly packed on each side of the IVth ventricle (Descarries and Saucier, 1972). What is unusual about this nucleus is that the majority of the perikarya synthesize NE in contrast to the traditionally defined nuclei (e.g. lateral reticular nucleus) in which the noradrenergic neurons are interspersed with nonadrenergic neurons (Dahlström and Fuxe, 1964). The histochemical studies of Ungerstedt (1971) and Olson and Fuxe (1971) have suggested that locus neurons send fibers in a *descending pathway* to the lower brainstem, through a *lateral pathway* that enters the cerebellum and gives rise to the noradrenergic terminals there and, finally, through an *ascending pathway*, the dorsal bundle, which innervates limbic and neocortex. The ascending pathway, which is partly crossed (Loizou, 1969), also gives off branches to the geniculate bodies and the thalamic nuclei as well as the hypothalamus, amygdala, and some basal-cortical regions. There is indirect evidence that a single neuron of the locus coeruleus may send collateral branches widely ramified into cerebellum and cerebrum (Olson and Fuxe, 1971; Hoffer *et al.*, 1973). Thus one nerve cell of the locus coeruleus can influence very wide-ranging areas of the brain.

B. ANTEROGRADE CHANGES IN CENTRAL NORADRENERGIC NEURONS

In the CNS, transection of ascending axons of noradrenergic neurons, produced either by lesions of the lateral hypothalamus or of cells of origin in the locus coeruleus, results in a gradual decline in the concentration of neurotransmitter as well as of the synthetic enzymes TH, DDC, and DBH in the fields of innervation (Heller and Moore, 1968; Reis and Molinoff, 1972; Ross *et al.*, 1973) (Fig. 1). The major differences between the anterograde

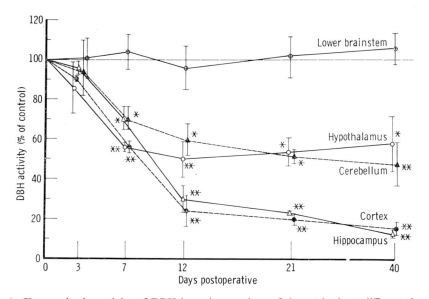

FIG. 1. Changes in the activity of DBH in various regions of the rat brain at different days following a unilateral electrolytic lesion of the locus coeruleus. Each point represents mean ± SEM of 8–12 animals expressed as percent of activity in unoperated controls. *$p < 0.01$; **$p < 0.001$. (From Ross *et al.*, 1973.)

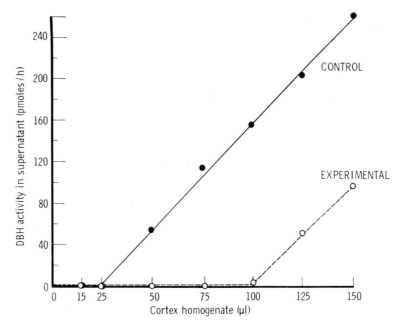

Fig. 2. Immunoprecipitation by a specific antibody to DBH of enzyme protein in homogenates of cerebral cortex from lesioned and control animals. In this experiment increasing amounts of a homogenate of frontal cortex (enzyme) ipsilateral to a 40-day-old hypothalamic lesion or from control animals were added to a constant amount of a specific antibody to DBH. The amount of enzyme in the lowest dilution of cortex is precipitated by available antibody and hence no enzyme activity is detectable in the supernatant. As more tissue homogenate is added the antibody is saturated and enzyme activity appears in the supernatant. The point at which enzyme activity first appears in the supernatant is called the equivalence point (Feigelson and Greengard, 1962) and represents the amount of enzyme (in microliters of homogenate) required to saturate the antibody. In this experiment it may be seen that the equivalence point for enzyme in the lesioned (experimental) cortex is shifted to the right of control. Four times as much tissue from the lesioned cortex is required to reach the equivalence point. Each curve was derived from pooled frontal cortex from 6 to 8 rats. Enzyme activity in samples measured individually from the lesioned animals was approximately 25 % of control. Thus the reduction of enzyme activity in the cerebral cortex as a consequence of hypothalamic lesions is entirely attributable to a loss of specific enzyme protein and not to any increase in enzyme inhibitors.

responses of central and peripheral noradrenergic neurons is that the rate at which the contents of severed axons disappear centrally is considerably prolonged, taking 2 weeks to reach a nadir (Fig. 1). This contrasts with the rapid rate of decline of these compounds in the peripheral nervous system where the fall of transmitter and enzymes occurs over only 1 or 2 days (Malmfors and Sachs, 1965; Kopin and Silberstein, 1972). The fall of enzyme activity during the anterograde response is due to loss of specific enzyme protein in the innervated brain region and not to inhibition of enzyme activity as can be seen in the immunoprecipitation experiment depicted in Fig. 2.

At one time it was proposed that the slow decline of transmitter in the cerebral cortex was a transsynaptic event and a consequence of the denervation of unidentified nor-adrenergic neurons lying rostral to the lesion. This concept has been abandoned, for the most part, for several reasons. Firstly, no noradrenergic neurons have been localized above the midbrain (Ungerstedt, 1971). Secondly, if the cell bodies of noradrenergic neurons within the locus coeruleus are directly lesioned, the rate of the decline of DBH is the same in all fields of innervation (Fig. 1). Conceivably the slow rate of decline reflects the incorporation of vesicles and their contents into reactive glial cells within the brain, the vesicles remaining viable over more days than they would in the periphery. In support is the observation that during degeneration dense core vesicles can be seen relatively intact in the glia from 7 to 14 days after lesions of the lateral hypothalamus (Field *et al.*, 1973) (Fig. 3). However, the fact remains that following unilateral hypothalamic lesions the concentration of neurotransmitter and the activities of the enzyme distal to the lesion never entirely disappear. Whether this reflects bilateral innervation or the presence of small noradrenergic interneurons, remains to be determined.

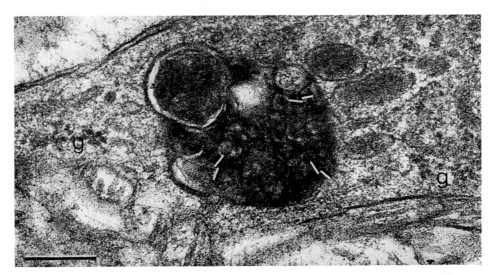

FIG. 3. Sequestration of degenerating axon terminal and dense core vesicles (arrows) within an astrocyte (note glycogen, g) in the bed nucleus of the stria terminalis 7 days following ipsilateral lesion of the posterolateral hypothalamus. Scale bar $= 0.5 \mu$. (Field *et al.*, 1973.)

C. THE RETROGRADE REACTION IN CENTRAL NORADRENERGIC NEURONS

1. *Morphological Changes*

There is little detailed information about the retrograde reaction of central noradrenergic neurons to injury. The available studies are based on changes in fluorescence histochemistry. These have demonstrated that within a day or two following axon injury there is an increased accumulation of NE in cell bodies of noradrenergic neurons (Dahlström and Fuxe, 1965; Andén *et al.*, 1966; Olson and Fuxe, 1971). The augmented fluorescence may persist for many days following the lesion. The classical chromatolytic response has been claimed to parallel this increase in fluorescence in cells of the locus coeruleus after lesions of ascending pathways (Andén *et al.*, 1966) or cerebellectomy (Olson and Fuxe, 1971). In the afore-mentioned studies massive lesions have been produced in very young animals, perhaps thereby producing an intense response. Ultimate recovery was not determined. At the present time Dr. Pauline Field in our laboratory has been unable to find any evidence at the light or electron microscopic level of chromatolytic changes in neurons in the locus coeruleus of adult animals following large lesions of the median forebrain bundle even though the neurons undergo the biochemical changes associated with a retrograde reaction (Reis and Ross, 1973). The falling out of locus neurons as a consequence of cell death induced by 6-hydroxydopamine has been described by Descarriers and Saucier (1972).

2. Biochemical Changes in the Retrograde Reaction

(a) *Norepinephrine*. The concentration of NE in the whole lower brainstem has not been observed to change during the retrograde reaction (Heller and Moore, 1968). The relative insensitivity of methods for measuring NE in the past have not provided data on the possible changes of the concentrations of the transmitter within discreet areas containing reactive cell bodies.

(b) *Brain DBH in the retrograde reaction*. Biochemically, perhaps, the most intensive study to address itself to the changes of central noradrenergic neurons during the retrograde reaction has been the study by Reis and Ross (1973) on the changes of DBH which occur following a lesion of the medial forebrain bundle. This enzyme, which catalyzes the conversion of dopamine to NE, is a unique marker of noradrenergic neurons. It also has other advantages as a biochemical marker for studying the retrograde reaction. Not only is it contained in biochemically specific and anatomically distinctive neurons, but it also is a specific protein produced by a specific group of cells, a protein whose function is known and which produces a product with known physiological activity, and a marker of the NE-storage vesicle wherein it is stored, partly in soluble form, and released along with the transmitter during nerve impulse activity (Axelrod, 1972). Hence it can be viewed as a specific protein produced for export by a specific species of neuron.

In our study we interrupted the axons of noradrenergic neurons by an electrolytic lesion unilaterally placed in the posterolateral hypothalamus, thereby interrupting the medial forebrain bundle (Fig. 4). By assaying enzyme activity in the ipsilateral cerebral cortex anterograde changes could be evaluated; by assaying enzyme activity in the lower brainstem or region of the locus coeruleus reactive changes in the retrograde response could be followed; by sampling of enzyme activity in the ipsilateral cerebellar hemisphere changes of enzyme activity in sustaining collaterals could be determined. Lesions placed anteriorly (Fig. 4, A) rather than posteriorly (Fig. 4, P) permitted assessment of the effects of the proximity of the lesion to the cell body.

Such a lesion resulted in a characteristic change of the activity of the enzyme in the brainstem and also within the locus coeruleus. Following the lesion there was a characteristic triphasic response in the brainstem in the activity of DBH (Fig. 5). Within the first 48 h, enzyme activity rose to 135% of control. Following this initial rise activity fell so that by day 7–14 enzyme activity remained at about 50% of control. Finally, the enzyme activity returned to normal by day 21 where it remained at normal levels through at least day 45. In the contralateral brainstem the response was similar in form but diminished in magnitude.

There are several reasons leading us to conclude that the complex changes in DBH activity in the brainstem and the locus coeruleus represented a retrograde reaction in the cell bodies of central noradrenergic neurons and not a transsynaptic effect due to interruption of fibers descending to synapse on noradrenergic cell bodies in the brainstem. This conclusion was based, in large measure, on comparisons with the behavior of peripheral sympathetic neurons and cholinergic motor neurons following axotomy and on the morphological changes in central neurons with identified transmitters. The arguments may be summarized as follows.

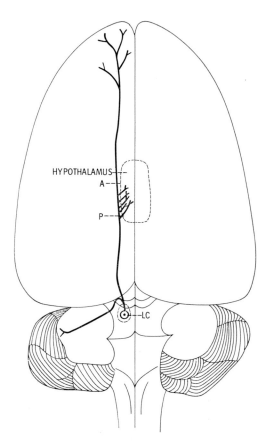

FIG. 4. Schematic horizontal view of rat brain portraying a representative neuron in the locus coeruleus (LC), its ascending projections through frontal cortex, and collateral branches the hypothalamus and cerebellum. Lesions placed in the medial forebrain bundle posteriorly in the lateral hypothalamus (P) will interrupt the axon before most hypothalamic collaterals leave the parent axon. A lesion placed anteriorly (A) will lie distal to emergence of collaterals. (From Reis and Ross, 1973.)

Firstly, the initial increase in DBH activity 48 h following a hypothalamic lesion parallels in direction and timing the increased fluorescence ("piling up") seen in cell bodies of central noradrenergic neurons following axotomy (Dahlström and Fuxe, 1964). It is also similar to the increased concentrations of DBH and TH in peripheral sympathetic neurons after interference with axonal transport (Kopin and Silberstein, 1972). In contrast, this initial increase in DBH does not occur after preganglionic denervation in sympathetic ganglia (Brimijoin and Molinoff, 1971).

Secondly, a decrease in the activity of DBH after a latency of several days parallels the observations of others made in peripheral sympathetic ganglia (Brimijoin and Molinoff, 1971; Kopin and Silberstein, 1972) following lesions of the axon terminals. It also mirrors the time course for the onset of retrograde changes in morphology and in protein synthesis of neurons following axotomy (Brattgård et al., 1957, 1958; Watson, 1965).

A third feature of the brainstem response is its reversibility. Reversible changes in the biosynthesis of NE in sympathetic ganglia, as estimated by accumulation behind a ligature,

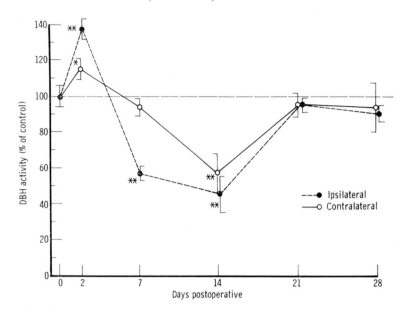

FIG. 5. Time course of changes in DBH activity in brainstem of rat following a unilateral lesion of the posterolateral hypothalamus. Enzyme activity is expressed as a percent of activity of mean activity in at least six matched unoperated controls. Each point represents mean ± SEM of 16–24 animals except for day 28 in which the n is 6. Ipsilateral brainstem is represented by solid circles (● – – – ●), contralateral brainstem by open circles (○——○). *$p < 0.05$; **$p < 0.001$. (From Reis and Ross, 1973.)

has been observed by Boyle and Gillespie (1970) after nerve injury. In cholinergic motor neurons a similar reversible decrease in the activity of the enzymes cholinacetyltransferase (Hebb and Waites, 1956) in sciatic nerve and cholinesterase (Swarzacher, 1958) in hypoglossal neurons, has been noted during the period of retrograde cell reaction induced by ligation or transection of the appropriate motor nerves.

On the other hand, the transsynaptic decrease in enzyme activity in peripheral sympathetic ganglia, caused by destruction of preganglionic neurons, is irreversible in the absence of reinnervation. Likewise, in the CNS transsynaptic degeneration is permanent.

Like all other types of retrograde neuronal changes induced by axonal transection, the effects of DBH activity in brainstem depend upon the proximity of the lesion to the noradrenergic cell bodies. This in turn may reflect the number of collateral sprouts from the parent axon which are spared by the lesion, i.e. sustained collaterals (Fry and Cowan, 1972). Thus interruption of ascending noradrenergic axons by lesions of the anterolateral hypothalamus (Fig. 4, A) do not alter brainstem DBH levels, as do posteriorly placed lesions interrupting the same axons (Fig. 4, P). A likely explanation for the efficacy of posterior lesions in influencing brainstem DBH activity is that many axon collaterals peel off from the ascending axon or brainstem norepinephrine neurons at the level of the hypothalamus (Ungerstedt, 1971). Posterior lesions will therefore interrupt the axons proximal while anterior lesions will interrupt axons distal to the collateral branchings. The preservation of sustaining collaterals therefore appears sufficient to preserve most brainstem neurons from retrograde changes in DBH activity.

The fifth argument against interpreting the observed fall in brainstem DBH as being the result of transsynaptic rather than retrograde changes is the fact that there is, as yet, no compelling anatomical evidence of fibers originating in or passing through the lateral hypothalamus which project into the lower brainstem particularly into the locus coeruleus (Millhouse, 1969).

Finally, there is a parallel decrease in DBH activity in collateral fibers of neurons of locus coeruleus in the cerebellum (see below).

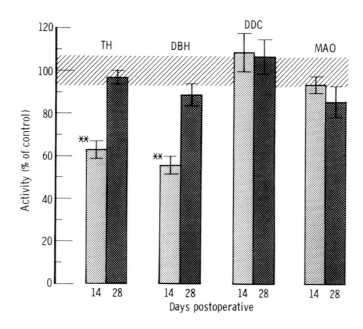

FIG. 6. Changes in the activities of tyrosine hydroxylase (TH), dopamine-β-hydroxylase (DBH), dopa decarboxylase (DDC), and monoamine oxidase (MAO) in the region of the ipsilateral locus coeruleus at 14 (light stipple) and 28 days (dark stipple) following a postero-lateral electrolytic lesion of the lateral hypothalamus in rat. Activity expressed as percent of unlesioned control ± SEM ($n = 6$–12). ** $P < 0.001$.

D. CHANGES IN THE ACCUMULATION OF TYROSINE HYDROXYLASE PROTEIN DURING THE RETROGRADE REACTION

Recently we have investigated the changes in the activity of TH, the rate-limiting enzymatic step in the biosynthesis of catecholamines (Levitt *et al.*, 1965), in neurons of the locus coeruleus during the retrograde reaction. Particularly we have sought to determine if there is a reversible decrease in the activity of this enzyme and, secondly, by the use of a specific antibody (Joh *et al.*, 1973) to determine if it reflects a reduced accumulation of enzyme protein.

During the retrograde reaction in the locus coeruleus the activity of TH is reversibly reduced with a time course similar to that of DBH. By day 14 (Fig. 6) the activity of the enzyme has fallen to about 60% of control returning to normal by day 28. Immuno-precipitation of the enzyme in the locus coeruleus taken 14 days after the lesion (Fig. 7) demonstrates that the decline of enzyme activity is the result of a reduction in the amount of precipitable enzyme protein exactly corresponding to the magnitude in the decrease of enzyme activity.

Thus the reduction of TH (and probably DBH) activity during the retrograde reaction is entirely the result of reduced accumulation of specific enzyme protein. Whether the reduction is due to an increased degradation or a decreased synthesis of the enzyme remains to be determined.

It is of considerable interest that in peripheral sympathetic ganglia during the retrograde reaction there is a marked increase in the number of lysosomes (Matthews and Raisman, 1972) and lysosomal activity (Huikuri, 1966). These findings suggest that there may be an

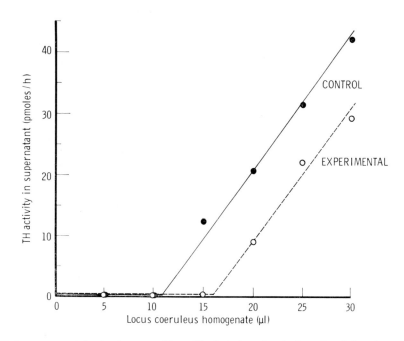

FIG. 7. Immunoprecipitation by a specific antibody to tyrosine hydroxylase of region of the locus coeruleus ipsilateral to a lateral hypothalamic lesion placed 14 days earlier. Each curve represents the pooled tissue from 8 to 10 animals. Measurement of enzyme activity in samples measured individually from lesioned animals was approximately 65% of control. Hence the reduction of enzyme protein in the locus coeruleus during the retrograde response is entirely attributable to reduced accumulation of specific enzyme protein and not to increase in enzyme inhibitors.

increase in the intracellular degradative processes. The quantity of the synthetic enzymes in reactive neurons may be regulated by degradation rather than synthesis. However, at the present time we have been unable to detect any changes in multivesicular bodies or lysosomes within neurons of the locus coeruleus at the time of maximal reduction of enzyme accumulation (Field et al., 1973). Conceivably this could reflect a difference in intracellular regulation of enzyme accumulation between central and peripheral noradrenergic neurons.

The accumulation of TH and DBH within neurons of the locus appear to be relatively specific. At the time at which there is maximal reduction in the accumulation of these enzymes no changes in the activities of DDC and MAO can be observed (Fig. 6). Although DDC and MAO subserve roles in the metabolism of the catecholamines, they are both more ubiquitously distributed enzymes and relatively nonspecific.

E. CHANGES IN COLLATERALS OF REACTIVE NEURONS DURING THE RETROGRADE REACTION

There is evidence that the intact (sustaining) collateral branches of neurons undergoing retrograde reaction may in some manner reflect the biochemical changes manifested in their parent neuron. Following lesions of noradrenergic axons within the hypothalamus, for example, the activity of DBH in the cerebellum is reversibly reduced with a similar time course to that seen in the perikarya of noradrenergic neurons in the brainstem (Fig. 8) (Reis and Ross, 1973). The magnitude of change is not as great as that of the brainstem,

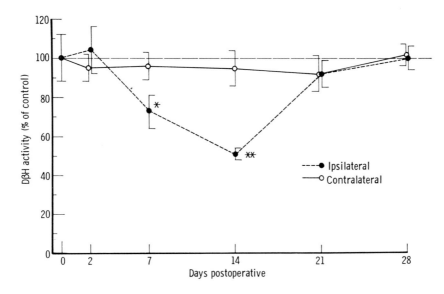

Fig. 8. Time course of changes in DBH activity in cerebellar hemisphere of rat following unilateral lesion of posterolateral hypothalamus. Enzyme activity is expressed as a percent of mean activity in at least six matched unoperated controls. Each point represents mean ± SEM of 6–12 animals. Ipsilateral cerebellum is represented by solid circles (● − − − ●); contralateral cerebellum by open circles (○——○). *$p < 0.05$; **$p < 0.001$. (From Reis and Ross, 1973.)

but in any individual case the magnitude of the decrease in the cerebellum is directly and linearly proportional to the decrease of enzyme activity in the brainstem. Since the adrenergic innervation of the cerebellum is derived from collaterals of locus neurons, some of whose axons are lesioned in the hypothalamus, the above finding suggests that a reduced accumulation of enzyme protein in noradrenergic neurons in the locus coeruleus results in a decreased quantity of enzyme transported by axoplasmic flow into collaterals still in continuity with the parent cell body. This finding also suggests that the persistence of NE in collaterals following axonal lesion (Hoffer et al., 1973) is probably not a consequence of the cells producing a constant amount of transmitter for fewer remaining collaterals. Perhaps the persistent level of NE in lesioned collaterals represents, as Hoffer has suggested, an impairment in the release of the transmitter by the injured nerve cell.

III. SOME GENERAL IMPLICATIONS

A. THE RETROGRADE REACTION IN RELATIONSHIP TO SPROUTING: CHROMATOLYSIS OF INTRINSIC NEURONS OF THE CNS REVISITED

It has been suggested that the retrograde reaction represents the biochemical and morphological concomitants of cellular regeneration rather than a response of the nerve to injury *per se* (Lieberman, 1971). The strongest evidence for this contention comes from studies by Brattgård *et al.* (1957) and Watson (1965, 1968, 1969, 1970) on the reaction of the hypoglossal nucleus to axonal injury (Brattgård *et al.*, 1957), treatment with botulinum (Watson, 1969) or in response to collateral sprouting of the otherwise uninjured axon to occupy denervate neuromuscular junctions (Watson, 1970). Simultaneously with sprouting, usually within 3–14 days after the stimulus, the biochemical and morphological characteristics of the retrograde response become evident. Functional reinnervation results in a return of neuron to normal.

A similar course of events appears to occur in peripheral sympathetic neurons. The peripheral sympathetic cell responds to axonal damage with energetic sprouting beginning within a few days after the injury paralleling the morphological signs of chromatolysis (Matthews and Raisman, 1972). The reduction in the activity and presumably accumulation of neurotransmitter synthesizing enzymes which parallels the traditional changes in cell morphology leads to the conclusion that the enzyme changes are events which coexist with, if they are in fact not intimately related to, the regenerative process.

On these assumptions, therefore, our findings of reversible changes of TH and probably DBH accumulation in central noradrenergic neurons during the retrograde response assumes a new significance. Taken with the recent demonstrations that central noradrenergic neurons respond to axonal damage by intensive sprouting (Katzman *et al.*, 1971; Björklund and Stenevi, 1971; Moore *et al.*, 1971) it leads to the inevitable conclusion that in noradrenergic neurons in brain, as in the periphery, a reversible reduction in the accumulation of neurotransmitter synthesizing enzymes are parallel and related events. This view is further reinforced by the fact that the time of maximal sprouting in central noradrenergic neurons in response to axonal injury occurs 8–15 days after injury (Katzman *et al.*, 1971; Moore *et al.*, 1971), the time of maximal change in enzymes.

Taken a step further, this logic leads to a conclusion of relevance to the whole problem of the reputed absence of reversible retrograde changes in intrinsic neurons of the CNS (Barron *et al.*, 1967; Cole, 1968; Lieberman, 1971). Unlike their peripheral counterparts, we have observed (Field *et al.*, 1973) that central noradrenergic neurons of locus coeruleus in adult rats fail to show evidence of chromatolysis either by light or semi-quantitative electron microscopy during the period of reduced accumulation of enzyme. This negative morphological finding suggests that the biochemical events of the retrograde reaction in at least central noradrenergic neurons may occur in the absence of the classical morphological changes. Thus the view that intrinsic neurons of the CNS do not show reversible changes of the retrograde reaction may not be entirely true. Central adrenergic neurons, at least, show the same biochemical changes as their peripheral counterparts as well as the capacity to respond to injury by regeneration. Thus it is only the morphological aspect of the retrograde response in the nerve cell body which is minimal in CNS and not the biochemical events nor sprouting.

B. ARE THERE SELECTIVE EFFECTS ON SPECIFIC PROTEINS IN THE RETROGRADE REACTION?

It is generally believed that during the retrograde reaction there is, in general, an increase in net protein and RNA biosynthesis in peripheral neurons including those of the sympathetic nervous system (Lieberman, 1971). Thus there is increased nuclear RNA synthesis, nucleolar RNA content, rate of passage of newly synthesized RNA from the nucleus to the cytoplasm, an increase in cytoplasmic RNA content, and an increase in cytoplasmic protein content and synthesis [as determined by the incorporation of labelled amino acid to TCA precipitable proteins (Brattgård *et al.*, 1957, 1958; Watson, 1965, 1968)]. These findings suggest, therefore, that the retrograde reaction is primarily an anabolic event and relates more to the attempts of the neuron to regenerate by sprouting than to degeneration. The observations of a decrease in the accumulation of catecholamine synthesizing enzymes in sympathetic ganglia, assuming they result from decreased synthesis of these enzymes, suggests that there may be a selective reordering of priorities for protein biosynthesis in the cell. These changes would be characterized by an increase of those proteins required for re-establishment of axonal membrane at the expense of those which are involved in the production of transmitter and possibly receptor functions of the neuron. Indeed, the changes of the pattern of protein biosynthesis in regenerating neurons have been suggested to reflect the reversion of the pattern of protein biosynthesis to that characteristic of immature nerve cells (Brattgård *et al.*, 1957; Griffith and La Velle, 1971).

C. THE ROLE OF SUSTAINING COLLATERALS IN SIGNALLING DAMAGE TO REMOTE AXONS: SOME POSSIBLE IMPLICATIONS

A final point of interest relates to the finding that the changes of enzyme accumulation in neurons of the locus coeruleus are reflected in the sustaining collaterals to the cerebellum. This observation indicates that the whole field of innervation of a neuron is "informed" of damage to a remote collateral. Thus the cerebellum knows that the hypothalamus is damaged through a process of *intraneuronal communication*. The biological significance of such widespread impairment of neuronal function is unknown. It could merely relate to a reduction in the activity of the neuron in transmission; collaterals thereby sharing in any decrease of nerve impulse activity. More intriguing, however, is the possibility that the biochemical changes at remote terminals might be of importance in the recovery of physiological function following brain damage, i.e. the transfer of function and activity from one brain area to another, leading to "compensation". Thus the distant terminal might share in the increased drive of the lesioned cell to sprout possibly forming new synapses at a distant site. Alternately, the altered release of macromolecules could be of significance. We believe this a problem of interest and worthy of future investigation.

ACKNOWLEDGEMENTS

This research was supported by a grant from the NIH (NS 06911) and the Harris Foundation.

REFERENCES

ACHESON, G., and REMOLINA, J. (1955) The temporal course of the effects of post-ganglionic axotomy on the inferior mesenteric ganglion of the cat. *J. Physiol.* **127**, 603–616.

ANDÉN, N. E., MAGNUSSON, T., and ROSENGREN, E. (1965) Occurrence of dihydroxyphenylalanine decarboxylase in nerves of the spinal cord and sympathetically innervated organs. *Acta physiol. scand.* **64**, 127–135.

ANDÉN, N. E., DAHLSTRÖM, A., FUXE, K., LARSSON, K., OLSON, L., and UNGERSTEDT, U. (1966) Ascending monoamine neurons to the telencephalon and diencephalon. *Acta physiol. scand.* **67**, 313–326.

AXELROD, J. (1972) Dopamine-β-hydroxylase: regulation of its synthesis and release from nerve terminals. *Pharmac. Rev.* **24**, 233–243.

BARRON, K. D., DOOLIN, P. F., and OLDERSHAW, J. B. (1967) Ultrastructural observations on retrograde atrophy of lateral geniculate body: I, Neuronal alterations, *J. Neuropath. Exp. Neurol.* **26**, 300–326.

BJÖRKLUND, A., and STENEVI, U. (1971) Growth of central catecholamine neurons into smooth muscle grafts in the rat mesencephalon. *Brain Res.* **31**, 1–20.

BOYLE, F. C., and GILLESPIE, J. S. (1970) Accumulation and loss of noradrenalin central to a constriction on adrenergic nerves. *Eur. J. Pharmac.* **12**, 77–84.

BRATTGÅRD, S. O., EDSTRÖM, J. E., and HYDÉN, H. (1957) The chemical changes in regenerating neurons. *J. Neurochem.* **1**, 316–325.

BRATTGÅRD, S. O., HYDÉN, H., and SJÖSTRAND, J. (1958) Incorporation of orotic acid-^{14}C and lysine-^{14}C in regenerating single nerve cells. *Nature, Lond.* **182**, 801–802.

BRIMIJOIN, W. S., and MOLINOFF, P. B. (1971) Effects of 6-hydroxydopamine on the activity of tyrosine hydroxylase and dopamine-β-hydroxylase in sympathetic ganglia of the rat. *J. Pharmac. Exp. Ther.* **178**, 417–424.

BROWN, G. L., and PASCOE, J. E. (1954) The effect of degenerative section of ganglionic axons on transmission through the ganglion. *J. Physiol.* **123**, 565–573.

CAUSEY, G., and STRATMANN, C. J. (1956) Changes in the nucleic acid content of ganglion cells during chromatolysis and after stimulation. *Biochem. J.* **64**, 29–32.

COLE, M. (1968) Retrograde degeneration of axon and soma in the nervous system. In *Structure and Function of Nervous Tissue*, (G. Bourne, ed.) vol. 1, Academic Press, London, pp. 269–298.

DAHLSTRÖM, A., and FUXE, K. (1964) Evidence for the existence of monoamine containing neurons in the central nervous system: I, Demonstration of monoamines in the cell bodies of brain stem neurons. *Acta physiol. scand.* **62**, Suppl. 232, 1–55.

DAHLSTRÖM, A., and FUXE, K. (1965) Experimentally induced changes in the intraneuronal amine levels of bulbospinal neuron systems. *Acta physiol. scand.* **64**, Suppl. 247, 1–36.

DESCARRIES, L., and SAUCIER, G. (1972) Disappearance of the locus coeruleus in the rat after intra-ventricular 6-hydroxydopamine. *Brain Res.* **37**, 310–316.

DIXON, J. S. (1970) Some fine structural changes in sympathetic neurons following axon section. *Acta anat.* **76**, 473–487.

ECCLES, J. C., LIBET, B., and YOUNG, R. R. (1958) The behavior of chromatolyzed motoneurons studied by intracellular recording. *J. Physiol.* **143**, 11–40.

FEIGELSON, P., and GREENGARD, O. (1962) Immunochemical evidence for increased titers of liver tryptophan pyrrolase during substrate and hormonal enzyme induction. *J. Biol. Chem.* **237**, 3714–17.

FIELD, P. M., ROSS, R. A., and REIS, D. J. (1973) In preparation.

FRY, F. J., and COWAN, W. M. (1972) A study of retrograde cell degeneration in the lateral mammillary nucleus of the cat with special reference to the role of axonal branching in the preservation of the cell. *J. Comp. Neurol.* **144**, 1–24.

FUXE, K., GOLDSTEIN, M., HÖKFELT, T., and JOH, T. H. (1971) Cellular localization of dopamine-β-hydroxylase and phenylethanolamine-N-methyl transferase as revealed by immunohistochemistry. In *Progress in Brain Research*, (O. Eranko, ed.) vol. 34, Elsevier, Amsterdam, pp. 127–138.

GEFFEN, L. B., and LIVETT, B. G. (1971) Synaptic vesicles in sympathetic neurons. *Physiol. Rev.* **51**, 98–157.

GRIFFITH, A., and LA VELLE, A. (1971) Developmental protein changes in normal and chromatolytic facial nerve nuclear regions. *Expl. Neurol.* **33**, 360–371.

HÄRKÖNEN, M. (1964) Carboxylic esterases, oxidative enzymes and catecholamines in the superior cervical ganglion of the rat and the effect of pre- and post-ganglionic nerve division. *Acta physiol. scand.* **63**, Suppl. 237, 1–94.

HEBB, C. O., and WAITES, G. M. H. (1956) Choline acetylase in antero- and retrograde degeneration of a cholinergic nerve. *J. Physiol.* **132**, 667–671.

HELLER, A., and MOORE, R. Y. (1968) Control of brain serotonin and norepinephrine by specific neural systems. *Adv. Pharmac. Chemother.* **6A**, 191–206.

HOFFER, B. J., SIGGINS, G. R., OLIVER, A. P., and BLOOM, F. E. (1973) Activation of the pathway from locus coeruleus to rat cerebellar Purkinje neurons: pharmacological evidence of noradrenergic central inhibition. *J. Pharmac. Exp. Ther.* **184**, 553–569.

HÖKFELT, T., JONSSON, G., and SACHS, C. (1972) Fine structure and fluorescence morphology of adrenergic nerves after 6-hydroxydopamine *in vivo* and *in vitro*. *Z. Zellforsch. mikrosk. Anat.* **131**, 529–543.

HUIKURI, K. T. (1966) Histochemistry of the ciliary ganglion of the rat and the effect of pre- and post-ganglionic nerve division. *Acta physiol. scand.* **69**, Suppl. 286, 1–83.

JACOBOWITZ, D., and WOODWARD, J. K. (1968) Adrenergic neurons in the cat superior cervical ganglion and cervical sympathetic nerve trunk. *J. Pharmac. Exp. Ther.* **162**, 213–226.

JOH, T. H., GEGHMAN, C., and REIS, D. J. (1973) Immunochemical evidence that reserpine increases the amount of specific tyrosine hydroxylase protein in adrenal gland and sympathetic ganglia. *Fed. Proc.* (In press.)

KAPELLER, K., and MAYOR, D. (1969) An electron microscopic study of the early changes proximal to a constriction in sympathetic nerves. *Proc. R. Soc. Lond.* **B, 172**, 39–51.

KATZMAN, R., BJÖRKLUND, A., OWMAN, C., STENEVI, U., and WEST, K. A. (1971) Evidence for regenerative axon sprouting of central catecholamine neurons in the rat mesencephalon following electrolytic lesions. *Brain Res.* **25**, 579–596.

KOPIN, I. J., and SILBERSTEIN, S. D. (1972) Axons of sympathetic neurons: transport of enzymes *in vivo* and properties of axonal sprouts *in vitro*. *Pharmac. Rev.* **24**, 245–254.

KUNO, M., and LLINAS, R. (1970) Alterations of synaptic action in chromatolyzed motoneurones of the cat. *J. Physiol.* **210**, 823–838.

LEVITT, M., SPECTOR, S. SJOERDSMA, A., and UDENFRIEND, S. (1965) Elucidation of the rate-limiting step in norepinephrine biosynthesis in the perfused guinea pig heart. *J. Pharmac. Exp. Ther.* **148**, 1–8.

LIEBERMAN, A. R. (1971) The axon reaction: a review of the principal features of perikaryal response to axon injury. *Int. Rev. Neurobiol.* **14**, 49–124.

LOIZOU, L. A. (1969) Projections of the nucleus locus coeruleus in the albino rat. *Brain Res.* **15**, 563–566.

MALMFORS, T. and SACHS, C. (1965) Direct studies on the disappearance of the transmitter and the changes in the uptake-storage mechanisms of degenerating adrenergic nerves. *Acta physiol. scand.* **64**, 211–223.

MATTHEWS, M. R., and RAISMAN, G. (1972) A light and electron microscopic study of the cellular response to axonal injury in the superior cervical ganglion of the rat. *Proc. R. Soc. Lond.* **B, 181**, 43–79.

MILLHOUSE, O. E. (1969) A golgi study of the descending medial forebrain bundle. *Brain Res.* **15**, 341–363.

MOORE, R. Y., BJÖRKLUND, A., and STENEVI, U. (1971) Plastic changes in the adrenergic innervation of the rat septal area in response to denervation. *Brain Res.* **33**, 13–35.

OLSON, L., and FUXE, K. (1971) On the projections from the locus coeruleus noradrenalin neurons: the cerebellar innervation. *Brain Res.* **28**, 165–171.

PILAR, G., and LANDMESSER, L. (1972) Axotomy mimicked by localized colchicine application. *Science* **177**, 116–118.

POTTER, L. T., COOPER, T., WILLMAN, V. L., and WOLFE, D. E. (1965) Synthesis, binding, release and metabolism of norepinephrine in normal and transplanted hearts. *Circ. Res.* **16**, 468–481.

REIS, D. J., and MOLINOFF, P. B. (1972) Brain dopamine-β-hydroxylase: regional distribution and effects of lesions and 6-hydroxydopamine on activity. *J. Neurochem.* **19**, 195–204.

REIS, D. J., and ROSS, R. A. (1973) Dynamic changes in brain dopamine-β-hydroxylase activity during anterograde and retrograde reactions to injury of central noradrenergic neurons. *Brain Res.* (In press.)

ROSS, R. A., SMITH, G. P., and REIS, D. J. (1973) Effects of lesions of locus coeruleus on regional distribution of dopamine-β-hydroxylase (DBH) and feeding and drinking behaviors in rat. *Fed. Proc.* (In Press).

SCHWARZACHER, H. G. (1958) Der cholinesterase-gehalt motorischer nervenzellen während der axonalen reacktion. *Acta anat.* **32**, 51–65.

SEDVALL, G. C., and KOPIN, I. J. (1967) Influence of sympathetic denervation and nerve impulse activity on tyrosine hydroxylase in the rat submaxillary gland. *Biochem. Pharmac.* **16**, 39–46.

UNGERSTEDT, U. (1971) Stereotaxic mapping of the monoamine pathways in the rat brain. *Acta physiol. scand.* **82**, Suppl. 367, 1–48.

WATSON, W. E. (1965) An autoradiographic study of the incorporation of nucleic acid precursors by neurons and glia during nerve regeneration. *J. Physiol. Lond.* **180**, 741–753.

WATSON, W. E. (1968) Observations on the nucleolar and total cell body nuclei acid of injured nerve cells. *J. Physiol.* **196**, 655–676.

WATSON, W. E. (1969) Some metabolic response of motor neurons to axotomy and to botulinum toxin after nerve transplantation. *J. Physiol. Lond.* **204**, 138.

WATSON, W. E. (1970) Some metabolic responses to axotomized neurons to contact between their axons and denervated muscle. *J. Physiol.* **210**, 321–343.

EFFECTS OF BRETYLIUM, RELATED QUATERNARY AMMONIUM COMPOUNDS, AND MITOSIS INHIBITORS ON THE DEGENERATION ACTIVITY IN THE SYMPATHETICALLY INNERVATED PERIORBITAL SMOOTH MUSCLE IN THE CONSCIOUS RAT

Dag Lundberg

Department of Pharmacology, University of Uppsala, and the Department of Anesthesia II, Sahlgrenska sjukhuset, Göteborg

SUMMARY

The results presented here emanate from pharmacological studies on the degeneration contraction of the sympathetically innervated periorbital smooth muscle in the rat. This transient degeneration activity is due to the release of stored transmitter from the degenerating nerve endings. Drugs from two pharmacologically different groups of substances were found to cause a real delay of the degeneration transmitter release. One of the groups consisted of the adrenergic neuron blocker bretylium and some other quaternary ammonium compounds. The delaying effect of these drugs was most prominent after injections given close to the expected onset of the degeneration transmitter release. The delaying action seems to be exerted in the distal parts of the neurons since the drugs are effective when given locally in the effector organ. The delaying effect is reduced by tricyclic antidepressants and indirect sympathomimetic amines. The other group of delaying drugs were the mitosis inhibitors colchicine, vinblastine, and vincristine which are known to inhibit the microtubular intra-axonal flow. These drugs delay the degeneration activity if given early after denervation. The delaying effect of colchicine decreases gradually with an increasing time interval between the denervation and the injection. The delaying effect of colchicine is absent after injections given 6 h or more after the denervation. Hypothetically, the mitosis inhibitors cause a delay by slowing down an "axotomy message" conveyed by the intra-axonal flow. The rate of transport of the signal seems to be about 4 mm/h. It is proposed that there are two latencies of the processes starting the degeneration transmitter release in the periorbital smooth muscle of the rat. One latency (about 5 h) is due to the transport of the axotomy message and is colchicine-sensitive. The other latency (about 8 h) which is due to the progress of local processes in the nerve endings is presumably bretylium-sensitive.

INTRODUCTION

The degeneration activity in the neuroeffector region of autonomically innervated organs which occurs during the early postdenervation period has evoked increasing interest during the last decade and has recently been reviewed (Emmelin and Trendelenburg, 1972). The spontaneous degeneration activity is due to temporary supraliminal release of stored transmitter from the degenerating axons (Emmelin and Strömblad, 1957; Sears and Bárány, 1960). The degeneration contraction of the periorbital smooth muscle of the rat which is a degeneration activity produced by excision of the superior cervical ganglion can easily be studied *in vivo* (Lundberg, 1969a, b, 1970a). The present paper mainly summarizes some studies on the ability of the adrenergic neuron blocker bretylium and related quaternary ammonium compounds and some mitosis inhibitors to delay the onset of the degeneration release of sympathetic transmitter in the rat's periorbital smooth muscle.

MATERIALS AND METHODS

EXPERIMENTAL ANIMALS

Male Sprague–Dawley rats weighing about 250 g were used.

SURGICAL PROCEDURE

If otherwise not stated, the right superior cervical ganglion was removed (denervation) and the left preganglionic trunk was cut (decentralization) under ether anesthesia.

MEASURING PROCEDURE

The width of the palpebral aperture is controlled by the tone of the sympathetically innervated periorbital smooth muscle (Müller's muscle). The aperture was measured in conscious rats using the method described in detail by Lundberg (1969a). The palpebral apertures of both eyes were measured simultaneously about once every hour during the experimental period. The difference in the mean width of aperture between the denervated and decentralized (control) side was plotted against time after denervation. The difference curve (the degeneration contraction curve) thus obtained was analyzed. The time corresponding to 50% of maximum effect on the ascending part of the curve was used as the time of start of the degeneration contraction (T_{50a}); the time of 50% peak effect on the descending phase was taken as the time of end of the contraction (T_{50d}). The height (the amplitude) of the contraction was the maximum value on the denervated side during the degeneration contraction, no regard being taken to the decentralized side.

DRUGS

The drugs were kindly donated by their manufacturers. The substances were dissolved in 0.9% NaCl just before use and usually injected s.c. Doses refer to salts.

Student's t-test was used for the analysis of significance.

RESULTS

The normal degeneration contraction of the periorbital smooth muscle is half-developed about 15 h and half relaxed about 23 h after denervation (Lundberg, 1969a) (Fig. 1). The degeneration contraction is most probably due to a release from the degenerating nerve endings of adrenergic transmitter synthesized before the time of denervation mainly since,

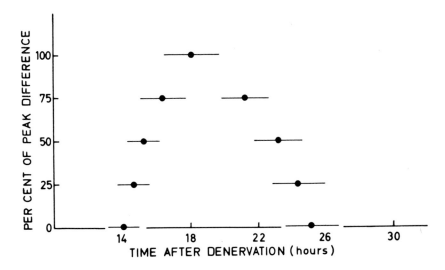

FIG. 1. The mean curve constructed from individual curves of 34 normal degeneration contractions in untreated rats. The difference plotted is the difference between the width of palpebral aperture on the denervated side and that of the decentralized side. For details of the method of construction, see Lundberg, 1969. Means and standard deviation are shown.

in the first place, it is prevented by reserpine and antagonized by phentolamine, secondly, it is not significantly changed by ganglionblockers or by inhibition of the rate-limiting step of the synthesis of noradrenaline (Lundberg, 1970a). The ascending limb of the degeneration contraction curve is steeper than the descending one. This asymmetry is probably due to the concomitant development of supersensitivity to noradrenaline (Treister and Bárány, 1970; Lundberg, 1972a).

EXPERIMENTS WITH BRETYLIUM

The observation made by Benmiloud and von Euler in 1963 that the neuron blocker bretylium was able to delay the postdenervation decline of endogenous noradrenaline from the submaxillary glands of the rat initiated the detailed studies of the actions of the drug in the present experimental system, some of which are presented here.

EFFECTS OF SINGLE INJECTIONS OF BRETYLIUM

Bretylium (4 mg/kg) was given to rats at different times after denervation. The results are shown in Table 1. If given at 6–11 h after denervation, which is more than 2 h before the expected onset of the degeneration contraction, bretylium delayed the start of the contraction without any greater change in appearance or magnitude. When bretylium was given close to the expected start of the contraction, i.e. at 12, 13, or 14 h after the operation, however, the effect of the drug was apparently changed. Firstly, the delaying effect was distinctly increased. Secondly, the delayed degeneration contraction often had a double hump instead of a normal single hump appearance. Moreover, there was a clearcut increase in the initial excitatory effect on the denervated side after injections of bretylium given at his period, i.e. an asymmetric sympathomimetic effect. When the drug was given at 16 h,

TABLE 1

Influence of the time interval between the denervation and the injection on the time course of the degeneration contraction and the asymmetric sympathomimetic effect after (4 mg/kg) bretylium. The asymmetric
sympathomimetic effect is the excess initial excitatory effect on the denervated side. The delay is the difference
in time between the half-maximum development of the contraction of the treated group (T_{50a}) and that of
the control group. The duration is the time interval between half-maximum development of the contraction
(T_{50a}) and the corresponding value on the descending phase (T_{50d}). Comparisons are between a treated
group and control group. The time of start and time of end of the contractions of all treated groups were
significantly different from those of the control group ($p < 0.001$). Values are means $\pm$ SEM if not otherwise
stated.

Time of injection (h)[a]	n	Delay (h)	Duration (h)	Type of curve	Asymmetric sympathomimetic effect[d]
6	5	3.3 ± 0.5	6.4 ± 0.8	Single hump	−
10	10	3.7 ± 0.4	$p < 0.05$		−
			8.1 ± 0.5	Single hump	
11	10	5.1 ± 0.2	7.1 ± 0.4	Single hump	−
			$p < 0.001$		
12	12	4.4 ± 0.4	10.3 ± 0.6	Double hump	+
13	10	5.5 ± 0.4	$9.5–11.3^{b}$	Single hump?	++
14	4	8.8 ± 0.5	$>9.1^{c}$	Double hump	+++
14	6	14.4 ± 0.5	$>1.5^{c}$	(?)	+++
Untreated rats (0.9% NaCl, 2 ml/kg)	21	0	7.0 ± 0.4	Single hump	−

[a] Hours after denervation.
[b] Range of the median.
[c] Median.
[d] −, absent; +, weak; ++, clear; +++, distinct.

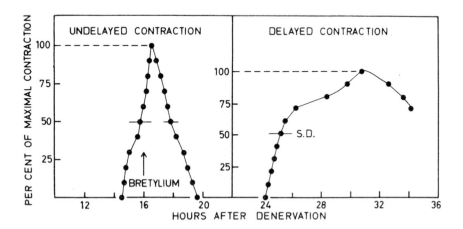

FIG. 2. Effect of bretylium given after the start of the degeneration contraction. Bretylium
(4 mg/kg) was given to the rats ($n=5$) at about 16 h after the denervation. The drug interrupted
the ongoing contraction and displaced the latter part. Mean curves for the two parts of the degeneration contraction are shown. For the method of construction of mean curves, see Lundberg, 1969a, b. S.D. = standard deviation.

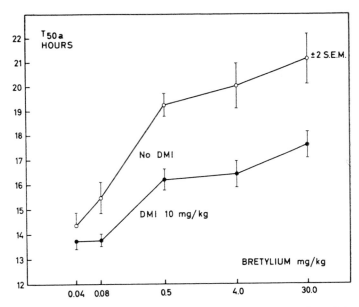

FIG. 3. Delaying effect of different doses of bretylium and the reducing effect of desmethylimi-pramine on the delay. Bretylium was given at 11 h and desmethylimipramine (or 0.9% NaCl) 13 h after denervation. T_{50a} is the time of half-maximum development of the degeneration contraction. There were five rats in each group.

when the degeneration contraction already had started, the result was different (Fig. 2). Firstly, the speed of the ongoing degeneration contraction seemed to be increased. Secondly, after full recovery of the contraction and after a period of ptosis, a second wave of degeneration activity was seen (Lundberg, 1970a).

Thus there seem to be three critical periods for the administration of bretylium: (1) well before the onset, (2) 1–3 h before the start of the degeneration contraction, and (3) after the contraction has started.

Different doses of bretylium given at period (1) cause a dose-dependent delay of the degeneration contraction (Fig. 3) (Lundberg, 1970b).

EFFECT OF REPEATED INJECTIONS OF BRETYLIUM

Rats were given injections of bretylium (4 mg/kg) every 4 h from 13 to 33 h after denervation. The results are shown in Fig. 4. In connection with the injections there was a sympathomimetic effect which was greater on the denervated than on the decentralized side. Until about 25 h this excitatory effect, however, was relatively small and shortlasting, but after that time it was distinctly increased, and in some rats there seemed to be spontaneous contraction going on despite the bretylium treatment. Thus bretylium seems to be able to delay the onset of the degeneration transmitter release until about 25 h but probably not further (Lundberg, 1970a).

INHIBITORS OF THE BRETYLIUM-INDUCED DELAY

The inhibitors of the axonal amine pump desmethylimipramine, protriptyline, and Lu 3-010, but not cocaine, distinctly reduced the bretylium-induced delay of the degeneration

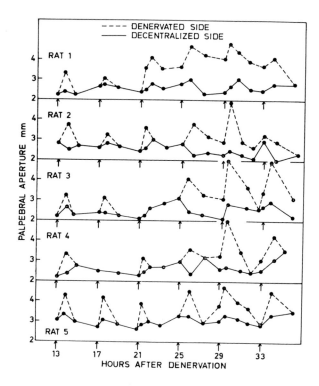

FIG. 4. Effect of repeated injections of bretylium on the degeneration contraction. Bretylium (4 mg/kg) was given every 4 h from 13 to 33 h after denervation. The injections are indicated by arrows. Readings in connections with injections were always made immediately preceding the latter.

contraction both when given before or after bretylium. Desmethylimipramine antagonized the delaying effect of bretylium in a dose-dependent fashion (Fig. 3), and the antagonism appears to be of the noncompetitive type (Lundberg, 1970b).

EXPERIMENTS WITH DRUGS RELATED TO BRETYLIUM

It seemed to be of interest to find out what kinds of substances possess the delaying effect in common with bretylium. Therefore sixteen drugs structurally and/or pharmacologically related to bretylium were tested, usually at two dose levels (4 mg/kg and 20 mg/kg). The ability of the drugs to induce ptosis in the intact animal (the adrenergic neuron-blocking effect) was tested before the degeneration experiment. Moreover, the tendency of the drugs to induce an asymmetric sympathomimetic effect was recorded. Some of the results are shown in Table 2 (for details see Lundberg, 1970e). A significant delaying effect was only seen among the quaternary ammonium compounds. Some of the best "delayers" were the simple compounds phenyltrimethylammonium (PTMA) and benzyltrimethylammonium (BTMA). The guanidine derivatives, such as bethanidine, however, which otherwise are closely related to bretylium pharmacologically by their local anesthetic effect, adrenergic neuron-blocking effect and monoamine oxidase-inhibiting effect (Boura and Green, 1965), lacked delaying effect. It is also notable that there did not seem to be any correlation between either the neuron-blocking effect or the asymmetric sympathomimetic effect and the delaying effect of the drugs.

However, PTMA has several actions at cholinergic sites (see, e.g., Wretlind, 1950), the delaying effect of PTMA could not be reduced by atropine, methylatropine, or mecamylamine (all drugs at 4 mg/kg) given before or after the delaying drug (Lundberg, 1970e).

BRETYLIUM-INDUCED DELAY OF DENERVATION SUPERSENSITIVITY TO NORADRENALINE

The denervation supersensitivity to noradrenaline, which depends on the deterioration of the axonal membrane amine pump, develops during the first few days after the denervation (Trendelenburg, 1969). Was bretylium able to delay this degeneration phenomenon too? To try to answer this question, rats were used which were treated with reserpine (2.5 mg/kg) at the time of operation in order to deplete the transmitter stores of the nerve endings and prevent the development of the degeneration contraction, which otherwise would interfere with the tests of the sensitivity of the periorbital smooth muscle to exogenous noradrenaline. The animals were given bretylium (4 mg/kg), bethanidine (4 mg/kg), or 0.9% NaCl at 12 h after denervation. The sensitivity to i.p. noradrenaline was tested at different time intervals after denervation (for details see text to Fig. 5). Bethanidine was used as a control substance since it shares several pharmacological effects with bretylium except the ability to delay the degeneration transmitter release. The results are shown in Fig. 5. There was an early transient increase in sensitivity to noradrenaline on both sides after bretylium and possibly after bethanidine. The reason is not quite clear. At 19–22 h the sensitivity in the bretylium group was low on both sides. However, this was not so in the bethanidine and the NaCl groups. In these groups there was a clearcut increase in sensitivity on the denervated side. At 27–30 h the sensitivity on the denervated side was increased also in the bretylium group. Hence, bretylium also seems to delay the onset of the denervation supersensitivity to noradrenaline, i.e. the deterioration of the axonal membrane pump mechanism (Lundberg, 1972a).

EXPERIMENTS WITH MITOSIS INHIBITORS

Somehow the distal parts of the neuron must be informed of the axotomy. It was tempting to think in terms of intra-axonal flow. Since the mitosis inhibitors colchicine, vincristine, and vinblastine are known to inhibit the flow of nerve constituents in adrenergic nerves (for references see Dahlström, 1971) it seemed natural to test them on the present experimental system. Colchicine given s.c. at the time of denervation delayed the start of the degeneration contraction in a dose-dependent manner (Lundberg, 1970f). In another experiment colchicine was given at a fixed dose (1 mg/kg) but at various times during the interval between the denervation and the expected onset of the degeneration contraction (Fig. 6) (Lundberg, 1972a, b). The contraction was delayed only if the drug was given within the first 6 h after the denervation and the delaying effect declined gradually with an increasing time interval between the denervation and the injection of colchicine. Vinblastine (1–4 mg/kg) or vincristine (1–2 mg/kg) given at the time of denervation also delayed the degeneration contraction (1–5 h).

TABLE 2

The influence on the degeneration contraction of some compounds related to bretylium and their sympathomimetic effects when given at 12 h after denervation. The table also shows the ability of the drugs to induce ptosis in the same rats while their innervation was still intact. The delay is the difference in time between the half maximum development of the contraction of the treated group and that of the control group. The duration is the time interval between the half maximum development of the contraction (T_{50a}) and the corresponding value on the descending phase (T_{50d}). Values are means ± SEM if not otherwise stated. The statistical difference between a treated group and the control group was tested only if the treated group contained at least four rats.
$* = p < 0.05$, $** = p < 0.01$, $*** = p < 0.001$.

Drug	Dose (mg/kg)	n	Delay (h)	Duration (h)	Ptosis-inducing effect	Sympathomimetic effect
Bretylium	4	12	***[d] 4.2 ± 0.4	*** 10.4 ± 0.7	++	+[f]
Benzyltrimethyl-ammonium (BTMA)	4	4	*** 3.8 ± 0.3	6.6 ± 0.5	−	++
Phenyltrimethyl-ammonium (PTMA)	4	4	*** 10.3 ± 0.7	4.5[c]	−	−
	4	3	m̄ = 5.9[e]	10.3[c] 11.3[c] 7.7[c]	−	−
Xylocholine	4	4	*** 2.5 ± 0.5	6.8 ± 0.3	+++	−
Guanethidine at 10 h[a]	25	3/5[b]	m̄ = 10.1	m̄ = 7.6	+++	++
Bethanidine at 11 h[a]	4	5	0.0 ± 0.5	7.2 ± 0.8	++	++
Hexamethonium	15	2	0.5 2.3	9.2 8.2	+++	−
Untreated rats (0.9% NaCl)	2 ml/kg	31	0	8.19 ± 0.2	−	−

[a] Hours after denervation.
[b] In 2 out of 5 rats there was no degeneration contraction.
[c] Median value
[d] − absent; + weak; ++ clear; +++ distinct.
[e] Indicates that the degeneration contraction was of the double hump type.
[f] Indicates that the sympathomimetic effect was asymmetric (denervated side > decentralized side).

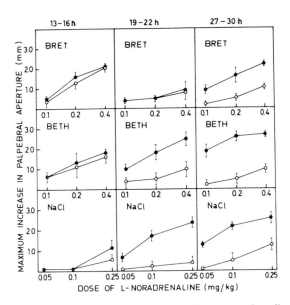

FIG. 5. Sensitivity of the periorbital smooth muscle to i.p. L-noradrenaline at different time intervals after denervation. The different noradrenaline doses of each test series were given 1 h apart. The first dose of the series was given at 13, 19, or 27 h respectively. The width of the palpebral aperture was measured just before each injection and after 15, 30, 45, and 60 min. The maximum effect of the injection was taken as the noradrenaline effect. There were four rats in each group. Means ± SEM are shown. Filled circles represent the denervated side, open circles the decentralized side.

DEGENERATION CONTRACTION AFTER "CHEMICAL DENERVATION" INDUCED BY LOCAL COLCHICINE OR VINBLASTINE

Rats were decentralized bilaterally and had their right superior cervical ganglions treated with either colchicine (injection of 100 μg in 5 μl. 0.6% NaCl) or vinblastine (soaking with 0.001 M in 0.9% NaCl with 10 I.E. per ml of testicular hyaluronidase, Hyalase^R). The left ganglion was treated in a corresponding manner with the solvents. There were degeneration contractions on the treated sides in all rats. The time of start, magnitude, or shape of these degeneration contractions did not significantly differ from those of "surgical" controls run simultaneously (Lundberg, 1972b).

DISCUSSION

Degeneration activity after sympathetic denervation has been studied in different organs of different species, e.g. in the eye and ear artery of the rabbit (Linnér and Prijot, 1955; Sears and Bárány, 1960; Emmelin and Ohlin, 1969; Bárány and Treister, 1970), salivary glands and nictitating membrane of the cat (Coats and Emmelin, 1962; Langer, 1966), vas deferens of the rat, guinea-pig, and mouse *in vitro* (Furness, 1970), the expensor secundarium of the chicken *in vitro* (Geffen and Hughes, 1971), the cerebral vessels of the mouse (Edvinsson *et al.*, 1971) and the rat periorbital smooth muscle, the latter being summarized in this paper. Findings from roughly comparable studies of the different degenerating systems are usually very congruent. This indicates that the processes which control the

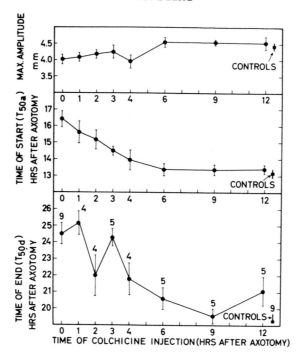

FIG. 6. Effect of single injections of colchicine (1 mg/kg) given at different time intervals after denervation (axotomy) on the degeneration contraction. The maximum amplitude is the peak aperture measured on the denervated side during the contraction (the height). T_{50a} is the time of half-maximum development of the contraction. T_{50d} is the corresponding time on the descending phase. The number of rats of each group is shown in the lowermost curve by the figure placed above the vertical bar. The vertical bars show SEM.

development of degeneration in adrenergic neurons follow regular courses. Studies of these processes may contribute information also about the physiological events in the neuro-effector area.

The main interest of the present study was at an early stage focused on earlier findings that the adrenergic neuron-blocker bretylium postponed the postdenervation disappearance of endogenous noradrenaline from the submaxillary glands of the rat (Benmiloud and von Euler, 1963) and that, β-TM10 delayed the onset of the degeneration contraction of the cat's nictitating membrane (Langer, 1966). The property of bretylium to interfere with degeneration events in adrenergic nerves was soon fully confirmed since the drug was found to be an efficient delayer of the start of the degeneration contraction of the rat's periorbital smooth muscle (Lundberg, 1969a). This effect was later studied in some detail.

The experiments with single doses of bretylium or PTMA (Lundberg, 1970c, e) given at different time intervals after denervation showed that there are three critical periods for the administration of the delaying drugs, namely, well before the onset of the expected degeneration contraction (period 1), 1–3 h before the expected start of the contraction (period 2) and some hours after the start of the contraction (period 3) during which the actions of the drugs differ with respect to delaying effect, influence on the appearance of the delayed degeneration contraction, and the sympathomimetic effect (cf. results). Histological studies by Malmfors and Sachs (1965) have shown that for each nerve ending the degeneration process is rapid but the development of the degeneration of the adrenergic innervation of a whole organ is slow because the time of start of degeneration differs in different fibers. The delaying effect of bretylium seems to be exerted in the periphery of the adrenergic neuron (Lundberg, 1970). Neuronal uptake and accumulation are probably prerequisites for the actions of bretylium (Brodie *et al.*, 1965; Haeusler *et al.*, 1969; Almgren and Lundberg, unpublished observation). It is thus likely that at different times during the development of degeneration there are groups of nerve endings which have reached different stages of degeneration and which react differently to bretylium, ranging from those which are unable to take up the drug and are thus insensitive to it, to those which still have an efficient capacity to take up and retain bretylium.

The mechanism of the delaying effect of bretylium in the rat is still obscure. There does not seem to be any correlation between the delaying action and any other known action of the drug such as its adrenergic neuron-blocking effect, monoamine oxidase-inhibiting activity, or its sympathomimetic activity (Lundberg, 1970c, d). Hypothetically, the location of the delaying activity, however, appears to involve intraneuronal sites in some way shared with tricyclic antidepressants and indirect sympathomimetic amines since such drugs reduce a bretylium-induced delay of the degeneration transmitter release (Lundberg, 1969b, 1970b). Despite the cholinergic "look" of the quaternary ammonium compounds, their delaying effect does not seem to involve any cholinergic site, since cholinergic activity is not a common feature among the delaying drugs and the bretylium-induced delay was not antagonized by anticholinergics (Lundberg, 1970e). The structurally simple compound benzyltrimethylammonium (BTMA) and phenyltrimethylammonium (PTMA) were found to be efficient delayers. The importance of the quaternary ammonium group (as a delaying principle) is demonstrated by comparing BTMA to bethanidine which did not delay. The two compounds differ mainly at the basic head of the molecule, BTMA having a quaternary ammonium group and bethanidine a guanidine group. Both are present as cations at physiological pH.

In the rat, bretylium not only delays the start of the degeneration transmitter release, but also the onset of the supersensitivity to exogenous noradrenaline *in vivo*, viz. the deterioration of the axonal amine pump mechanism (Lundberg, 1972a). This is not quite in accordance with findings of the Trendelenburg group who found that β-TM10 delayed the degeneration transmitter release in the cat but no other events of degeneration such as supersensitivity to noradrenaline *in vitro* or decrease in capacity to take up and retain noradrenaline *in vitro* (Pluchino *et al.*, 1970). This discrepancy, however, may well be due to species differences or the different methods used.

The distal parts of the neurons must be informed in one way or another of the axotomy and consequently the processes responsible for the initiation of the degeneration transmitter release be started. Emmelin (1967) showed that the shorter the distance between the site of axotomy and the nerve terminals the earlier the degeneration transmitter release starts. Hence the information that an axotomy has been performed, later referred to as "the axotomy message", is presumably transported along the neuron. The message could well rely on the function of the microtubular intra-axonal flow system. The mitosis inhibitors, colchicine, vinblastine, and vincristine are known to slow down the rate of intra-axonal transport in adrenergic nerves (for references, see Dahlström, 1971). In the present studies systemic colchicine given at the time of denervation was found to delay the onset of the degeneration contraction in a dose-dependent manner. The delaying effect decreased gradually with an increasing time interval between denervation and the injection of colchicine and it was absent when the drug was injected 6 h or more after the operation (Lundberg, 1972b). This may imply that the later colchicine was given, the longer the transport of information had advanced with its normal rate and the less is the chance of the drug to lengthen the total time needed for the transport by slowing down its rate. If this interpretation is correct, the nerve terminals should receive their information after about 5 h, but the degeneration release does not start until about 8 h later. Thus there seems to be two latencies—one which is due to transport of the "axotomy message" and one which relies on the progress of the processes of degeneration localized to the nerve endings. The first latency is colchicine-sensitive and the second tentatively bretylium-sensitive. If the "axotomy message" starts from the site of axotomy immediately and if the distance between the superior cervical ganglion and the periorbital smooth muscle is approximated to 20 mm, the rate of transport is 4 mm/h. This rate is roughly that calculated for the intra-axonal transport of amine storage granules in the rat sciatic nerve, i.e. 5 mm/h (Dahlström and Häggendal, 1966).

The axotomy message transported along the neuron could either be negative such as the absence of matter usually transported or positive consisting of substance formed at the site of axotomy. So far no experiments seem to have solved this problem but both kinds of information may well be conveyed by the microtubular intra-axonal flow system.

REFERENCES

ALMGREN, O., and LUNDBERG, D. (1973) To be published.

BÁRÁNY, E. H., and TREISTER, G. (1970) Time relations of degeneration mydriasis and degeneration vasoconstriction in the rabbit ear after sympathetic denervation: effect of bretylium. *Acta Physiol. scand.* **80**, 79.

BOURA, A. L. A., and GREEN, A. F. (1965) Adrenergic neurone blocking agents. *A. Rev. Pharmac.* **5**, 183.

BRODIE, B. B., CHANG, C. C., and COSTA, E. (1965) On the mechanism of action of guanethidine and bretylium. *Br. J. Pharmac.* **25**, 171.

COATS, D. A., and EMMELIN, N. (1962) The short-term effects of sympathetic ganglionectomy on the cat's salivary secretion. *J. Physiol. Lond.* **162**, 282.

DAHLSTRÖM, A. (1971) Axoplasmic transport. *Phil. Trans.* B, 261.

DAHLSTRÖM, A., and HÄGGENDAL, J. (1966) Studies on the transport and lifespan of amine storage granules in a peripheral adrenergic nerve system. *Acta physiol. scand.* **67**, 278.

EDVINSSON, L., OWMAN, CH., and WEST, K. A. (1971) Changes in cerebral blood volume of mice at various time-periods after superior cervical sympathectomy. *Acta physiol. scand.* **82**, 521.

EMMELIN, N. (1967) Parotid secretion after cutting the auriculotemporal nerve at different levels. *J. Physiol. Lond.* **188**, 44–45P.

EMMELIN, N., and STRÖMBLAD, R. (1957) A transient periodic secretion from the parotid gland after postganglionic, parasympathetic denervation. *J. Physiol. Lond.* **140**, 21–22P.

EMMELIN, N., and OHLIN, P. (1969) Skin temperature of the rabbit ear during degeneration of its sympathetic nerve supply. *Q. J. Exp. Physiol.* **54**, 207.

EMMELIN, N., and TRENDELENBURG, U. (1972) Degeneration activity after parasympathetic or sympathetic denervation. *Rev. Physiol.* **66**, 147.

FURNESS, J. B. (1970) The excitatory input to a single smooth muscle cell. *Pflügers Arch.* **314**, 1.

GEFFEN, L. B., and HUGHES, C. C. (1971) Degeneration of sympathetic nerves *in vitro* and development of smooth muscle supersensitivity to noradrenaline. *J. Physiol. Lond.* **221**, 71.

HAEUSLER, G., HAEFELY, W., and HUERLIMANN, H. (1969) On the mechanism of the adrenergic nerve blocking action of bretylium. *Naunyn-Schmiedeberg's Arch. exp. Path. Pharmak.* **265**, 260.

LANGER, S. Z. (1966) The degeneration contraction of the nictitating membrane in the unanesthetized cat. *J. Pharmac. Exp. Ther.* **151**, 66.

LINNÉR, E. and PRIJOT, E. (1955) Cervical sympathetic ganglionectomy and aqueous flow. *Archs. Ophthal.* **54**, 831.

LUNDBERG, D. (1969a) Adrenergic neuron blockers and transmitter release after sympathetic denervation studied in the conscious rat. *Acta physiol., scand.* **75**, 415.

LUNDBERG, D. (1969b) Effects of some drugs on the bretylium-induced delay of the degeneration release of sympathetic transmitter. *Acta physiol. scand.*, Suppl. 330, 66.

LUNDBERG, D. (1970a) Some aspects of the pharmacology of the degeneration contraction of rat periorbital smooth muscle after sympathetic denervation. *Abstr. Uppsala Diss. Med.* 79.

LUNDBERG, D. (1970b) Interactions between inhibitors of the axonal amine pump and bretylium in the degeneration release of transmitter. *Acta physiol. scand.* **78**, 503.

LUNDBERG, D. (1970c) Bretylium and the degeneration contraction of the sympathetically innervated periorbital smooth muscle in the rat. *Acta physiol. scand.* **79**, 411.

LUNDBERG, D. (1970d) The degeneration contraction of a sympathetically innervated smooth muscle in the rat after reserpine, inhibition of monoamine oxidase or tyrosine hydroxylase. *Acta physiol. scand.* **80**, 107.

LUNDBERG, D. (1970e) Effects of some adrenergic neuron blockers, related quaternary ammonium compounds and guanidine derivatives on degenerating adrenergic nerves in the conscious rat. *Acta physiol. scand.* **80**, 323.

LUNDBERG, D. (1970f) Colchicine-induced delay of the degeneration release of sympathetic transmitter in the conscious rat. *Acta physiol. scand.* **80**, 430.

LUNDBERG, D. (1972a) Bretylium and the supersensitivity to exogenous noradrenaline after sympathetic denervation studied in the conscious rat. *Acta physiol. scand.* **84**, 500.

LUNDBERG, D. (1972b) Effects of colchicine, vinblastine and vincristine on degeneration transmitter release after sympathetic denervation studied in the conscious rat. *Acta physiol. scand.* **85**, 91.

MALMFORS, T., and SACHS, C. (1965) Direct studies on the disappearance of the transmitter and changes in the uptake-storage mechanisms of degenerating adrenergic nerves. *Acta physiol. scand.* **64**, 211.

PLUCHINO, S., VAN ORDEN, L. S. III, DRASKOCZY, P. R., LANGER, S. Z., and TRENDELENBURG, U. (1970) The effect of beta-TM 10 on the pharmacological, biochemical and morphological changes induced by denervation of the nictitating membrane of the cat. *J. Pharmac. Exp. Ther.* **151**, 87.

SEARS, M. L., and BÁRÁNY, E. H. (1960) Outflow resistance and adrenergic mechanisms. *Archs. Ophthal.* **64**, 839.

TREISTER, G., and BÁRÁNY, E. H. (1970) The effect of bretylium on the degeneration mydriasis and intraocular pressure decrease in the conscious rabbit after unilateral cervical ganglionectomy. *Invest. Ophthal.* **9**, 343.

TRENDELENBURG, U. (1969) The pharmacological importance of the uptake mechanism for sympathomimetic amines. *Progr. Brain. Res.* **31**, 73.

WRETLIND, K. A. J. (1950) Studies on the pharmacological effects of trimethyl-, methylethyl-, and triethyl-phenylammonium. *Acta physiol. scand.* **20**, 221.

NORADRENALINE NERVE TERMINALS IN THE RAT CEREBRAL CORTEX FOLLOWING LESION OF THE DORSAL NORADRENALINE PATHWAY: A STUDY ON THE TIME COURSE OF THEIR DISAPPEARANCE

PETER LIDBRINK

Department of Histology, Karolinska Institutet, Stockholm, Sweden

THE nucleus locus coeruleus in the dorsolateral tegmentum of the pons is mainly composed of noradrenaline (NA) containing nerve cells (Dahlström and Fuxe, 1964). These nerve cells send fibers ascending through the mediodorsal reticular formation in the mesencephalon, where they are assembled in the "dorsal NA pathway" (Ungerstedt, 1971; Olson and Fuxe, 1971; Maeda and Shimizu, 1972). The fibers end among other places in the cerebral cortex with a diffuse network of NA containing terminals (Fuxe *et al.*, 1968; Ungerstedt, 1971).

When 6-hydroxydopamine (6-OH-DA) is introduced into the brain close to catecholamine (CA) axons, this drug may produce a rather specific axotomy of CA neurons (Ungerstedt, 1968), and such a lesion of the dorsal NA pathway leads to a complete disappearance of the NA nerve terminals of the cerebral cortex (Ungerstedt, 1971) as seen histochemically in smear preparations from that area.

An analysis of the acute and chronic effects on uptake, storage, and synthesizing properties of the cortical NA nerve terminals after axotomy with 6-OH-DA has now been made. It was also of interest to compare the different methods in estimating the effects of lesions of the dorsal NA pathway.

About 2 weeks after the injection of 6-OH-DA (8 μg/4 ml) into or in the close vicinity of the dorsal NA pathway, the green fluorescent CA varicosities can no longer be detected in smear preparations from the ipsilateral neocortical areas (mainly the parietal, temporal, and occipital regions) (Fig. 1c). No changes are seen in the hypothalamus or the preoptic area. The disappearance of fluorescent varicosities is accompanied by a reduction of the NA content by about 90% as compared to the intact side (Fig. 2, left), whereas a bilateral lesion of the dorsal NA pathway produces an almost 80% reduction of the NA content in the whole forebrain (tel- and diencephalon) (Fig. 2, right). These results show that the

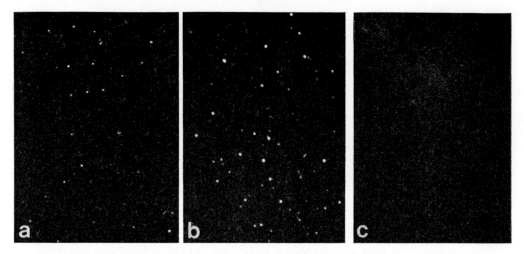

FIG. 1. Smears from the cerebral cortex prepared for fluorescence histochemistry (see Olson and Ungerstedt, 1970). (a) Control rat. Many green fluorescent varicosities evenly spread out over the smear can be seen. (×180.) (b) Lesioned rat acute. The smear exhibits an increased number and intensity of green fluorescent varicosities. (×180.) (c) Lesioned rat chronic. Green fluorescent varicosities can no longer be detected. (×180.)

NA AFTER 6-OH-DA INDUCED LESIONS OF THE DORSAL NA PATHWAY

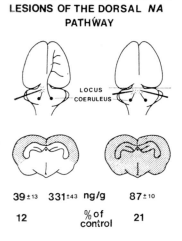

FIG. 2. Determination of NA in the forebrain after 6-OH-DA. The upper part shows the approximate place of injection of 6-OH-DA (8 μg per 4 μl); the NA pathway from the locus coeruleus is lesioned unilaterally and bilaterally respectively. The transverse sections below depict the areas taken for the determination of NA in each case, and on the bottom the concentration of NA after respective treatment.

major portion of the NA neurons in the forebrain probably travel via the dorsal pathway and originate in the locus coeruleus.

The site of injection of 6-OH-DA in the mesencephalic reticular formation was examined both with fluorescence histochemistry and with ordinary histology. With the former method it is possible to study the effects primarily in the acute stage when the unspecific damage to the brain tissue produced by 6-OH-DA and the specific effects on the NA containing axons

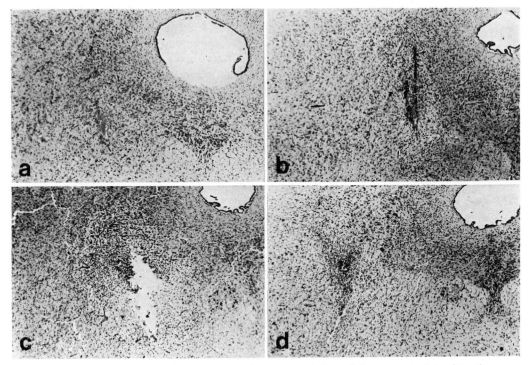

FIG. 3. Site of injection of 6-OH-DA in the mesencephalon of the rat ventrolateral to the central grey area; (a) From a rat which had received 6-OH-DA (8 μg/4 μl) 2 days earlier. Only the end of the needle trace can be detected. (b) Same procedure as in (a). More tissue has been engaged and shows degenerative signs and microglial infiltration especially along the needle trace. Most animals show this degree of tissue damage after 6-OH-DA injection. (c) Same procedure as in (a). A rather large cavity surrounded by necrotic tissue is observed in a few animals. (d) Taken from a rat which received 6-OH-DA (16 μg/8 μl) about a month earlier. Despite this quite large dose of 6-OH-DA, the remaining scar from the unspecific necrotizing effects of the drug is minimal and shows a small area with dense gliosis.

are seen. The unspecific necrosis generally consists of a small hole surrounded by auto-fluorescent pigments and some degenerating nerve cells. Caudally to the lesion the axons exhibit a strong green fluorescence due to pile up of NA. The axons can be traced back to the locus coeruleus. In the chronic animals, these phenomena have disappeared, and the effects of the 6-OH-DA injection can no longer be observed. The unspecific effects are more readily seen on cresyl-violet-stained sections. Generally, a small area with microglial infiltration, red blood corpuscles, and necrosis of the tissue is observed (Fig. 3a, b). Often the trace of the injection needle is also seen. Sometimes the injection produces a quite large lesion although the same concentration and volume of 6-OH-DA is used (Fig. 3c). This also occurs at other injection sites, since Hökfelt and Ungerstedt (1973) have reported such variability in unspecific effects after injection of 6-OH-DA into the substantia nigra. In chronic animals the lesion always looks very small with gliosis and disappearance of some nerve cells (Fig. 3d). Whereas Poirier *et al.* (1972) presented great unspecific effects of 6-OH-DA when injected intracerebrally in the cat, the results of this study and that of Hökfelt and Ungerstedt (1973) show that in most cases degeneration of CA axons and terminals can be obtained with very limited unspecific effects in the rat.

The time course of the degeneration of the NA nerve terminals in the cortex after a unilateral lesion of the dorsal NA pathway was followed by studying the decline in amine storage capacity and membrane pump function in three different ways.

(1) *Visualization of the cortical NA nerve terminals* with the fluorescence histochemical technique of Falck and Hillarp (Falck *et al.*, 1962) on tissue smears from various cortical regions (Olson and Ungerstedt, 1970; Lidbrink and Jonsson, 1971). The number and intensity of the varicosities were estimated.

(2) *Endogenous content of NA*, measured at various time intervals after the lesion with the enzymatic method of Saelens *et al.* (1967) or with a fluorimetric method (Bertler *et al.*, 1958).

(3) *Uptake of ^{3}H-NA* into slices of various regions of the cerebral cortex (Lidbrink and Farnebo, 1973).

ESTIMATION OF FLUORESCENCE IN CORTICAL SMEARS AFTER UNI-LATERAL *6-OH-DA* INDUCED LESIONS OF THE DORSAL *NA* PATHWAY

TIME AFTER LESION	INTACT SIDE	LESIONED
4h	3+	4+
2d	3+	4+
5d	3+	3+
10d	3+	1+
15d	3+	0
90d	3+	0

FIG. 4. 3+ = normal fluorescence of the controls. 4+ = increased number and intensity of green fluorescent varicosities. 1+ = a few remaining green varicosities. 0 = no or practically no green fluorescent varicosities observed.

At least two of the methods were employed on the same animal, either fluorescence histochemistry and NA determinations, or fluorescence histochemistry and NA uptake.

The estimation of fluorescence in smears from the cerebral cortex (mostly the parietal and temporal regions) reveals that acutely after the lesion there is an increased fluorescence intensity in the NA varicosities on the ipsilateral side of the lesion (Figs. 1b and 4). Gradually, the number of green fluorescent dots decrease, and after 15 days no terminals can be observed. These changes are accompanied by corresponding changes in the endogenous levels of NA. During the acute phase an increased concentration of NA is seen, and thereafter, due to the degeneration, the content of NA falls down to about 10% (Fig. 5).

The effect of the lesion on uptake of ^{3}H-NA (10^{-7} M, 5 min) is evident already after 5 days (Fig. 6). After 15 days the uptake of ^{3}H-NA is about 35% of the contralateral control side and remains at this value up to 50 days. The uptake of ^{3}H-metaraminol (MA) (10^{-7} M, 5 min), however, is only affected in the chronic animal and is then decreased to about 60–70% of the control. No effect or a slight enhancement of the uptake of ^{3}H-5-hydroxytryptamine (5-HT) (10^{-7} M, 5 min) is seen.

Based on these curves, two phases of the degeneration can be distinguished: the acute (up to 2 day) and the chronic (15 days or more).

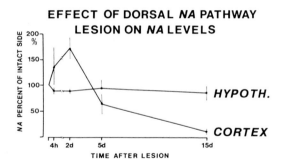

FIG. 5. NA was determined according to the method of Saelens *et al.* (1967). Vertical bars = SEM.

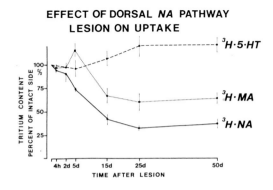

FIG. 6. Slices from the cerebral cortex of unilaterally lesioned animals were preincubated in Krebs–Ringer bicarbonate buffer for 10 min before either of ^{3}H-5-HT, ^{3}H-NA, or ^{3}H-MA was added to make a final concentration of 10^{-7} M. After 5 min, incubation was terminated and total tritium determined. Vertical bars = SEM.

The acute increase in concentration of NA in the cortical NA neurons after axotomy is similar to that found in other CA neurons, e.g. in adrenergic neurons (Sedvall, 1964) or in central DA neurons Andén *et al.*, 1972). Korf *et al.* (1973) have also recently observed such an elevation of NA levels in the cortex acutely after a mechanical lesion involving the dorsal NA pathway.

Although the three methods for estimating the disappearance of NA nerve terminals in the cortex give similar results, there is a certain discrepancy as to the absolute value. Whereas practically no green fluorescent varicosities can be detected in smears and the concomitant determination of NA yields only 10–15% of the control, the uptake of ^{3}H-NA into cortical slices is about 35% as compared to the control. Does this residual uptake depict remaining NA nerve terminals or does it take place in other structures? To test these possibilities several different experiments have been performed.

It is known that 5-HT terminals exist in the cortex (Fuxe, 1965), and these may interfere with the uptake of NA, but when performing uptake studies like these, little NA will enter 5-HT terminals and vice versa provided that the concentration of the amines is low (Shaskan and Snyder, 1970; Lidbrink *et al.*, 1971). This is partly corroborated by the finding that lesion of the dorsal NA pathway does not decrease the uptake of 5-HT (Fig. 6). Furthermore, chlorimipramine, which strongly inhibits the uptake of 5-HT, is only a weak inhibitor of NA uptake into slices from the cortex lacking NA nerve terminals. These results make it unlikely that the remaining uptake of NA takes place in 5-HT nerve terminals.

Since the total tritium generally has been calculated in the uptake studies, it is possible that the labeled NA taken up into the denervated slices in fact represents metabolites. This can be ruled out, however, since separation on thin layer chromatography reveals that 80–90% of the total tritium content represents unchanged NA both in denervated and in intact slices.

If slices from the cerebral cortex are incubated with labeled NA for a longer period of time (30 min) followed by rinsing in NA-free media, this will give an index of the capacity of the nerve terminals to accumulate and retain NA. Figure 7 shows that in the chronically denervated cortex, this ability is decreased as compared to the control, since the wash out of NA is more rapid. This suggests that in the denervated slices at least some of the NA taken up is differently bound.

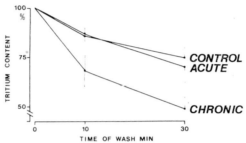

RETENTION OF $^3H \cdot NA$ AFTER LESION OF THE DORSAL *NA* PATHWAY

FIG. 7. Slices from the cerebral cortex of unilaterally lesioned animals were preincubated (10 min), incubated in ^{3}H-NA (10^{-7} M) for 30 min and then washed in fresh buffer for 10 or 30 min to let the slices spontaneously release tritium. The remaining tritium in the slices was determined and calculated as per cent of the tritium at the beginning of wash. Vertical bars = SEM.

If denervated and intact cortical slices are incubated with tritium labeled DA or tyrosine for 30–60 min, it is possible to study the formation of ^{3}H-NA from ^{3}H-DA and ^{3}H-NA and ^{3}H-DA from ^{3}H-tyrosine respectively. When labeled DA is used, the uptake of DA into slices from the parietal region is not affected by a dorsal NA pathway lesion, while the formation of NA from DA is only about 15% of the control. This value corresponds to the endogenous content of NA (Fig. 5). The same degree of formation of NA in the parietal cortex is also obtained from tyrosine.

This further indicates that the value obtained by incubating denervated slices for 5 min in ^{3}H-NA (35% of control) does not truly represent the amount of remaining NA nerve terminals. Part of it is probably located in other structures, e.g. non-NA nerve terminals or extraneuronal sites capable of loosely binding NA.

In agreement, desmethylimipramine (DMI), which strongly inhibits the uptake of NA into NA nerve terminals, is much less potent as an inhibitor of NA uptake in denervated slices than it is in intact.

Recently, Thierry *et al.* (1973) have proposed the existence of DA nerve terminals in the cortex on the basis of biochemical findings, and by means of certain pharmacological models, which rather selectively allows the visualization of DA neurons and terminals

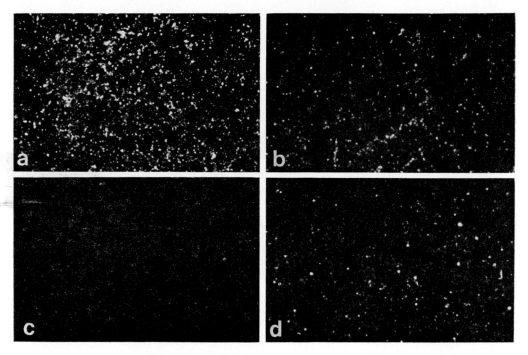

FIG. 8. Smears prepared from slices from reserpine-pretreated rats (10 mg/kg, 16–20 h). The slices were incubated in Krebs–Ringer bicarbonate buffer containing DL-NA HCl (10^{-5} M). For details, see Lidbrink et al. (1974). (a) Caudate nucleus. A very high density of green fluorescent varicosities can be seen. ($\times$180.) (b) Cingulate gyrus. Many green fluorescent varicosities are seen. ($\times$180.) (c) Parietal cortex. Only a few varicosities with green fluorescence can be detected. ($\times$180.) (d) Entorhinal cortex. A moderate number of green fluorescent varicosities are present. (From Lidbrink et al., 1974.)

histochemically, DA nerve terminals have been found in certain regions of the cortex (Fuxe et al., 1973; Lidbrink et al., 1974). The latter studies suggest that the cortical DA nerve terminals are most numerous in the phylogenetically older cortices (e.g. cingulum, pre-pyriform, and amygdaloid cortex and the hippocampal formation), while they are relatively few in the neocortical regions (Fig. 8).

Thus it is possible that part of the uptake of NA resistant to dorsal NA pathway lesions takes place in cortical DA nerve terminals. It should be pointed out, however, that neo-cortical smears prepared for fluorescence histochemistry from lesioned animals show practically no green varicosities (Figs. 1c and 4), whereas smears from the cingulate gyrus or the entorhinal cortex show many such varicosities. These terminals may contain DA in view of the findings of Fuxe et al. (1973) and Lidbrink et al. (1974).

To conclude, the transection of the axons from the NA containing cells of the locus coeruleus at the level of the dorsal NA pathway with intracerebrally administered 6-OH-DA is associated with certain changes in the levels of NA in the cerebral cortex. Acutely, the NA concentration rise before it gradually decreases as a consequence of the anterograde degener-ation. The degeneration appears to be completed after about 2 weeks. Also due to the degeneration, the uptake of tritium labeled NA into slices from the cerebral cortex pro-gressively decrease. This decrement is, however, not as pronounced as the fall in NA levels, suggesting the existence of other structures capable to take up NA, possibly cortical DA nerve terminals.

By applying fluorescence histochemistry, biochemical assay of NA or determination of uptake capacity of NA in certain defined regions of the cortex it is possible to get a good picture on the degree of and extent of the effects on NA nerve terminals produced by lesion of the dorsal NA pathway.

ACKNOWLEDGEMENTS

This investigation has been supported by research grants from the Swedish Medical Research Council (04X-715, 14X-2295) and Karolinska Institutets Forskningsfonder. The skilful work of Mrs. Agneta Eliasson and Miss Beth Hagman is gratefully acknowledged.

REFERENCES

ANDÉN, N.-E., BÉDARD, P., FUXE, K., and UNGERSTEDT, U. (1972) Early and selective increase in brain dopamine levels after axotomy. *Experientia* **28**, 300–301.

BERTLER, Å., CARLSSON, A., and ROSENGREN, E. (1958) A method for the fluorimetric determination of adrenaline and noradrenaline in tissues. *Acta physiol. scand.* **44**, 273–292.

DAHLSTRÖM, A., and FUXE, K. (1964) Evidence for the existence of monoamine containing neurons in the central nervous system: I, Demonstration of monoamines in the cell-bodies of brain stem neurons. *Acta physiol. scand.* **62**, Suppl. 232.

FALCK, B., HILLARP, N.-Å., THIEME, G., and TORP, A. (1962) Fluorescence of catecholamines and related compounds condensed with formaldehyde. *J. Histochem. Cytochem.* **10**, 348–354.

FUXE, K. (1965) Evidence for the existence of monoamine neurons in the central nervous system. IV. Distribution of monoamine nerve terminals in the central nervous system. *Acta physiol. scand.* **64**, Suppl. 247, 27–85.

FUXE, K., HAMBERGER, B., and HÖKFELT, T. (1968) Distribution of noradrenaline nerve terminals in cortical areas of the rat. *Brain Res.* **8**, 125–131.

FUXE, K., GOLDSTEIN, M., HÖKFELT, T., JONSSON, G., and LIDBRINK, P. (1973) Dopaminergic involvement in hypothalamic function: extrahypothalamic and hypothalamic control: a neuroanatomical analysis. Conference on Parkinson's Disease, Princeton, 1973.

HÖKFELT, T., and UNGERSTEDT, U. (1973) Specificity of 6-hydroxydopamine induced degeneration of central monoamine neurons: an electron and fluorescence microscopic study with special reference to intercerebral injection on the nigro-striatal dopamine system. *Brain Res.* **60**, 269–297.

KORF, J., ROTH, R. H., and AGHAJANIAN, G. K. (1973) Alteration in turnover and endogenous levels of norepinephrine in cerebral cortex following electrical stimulation and acute axotomy of cerebral noradrenergic pathways. *Eur. J. Pharmac.* **23**, 276–282.

LIDBRINK, P., and JONSSON, G. (1971) Semiquantitative estimation of formaldehyde-induced fluorescence of noradrenaline in central noradrenaline nerve terminals. *J. Histochem. Cytochem.* **19**, 747–757.

LIDBRINK, P., and FARNEBO, L.-O. (1973) Uptake and release of noradrenaline in rat cerebral cortex *in vitro*: no effect of benzodiazepines and barbiturates. *Neuropharmacol.* **12**, 1087–1095.

LIDBRINK, P., JONSSON, G., and FUXE, K. (1971) The effect of imipramine-like drugs and antihistamine drugs on uptake mechanisms in the central noradrenaline and 5-hydroxytryptamine neurons. *Neuropharmacology* **10**, 521–536.

LIDBRINK, P., JONSSON, G., and FUXE, K. (1974) Selective reserpine-resistant accumulation of catecholamines in central dopamine neurons after DOPA administration. *Brain Res.* **67**, 439–456.

MAEDA, T., and SHIMIZU, N. (1972) Projections ascendantes du locus coeruleus et d'autres neurones aminergiques pontiques au niveau du prosencéphale du rat. *Brain Res.* **36**, 19–35.

OLSON, L., and UNGERSTEDT, U. (1970) Monoamine fluorescence in CNS smears: sensitive and rapid visualization of nerve terminals without freeze-drying. *Brain Res.* **17**, 343–347.

OLSON, L., and FUXE, K. (1971) On the projections from the locus coeruleus noradrenaline neurons: the cerebellar innervation. *Brain Res.* **28**, 165–171.

POIRIER, L. J., LANGELIER, P., ROBERGE, A., BOUCHER, R., and KITSIKIS, A. (1972) Non-specific histopathological changes induced by the intracerebral injection of 6-hydroxydopamine (6-OH-DA). *J. Neurol. Sci.* **16**, 401–416.

SAELENS, J. K., SCHOEN, M. S., and KOVACSICS, G. B. (1967) An enzyme assay for norepinephrine in brain tissue. *Biochem. Pharmac.* **16**, 1043–1049.

SEDVALL, G. (1964) Noradrenaline storage in skeletal muscle. *Acta physiol. scand.* **60**, 39–50.

SHASKAN, E. G., and SNYDER, S. H. (1970) Kinetics of serotonin accumulation into slices from rat brain: Relationship to catecholamine uptake. *J. Pharmac. Exp. Ther.* **175**, 404–418.

THIERRY, A. M., STINUS, L., BLANC, G., and GLOWINSKI, J. (1973) Some evidence for the existence of dopaminergic neurons in the rat cortex. *Brain Res.* **50**, 230–234.

UNGERSTEDT, U. (1968) 6-hydroxydopamine induced degenerations of central monoamine neurons. *Eur. J. Pharmac.* **5**, 107–110.

UNGERSTEDT, U. (1971) Stereotaxic mapping of the monoamine pathways in the rat brain. *Acta physiol. scand.*, Suppl. 367, 1–48.

DEGENERATION PROCESSES IN PERIPHERAL AND CENTRAL NEURONS

SESSION II

Chairman: O. ERÄNKÖ

STUDIES ON THE NEUROTOXIC PROPERTIES
OF HYDROXYLATED TRYPTAMINES

H. G. Baumgarten, A. Björklund, A. S. Horn,
and H. G. Schlossberger

Department of Neuroanatomy, University of Hamburg, W. Germany; Department of Histology, University of Lund, Lund, Sweden; MRC Neurochemical Pharmacology Unit, Department of Pharmacology, Cambridge, England;
Max-Planck-Institut für Biochemie, Martinsried bei München, W. Germany

A. INTRODUCTION

Porter *et al.* (1963) originally demonstrated that the hydroxyderivative of dopamine 3,4,6-trihydroxyphenylethylamine (6-hydroxydopamine, 6-OH-DA) caused—following its intraperitoneal injection—a long-lasting depletion of noradrenaline (NA)† from the sympathetically innervated mouse heart. Their observations were confirmed and extended by Laverty *et al.* (1965) who also reported a transitory depletion of hypothalamic NA after systemic application of this compound in the kitten. The remarkable, long-lasting action of 6-OH-DA remained unexplained until Thoenen and Tranzer (1968) showed with the electron microscope that 6-OH-DA caused degeneration of adrenergic nerve terminals in several organs without causing concomitant damage to intermingled cholinergic nerve fibers. Subsequently, Ungerstedt (1968) and Uretsky and Iversen (1969) applied 6-OH-DA to the brain ventricles and gained morphological and chemical evidence for a similar, selective toxic effect of 6-OH-DA on central catecholamine (CA) neurons in the rat. These findings provided the basis for a new, exciting approach to study the anatomy and function of defined neuronal systems in the brain and in peripheral organs of experimental animals: the method of selective lesioning of neurons characterized by individual, defined transmitters. Especially in the brain where mechanical interruption of pathways is never selective—due to intricate intermingling of axons of different origin, destination, and transmitter type—this new technique offers highly interesting possibilities for correlative studies on projection of individual CA neurons and their role in brain-controlled body functions and on neuronal interrelationships and functional interdependence in the central nervous system itself.

†Abbreviations: Catecholamine, CA; dopamine, DA; noradrenaline, NA; dihydroxytryptamine, DHT; hydroxytryptamine, HT; indoleamine, IA.

Considerations of the chemical properties of 6-OH-DA lead us to design comparable hydroxylated tryptamine derivatives that might more or less selectively damage 5-hydroxy-tryptamine-containing (5-HT; serotonin) neurons. From all the potentially neurotoxic dihydroxylated indole-amines (4,5, 5,6-, 6,7-, 4,6-, 4,7-, and 5,7-DHT), those sharing with serotonin the hydroxyl group in position 5 of the indole nucleus were supposed to be the most selective compounds (4,5-, 5,6-, and 5,7-DHT). Among these, 5,6-DHT was hypo-thesized to be the most suitable for the induction of selective disintegration of 5-HT neurons, since 6-HT had earlier been shown to have a good affinity for the membrane-bound mono-amine uptake system of 5-HT neurons (Jonsson et al., 1969) and would thus presumably not severely interfere with the uptake properties of the 5-hydroxyl group in the 5,6-DHT molecule.

The administration of 5,6-DHT to the lateral ventricle of rats led to the discovery by Baumgarten et al. (1971) of a rather selective and long-lasting depletion of 5-HT from various brain regions and from the spinal cord, a finding which was confirmed in a separate investigation of brain monoamine and 5-hydroxyindole acetic acid content, amine uptake inhibition and tyrosine hydroxylase activity in the rat CNS by Baumgarten et al., (1972b).

Parallel studies on the morphology of IA-containing neurons in the rat brain (Baum-garten and Lachenmayer 1972a; Baumgarten et al., 1972a,c; Björklund et al., 1973b) revealed degenerative events in terminal, and signs of a toxic reaction in non-terminal, IA axons following the application of 5,6-DHT.

The careful and extensive chemical and morphological work on the effects of 5,6-DHT on brain and spinal cord (literature cited above) revealed certain limitations in the applic-ability of 5,6-DHT as a tool for degeneration of IA neurons in brain. Firstly, 5,6-DHT was found to be selective for IA neurons only in a restricted dose range (10–75 μg). Secondly, doses higher than 75 μg caused damage to central NA and DA neurons in addition to IA ones and were severely toxic, provoking convulsions, limb paralysis, and tremor in the pre-treated animals. Thirdly, all doses of 5,6-DHT tested (25, 50, 75, and 100 μg) induced moderate to severe damage to myelinated axons, either confined to the brain regions surrounding the tip of the injection cannula (all doses) or to myelinated tracts near the surface (e.g. the pyramidal tract and decussation at the ventral aspect of the medulla oblongata, with 75 or 100 μg; see Nobin et al., 1973). Finally, part of the drug was found to be prevented from reaching specific uptake sites in brain due to rapid conversion of 5,6-DHT into a brownish pigment soon after its intraventricular injection. As will be discussed in further detail below (paragraph 7), this chemical lability probably provides 5,6-DHT with rather limited diffusion capacity, an assumption which receives support from studies on the penetration and fate of labeled 5,6-DHT in brain (Baumgarten et al., unpublished ob-servations). The chemical data on the depletion of 5-HT in individual brain regions also suggest that part of the 5-HT neurons in brain are not reached by 5,6-DHT in doses up to 75 μg. Thus a near total destruction of 5-HT axons cannot be accomplished with 5,6-DHT after its intraventricular administration. This limitation to the intraventricular administra-tion of 5,6-DHT is, however, largely overcome when the drug is injected directly into the brain parenchyma, close to the indoleamine fiber bundles (Björklund et al., 1973c). With such local injections more complete denervation can be achieved with 5,6-DHT without the production of any substantial unspecific damage. Moreover, the regeneration of IA axons, which is very prominent after intraventricular injections (Baumgarten et al., 1973b; Björklund et al., 1973a), is probably much slower and more limited after the local, intra-cerebral injections.

These studies prompted us to test other dihydroxyindoles for their potential neurotoxicity against CNS monoamine neurons that might not be complicated by the drawbacks noted with 5,6-DHT. In addition, several monohydroxytryptamines were investigated with the same methods in order to clarify whether or not two hydroxyl substituents on the benzene nucleus of the indole molecule are required for toxicity against CNS monoamine neurons.

B. EVALUATION OF THE SELECTIVE TOXICITY OF HYDROXYINDOLES AGAINST DIFFERENT MONOAMINE NEURONS

1. UPTAKE SITE AFFINITY, STUDIED *IN VITRO* AS INHIBITION OF UPTAKE

The selectivity of action of the transmitter analogs tested for their potential neurotoxicity in all probability depends on their active uptake, concentration, and retention by the different monoamine neurons. The absorption and accumulation of the neurotransmitter analogs are mediated by the membrane-bound, energy-dependent transport mechanism which has—at low concentrations of the amine—a high degree of selectivity for the natural substrate. Thus exogenous 5-HT is preferentially taken up and accumulated by 5-HT neurons when added *in vitro* to slices of rat hypothalamus in concentrations of 1×10^{-7} M or less (see Shaskan and Snyder, 1970) despite the presence of considerable amounts of NA and DA terminals in the same tissue. Since uptake occurs mainly into nerve terminals it can be measured also in synaptosome fractions (see Coyle and Snyder, 1969) of homogenates from hypothalamus (for 5-HT and NA uptake) or striatum (for DA uptake), where little metabolism takes place and uptake increases linearly at least during the first 10 min of incubation. For 5-HT uptake, the IC-50 values (concentration of indoleamine causing a 50% inhibition of the uptake of radioactive 5-HT) were measured. These are approximately equal to the Ki values when a low concentration of 1×10^{-7} M ^{3}H-5-HT is used (Table 1). For NA and DA uptake, the analogs were tested at a fixed concentration of 1×10^{-6} or 1×10^{-5} M, using 1×10^{-7} M ^{3}H-CA (Table 2) (for details, see Horn, 1973; Horn *et al.*, 1973).

The results shown in the Table 1 reveal that of the compounds tested, 5,6-DHT is the most selective inhibitor of ^{3}H-5-HT uptake into synaptosomes of rat hypothalamus. Similar

TABLE 1. AFFINITY OF VARIOUS HYDROXYLATED TRYPTA-
MINES FOR THE 5-HT UPTAKE SITES, MEASURED AS THE
CONCENTRATION OF THE COMPOUND CAUSING 50% INHIBI-
TION OF THE ^{3}H-5-HT UPTAKE BY SYNAPTOSOMES
PREPARED FROM RAT HYPOTHALAMUS
Data from Horn *et al.* (1973) and unpublished results

Compound	5-HT uptake IC-50
5,6-DHT	6.0×10^{-7} M
6-HT	8.0×10^{-7} M
4,5-DHT	1.7×10^{-6} M
7-HT	2.8×10^{-6} M
5,7-DHT	4.0×10^{-6} M
6,7-DHT	4.4×10^{-6} M
4-HT	4.5×10^{-6} M
4-OH-5-CH$_3$O-T	5.6×10^{-6} M

results have been obtained on slices of rat hypothalamus by Baumgarten *et al.* (1972b) and Heikkila and Cohen (1973). 5,6-DHT is closely followed by 6-HT, which has been suggested as a marker for serotonergic neurons by Jonsson *et al.* (1969). 4,5-DHT has quite a good affinity for the 5-HT uptake sites, whereas 5,7-DHT is more than six times less potent than 5,6-DHT. 7-HT competes for uptake sites in 5-HT neurons only slightly better than 5,7-DHT and both are more potent in inhibiting 5-HT uptake than 4-HT and 6,7-DHT. Methylation of the 5-hydroxyl group in 4,5-DHT, which gives 4-hydroxy-5-methoxy-tryptamine (4-OH-5-CH$_3$OT), results in a more than threefold decrease in uptake site affinity. This compound, which is highly interesting since it is the only monohydroxylated tryptamine that causes almost selective toxic damage to CNS 5-HT neurons (Baumgarten and Lachenmayer, unpublished), inhibits the uptake of ^{3}H-5-HT only very weakly.

Some important conclusions regarding the specificity of action and the molecular mechanism of action of toxic and nontoxic IAs can be drawn from these findings. None of the tryptamine derivatives tested has such a high affinity for the 5-HT uptake system as exogenous 5-HT itself. The most specific compound with a Ki close to 5-HT is 5,6-DHT, which according to the theoretical considerations, was presumed to be the most favorable drug for chemical degeneration of serotonin neurons. For optimum binding to the membrane transport system, the presence of a 5-hydroxyl group is an important prerequisite in the DHTs as revealed, e.g., by the significantly decreased uptake site affinity of the 5-*O*-methylated analog 4-OH-5-CH$_3$OT in comparison to 4,5-DHT, or as noted by the comparatively low inhibition of 5-HT uptake by 6,7-DHT. A catechol-like, *ortho* arrangement of the hydroxyl groups in 5,6- and 4,5-DHT seems to favor uptake site affinity, whereas a *meta* substitution of the hydroxyl groups, realized in, e.g., 5,7-DHT, decreases uptake affinity despite the presence of one of the OH groups in the optimum position (5-position). The observation of a progressive decrease in uptake site affinity with the OH-group being increasingly displaced from the 5-position (5-HT > 6-HT > 7-HT) suggests that the 5-OH group is an important factor in the binding of the indole molecule to the 5-HT uptake sites. As seen from Table 2, all tryptamine derivatives compete more or less well for uptake sites in NA or DA neurons, and the difference in binding affinity of a given compound for 5-HT uptake, on the one hand, and NA or DA uptake, on the other hand, is sometimes rather small.

TABLE 2. RELATIVE AFFINITY OF VARIOUS HYDROXYLATED TRYPTAMINES FOR THE 5-HT, NA, AND DA UPTAKE SITES, MEASURED AS THE PERCENTAGE INHIBITION CAUSED BY THE COMPOUNDS AT A FIXED CONCENTRATION (10^{-6} or 10^{-7} M).
The uptake was measured into synaptosomes prepared from rat hypothalamus (^{3}H-5-HT and ^{3}H-NA) or striatum (^{3}H-DA). In the table the order is for decreasing potency (IC 50 values) in inhibiting 5-HT uptake. Data from Horn *et al.* (1973).

Concentration of hydroxylated tryptamine		% inhibition of uptake		
		5-HT (hypothalamus)	NA (hypothalamus)	DA (corpus striatum)
1 μM	5,6	59.0	43.3	44.7
10 μM	4,5	74.4	32.0	34.3
1 μM	7	32.5	60.8	51.1
1 μM	5,7	25.7	32.5	15.4
10 μM	6,7	67.5	30.1	15.6
10 μM	4	71.7	43.0	15.3
10 μM	4,5-methoxy	54.1	36.6	8.3

This implies that most tryptamines in general have a rather good affinity for CA-uptake sites and are not as selective for 5-HT uptake as CA analogs are for NA uptake (e.g. 6-OH-DA). Therefore, specific effects of tryptamines on 5-HT neurons can be expected only in a very limited dose range and unselective side effects on CA neurons are more likely to occur than with toxic CA analogs at 5-HT neurons (e.g. no inhibition of uptake of ^{3}H-5-HT by 6-OH-DA at 10^{-7} to 10^{-4} M: Heikkila and Cohen, 1973).

2. UPTAKE IMPAIRMENT AS A MEASURE OF POTENTIAL TOXICITY AGAINST MONOAMINE NEURONS, STUDIED *IN VITRO*

Short-term exposure to ^{3}H-5-HT of brain slices that have been preincubated with the tryptamine derivatives for 30 min has been used in a study by Djörklund *et al.* (1973d) as a means of evaluating the direct potential neurotoxicity of the compounds, since neuronal uptake is known to be a sensitive indicator of the functional integrity of monoamine neurons. Uptake impairment under these experimental conditions will be indicated by a reduction in uptake and retention of ^{3}H-5-HT or ^{3}H-NA by the tissue slices in a subsequent 10 min incubation, whereas nontoxic competition to uptake is not measured due to a thorough washout of the tested compounds prior to the ^{3}N-5-HT or ^{3}H-NA incubation (for methodological details, see Björklund *et al.*, 1973d).

No reduction in the short-term uptake of ^{3}H-5-HT is seen on preincubation in 10^{-5} M cold 5-HT, 4-HT, 6-HT, or 4-OH-5-CH$_3$OT, whereas a significant impairment of ^{3}H-5-HT retention is observed with 10^{-5} M 6,7-, 5,6-, 5,7-, and 4,5-DHT (Table 3). At either 10^{-5} or 10^{-6} M, 5,7-DHT proves to be the most potent drug to impair the subsequent ^{3}H-5-HT uptake, closely followed by 5,6-DHT. The difference in percentage uptake impairment between 10^{-6} and 10^{-5} M is negligible with both compounds, indicating that they exert toxic effects on the membrane-bound uptake mechanism of 5-HT neurons already at low concentrations. This is clearly different from 6,7- and 4,5-DHT which both impair 5-HT uptake to a substantial degree only at a concentration of 10^{-5} M in the preincubation medium.

As already suggested by the data on the relative uptake site affinity of the various HTs for CA uptake systems, the DHTs also impair the NA uptake mechanism, at either concentration tested (10^{-6} or 10^{-5} M), except 5,6-DHT which thus proves to be remarkably selective also in this respect. Also with the other DHTs tested, 6,7-, 5,7-, and 4,5-DHT, the impairment of ^{3}H-NA uptake is lower than the impairment of ^{3}H-5-HT uptake, implying a preferential action on 5-HT neurons.

The figures obtained in this study therefore suggest that all DHTs investigated so far are candidates for a direct chemical degeneration of 5-HT neurons (and to a variable extent also NA neurons). If we compare the order of potency for uptake site competition of the DHTs (5,6-DHT > 4,5-DHT > 5,7-DHT > 6,7-DHT) with that of uptake impairment (5,7-DHT > 5,6-DHT > 6,7-DHT > 4,5-DHT) with respect to ^{3}H-5-HT uptake, it becomes evident that the two orders do not agree. This is furthermore supported by the morphological finding of 4-OH-5-CH$_3$OT as a compound which induces selective alterations in 5-HT axons suggestive of damage, a finding not expressed in either the data on relative uptake affinity nor on uptake impairment. Thus each of the two parameters evidently does not serve as an entirely reliable measure of the potential toxic action of the HTs on monoaminergic neurons *in vivo*. This becomes even clearer when we analyze the *in vivo* effects of the tryptamine derivatives on the CNS 5-HT, NA, and DA concentrations, and when we consider the morphology of CNS monoamine neurons.

3. MONOAMINE DEPLETION IN BRAIN AND SPINAL CORD

Evaluation of the changes in regional 5-HT, NA, and DA concentrations of rat brain and spinal cord has proven to give a very informative picture about the effect of the various tryptamines on CNS monoamine neurons, and to nicely correspond to and supplement the morphological alterations seen in these neurons after the intraventricular application of neurotoxic indoleamines. Extensive data on the time course of response of CNS 5-HT, NA, and DA concentrations are so far available for both 5,6- and 5,7-DHT (see Baumgarten et al., 1971, 1972b, 1973a). These biochemical findings supported the idea that both drugs cause acute direct toxic disintegration of ventricle- and surface-near 5-HT terminal systems and indirect, anterograde, protracted degeneration of additional terminal systems, that belong to non-terminal axons primarily damaged by either 5,6- or 5,7-DHT (for details, see also paragraph 5, below). This retarded degeneration process resulted in transient minimum levels of 5-HT (with 5,6- or 5,7-DHT) and NA (with 5,7-DHT) at 10 days after drug administration.

In order to compare the effect of various indoleethylamines on CNS monoamine content, brain and spinal cord samples were analyzed 10 days after the application of 50 μg 4,5-, 5,6-, 5,7-, 6,7-DHT, of 4-OH-5-CH$_3$OT, or of 7-, 6-, or 4-HT (Table 4). The most potent compound in depleting 5-HT from brain and spinal cord is 5,7-DHT, followed by 5,6-DHT, 5,6-diacetoxy-tryptamine (5,6-DAcOT) and 6,7-DHT. The two latter compounds have, however, less effect on 5-HT in spinal cord than 5,6-DHT. The long-term depletion of 5-HT is clearly less after treatment with 4,5-DHT or 4-OH-5-CH$_3$OT. The data for the NA and DA concentrations reveal that 5,6-DHT causes small but significant reductions of both amines, and appears in this respect to be less selective than 5,6-DAcOT. 5,7-DHT markedly affected also brain and spinal cord NA, and in fact the reduction obtained with the present dose (50 μg) was similar for NA and 5-HT in the brain. 4,5-DHT, finally, had its greatest effects on NA in brain and 5-HT in spinal cord, a finding that may be related to the very limited diffusion of this compound in the brain tissue (see below). A comparison of the results on impairment of ^{3}H-5-HT uptake with those on the percentage depletion of 5-HT in brain and spinal cord (Tables 3 and 4) reveals a good correspondence and documents the value of both techniques in studies on the mechanism of action of toxic hydroxyindoles.

TABLE 3. EFFECT OF PREINCUBATION OF THIN SLICES OF RAT CORTEX FOR 30 MIN AT $+37°C$ IN THE PRESENCE OF VARIOUS HYDROXYLATED TRYPTAMINES (10^{-6} OR 10^{-5} M) ON THE UPTAKE OF ^{3}H-5-HT (0.5×10^{-7} M) OR ^{3}H-NA (10^{-7} M) DURING A SUBSEQUENT INCUBATION FOR 10 MIN AT $+37°C$.

The slices were washed in fresh buffer for 20 min at $+37°C$ (buffer changed 3 times) between the two incubations to wash out the cold hydroxylated tryptamines. Data from Björklund et al. (1973d).

Compound	^{3}H-5-HT		^{3}H-NA	
	10^{-5} M	10^{-6} M	10^{-5} M	10^{-6} M
5,7-DHT	-72%	-69%	-15%	-24%
5,6-DHT	-64%	-60%	$+3\%$	$+6\%$
6,7-DHT	-42%	-19%	-12%	-10%
4,5-DHT	-36%	$+21\%$	-13%	-6%
4-OH-5-CH$_3$OT	0%			

TABLE 4. COMPARISON OF THE EFFECTS OF VARIOUS HYDROXYLATED TRYPTAMINES ON WHOLE RAT BRAIN AND SPINAL CORD 5-HT, NA, AND DA CONCENTRATIONS.

The compounds were all injected in a single injection of 50 μg into the lateral ventricle and the animals were killed 8–10 days after injection. Values expressed as percentage of control. Differences from control values: * $= 0.05 > p > 0.01$; ** $= 0.01 > p > 0.001$; *** $= p < 0.001$. Student's t-test.

Compound	Amine concentrations in % of control				
	Brain			Spinal cord	
	5-HT	NA	DA	5-HT	NA
5,6-DHT	56 ± 3***	84 ± 3*	70 ± 3**	12 ± 3***	121 ± 2**
5,7-DHT	48 ± 2***	52 ± 2***	91 ± 10	12 ± 1***	47 ± 6***
4,5-DHT	87 ± 11	52 ± 12***	84 ± 8	42 ± 5***	100 ± 13
6,7-DHT	79 ± 6*	67 ± 4***	103 ± 17	54 ± 7***	95 ± 5
5,6-DAcOT[1]	59 ± 3***	117 ± 5*	93 ± 14	21 ± 3***	158 ± 10*
4-OH-5-CH$_3$OT	85 ± 3**	86 ± 4*	89 ± 16	79 ± 11	126 ± 4*
4-HT	121 ± 7*	105 ± 4	116 ± 15	146 ± 11**	126 ± 13
6-HT	116 ± 6	124 ± 3**	150 ± 11***	125 ± 13	126 ± 5*
7-HT	137 ± 16	100 ± 6	125 ± 9	136 ± 16*	126 ± 11

[1] 5,6-DAcOT = 5,6-diacetoxytryptamine.

4. EFFECT ON CNS TRYPTOPHAN HYDROXYLASE

The most specific enzyme marker for serotoninergic neurons is tryptophan hydroxylase which catalyzes the first step in 5-HT synthesis. Pharmacological blockade of this enzyme, e.g. by *para*-chlorophenylalanine, causes a pronounced decrease in brain 5-HT content since there is, under physiological circumstances, practically no supply of 5-hydroxy-tryptophan to the brain that could compensate for the impairment of tryptophan hydroxylation. Degeneration of 5-HT neurons should—in the event that this enzyme is selectively localized in serotonin neurons—result in a drop in enzyme activity (or loss of enzyme) that roughly parallels the number of neurons, axons, or terminals destroyed by the drug. Conversely, recovery of enzyme activity after a long latency may be compatible with a regeneration of severed 5-HT neurons. Demonstration of a drop in enzyme activity following the application of neurotoxic drugs was therefore regarded as a critical piece of information that would support the idea of neuronal damage by toxic hydroxyindoleamines. In addition, tryptophan hydroxylase was supposed to be a more sensitive and reliable indicator of the number of neurons damaged than 5-HT content, since the apparent serotonin concentration measured is strongly influenced by a number of factors, such as substrate supply, enzyme activity levels, storage capacity and conditions, and metabolism of the transmitter.

The effect of intraventricularly administered 5,6- and 5,7-DHT on regional tryptophan hydroxylase was analyzed in rat brain and spinal cord (Baumgarten *et al.*, 1973b; Victor *et al.*, 1973, 1974). Time-course patterns of activity of tryptophan hydroxylase have been analyzed after one injection of 75 μg 5,6-DHT. With 5,7-DHT, measurements that can be evaluated statistically have been performed so far only 2 and 12 days after the injection of the drug.

The pattern of depletion and recovery of tryptophan hydroxylase varies in different CNS regions. Despite these differences, two principal types of time-course pattern have been distinguished. (1) A gradual protracted drop in enzyme activity between the first and twelfth day that follows an initial rapid reduction in tryptophan hydroxylase activity at 1 h. This simple pattern of response, seen only in the spinal cord after 5,6-DHT, conforms to the pattern of loss of 5-HT from the same region after either 5,6- or 5,7-DHT. Since this pattern of depletion resembles that of 5-HT or enzyme activity in the spinal cord after a mechanical transection of the descending serotonin pathways at a high cervical level (Carlsson et al., 1964; Clineschmidt et al., 1971), it may be explained as signifying a retarded, anterograde degeneration of the spinal cord 5-HT terminal systems due to a primary damage to the nonterminal 5-HT axons. The validity of this explanation has been tested in a detailed fluorescence histochemical study on the bulbospinal indoleamine neuron system, following the intraventricular injection of 5,6-DHT (Nobin et al., 1973). (2) The remaining regions exhibited a complicated, biphasic pattern of enzyme inactivation (or loss of enzyme) and recovery which consists of a rapid, early decline to temporary minimum levels at either 1 h (septum, hypothalamus, mesencephalic tegmentum), 1 day (pons-medulla oblongata, mesencephalic tectum), or 2 days (striatum, forebrain rest sample). This is followed by an early recovery period (between 1 h, 1 day or 2 days, and 4–6 days), a second reduction phase between 4–6 and 9–12 days (late minimum levels), and a late recovery phase (between 9–12 and 60 days; not apparent in all regions, however). This complicated type of drug response probably reflects mutual overlapping and a sequence of different processes occurring at different parts of the indoleamine neurons. The early drop in activity at 1 h may be explained by a direct toxic inactivation of the enzyme by the injected 5,6-DHT. This interpretation is supported by in vitro studies on the effect of 5,6-DHT on partially purified tryptophan hydroxylase (Victor et al., unpublished observations). Minimum levels at either 1 or 2 days are presumably caused by a degeneration of ventricle-near (or surface-near) 5-HT terminal systems, damaged directly by high concentrations of the drug. The intermediate recovery of activity levels noted in all regions except the spinal cord between 1–2 and 4–6 days may signify recovery of enzyme activity from a temporary, initial, and direct inhibition caused by 5,6-DHT itself (or of a metabolite) and increased down-transport of newly synthesized enzyme in nonsevered neurons and their axons. The second retarded phase of decline in enzyme activity (between 4–6 and 9–12 days) is most probably due to a loss of enzyme from a late anterograde degeneration of terminals, the preterminal axons of which have been initially damaged by the drug. Finally, the late recovery observed in some regions of the rat CNS, which parallels the rise in 5-HT levels (Baumgarten et al., 1973b), is caused by intense regenerative sprouting from the lesioned 5-HT axons (see Nobin et al., 1973, Björklund et al., 1973a).

The tryptophan hydroxylase values obtained for 5,7-DHT (150 μg) are very different from those gained with 5,6-DHT (75 μg), and the differences cannot be explained solely by the different doses applied. Assuming that both drugs are roughly equipotent (as suggested by the uptake impairment data and the data on 5-HT depletion in whole brain), the percentage drop in enzyme activity following 150 μg 5,7-DHT should be less than that actually found in most regions (for details, see Baumgarten et al., 1973b). This points to differences in the mode of action and in the efficiency of 5,6- and 5,7-DHT that will be further dealt with below (paragraph C).

5. EFFECTS ON MONOAMINE UPTAKE

Another important parameter of actual axonal degeneration after treatment with the dihydroxylated tryptamines *in vivo* is the capacity for active uptake of 5-HT or catecholamines. The initial rate of uptake—measured during a short incubation of the tissue *in vitro*—can be taken as a measure of the number of uptake sites in the tissue, and for a homogeneous population of monoamine terminals this is a useful index of the integrity of the terminal axonal networks (see Iversen, 1972). The effects of DHTs *in vivo* on the capacity for uptake of ^{3}H-5-HT and ^{3}H-NA have been studied for 5,6-DHT (Björklund *et al.*, 1973a,b) and 5,7-DHT (Baumgarten *et al.*, 1973a) at 9–12 days after a single injection of 75 or 200 μg respectively. The uptake was measured on thin slices from cortex, hypothalamus, and spinal cord incubated for 10 min in ^{3}H-5-HT (0.5×10^{-7} M) or ^{3}H-NA (1×10^{-7} M).

Seventy-five μg 5,6-DHT caused a strong reduction in the uptake of ^{3}H-5-HT in all regions tested (40–50% in hypothalamus and cortex and 85% in spinal cord), whereas the ^{3}H-NA uptake was unaffected in hypothalamus and spinal cord, and only slightly reduced (about 35% reduction) in cortex. In contrast, 200 μg 5,7-DHT caused significant reductions in both ^{3}H-5-HT and ^{3}H-NA uptake in all these regions. The effect was considerably greater on the ^{3}H-5-HT uptake, and while the reduction in ^{3}H-NA uptake varied between 40 and 57%, it was 85–90% in ^{3}H-5-HT uptake.

These results are consistent with an extensive axonal degeneration caused by the 5,6-DHT and the 5,7-DHT treatment, and after 5,6-DHT the degeneration seemed to be largely confined to the IA neurons.

6. MORPHOLOGICAL FINDINGS

Since the morphological alterations in central and peripheral monoamine neurons following the application of 5,6- or 5,7-DHT have been described in detail (Baumgarten and Lachenmayer, 1972a, b, 1973; Baumgarten *et al.*, 1972a, c, 1974; Björklund *et al.*, 1973a, b; Nobin *et al.*, 1973; Lachenmayer and Groth, 1973), only a short summary will be presented and some unpublished observations on the effects of the remaining hydroxyindoles will be mentioned that help one to understand their effect on CNS monoamine concentrations. 5,6- and 5,7-DHT, when given to rat brain via the lateral ventricle in doses of 50 or 75 μg (5,6- or 5,7-DHT) or of 100–300 μg (5,7-DHT), cause a rapid disappearance in the fluorescence microscope of ventricle-near IA fibers (e.g. from the suprachiasmatic nucleus and the subcommissural organ), and it seems likely that this is due, at least partly, to an acute drug-induced disintegration of axon terminals that has been demonstrated electronmicroscopically. IA terminals located deeper in brain or spinal cord initially escape the direct toxic effect of medium or low doses of 5,6- or 5,7-DHT (10–50 μg) (e.g. those in the gray matter of the spinal cord; see Nobin *et al.*, 1973). Higher doses of 5,7-DHT, however, appear to provoke a direct toxic disintegration of all ventricle-near and many of the ventricle-distant IA terminals (see Baumgarten and Lachenmayer, 1972b), indicating that this dihydroxyindoleamine readily diffuses into the brain tissue without substantial inactivation. Two to 4 days after the application of 5,6- or 5,7-DHT, the initially surviving IA terminals situated in deeper parts of the rat CNS are no longer detectable in the fluorescence microscope, suggesting that they have become involved in degeneration processes secondary to drug-induced lesions of nonterminal axon parts or cell bodies. Since the IA cell bodies remain largely unaffected (except for an initial transmitter depletion and a temporary, supranormal increase in fluorescence intensity by 2 days), the site of the primary action of 5,6- or 5,7-DHT must, with respect to the slowly disappearing terminal systems, be the nonterminal axons (see Nobin et al., 1973). This is reflected in the development of numerous highly fluorescent, distorted, and enlarged axon sections that resemble the droplet fiber formations described by Björklund (1968) as regular features of part of the tuberohypophysial DA fibers. Similar enlargements occur in axons of mono-amine-containing neurons subjected to different kinds of surgical injury (Dahlström and Fuxe, 1965; Björklund et al., 1971). The amine-filled axonal distensions indicate an arrest of proximo-distal axonal flow of transmitter organelles that pile up due to axonal damage. Following treatment with the neurotoxic DHTs, they appear first 12–24 h after injection and increase in number, size, and fluorescence intensity up to the second to fourth day. Thereafter, they decrease in size and number, and, by the tenth day, if not earlier, small varicose axons are observed to grow out from the distended axons, invading the surrounding tissue (see Baumgarten and Lachenmayer, 1972b, 1973; Björklund et al., 1973a; Nobin et al., 1973). This sprouting phenomenon continues over weeks and months until systems of newly formed IA-containing varicose fibers occupy areas of the brain that either were initially denervated by the drug or that normally do not seem to receive significant IA innervations (Nobin et al., 1973; Björklund et al., 1973a). The regeneration process is not complete, however, and in some regions the denervation thus seems to be permanent (Nobin et al., 1973; Björklund et al., 1973a).

Besides IA-containing axons and terminals, 5,6-DHT also damages ventricle-near DA terminals of the head of the caudate nucleus, but leaves the NA terminals largely unaffected. This is different with 5,7-DHT which causes pronounced lesions, e.g. to the dorsal NA bundle and its projections, and to part of the periventricular NA terminals (see Baumgarten and Lachenmayer, 1972b; Baumgarten et al., 1973a). Of all the new HTs investigated, only the dihydroxyderivatives and the monohydroxy compound 4-OH-5-CH$_3$OT provoke observable toxic damage to CNS monoamine neurons (besides unspecific toxic side effects) in the fluorescence microscope.

Both 6,7- and 4,5-DHT induce extensive piling-up of fluorescence in grotesquely dilated and distorted preterminal sections of IA axons at sites where they approach the brain surface (at the junction of the medulla oblongata and spinal cord) or the ventricular ependyma (e.g. in the anterior part of the mesencephalon and the rostral septum; Baumgarten and Lachenmayer, unpublished). It is important to note that the axonal lesions after 4,5- or 6,7-DHT appear to be more severe and the lesioned axons are more dilated and distorted than after either 5,6- or 5,7-DHT, and the morphological features suggest a profound disorganization of the axonal ultrastructure. The penetration capacity of these two drugs seems rather limited, however, as indicated by the amount and distribution of the lesioned 5-HT axons in brain. Besides IA terminals and axons in ventricle-near locations, also scattered droplet fiber formations are observed in some tract systems known to comprise NA axons.

Similar phenomena are seen after intraventricular injection of 4-OH-5-CH$_3$OT, but the morphological alterations in the IA axons differ strikingly from those after all the DHTs. The acute axonal damage induced by 4-OH-5-CH$_3$OT results in an alteration of the morphology of the preterminal fibers which is characterized by an increased number of seemingly normal varicose swellings that fluoresce with clearly enhanced intensity. Not even the ventricle-near IA terminals are affected initially, in contrast to what is documented after the DHTs. 4-OH-5-CH$_3$OT thus probably induces a very discrete type of axonal injury that may be difficult to distinguish from fluorescence phenomena in normal monoaminergic axons. The remaining monohydroxytryptamines tested (4-HT, 6-HT, and 7-HT) do not cause similar signs of injury to monoamine axons although there is fluorescence microscopical evidence for their accumulation into monoamine neurons shortly after their intraventricular injection.

C. UNSPECIFIC TOXIC EFFECTS AND MOLECULAR MECHANISM OF ACTION

The effects of all the DHTs are complicated by their potential unspecific toxicity, which limits their applicability for selective lesioning of central (or peripheral) monoamine neurons. Unspecific toxicity is reflected in severe behavioral alterations, such as, e.g., convulsions, limb tremor and limb paralysis, persistent piloerection, or reduction in body weight (after intraventricular application) and intense peripheral vasoconstriction, heart failure, acute edema of the lungs, or urinary retention (after i.p. or i.v. administration). Pigmentation of the ventricular ependyma and adjacent brain tissue is observed following, e.g., 5,6-DHT, and precipitation of a colored polymer in the ventricles and brain wall occurs after 4,5-DHT. Morphically, there is evidence for focal or widespread demyelination in ventricle-near or surface-near brain regions following the application of 5,6-DHT (Baumgarten et al., 1972a; Nobin et al., 1973), 4,5-DHT or 6,7-DHT (Baumgarten, unpublished observations), but after 5,7-DHT the effects on myelinated axons seem to be limited to a transient swelling and temporary, reversible myelin disorganization. Glial cell reactions develop synchronously with the myelin damage and breakdown of degenerated unmyelinated axons. Furthermore, shortly after the intraventricular application of 4,5-, 5,6-, or 6,7-DHT, a partial desquamation of the ventricular ependyma may occur, which is, however, rapidly repaired.

When compared on a molar basis, the dihydroxyindoles characterized by a catechol-type substitution (i.e. an ortho arrangement) of their hydroxyl groups are more generally toxic than 5,7-DHT which has a noncatechol distribution (meta arrangement) of its hydroxyls. The order of potency in causing unspecific tissue damage (according to the criteria listed above) among the former compounds is 4,5-DHT > 6,7-DHT > 5,6-DHT. The same order holds true also concerning the rate at which these compounds are oxidized in aqueous solution at neutral pH in the presence of oxygen. This oxidation, which is recognized as a change in colour of the solution, initially gives rise to compounds of semiquinoid (one electron transfer) or quinoid (two electron transfers) structures. Drugs of this kind are known to be provided with a high reactivity, giving rise to different substitution or addition reactions with low or high molecular compounds at biological pH. The results obtained in the present study show that the rate of oxidation of the individual DHTs roughly corresponds to their degree of unspecific toxic effects exerted on the CNS, whereas their selective neurotoxicity against monoaminergic structures is influenced by additional factors, e.g. active uptake and metabolism. It is probably also the rate of auto-oxidation of a given ortho-DHT that determines its diffusion capacity and thus limits its potential effect on CNS monoamine neurons. It is important to note in this context that only the unmetabolized DHTs are substrates for the membrane-bound monoamine uptake mechanism, not their corresponding indolequinones. This can be shown by applying oxidized solutions of each compound to the brain ventricles. Such solutions fail to produce any detectable fluorescence microscopical change in monoamine-containing neurons, while they cause tremendous signs of unspecific toxic damage, e.g. severe convulsions and early death of the injected animals.

The unspecific toxic effects of, e.g., 5,6-DHT, can be dramatically increased by pretreatment of animals with a monoamine oxidase inhibitor prior to the administration of 5,6-DHT. This is easily understandable when considering that 5,6-DHT is a good substrate for monoamine oxidase (Schlossberger and Kuch, 1963). After monoamine oxidase inhibition unmetabolized 5,6-DHT, which has not been accumulated into monoaminergic neurons, can therefore accumulate unselectively in any structure of the brain and convert to a toxic o-quinone to a much greater extent under these conditions.

The mechanism of action of the DHTs responsible for the induction of selective chemical degeneration is still unknown. Considerations on the mechanism of action of 6-hydroxydopamine by Saner and Thoenen (1971) have led to the hypothesis that 6-OH-DA causes neuronal degeneration by irreversible covalent binding of quinone-metabolites (most probably indole-quinones) to macromolecules of the neuron. A similar mechanism of action may be postulated also for the DHTs. Theoretically, dehydration of the ortho-DHTs may either yield o-quinones, or o- and p-quinoneimines. A quinoid oxidation product derived from 5,7-DHT—in contrast to those obtained from the o-substituted tryptamines—can only be o- or p-quinoneimines. This difference in the initial oxidation of o- and m-DHTs may in part be responsible for the differences in the rate of auto-oxidation and the degree of selective and unselective toxicity. In the event that the mechanism of neurotoxic action of the HTs is dependent on quinoid intermediary products, knowledge of the redox potentials of the different compounds would assist in understanding their different degree of selective versus unselective toxicity.

The fact that besides all the DHTs a monohydroxyindoleamine is also capable of damaging monoamine neurons is not entirely unexpected in view of the theory that quinone-like compounds are necessary for toxic damage. This monohydroxyindoleamine, 4-hydroxy-5-methoxytryptamine, is easily oxidized already at slightly acid pH in the presence of oxygen. Considerations on the molecular structure of 4-OH-5-CH$_3$OT reveal that it can undergo oxidation by forming a quinoid system, similar to 4-HT which is, however, comparatively much more stable. The formation of a quinoid or semiquinoid oxidation product from 4-OH-5-CH$_3$OT is promoted by the additional, electron-displacing substituent in position 5 which 4-HT is lacking. A subsequent nucleophilic substitution of the methoxy group would be likely to occur in this quinoid system.

From these considerations it seems that the common structural requirement for selective neurotoxicity is not the o- or m-grouping of the hydroxyl in the benzene nucleus of the indole, but rather the potential of the HTs to form any type of quinoid system within a critical time once incorporated into the neurons.

Although there is much evidence that the selectivity of the neurotoxic effects of hydroxylated tryptamines on the monoamine neurons is due to the intraneuronal accumulation of the drug, it is evident that the affinity of the uptake mechanism of the neuron is not the only factor that determines the neurotoxicity. This is readily shown when the affinity of 5,7-DHT for the monoamine uptake sites is contrasted with its actual, measurable toxic effects on CNS 5-HT and NA neurons. According to the uptake affinity data, 5,7-DHT should accumulate in NA neurons to a greater extent than in 5-HT neurons, but the direct toxic effects—as determined in the uptake impairment experiments in vitro—are significantly greater on the 5-HT neurons (Björklund et al., 1973d). This higher susceptibility of the IA neurons to 5,7-DHT has been observed also in vivo after local intracerebral injections (Björklund et al., 1973c). After intraventricular injection, the long-term action on whole brain NA is stronger than on whole brain 5-HT only at a dose of 25 or 50 μg, and the situation is reversed after doses higher than 50 μg (see Baumgarten *et al.*, 1973a). This discrepancy between high and low doses after intraventricular injection can partly be explained by differences in the anatomical distribution of both types of neurones in the brain, giving the drug better access to NA terminal systems due to their ventricle-near arrangement. But since we are dealing with a compound of low auto-oxidability that can readily diffuse into brain tissue it seems probable that at higher doses the drug will reach 5-HT and NA axons equally well. Several factors have to be considered that determine the unexpected, much larger effect of 5,7-DHT on CNS 5-HT neurons. Such factors, yet unknown, can perhaps be found in differences in the rate of metabolism, storage, and release or in differences in the subcellular distribution of the accumulated transmitter analogues in NA and 5-HT neurons, and perhaps also in differences in the effect of toxic metabolites from 5,7-DHT on functionally important structures of the neurons. For example, *O*-methylation of 5,7-DHT to an inert (or less potent) monohydroxyderivative could hypothetically occur to a much larger extent in NA than in 5-HT neurons, where monoamine oxidase has been found to be a primary catabolizing enzyme. It is interesting to note that monoamine oxidase inhibition can strikingly reduce the damage caused by 5,7-DHT in noradrenaline neurons (Lundström *et al.*, 1973). Thus the difference in susceptibility of NA and 5-HT neurons towards toxic effects of 5,7-DHT may very well be due to a different handling of the false transmitter. Studies on neuronal enzymes and studies on the fate of labelled 5,6- and 5,7-DHT hopefully will assist in answering these interesting questions in the future.

ACKNOWLEDGEMENTS

These investigations were supported by grants from The Deutsche Forschungsgemeinschaft and the National Institutes of Health USPHS (NS 06701-07), and were partly carried out within a research organization sponsored by the Swedish Medical Research Council (Nos. 14X-712 and 14X-56).

REFERENCES

BAUMGARTEN, H. G., and LACHENMAYER, L. (1972a) Chemically induced degeneration of indoleamine-containing nerve terminals in rat brain. *Brain Res.* **38**, 228–232.

BAUMGARTEN, H. G., and LACHENMAYER, L. (1972b) 5,7-dihydroxytryptamine: Improvement in chemical lesioning of indoleamine neurons in the mammalian brain. *Z. Zellforsch.* **135**, 399–414.

BAUMGARTEN, H. G., and LACHENMAYER, L. (1973) Falsche Überträgerstoffe im Gehirn. Selektive, chemisch-induzierte Degeneration monoaminerger Neuronensysteme: Eine neue Methode für die Neuroanatomie und Neuropharmakologie. *Dt. med. Wschr.* **98**, 574–577.

BAUMGARTEN, H. G., BJÖRKLUND, A., LACHENMAYER, L., NOBIN, A., and STENEVI, U. (1971) Long-lasting selective depletion of brain serotonin by 5,6-dihydroxytryptamine. *Acta physiol. scand.*, Suppl. 373, 1–15.

BAUMGARTEN, H. G., BJÖRKLUND, A., HOLSTEIN, A. F., and NOBIN, A. (1972a) Chemical degeneration of indoleamine axons in rat brain by 5,6-dihydroxytryptamine: an ultrastructural study. *Z. Zellforsch.* **129**, 256–271.

BAUMGARTEN, H. G., EVETTS, K. D., HOLMAN, R. B., IVERSEN, L. L., VOGT, M., and WILSON, G. (1972b) Effects of 5,6-dihydroxytryptamine on monoaminergic neurons in the central nervous system of the rat. *J. Neurochem.* **19**, 1587–1597.

BAUMGARTEN, H. G., LACHENMAYER, L., and SCHLOSSBERGER, H. G. (1972c) Evidence for a degeneration of indoleamine-containing nerve terminals in rat brain, induced by 5,6-dihydroxytryptamine. *Z. Zellforsch.* **125**, 553–569.

BAUMGARTEN, H. G., BJÖRKLUND, A., LACHENMAYER, L., and NOBIN, A. (1973a) Evaluation of the effects of 5,7-dihydroxytryptamine on brain serotonin and catecholamine neurons in the rat CNS. *Acta physiol scand.*, Suppl. 391, 1–22.

BAUMGARTEN, H. G., LACHENMAYER, L., BJÖRKLUND, A., NOBIN, A., and ROSENGREN, E. (1973b) Long-term recovery of serotonin concentrations in the rat CNS following 5,6-dihydroxytryptamine. *Life Sci.* **12,** 357–364.

BAUMGARTEN, H. G., GROTH, H.-P., GÖTHERT, M., and MANIAN, A. A. (1974a) The effect of 5,7-dihydroxytryptamine on peripheral adrenergic nerves in the mouse. *Naunyn-Schmiedebergs Arch. exp. Path. Pharmak.* (In press.)

BAUMGARTEN, H. G., BJÖRKLUND, A., ROSENGREN, E., and SCHLOSSBERGER, H. G. (1974b) Effect of various tryptamine derivatives on central monoamine neurons in the rat. (In preparation.)

BAUMGARTEN, H. G., LACHENMAYER, L., ROSENGREN, E., and SCHLOSSBERGER, H. G. (1973d) Effect of 4-HT, 4,5-DHT and 4-OH-5-CH$_3$OT on central monoamine neurons in the rat. (In preparation.)

BAUMGARTEN, H. G., VICTOR, J. S., and LOVENBERG, W. (1973e) Effect of intraventricular injection of 5,7-dihydroxytryptamine on regional tryptophan hydroxylase of rat brain. *J. Neurochem.* **21,** 251–253.

BJÖRKLUND, A. (1968) Monoamine-containing fibres in the neuro-intermediate lobe of the pig and rat. *Z. Zellforsch.* **89,** 573–589.

BJÖRKLUND, A., KATZMAN, R., STENEVI, U., and WEST, K. A. (1971) Development and growth of axonal sprouts from noradrenaline and 5-hydroxy-tryptamine neurones in the rat spinal cord. *Brain Res.* **31,** 21–33.

BJÖRKLUND, A., NOBIN, A., and STENEVI, U. (1973a) Regeneration of central serotonin neurons after axonal degeneration induced by 5,6-dihydroxytryptamine. *Brain Res.* **50,** 214–220.

BJÖRKLUND, A., NOBIN, A., and STENEVI, U. (1973b) Effects of 5,6-dihydroxytryptamine on nerve terminal serotonin and serotonin uptake in the rat brain. *Brain Res.* **53,** 117–127.

BJÖRKLUND, A., NOBIN, A., and STENEVI, U. (1973c) The use of neurotoxic dihydroxytryptamines as tools for morphological studies and localized lesioning of central indolamine neurons. *Z. Zellforsch.* **145,** 479–501.

BJÖRKLUND, A., BAUMGARTEN, H. G., NOBIN, A., and SCHLOSSBERGER, H. G. (1973d) *In vitro* studies on the neurotoxic potency of hydroxylated tryptamines on central monoamine axons. (In preparation.)

CARLSSON, A., FALCK, B., FUXE, K., and HILLARP, N. A. (1964) Cellular localization of monoamines in the spinal cord. *Acta physiol. scand.* **60,** 112–119.

CLINESCHMIDT, B. V., PIERCE, J. E., and LOVENBERG, W. (1971) Tryptophan hydroxylase and serotonin in spinal cord and brain stem before and after chronic transection. *J. Neurochem.* **18,** 1593–1596.

COYLE, J. T., and SNYDER, S. H. (1969) Catecholamine uptake by synaptosomes in homogenates of rat brain: stereospecificity in different areas. *J. Pharmac. Exp. Ther.* **170,** 212–231.

DAHLSTRÖM, A., and FUXE, K. (1965) Evidence for the existence of monoamine neurons in the central nervous system: II, Experimentally induced changes in the intraneuronal amine levels of bulbospinal neuron systems. *Acta physiol. scand.* **64,** Suppl. 247, 1–36.

HEIKKILA, R. E., and COHEN, G. (1973) The inhibition of 3H-biogenic amine uptake by 5,6-dihydroxytryptamine: comparison with the effects of 6-hydroxydopamine. *Eur. J. Pharmac.* **21,** 66–69.

HORN, A. S. (1973) Structure-activity relations for the inhibition of catecholamine uptake into synaptosomes from noradrenaline and dopaminergic neurones in rat brain homogenates. *Br. J. Pharmac.* **47,** 332–338.

HORN, A. S., BAUMGARTEN, H. G., and SCHLOSSBERGER, H. G. (1973) Inhibition of the uptake of 5-hydroxytryptamine, noradrenaline and dopamine into rat brain homogenates by various hydroxylated tryptamines. *J. Neurochem.* **21,** 233–236.

IVERSEN, L. L. (1972) Methods involved in studies of the uptake of biogenic amines. In *Methods of Investigative and Diagnostic Endocrinology* (S. A. Berson, ed.), Vol. 1. *The Thyroid and Biogenic Amines* (J. E. Rall and I. J. Kopin, eds.), North-Holland, Amsterdam, pp. 569–603.

JONSSON, G., FUXE, K., HAMBERGER, B., and HÖKFELT, T. (1969) 6-hydroxytryptamine—a new tool in monoamine fluorescence histochemistry. *Brain Res.* **13,** 190–195.

LACHENMAYER, L., and GROTH, H.-P. (1973) De- and regeneration of the adrenergic nerves in the rat iris induced by dihydroxytryptamines. *Virchows Arch.*, Abt. B, Cell Pathology. (In press.)

LAVERTY, R., SHARMAN, D. F., and VOGT, M. (1965) Action of 2,4,5-trihydroxyphenylethylamine on the storage and release of noradrenaline. *Br. J. Pharmac.* **24,** 549–560.

LUNDSTRÖM, J., MCNEAL, E. T., DALY, J. W., and CREVELING, C. R. (1973) Acute and chronic effects of trihydroxyphenylethylamines and dihydroxytryptamines on adrenergic mechanisms in the murine heart. *Fed. Proc.* **32** (3126) 3.

NOBIN, A., BAUMGARTEN, H. G., BJÖRKLUND, A., LACHENMAYER, L., and STENEVI, U. (1973) Axonal degeneration and regeneration of the bulbospinal indolamine neurons after 5,6-dihydroxytryptamine treatment. *Brain Res.* **56,** 1–24.

PORTER, C. C., TOTARO, J. A., and STONE, C. A. (1963) Effects of 6-hydroxydopamine and some other compounds on the concentration of norepinephrine in the hearts of mice. *J. Pharmac. Exp. Ther.* **140,** 308–316.

SANER, A., and THOENEN, H. (1971) Model experiments on the molecular mechanism of action of 6-hydroxydopamine. *Molec. Pharmac.* **7,** 147–154.

SCHLOSSBERGER, H. G., and KUCH, H. (1963) Synthèse von 5,6-dihydroxytryptophan und verwandten Verbindungen. *Liebig's Annalen Chemie* **662,** 132–138.

SHASKAN, E. G., and SNYDER, S. H. (1970) Kinetics of serotonin accumulation into slices from rat brain: relationship to catecholamine uptake. *J. Pharmac. Exp. Ther.* **175,** 404–418.

THOENEN, H., and TRANZER, J. P. (1968) Chemical sympathectomy by selective destruction of adrenergic nerve endings with 6-hydroxydopamine. *Naunyn-Schmiedeberg's Arch. exp. Path. Pharmak.* **261,** 271–288.

UNGERSTEDT, U. (1968) 6-hydroxydopamine induced degeneration of central monoamine neurons. *Eur. J. Pharmac.* **5,** 107–110.

URETSKY, N. J., and IVERSEN, L. L. (1969) Effects of 6-hydroxydopamine on noradrenaline-containing neurons in the rat brain. *Nature* **221,** 557–559.

VICTOR, S. J., BAUMGARTEN, H. G., and LOVENBERG, W. (1973) Effect of intraventricular administration of 5,6- and 5,7-dihydroxytryptamine on regional tryptophan hydroxylase activity in rat brain. *Fed. Proc.* **32** (1954) 3.

VICTOR, J. S., BAUMGARTEN, H. G., and LOVENBERG, W. (1974) Depletion of tryptophan hydroxylase by 5,6-dihydroxytryptamine in rat brain. Time course and regional differences. *Brain Res.* (In press.)

STUDIES ON CENTRAL 5-HYDROXYTRYPTAMINE NEURONS USING DIHYDROXYTRYPTAMINES: EVIDENCE FOR REGENERATION OF BULBOSPINAL 5-HYDROXYTRYPTAMINE AXONS AND TERMINALS

KJELL FUXE, GÖSTA JONSSON, LARS-GÖRAN NYGREN, AND LARS OLSON

Department of Histology, Karolinska Institutet, Stockholm, Sweden

SUMMARY

The present study provides morphological, biochemical, and functional evidence that after a lesion of descending bulbospinal 5-hydroxytryptamine (5-HT) neurons induced by 5,6-HT, there occurs an almost complete degeneration followed by a relatively complete reinnervation at all levels of the spinal cord. The reinnervation is probably accomplished at least partly by downgrowth of new axons from the surviving proximal ends close to the apparently undamaged cell bodies. These downgrowing axons in turn give rise to the new terminal networks with a seemingly normal distribution pattern probably restoring functional integrity to the descending 5-HT pathway. Thus the supersensitivity of the 5-HT receptor that has developed in response to the degeneration disappears as the new 5-HT networks are being formed, suggesting that the 5-HT boutons are localized at the proper sites to restore 5-HT neurotransmission.

INTRODUCTION

The neurotoxic action of 5,6-dihydroxytryptamine (5,6-HT) on central 5-HT neurons leading to their degeneration is now well established (Baumgarten *et al.*, 1971, 1972a, b; Daly *et al.*, 1972, 1973). In a proper dose-range the damage to the central catecholamine (CA) neurons is slight after intraventricular or intracerebral injections of 5,6-HT pointing to a rather selective action on 5-HT neurons. The data accumulated so far have clearly shown that 5,6-HT provides a useful tool in the morphological and functional analysis of the central 5-HT neurons. However, unspecific damage of brain tissue can occur close to the site of injection after local intracerebral injections and also in ventricle-near regions after intraventricular injections. Some myelinated bundles seem to be particularly sensitive, and occasionally certain myelinated fibre tracts become strongly autofluorescent (emission maximum around 500 nm). It is not known, however, whether this 5,6-HT induced autofluorescence is associated with a degeneration and functional damage of the fibers. The unspecific damage seems to be less pronounced with 5,7-HT which recently has been shown to cause degeneration of central 5-HT neurons (Baumgarten and Lachenmayer, 1972; Fuxe *et al.*, 1973). In addition, it has been found that 5,7-HT is a more potent neurotoxic agent on 5-HT neurons than is 5,6-HT, although 5,7-HT has the disadvantage of being less selective due to a somewhat higher neurotoxic action on the central CA neurons.

In the present study 5,6-HT was given intraventricularly to cause a more or less complete degeneration of the 5-HT axons and terminals of the spinal cord (cf. Daly *et al.*, 1973), after which possible morphological, biochemical, and functional signs of regeneration have been investigated. The evidence suggests that with the dose of 5,6-HT used (50 μg) a regrowth of 5-HT axons occurs all the way down to the lumbosacral part giving rise to new 5-HT nerve terminal plexa with an apparently normal distribution pattern with a concomitant functional recovery as revealed by studies on receptor sensitivity. The reinnervation appears to be completed within 3–4 months after the 5,6-HT-induced lesion.

EXPERIMENTAL DESIGN

Male Sprague–Dawley rats (150 g body weight) were given intraventricular injections of 5,6-HT (50 μg in 20 μl Ringer solution injected during 2 min) and sacrificed 2, 4, 8, 12, and 14 days, 1, 2, 3, and 4 months after the 5,6-HT injection together with Ringer injected controls. Figure 1 illustrates the design of the experiments.

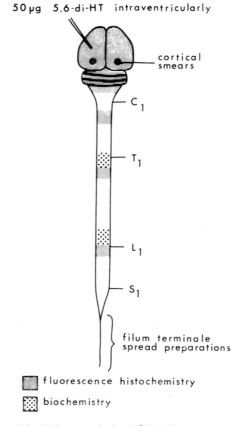

FIG. 1. Design of the combined histochemical and ^{3}H-5-HT uptake studies used to follow de- and regeneration of the bulbospinal 5-HT nerve tracts.

For each experiment, the rats were first tested for possible changes of the 5-HT receptors, following 5,6-HT-induced denervation and possible reinnervation. This was evaluated by studying the effects of L-tryptophan (50 mg/kg i.v.) on the *extensor hindlimb reflex* of acutely spinalized (midthoracic) rats pretreated with nia'amide (500 mg/kg i.p., 1 h; Andén, 1968; Andén *et al.*, 1971). The potent 5-HT receptor stimulating agent 5-methoxy-*N,N*-dimethyltryptamine (5-MeO-DMT, 0.5, 1, and 2 mg/kg i.p.; Fuxe *et al.*, 1972) was also tested in this model. The strength of the reflex was evaluated semiquantitatively on coded animals, and the test period lasted for 1 h. For experimental details see Figs. 6 and 7.

Thereafter the animals were sacrificed and pieces from the cervical, thoracic, and lumbar part of the spinal cord were taken for *fluorescence histochemistry* according to the technique of Falck and Hillarp (Falck *et al.*, 1962; Corrodi and Jonsson, 1967; see also Fuxe *et al.*, 1970; Fuxe and Jonsson, 1973) using freeze-drying (Olson and Ungerstedt, 1970). 5-HT nerve terminals were also studied in the filum terminale using a spread preparation (Olson and Nygren, 1972). The number of 5-HT nerve terminals in the gray matter of the ventral horn and sympathetic lateral column was evaluated on transverse sections of the spinal cord using coded slides and a semi-quantitative scale. For further details see Nygren *et al.* (1973). Adjacent tissue pieces of the thoracic and lumbar region were taken for recording of the *in vitro* uptake of ^{3}H-5-HT. These pieces (approximately 50 mg) were weighed and homogenized in cold 0.5 ml 0.25 M sucrose of which aliquots were taken for *in vitro* incubation in ^{3}H-5-HT (0.5×10^{-8} M, 5 min). Radioactivity was determined by liquid scintillation spectrometry. For details see Table 1.

FLUORESCENCE HISTOCHEMISTRY

The results from the thoracic and lumbar regions are summarized in Fig. 2. A maximum decrease in number of 5-HT nerve terminals almost down to zero was observed 8–14 days following the 5,6-HT injection. The same time course of degeneration is observed following axotomy of the 5-HT axons (Carlsson *et al.*, 1964; Dahlström and Fuxe, 1965). Therefore it is likely that the disappearance of 5-HT fluorescence is mainly the result of a neurotoxic action of 5,6-HT on the descending 5-HT fibers. They occupy superficial positions in the white matter of the spinal cord where they are presumably affected by 5,6-HT coming from the subarachnoidal space. Direct evidence for this view is given by the fact that marked accumulations of 5-HT fluorescence occurred in these axons 1–2 days following the injection (Baumgarten *et al.*, 1972a, b; Daly *et al.*, 1972, 1973; Nobin *et al.*, 1973).

At 1 month the density of 5-HT nerve terminals in the cervical segment showed a peak value of about 100%, so that no difference could be observed between treated animals and controls. A similar, although much smaller peak was observed in the thoracic region (Fig. 2a). During the following 3 months recovery of the nerve density took place in a gradual fashion with respect both to time and to distance from nerve cell bodies. Thus the cervical segment became reinnervated faster than the lumbar region.

At 3 months there was a clearcut reappearance of fluorescent 5-HT nerve terminals in all parts of the spinal cord including the lumbosacral region and the filum terminale. The distribution of these terminals, which probably were newly formed, was similar to that found in the normal animal with a rich innervation of the sympathetic lateral column and the ventral horn, especially of the α-motor neurons in the lumbar region.

Simultaneous studies by Nobin *et al.* (1973) have failed to show any appreciable reinnervation of the spinal cord following intraventricular 5,6-HT injections with the excep-

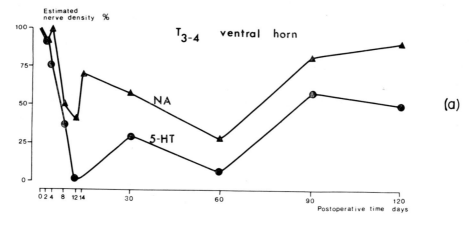

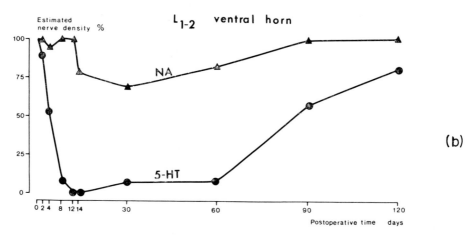

FIG. 2. Time course of degeneration and regeneration of 5-HT and NA nerve terminals in the ventral horn of the gray matter in the spinal cord following intraventricular 5,6-HT. (a) Thoracic region; (b) lumbar region. The nerve density was estimated semiquantitatively (on a 0–4 scale) in controls and treated animals on a blind basis. The mean estimations for treated animals were then expressed as percent of the mean estimations for the controls at each time point. Each point represents at least 4 + 4 animals.

tion of the most cranial part of the spinal cord. These authors found a re-establishment of the 5-HT innervation pattern in certain areas, but in addition an abnormal supply to areas where few or no 5-HT fibers can be seen normally. The explanation for this difference is not clear, but might be related to the dose of 5,6-HT (75 μg) used. The same group, however, has found a long-term recovery of 5-HT concentrations in various regions of the brain and also fluorescence histochemical signs of 5-HT reinnervation in the brain (Björklund et al., 1973). It should be underlined that it is difficult to differentiate between collateral accumulations of 5-HT and true outgrowth of new 5-HT terminals, e.g. in the lower brain stem. An example of this is the increased number of fluorescent 5HT nerve terminals found in the inferior olivary complex 1–3 months following intraventricular 5,6-HT injection (Fuxe and Jonsson, unpublished data; Nobin et al., 1973).

Figures 3–5 illustrate the 5-HT de- and reinnervation of the spinal cord as seen in the fluorescence microscope.

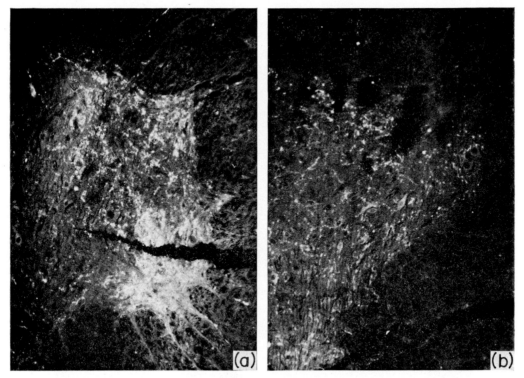

FIG. 3. Ventral horn of the spinal cord (upper lumbar segment) from rats injected intraventricularly 8 days earlier with Ringer and 5,6-HT respectively. Transverse sections. Fluorescence microphotographs. ($\times$140.) (a) Ringer-treated rat. Dense pattern of NA and 5-HT nerve terminals. (b) 5,6-HT-treated rat. The sparse distribution of terminals seen depends on a complete absence of 5-HT and a slight decrease in number of NA terminals.

As seen from Fig. 1a, certain reduction in number of NA nerve terminals is also present after 5,6-HT. It is interesting to note that the reduction is greater in the thoracic part than in the lumbar region which may suggest that the NA axons to the thoracic region are more superficially located and therefore more easily damaged. After 2–3 months there is a clear-cut recovery back towards normal also in the number of NA nerve terminals, suggesting that also new NA networks are being formed. These findings are in agreement with Nygren et al. (1971), demonstrating NA reinnervation of the spinal cord following 6-OH-DA induced lesions of the NA tracts.

^{3}H-5-HT UPTAKE

See Table 1. Since the initial rate of ^{3}H-5-HT uptake was measured, the uptake results will reflect the number of transport sites which is related to the axonal area. In view of the extensive arborization of the terminal parts of the 5-HT neurons, the ^{3}H-5-HT uptake data are a measurement of the relative density or number of 5-HT nerve terminals (see Jonsson and Sachs, 1972).

In agreement with the fluorescence histochemical findings there is a marked decrease of ^{3}H-5-HT uptake in the thoracic and lumbar part of the spinal cord 1–2 weeks after 5,6-HT injection. Here also the time-course of the 5,6-HT induced reduction of ^{3}H-5-HT uptake

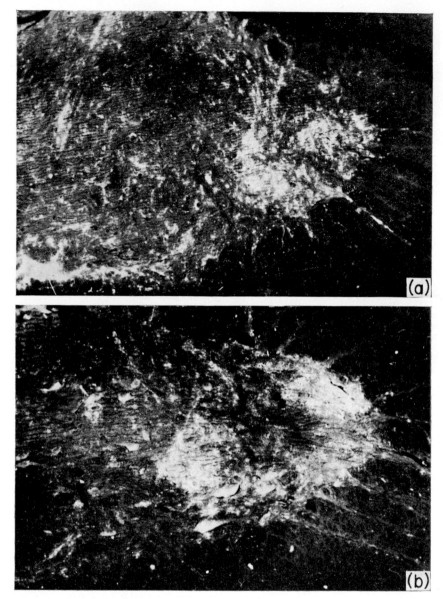

Fig. 4. Ventral horn of the spinal cord (upper lumbar segment) from rats injected intraventricularly 3 months earlier with Ringer or 5,6-HT respectively. Transverse sections.
Fluorescence microphotographs. (×140.) (a) Ringer-treated rat. Dense pattern of both NA
and 5-HT terminals. (b) 5,6-HT-treated rat. The number of NA and 5-HT terminals is similar
to the control rat above.

support the view of an anterograde degeneration pattern. A gradual recovery of ^{3}H-5-HT
uptake thereafter occurs, and 3 months following the lesion the uptake in both the thoracic
and the lumbar part has recovered to approximately 80% of control values. In agreement
with our view that a true downgrowth of 5-HT axons occurs, the recovery of ^{3}H-5-HT
uptake was consistently found to be somewhat more rapid in the thoracic part than in the

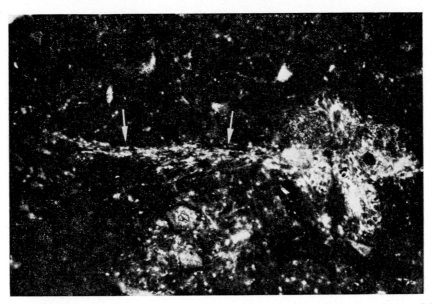

FIG. 5. Large 5-HT bundle (↑) innervating an internal motor nucleus in the ventral horn of the spinal cord upper lumbar segment. Rat treated with 5,6-HT intraventricularly 4 months earlier. Transverse section. Fluorescence microphotograph. (×210.)

lumbar part, although both parts showed a similar maximal reduction of uptake 14 days after 5,6-HT, indicating that the two regions were equally efficient denervated initially. In a separate experiment it has been found that 4 months after the 5,6-HT injection the uptake of ^{3}H-5-HT was restored back to normal. Fluorescence histochemical analysis also revealed an apparently normal amount of 5-HT nerve terminals in this experiment.

TABLE 1. TIME COURSE OF THE EFFECT OF 5,6-HT (50 μg) INJECTED INTRAVENTRICULARLY ON THE *in vitro* UPTAKE OF ^{3}H-5-HT (5×10^{-8} M, 5 MIN) IN HOMOGENATES FROM THORACIC AND LUMBAR REGION OF THE SPINAL CORD.

	Time (week)	n	^{3}H-5-HT uptake thoracic (%)	Lumbar (%)
Control	—	18	100 ± 8	100 ± 8
5,6-HT	1	4	49 ± 6	35 ± 7
	2	4	27 ± 11	22 ± 12
	4	4	71 ± 10	31 ± 5
	8	4	60 ± 9	42 ± 6
	12	6	84 ± 20	74 ± 15

About 50 mg spinal cord tissue was homogenized in 0.5 ml 0.25 M sucrose and centrifuged 1000 g, 10 min. An aliquot (100 μl) of the homogenate was added to 1.9 ml Krebs–Ringer bicarbonate buffer. After 10 min preincubation at +37°C, ^{3}H-5-HT was added giving a concentration of 5×10^{-8} M and the incubation continued for another 5 min. After centrifugation (10,000 g, 10 min), the radioactivity was extracted from the pellet and the radioactivity determined by liquid scintillation spectrometry (cpm/mg wet weight of the tissue). Extraneuronal uptake was determined by performing the incubation at 0°C, which values were subtracted from the values obtained at +37°C (= active uptake). The values represent the mean ±SEM and are expressed as percent of control value.

A good correlation was generally found between ^{3}H-5-HT uptake and nerve density estimations when comparing adjacent pieces of the spinal cord from individual animals. However, when mean values of uptake and nerve density estimations at various times were compared, two important dissociations between histochemistry and biochemistry were found. After 1 month histochemistry tended to indicate more nerves in the thoracic region than the uptake values, and although no ^{3}H-5-HT uptake data were available from the cervical region, histochemistry here showed an approximately normal amount of nerve terminals. On the other hand, the uptake studies demonstrated higher values after 3 months in the lumbar region than could be accounted for by histochemistry. These two discrepancies are explainable when considering that the histochemistry mainly reflects amine storage, while the uptake measurements mainly reflect the surface area of the nerve membrane. Thus the 5,6-HT induced axotomics causes transient increases in the 5-HT storage capacity in the most proximal parts of the spinal cord at 1 month, thereby increasing the number of detectable remaining nerve terminals without increasing the membrane surface area. These phenomena may be related to a less nerve terminal volume in this phase of the outgrowth with an intact or maybe increased synthesis of storage granules.

On the other hand, the newly formed nerve fibers in the distal parts of the spinal cord observed after 3 months may be assumed to have a normal membrane pump but a 5-HT content less than normal probably explaining the discrepancy between histochemistry and ^{3}H-5-HT uptake. In line with this interpretation is the fact that the storage granule capacity of growing CA fibers in the CNS during ontogeny lags behind the development of the membrane uptake mechanism (Coyle and Axelrod, 1971). Identical conclusions have been obtained from studies on regenerating sympathetic adrenergic nerves (Jonsson and Sachs, 1972).

Evidence from two approaches thus suggest that in the spinal cord following an intraventricular 5,6-HT injection, there occurs a relatively complete 5-HT denervation followed by a regeneration phase of several months characterized by outgrowth of 5-HT fibers and the formation of new networks of 5-HT terminals with a seemingly normal distribution pattern all over the spinal cord from the cervical to the lumbar region.

HINDLIMB EXTENSOR REFLEX

As seen in Fig. 6, there occurred a marked potentiation of the hindlimb extensor reflex response to tryptophan treatment after MAO inhibition 8 days after the 5,6-HT injection: 1–4 months following the 5,6-HT injection there was a gradual reduction of the response back to control values. These results indicate that in relation to the degeneration of the 5-HT nerve terminals, the 5-HT receptors develop a supersensitivity. This supersensitivity in the 5-HT receptor then gradually disappears as the new terminal system grows in to replace the systems that have degenerated and disappeared.

In relation to the anterograde degeneration of the 5-HT terminals also, the tryptophan hydroxylase activity disappears (Baumgarten, this symposium). It therefore seems likely that the increased response to tryptophan is due to formation of tryptamine in the capillary walls which then by diffusion reach the supersensitive 5-HT receptor and increases receptor activity. It is known that tryptamine is a weak 5-HT receptor stimulating agent (Andén et al., 1971). This hypothesis needs further investigations.

In agreement with the view given above for the development of a post-synaptic supersensitivity, it was also found that the extensor reflex response to 5-MeO-DMT was enhanced

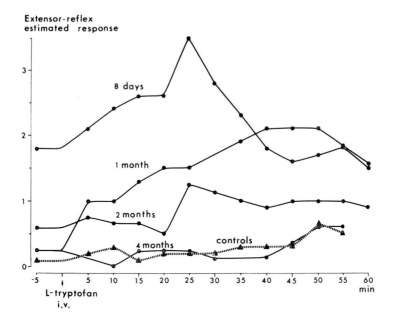

FIG. 6. Tryptophan-induced increase in hindlimb extensor reflex activity after nialamide pretreatment (500 mg/kg i.p., 1 h before L-tryptophan). The dose of L-tryptophan was 50 mg/kg given i.v. Subjective semiquantitative estimations with a scale from 0 to 4 were used. The estimations were performed on a blind basis at various times after intraventricular 5,6-HT. The rats were spinalized immediately before nialamide treatment at the midthoracic level. Each point represents the mean of at least four rats.

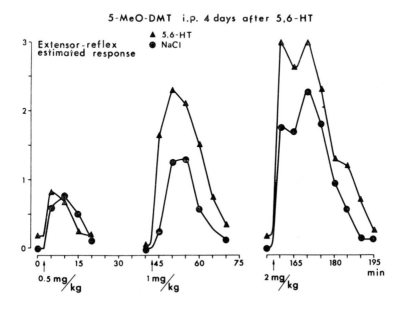

FIG. 7. Demonstration of the supersensitivity of the 5-HT receptor to the 5-HT receptor stimulating drug 5-MeO-DMT, present 4 days after intraventricular 5,6-HT. The hindlimb extensor reflex was evaluated as in Fig. 6. A clear difference between 5,6-HT treated and saline treated rats is seen using 1 or 2 mg/kg of 5-MeO-DMT.

already 4 days after 5,6-HT-induced degeneration of 5-HT neurons (Fig. 7) when the anterograde degeneration is not yet completed.

ACKNOWLEDGEMENTS

This work has been supported by grants from the Swedish Medical Research Council (04X-715, 04X-3185, 04X-2985) and by grants from the Karolinska Institute and Magn. Bergvalls Stiftelse. For excellent technical assistance we thank Mrs. M. Baidins, Mrs. A. Eliasson, Miss M. Eliasson, Mrs. U.-B. Finnman, Miss B. Hagman, and Miss I. Strömberg.

REFERENCES

ANDÉN, N.-E. (1968) Discussion of serotonin and dopamine in the extrapyramidal system. *Adv. Pharmac.* **64**, 347–349.

ANDÉN, N.-E., CORRODI, H., and FUXE, K. (1971) Hallucinogenic drugs of the indolealkylamine type and central monoamine neurons. *J. Pharmac. Exp. Ther.* **179**, 236–249.

BAUMGARTEN, H. G., and LACHENMAYER, L. (1972) 5,7-Dihydroxytryptamine: improvement in chemical lesioning of indoleamine neurons in the mammalian brain. *Z. Zellforsch.* **135**, 399–414.

BAUMGARTEN, H. G., BJÖRKLUND, A., LACHENMAYER, L., NOBIN, A., and STENEVI, U. (1971) Long-lasting selective depletion of brain serotonin by 5,6-dihydroxytryptamine. *Acta physiol. scand.*, Suppl. 373.

BAUMGARTEN, H. G., BJÖRKLUND, A., HOLSTEIN, A. F., and NOBIN, A. (1972a) Chemical degeneration of indolamine axons in rat brain by 5,6-dihydroxytryptamine. An ultrastructural study. *Z. Zellforsch.* **129**, 256–271.

BAUMGARTEN, H. G., LACHENMAYER, L., and SCHLOSSBERGER, H. G. (1972b) Evidence for a degeneration of indoleamine containing nerve terminals in rat brain induced by 5,6-dihydroxytryptamine. *Z. Zellforsch.* **125**, 553–569.

BJÖRKLUND, A., NOBIN, A., and STENEVI, U. (1973) Regeneration of central serotonin neurons after axonal degeneration induced by 5,6-dihydroxytryptamine. *Brain Res.* **50**, 214–220.

CARLSSON, A., FALCK, B., FUXE, K., and HILLARP, N.-Å. (1964) Cellular localization of monoamines in the spinal cord. *Acta physiol. scand.* **60**, 112–119.

CORRODI, H., and JONSSON, G. (1967) The formaldehyde fluorescence method for the histochemical demonstration of biogenic monoamines: a review on the methodology. *J. Histochem. Cytochem.* **15**, 65–78.

COYLE, J. T., and AXELROD, J. (1971) Development of the uptake and storage of L-(^{3}H)norepinephrine in the rat brain. *J. Neurochem.* **18**, 2061–2075.

DAHLSTRÖM, A., and FUXE, K. (1965) Evidence for the existence of monoamine neurons in the central nervous system: II, Experimentally induced changes in the intraneuronal amine levels of bulbo-spinal neuron systems. *Acta physiol. scand.* **64**, Suppl. 247, 1–36.

DALY, J., FUXE, K., and JONSSON, G. (1972) 5,6-Dihydroxytryptamine: a new tool in the mapping out of central 5-HT neurons. In *Proc. 4th Int. Congr. Histochem. Cytochem.* (T. Takeuchi, K. Ogawa, and S. Fujita, eds.), Nakanishi Print. Co., Kyoto, Japan.

DALY, J., FUXE, K., and JONSSON, G. (1973) Effects of intracerebral injections of 5,6-dihydroxytryptamine on central monoamine neurons: evidence for selective degeneration of central 5-hydroxytryptamine neurons. *Brain Res.* **49**, 476–482.

FALCK, B., HILLARP, N.-Å., THIEME, G., and TORP, A. (1962) Fluorescence of catecholamines and related compounds condensed with formaldehyde. *J. Histochem. Cytochem.* **10**, 348–354.

FUXE, K., and JONSSON, G. (1973) The histochemical fluorescence method for the demonstration of catecholamines: theory, practice and application. *J. Histochem. Cytochem.* **21**, 293–311.

FUXE, K., HÖKFELT, T., JONSSON, G., and UNGERSTEDT, U. (1970) Fluorescence microscopy in neuroanatomy. In *Contemporary Research Methods in Neuroanatomy* (W. Nauta and S. Ebbesson, eds.), Springer-Verlag, Berlin.

FUXE, K., HOLMSTEDT, B., and JONSSON, G. (1972) Effects of 5-methoxy-*N*,*N*-dimethyltryptamine on central monoamine neurons. *Eur. J. Pharmac.* **19**, 25–34.

FUXE, K., JONSSON, G., and DALY, J. (1973) The effect of 5,7-HT on central monoamine neurons. (To be published.)

JONSSON, G., and SACHS, CH. (1972) Neurochemical properties of adrenergic nerves regenerated after 6-hydroxydopamine. *J. Neurochem.* **19**, 2577–2585.

JONSSON, G., FUXE, K., and DALY, J. (1972) Intracerebral injections of 5,6-dihydroxytryptamine (5,6-HT): evidence for selective degeneration of central 5-hydroxytryptamine (5-HT) neurons. *Acta pharmac. tox.* **31**, Suppl. 1.

NOBIN, A., BAUMGARTEN, H. G., BJÖRKLUND, A., LACHENMAYER, L., and STENEVI, U. (1973) Axonal degeneration and regeneration of the bulbospinal indoleamine neurons after 5,6-dihydroxytryptamine treatment. *Brain Res.* **56**, 1–24.

NYGREN, L.-G., OLSON, L., and SEIGER, Å. (1971) Regeneration of monoamine-containing axons in the developing and adult spinal cord of the rat following intraspinal 6-OH-dopamine injections or transections. *Histochemie* **28**, 1–15.

NYGREN, L.-G., FUXE, K., JONSSON, G., and OLSON, L. (1973) Functional regeneration of 5-hydroxytryptamine nerve terminals in the rat spinal cord following 5,6-dihydroxytryptamine induced degeneration. (To be published).

OLSON, L., and UNGERSTEDT, U. (1970) A simple high capacity freeze-drier for histochemical use. *Histochemie* **22**, 8–19.

OLSON, L., and NYGREN, L.-G. (1972) A new model for fluorescence histochemical studies of central 5-hydroxytryptamine and noradrenaline nerve fibers: The filum terminale spread preparation. *Histochemie* **29**, 265–273.

EFFECTS OF DRUGS ON SYMPATHETIC NERVE CELLS AND SMALL INTENSELY FLUORESCENT (SIF) CELLS

Olavi Eränkö and Liisa Eränkö

Department of Anatomy, University of Helsinki, Siltavuorenpenger, Helsinki 17, Finland 00170

SUMMARY

Administration of 6-hydroxydopamine or guanethidine causes in newborn rats irreversible destruction of sympathetic nerve cells. 6-Hydroxydopamine does not affect the number of small intensely fluorescent (SIF) cells/ganglion, and guanethidine causes an increase in their number. In cultures of sympathetic ganglia, higher concentrations of 6-hydroxydopamine or guanethidine are required to observe nerve cell damage, and individual neurons show greatly varying sensitivity. Bretylium tosylate and ascorbic acid also show some neurotoxicity. Glucocorticoids have little effect on adult ganglia but cause in newborn rats and in cultures a dramatic increase in the number of SIF cells, in the histochemically demonstrable catecholamine content of these cells and in the number of granular vesicles in them. Sympathetic nerve cells grow in cultures undisturbed by the presence of 1% of ethanol but become damaged when the concentration is increased to 2%.

INTRODUCTION

A large number of studies have been published on the effects of drugs on sympathetic nerve cells, and it is obvious that only some aspects of this topic can be discussed in this paper. Therefore the presentation is limited to morphological and histochemical observations, and special attention will be paid to the small intensely fluorescent (SIF) cells in developing sympathetic ganglia. These cells were described by Eränkö and Härkönen (1963, 1965). For the general characteristics, fine structure and functional significance of these cells the reader is referred to recent papers by Matthews and Raisman (1969), Williams and Palay (1969), Jacobowitz (1970), as well as Eränkö and Eränkö (1971b). Studies on sympathetic ganglia cultured *in vitro* have as yet been relatively few, although organ cultures make it possible to observe the effect of drugs on the structure of living cells under the microscope. Discussion of such observations is another special feature of this article.

6-HYDROXYDOPAMINE

While administration of 6-hydroxydopamine causes in adult rats a reversible destruction of terminal adrenergic nerve fibers (Tranzer and Thoenen, 1968), in newborn rats it results

181

in an irreversible destruction of most sympathetic nerve cells (Angeletti and Levi-Montalcini, 1970a). However, this "chemical sympathectomy" is almost, but not quite, complete, a small number of sympathetic nerve cells remaining in the residual nodules (Eränkö and Eränkö, 1972a). As can be seen by comparing a fluorescence photomicrograph of a control ganglion (Fig. 1) with another taken of the residual ganglion nodule of a rat treated with 50 mg/kg b.w. of 6-hydroxydopamine daily for 8 days after birth and killed at the age of 1 month (Fig. 2), the number of cells per unit of section area is reduced but they appear approximately normal. In fact all cell organelles show a normal fine structure in such cells with well-developed endoplasmic reticulum and Golgi apparatus, as well as mitochondria with numerous cristae; if anything, these cells are larger and contain larger than normal cytoplasmic organelles (Eränkö and Eränkö, 1972a). As can be seen in Fig. 2, the wide spaces between the nerve cell perikarya contain numerous fluorescent cell processes.

Besides some sympathetic nerve cells, all SIF cells survive the treatment with 6-hydroxydopamine. Their mean number was 472 per ganglion in the experimental group, while the corresponding figure for untreated controls was 466 SIF cells per ganglion (Eränkö and Eränkö, 1972a). It is likely that at least some of the fluorescent nerve fibres in the intercellular spaces originate from the SIF cells, even if the surviving, enlarged, ordinary sympathetic nerve cells may also have grown new processes with fluorescent boutons.

Exposure of cultures of neuroblastoma cells for 1 h to a concentration of 50 mg/l of 6-hydroxydopamine results in marked degenerative changes in these cells and three consecutive exposures kill all neuroblastoma cells (Angeletti and Levi-Montalcini, 1970b). Approximately similar sensitivity of sympathetic neurons to 6-hydroxydopamine has been demonstrated in cultures of rat and chicken sympathetic ganglia (Hill et al., 1973). However, individual neurons exhibit marked differences in the susceptibility to 6-hydroxydopamine. Thus while exposure for 1.5 h to 40 mg/l of this drug causes in a few hours fragmentation of nerve fibres and death of some nerve cells, other nerve cells survive the exposure for 20 h to twice that concentration of the drug and regenerate new processes thereafter.

For the mechanisms and sequence of morphological changes due to 6-hydroxydopamine, the reader is referred to the recent volume edited by Malmfors and Thoenen (1971). Suffice it to say here that mitochondria in the nerve cells are the first to show extensive alterations (Angeletti and Levi-Montalcini, 1970a).

ASCORBIC ACID

Ascorbic acid is commonly used to prevent oxidation of 6-hydroxydopamine when making solutions for injection or culture medium (Angeletti and Levi-Montalcini, 1970b). It is therefore of some interest that exposure to 200 mg/l of ascorbic acid for 1 h causes fragmentation of nerve fibres in cultures of rat sympathetic ganglia, and exposure to the same concentration for 20 h results in damage and death of many nerve cells (Hill et al., 1973). Thus ascorbic acid is toxic to nerve cell cultures in a concentration which is not very much higher than the toxic concentration of 6-hydroxydopamine.

GUANETHIDINE

Daily intraperitoneal injections of 20 mg/l of guanethidine sulphate cause in 2 weeks degenerative changes in sympathetic nerve cells and a round cell infiltration of the sympathetic ganglia of adult rats (Jensen-Holm and Juul, 1970). In newborn rats, the same

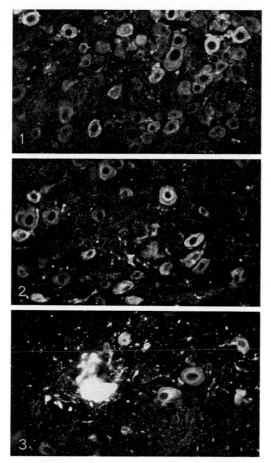

Fig. 1. Formaldehyde-induced fluorescence due to catecholamines in the superior cervical
ganglion of a 1-month-old control rat. No SIF cells are visible. (×175.)

Fig. 2. Similar photograph of a rat injected after birth daily with 6-hydroxydopamine for 8
days. Observe the large distances between the ganglion cell bodies. (×175.)

Fig. 3. Photomicrograph obtained under similar conditions of a surviving nodule in the
superior cervical ganglion of a 1-month-old rat given 8 daily injections of guanethidine after
birth. Note the overexposed cluster of SIF cells in the centre and the numerous fluorescent
nerve fibres. (×175.)

daily dose on 8 consecutive days results in an almost complete destruction of nerve cells in
the sympathetic ganglia (Eränkö and Eränkö, 1971a, b; Angeletti *et al.*, 1972). However,
again some nerve cell bodies survive; they can be seen in the ganglion remnants surrounded
by a surprisingly large number of fluorescent nerve fibres, some of which are apparently
terminal fibres, showing beadings with stronger fluorescence (Fig. 3). In accordance with
the survival of some nerve cell bodies, peripheral organs such as the iris occasionally show
some fluorescent nerve fibres when a recovery period is allowed after guanethidine treatment (Eränkö and Eränkö, 1971c).

   The SIF cells not only survive but show a significant increase in number after guanethidine treatment. In the superior cervical ganglion the mean number of SIF cells per gang-

lion increased from 479 to 1427, while the corresponding figures for the coeliac ganglion were 198 and 1071; this was due to an increase in the number of SIF cells in each cluster rather than to appearance of new clusters (Eränkö and Eränkö, 1971a). Because the SIF cells observed after guanethidine treatment apparently send even more numerous processes than those in normal ganglia, it is likely that they essentially contribute to the rich net of fluorescent fibres between the cell bodies. Since the total number of nerve cells and SIF cells together is very small as compared with the number of nerve cells in an intact ganglion, the large number of these fibres is somewhat puzzling. However, it seems likely that not only do the surviving neurons and SIF cells regenerate a larger number of processes than those present in normal cells but, because of the derangement caused by the death of most nerve cells in the ganglion, the nerve fibres may not reach their normal destinations but perhaps remain inside the ganglion remnant and coil in the same manner as fibres in an amputation neurinoma.

When the daily dose of guanethidine is increased and/or the length of the treatment prolonged to several weeks, adrenergic neurons can be irreversibly destroyed also in adult animals (Burnstock et al., 1971; Juul and McIsaac, 1973), in whose ganglia an increase in the number of fluorescent processes is likewise seen between the scattered nerve cell bodies (Heath et al., 1972). Damaged mitochondria and dilatation of the cisternae of endoplasmic reticulum are typical fine structural changes after guanethidine administration to newborn (Angeletti et al., 1972) or adult (Jensen-Holm and Juul, 1971; Heath et al., 1972) rats, the mitochondria apparently being the primary target.

While a daily dose of 20 mg/l of guanethidine sulphate is highly toxic in vivo, when the concentration of this drug in the tissue culture medium is from the beginning kept as high as 36 mg/l, explants of rat sympathetic ganglia in vitro not only survive but form a nerve fibre network at about the same rate as in control cultures (Eränkö et al., 1972a). On the other hand, when the drug is later added to ganglion cultures which have first grown in a control medium, some growth inhibition is already seen in a concentration of 10 mg/l of guanethidine sulphate, and fragmentation of nerve fibres and nerve cell death are observed at a concentration of 50 mg/l. However, even after exposure for 3 days to a concentration of 100 mg/l of this drug, regeneration of new nerve fibres from some neurons can be observed. While a very wide range of susceptibility of individual sympathetic nerve cells makes it understandable that some nerve cells are affected at a concentration one-tenth of that of other nerve cells, it is not so easy to explain the great difference between the toxicity of guanethidine in vivo and in vitro (Hill et al., 1973).

The number of SIF cells increases in guanethidine-containing cultures of sympathetic ganglia (Eränkö et al., 1972c) but the number of amine-storing granular vesicles is decreased in the cytoplasm of these cells, as compared with control cultures, presumably because of depletion of catecholamines by guanethidine from the SIF cells (Heath et al., 1973).

BRETYLIUM TOSYLATE

When bretylium tosylate is injected every other day to developing rats for 1–2 weeks beginning 1 day after birth, degenerative changes develop in numerous sympathetic nerve cells, which show dramatic swelling of the mitochondria but well preserved other cell organelles (Caramia et al., 1972). No information is available on the fate of SIF cells under the influence of this drug, neither has its effect been studied on cultures of sympathetic cells.

GLUCOCORTICOIDS

While the drugs hitherto described exert dramatic effects on the sympathetic nerve cells, glucocorticoids little affect the appearance of the nerve cells but cause a dramatic increase in the number of SIF cells in the sympathetic ganglia of newborn, but not adult rats (Eränkö, and Eränkö, 1972b). Figure 4 is a fluorescence photomicrograph of a 6-day-old control rat showing weakly or moderately fluorescent sympathicoblasts and young nerve cells. No SIF cells are visible in this field, although clusters of them can be found in the sympathetic

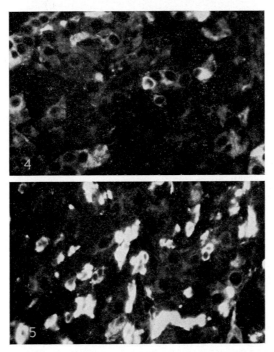

Fig. 4. Amine fluorescence in the superior cervical ganglion of a 6-day-old control rat. No SIF cells are visible. The developing nerve cells show weak to moderate fluorescence. (×260.)

Fig. 5. Fluorescence photomicrograph of the superior cervical ganglion of a rat injected with hydrocortisone. There are numerous SIF cells all over the field. (×260.)

ganglia of newborn rats (Eränkö, 1972). Figure 5 is of the same ganglion of a littermate who had been given 40 mg/kg b.w. of hydrocortisone acetate daily since birth; it is a view typical of the sympathetic ganglion of hydrocortisone-injected rats which contains numerous small clusters and individual SIF cells throughout the ganglion. Since control rats show only a limited number of SIF cell clusters, between which large areas contain only developing nerve cells, the thought appears reasonable that the increase in the number of SIF cells is due to differentiation from less mature sympathetic cell elements.

Ciaranello et al. (1973) confirmed our observation using dexamethasone as glucocorticoid and showed, furthermore, that there was an approximately tenfold increase in the phenyl-ethanolamine N-methyltransferase activity of the sympathetic ganglia. They proposed the possibility that increased numbers of SIF cells may be derived from preexisting ganglion cell bodies rather than undifferentiated stem cells. Since all cells of the sympathetic ganglia

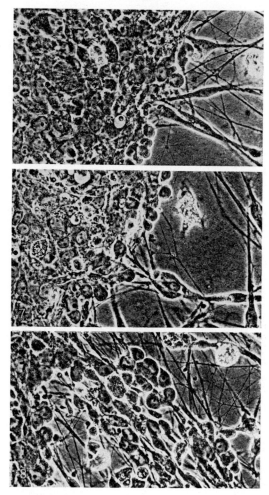

FIG. 6. Phase contrast photomicrograph of nerve cell bodies and nerve fibres of a ganglion explant cultured for 3 days in the control medium. (×325.)

FIG. 7. The same field photographed 6 h after culture in a medium containing 1% ethanol. (×325.)

FIG. 8. The same field after culture for 50 h in a medium containing 1% ethanol. Note the apparently normal nerve cells and the dense nerve fibre network. (×325.)

of the newborn rat are yet at an early developmental stage (Eränkö, 1972), the difference between these two possibilities is mainly a matter of definition. Hervonen *et al.* (1972) also demonstrated an increase in the number of SIF cells in the paracervical ganglion of the rat uterus using prednisolone or hydrocortisone.

While SIF cells of adult rats all show an intense fluorescence and do not essentially change after glucocorticoid treatment (Eränkö and Eränkö, 1972b), glomus cells of the carotid body of adult rats, which normally range from nonfluorescent to intensely fluorescent, respond to treatment with methylprednisolone by an increase in the intensity of the fluorescence (Korkala *et al.*, 1973). It is pertinent to state here that Lempinen (1964) was the first

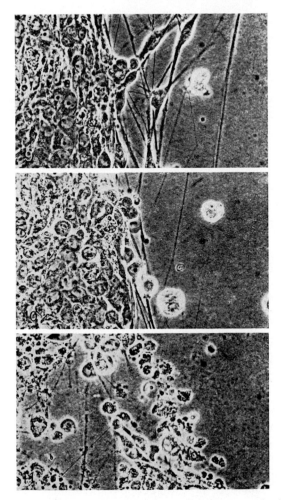

FIG. 9. Explant and outgrowth of sympathetic ganglion in a control culture. ($\times$325.)

FIG. 10. The same field as that in Fig. 9 1 h after culture in a medium containing 2% of ethanol. ($\times$325.)

FIG. 11. The same field after culture with 2% of ethanol for 26 h. Note the destruction of nerve cells and the disappearance of the fibre network. ($\times$325.)

to observe, in the abdominal paraganglia of newborn rats, a dramatic increase in the number of chromaffin cells after treatment with cortisone or hydrocortisone.

In electron microscopic preparations, the SIF cells correspond to small cells with granular vesicles (Eränkö and Härkönen, 1965; Matthews and Raisman, 1969). After hydrocortisone administration to newborn rats, the number of such small cells increases in sympathetic ganglia, as does the number of granular vesicles in each cell (Eränkö et al., 1973).

The number of SIF cells dramatically increases also in sympathetic ganglia cultured *in vitro* when hydrocortisone is added to the culture medium; the intensity of the fluorescence in the cytoplasm of the SIF cells increases as well, and there is a shift in the colour of the formaldehyde-induced fluorescence of these cells from green through yellow to reddish (Eränkö *et al.*, 1972a). The number of granular vesicles in each cell also increases *in vitro* under the influence of hydrocortisone; moreover, many such cells show unusually large vesicles with large granules of variable electron density after fixation in glutaraldehyde and osmium tetroxide (Eränkö *et al.*, 1972b). Granules of low density are not found in the normal SIF cells *in vivo* or *in vitro*; they may contain adrenaline formed owing to increased activity of phenylethanolamine *N*-methyltransferase due to glucocorticoids (see above).

ETHANOL

In addition to the drugs hitherto discussed in this paper, it appeared to be of interest to add some recent observations on the effect of ethanol on sympathetic ganglia cultured *in vitro*. These studies have been carried out in collaboration with Anneli Nikkinen. They serve to illustrate the extreme tolerance of sympathetic nerve cells towards this popular poison.

Figure 6 shows a 3-day-old culture of a sympathetic chain ganglion from a newborn rat immediately before the culture medium was replaced by a medium containing 1 % (v/v) of spectrographically pure ethanol. Figure 7 is of the same region of the same culture 6 h later, and Fig. 8 again the same region but 50 h later. The relatively high ethanol concentration (7.890 mg/l) has little effect on the microscopic appearance of the nerve cells and fibres. Moreover, outgrowth of nerve fibres and migration of nerve cells proceeds essentially as in control cultures.

Doubling the ethanol concentration in a similar experiment provides different results. Figure 9 is a culture with a normal medium. Figure 10 is of the same region 1 h after replacing the medium with one containing 2 % (v/v) of ethanol. The number of fibres emerging from the explant is reduced, and there is a change in the appearance of the nerve cells in the explant. Figure 11 shows the same region after exposure to 2 % ethanol for 26 h; there is an obvious destruction of the cultured ganglion.

Without further going to the extensive literature on the effects of ethanol on nervous systems, it may be adequate to note that ethanol does affect impulse transmission and metabolism of the nervous tissue (Wallgren and Barry, 1970). The study by Corrodi *et al.* (1966) deserves special mention. These authors histochemically demonstrated an accelerated loss of noradrenaline from adrenergic synapses of the brain after inhibition of enzymes synthesizing dopamine and noradrenaline and ethanol treatment.

Our studies on the effects of ethanol on cultured nervous tissue will be continued to cover observations of histochemically demonstrable catecholamines and fine structure of the nerve cells and SIF cells. It is here of interest to observe that differences in the sensitivity towards ethanol of individual neurons can be observed, in principle in the same manner as towards 6-hydroxydopamine or guanethidine.

ACKNOWLEDGEMENTS

This study has been supported by grants from the Sigrid Jusélius Foundation, the Emil Aaltonen Foundation and the Alcohol Research Foundation of Finland.

The tissue culture studies dealing with the effect of alcohol were carried out in collaboration with Miss Anneli Nikkinen, Ph.M. The authors gratefully acknowledge skilful technical assistance by Mrs. Paula Hasenson.

REFERENCES

ANGELETTI, P. U., and LEVI-MONTALCINI, R. (1970a) Sympathetic nerve cell destruction in newborn mammals by 6-hydroxydopamine. *Proc. Natn. Acad. Sci. USA* **65**, 114–121.

ANGELETTI, P. U., and LEVI-MONTALCINI, R. (1970b) Cytolytic effect of 6-hydroxydopamine on neuroblastoma cells. *Cancer Res.* **30**, 2863–2869.

ANGELETTI, P. U., LEVI-MONTALCINI, R., and CARAMIA, F. (1972) Structural and ultrastructural changes in developing sympathetic ganglia induced by guanethidine. *Brain Res.* **43**, 515–525.

BURNSTOCK, G., EVANS, B., GANNON, B. G., HEATH, J. W., and JAMES. V. (1971) A new method of destroying adrenergic nerves in adult animals using guanethidine. *Br. J. Pharmac.* **43**, 295–301.

CARAMIA, F., ANGELETTI, P. U., LEVI-MONTALCINI, R., and CARRATELLI, L. (1972) Mitochondrial lesions of developing sympathetic neurons induced by bretylium tosylate. *Brain Res.* **40**, 237–246.

CIARANELLO, R. D., JACOBOWITZ, D., and AXELROD, J. (1973) Effect of dexamethasone on phenylethanolamine *N*-methyltransferase in chromaffin tissue of the neonatal rat. *J. Neurochem.* **20**, 799–805.

CORRODI, H., FUXE, K., and HÖKFELT, T. (1966) The effect of ethanol on the activity of central catecholamine neurones in rat brain. *J. Pharm. Pharmac.* **18**, 821–823.

ERÄNKÖ, L. (1972) Ultrastructure of the developing sympathetic nerve cell and the storage of catecholamines. *Brain Res.* **46**, 159–175.

ERÄNKÖ, L. and ERÄNKÖ, O. (1971a) Effect of guanethidine on nerve cells and small intensely fluorescent cells in sympathetic ganglia of newborn and adult rats. *Acta pharmac. tox.* **30**, 403–416.

ERÄNKÖ, L., and ERÄNKÖ, O. (1972a) Effect of 6-hydroxydopamine on the ganglion cells in the superior cervical ganglion of the rat. *Acta physiol. scand.* **84**, 115–124.

ERÄNKÖ, L., and ERÄNKÖ, O. (1972b) Effect of hydrocortisone on histochemically demonstrable catecholamines in the sympathetic ganglia and extra-adrenal chromaffin tissue of the rat. *Acta physiol. scand.* **84**, 125–133.

ERÄNKÖ, L., HILL, C., ERÄNKÖ, O., and BURNSTOCK, G. (1972c) Lack of toxic effect of guanethidine on nerve cells and small intensely fluorescent cells in cultures of sympathetic ganglia of newborn rats. *Brain Res.* **43**, 501–513.

ERÄNKÖ, O., and ERÄNKÖ, L. (1971b) Small, intensely fluorescent granule-containing cells in the sympathetic ganglion of the rat. In *Histochemistry of Nervous Transmission* (O. Eränkö, ed.), *Progr. Brain Res.*, vol. 34, Elsevier, Amsterdam, London, and New York, pp. 39–51.

ERÄNKÖ, O., and ERÄNKÖ, L. (1971c) Histochemical evidence of chemical sympathectomy by guanethidine in newborn rats. *Histochem. J.* **3**, 451–456.

ERÄNKÖ, O., and HÄRKÖNEN, M. (1963) Histochemical demonstration of fluorogenic amines in the cytoplasm of sympathetic ganglion cells of the rat. *Acta physiol. scand.* **58**, 285–286.

ERÄNKÖ, O., and HÄRKÖNEN, M. (1965) Monoamine-containing small cells in the superior cervical ganglion of the rat and an organ composed of them. *Acta physiol. scand.* **63**, 511–512.

ERÄNKÖ, O., ERÄNKÖ, L., HILL, C., and BURNSTOCK, G. (1972a) Hydrocortisone-induced increase in the number of small intensely fluorescent cells and their histochemically demonstrable catecholamine content in cultures of sympathetic ganglia of the rat. *Histochem. J.* **4**, 49–58.

ERÄNKÖ, O., HEATH, J. W., and ERÄNKÖ, L. (1972b) Effect of hydrocortisone on the ultrastructure of the small, intensely fluorescent, granule-containing cells in cultures of sympathetic ganglia of newborn rats. *Z. Zellforsch.* **134**, 297–310.

ERÄNKÖ, O., HEATH, J. W., and ERÄNKÖ, L. (1973) Effect of hydrocortisone on the ultrastructure of the small, granule-containing cells in the superior cervical ganglion of the newborn rat. *Experientia* **29**, 457–459.

HEATH, J. W., EVANS, B. K., GANNON, B. G., BURNSTOCK, G., and JAMES, V. B. (1972) Degeneration of adrenergic neurons following guanethidine treatment: an ultrastructural study. *Virchows Arch.*, Abt. B, Zellpath. **11**, 182-197.

HEATH, J. W., ERÄNKÖ, O., and ERÄNKÖ, L. (1973) Effect of guanethidine on the ultrastructure of the small, granule-containing cells in cultures of rat sympathetic ganglia. *Acta pharmac. tox.* **33**, 209–218.

HERVONEN, A., KANERVA, L., LIETZEN, R., and PARTANEN, S. (1972) Effects of steroid hormones on the differentiation of the catecholamine storing cells of the paracervical ganglion of the rat uterus. *Z. Zellforsch.* **134**, 519–527.

HILL, C. E., MARK, G., ERÄNKÖ, O., ERÄNKÖ, L., and BURNSTOCK, G. (1973) The use of tissue culture of sympathetic neurons to examine the mechanism of action of guanethidine and 6-hydroxydopamine. *Eur. J. Pharmac.* **23**, 162–174.

JACOBOWITZ, D. (1970) Catecholamine fluorescence studies of adrenergic neurons and chromaffin cells in sympathetic ganglia. *Fed. Proc.* **29**, 6, 1929–1944.

JENSEN-HOLM, J., and JUUL, P. (1970) The effects of guanethidine, pre- and post-ganglionic nerve division on the rat superior cervical ganglion: cholinesterases and catecholamines (histochemistry) and histology. *Acta pharmac. tox.* **28**, 270–282.

JENSEN-HOLM, J., and JUUL, P. (1971) Ultrastructural changes in the rat superior cervical ganglion following prolonged guanethidine administration. *Acta pharmac. tox.* **30**, 308–320.

JUUL, P. and MCISAAC, L. (1973) The effect of guanethidine on the noradrenaline content of the adult rat superior cervical ganglion. *Acta pharmac. tox.* **32**, 382–389.

KORKALA, O., ERÄNKÖ, O., PARTANEN, S., ERÄNKÖ, L., and HERVONEN, A. (1973) Histochemically demonstrable increase in the catecholamine content of the carotid body in adult rats treated with methylprednisolone or hydrocortisone. *Histochem. J.* **5**, 479–485.

LEMPINEN, M. (1964) Extra-adrenal chromaffin tissue of the rat and the effect of cortical hormones on it. *Acta physiol. scand.* **62**, Suppl. 231.

MALMFORS, T., and THOENEN, H. (eds.) (1971) 6-*Hydroxydopamine and Catecholamine Neurons*, North-Holland, Amsterdam and London.

MATTHEWS, M. R., and RAISMAN, G. (1969) The ultrastructure and somatic efferent synapses of small granule-containing cells in the superior cervical ganglion. *J. Anat. Lond.* **105**, 255–282.

TRANZER, J. P., and THOENEN, H. (1968) An electron microscopic study of selective, acute degeneration of sympathetic nerve terminals after administration of 6-hydroxydopamine. *Experientia* **24**, 155–156.

WALLGREN, H. and BARRY, H. (1970) *Actions of Alcohol*. Elsevier, Amsterdam, London and New York, vol. 1, 400 pp.

WILLIAMS, T. H., and PALAY, S. L. (1969) Ultrastructure of the small neurons in the superior cervical ganglion. *Brain Res.* **15**, 17–34.

THE EFFECT OF INDUSTRIAL SOLVENTS ON ADRENERGIC TRANSMITTER MECHANISMS

B. Holmberg† AND T. Malmfors‡

SUMMARY

In a preliminary study the effect of various industrial solvents on the adrenergic transmission has been studied. In order to make a first screening, two simple *in vitro* models were used; the mechanical response of mouse vas deferens and the uptake of noradrenaline (NA) by the adrenergic nerves. It was found that the effect of various solvents on these models was not closely related to their physical properties.

Several solvents, e.g. trichloroethylene, toluene, and benzyl chloride, had a marked potentiating effect on the adrenergic transmission. The main reason for this appeared to be an increased sensitivity of the effector cells to NA. However, other mechanisms of the adrenergic transmission seemed also to be affected. Preliminary studies have also indicated that some solvents affect the NA turnover in the central nervous system. This observation might offer a good possibility to evaluate the addictive effect of different solvents.

INTRODUCTION

In industry, organic chemicals used as solvents are present frequently and often in high amounts. They have various chemical composition, but they have more or less the same property in dissolving unpolar compounds as e.g. lipids. The workers are very often heavily exposed to the industrial solvents, as most of these compounds are considered rather a little toxic.

However, the knowledge about the toxicity of different industrial solvents varies quite considerably. Different types of biological effects have been reported. The general anesthetic effect is the most often observed and has been shown to be fairly well correlated to the liposolubility of the solvents. It has been proposed that the most probable site of the anesthetic effect is the plasma membrane of the nerve cells. Due to their physical properties the solvents should be able to accumulate in the lipoproteins in the membranes affecting the different functions of the membrane. With that theory in mind a study was undertaken in order to explore the possibility that industrial solvents affect membrane mechanisms involved in the adrenergic transmission as transmitter release, reuptake of the transmitter by the nerves, and stimulation of the effector cells by the transmitter.

† Section of Occupational Toxicology, Department of Occupational Health, National Board of Occupational Safety and Health, P.O. Box, S 100 26 Stockholm 34, Sweden.
‡ Astra Pharmaceutical AB, Toxicology Laboratories, S 151 85 Södertälje, Sweden.

The use of the adrenergic nerves for studying the effect of organic solvents on nerve cells does not only provide a more versatile system for the study but directs the attention to a very important type of neurons in the nervous system. It will not only be possible to elucidate the well-known sensitizing effect of some industrial solvents on the heart, but it will also be possible to estimate the total effect of these compounds on the adrenergic regulation via the sympathetic nervous system and the adrenal medulla of many important autonomic functions in, e.g., the cardiovascular system. Furthermore, as these compounds easily penetrate the blood–brain barrier, any effect observed on the peripheral adrenergic neurons must also take place in the corresponding monoamine neurons of the brain. As these neurons are strongly considered being involved in many important functions of the brain, as, e.g., regulation of the emotional status and other behavioral mechanisms, it is obvious that any effect of the industrial solvents on these neurons might have significant implications.

In this study a few *in vitro* methods have been used for screening a lot of different solvents belonging to different chemical groups. After that a few compounds have been studied more in detail.

MATERIALS AND METHODS

The animals used were Sprague–Dawley rats and NMRI mice.

The total effect of industrial solvents on the adrenergic transmission was studied by recording the mechanical response of mouse vas deferens elicited by transmural stimulation *in vitro* in the presence of different solvents (for details see Farnebo and Malmfors, 1971). In order to dissolve the solvent properly it was added to the Krebs–Ringer solution, then the solution was shaken vigorously in a closed vessel. This solution was then infused successively into the organbath from a preheating chamber. It was thus possible to get a homogeneous and repeatable exposure of the mouse vas deferens with the solvent. The mechanical response was recorded by a strain gauge and registered by a Grass polygraph. Both the maximal and integrated mechanical response was obtained. The preparation was normally stimulated with 10 impulses/s during 30 s.

In order to study the effect on the membrane of the adrenergic nerves, rat irides were incubated with ^{3}H-noradrenaline (NA) in the presence of different organic solvents in a Krebs–Ringer solution, and the uptake and accumulation of radioactivity—mainly ^{3}H-NA —by the irides was measured (see Jonsson et al., 1969). In order to avoid variation in the results due to evaporation of the solvents, the procedure was slightly modified by shortening the incubation time (10 min) and using incubation flasks with tight-fitting closures.

More detailed studies were performed using the mechanical response of the mouse vas deferens. By adding exogenous NA the effect of the solvents on the stimulation of the smooth muscle cells could be studied particularly when the adrenergic nerves were previously removed by giving the animals 6-hydroxy-dopamine (6-OH-DA) 300 mg/kg i.v., 20–24 h before. The amount of transmitter released by nerve stimulation was indirectly studied by measuring the amount of radioactivity released by field stimulation of a mouse vas deferens preincubated in ^{3}H-NA (see Farnebo and Malmfors, 1971).

The effect on the central monoamine neurons was studied by measuring indirectly the NA turnover in the brain of rats exposed to some industrial solvents. The animals were given H44/68, the methylester of α-methyl-*para*-tyrosine, 250 mg/kg i.p., and at the same time exposed to solvent vapors for 4 h. The animals were killed and the amount of NA in the brain was estimated.

RESULTS AND DISCUSSION

SCREENING OF VARIOUS SOLVENTS

In order to pick out the most interesting solvents or groups of solvents for further studies, two simple screening methods were used. The first one was considered to evaluate the overall effect on the adrenergic transmission in the peripheral nervous system. That involved recording the mechanical response from the smooth muscles of the vas deferens elicited by electric, transmural stimulation *in vitro* in the presence of various solvents. This *in vitro* technique should reveal the effect *in vivo* at the level of the sympathetic neural effector sites, where the nerve impulse releases the transmitter substance NA onto the receptors of the smooth muscle cells. There are thus several mechanisms which could be affected by the industrial solvents and cause a change of the adrenergic transmission; the transmitter release, the sensitivity of the smooth muscle cells, and the inactivation of transmitter. However, this *in vitro* model does not test the effect on impulse frequency or velocity. There are possibilities that the effects on the different events might counteract each other, but, on the other hand, this screening model should be adequate for the in-life situation.

The second way of screening various solvents deals with one of these events at the adrenergic transmission, namely the inactivation process by reuptake into the adrenergic nerves. It is known from earlier work (see Malmfors, 1965) that the main mechanism for the inactivation of released transmitter is localized to the axonal membrane, where the so-called membrane mechanism efficiently takes up NA from the extracellular space. By adding NA *in vitro* to rat iris preparation, incubated in industrial solvents, the influence of these compounds on the uptake mechanism can be studied. The suspected affinity of the solvents for lipids in membranes makes this screening model particularly attractive. It is difficult to transfer the results obtained in *in vitro* systems to *in vivo* situations. However, even if the quantitative aspects of the results are different *in vivo*, there is reason to believe that the qualitative dimensions of the results are valid. The relations between the effects of different solvents are also different *in vivo* compared to the *in vitro* situation, as the uptake, distribution, accumulation, biotransformation, and elimination is different for different solvents, due to among other things their various physical and chemical properties. Thus before final conclusions about the relative toxicity of industrual solvents are drawn, complementary *in vivo* studies have to be performed.

For simplicity only one concentration has been chosen (100 ppm), which must be looked upon as insufficient for a proper dose response determination. However, in this particular case, this procedure was considered satisfactory. Due to some variation between different preparations, the results are expressed as percent of the control, in the case of studies of the mechanical response the pre-exposure value and in the case of the NA-uptake controls ran at the same time. The mechanical response on mouse vas deferens (Fig. 1) varies quite considerably as far as shape is concerned. It was therefore decided to integrate the mechanical response during the whole stimulation period (30 s), and these figures are shown in Fig. 1.

The results of the screening experiments are shown in Table 1. Due to the insufficient amount of data only clear-cut deviation from the controls will be commented upon. Among the hydrocarbons tested, cyclohexane seems to have an inhibiting effect on the adrenergic transmission as well as an inhibiting effect on the NA uptake. Among solvents typical for different types of groups of solvents ethyl alcohol (500 ppm) seems to have a slight inhibiting effect on the mechanical response but no effect on the NA uptake. Formaldehyde as a representative for aldehydes was certainly very effective in both inhibiting the mechanical response and the NA uptake. This effect should, however, be disregarded in this case and shows only that a strongly corrosive compound as formaldehyde in an *in vitro* system can have effects, which will never occur *in vivo*, due to the impossibility for the substance to be present at the nerves at such a high concentration. Nitrobenzene showed an inhibiting effect on the adrenergic transmission, which in all probability also reflects an effect apart from what can be expected from just physical properties.

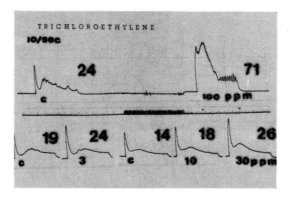

FIG. 1. The mechanical response to electric stimulation (10 per s) at different concentrations of trichloroethylene (3, 10, 30, and 100 ppm). The c tracing represent the preexposure control response. The stimulation period was 30 s. (Note: The numerical value of the integrated response is given in relative arbitrary units to the right of this and the following relevant figures.)

TABLE 1

	Mechanical response (% of controls)	Na uptake (% of controls)
n-Pentane	215 ± 20	—
n-Heptane	110 ± 19	119 ± 5
iso-Octane	80 ± 5	73 ± 10
Cyclohexane	36 ± 6	75 ± 6
Ethyl alcohol (500 ppm)	60 ± 10	104 ± 5
Formaldehyde	21 ± 3	42 ± 9
Cyclohexanon	90 ± 10	100 ± 10
Dioxan	80 ± 20	118 ± 7
Amylacetate	70 ± 19	—
Pyridine	90 ± 13	143 ± 12
Nitrobenzen	30 ± 6	—
Toluene	226 ± 21	92 ± 7
o-Xylene	173 ± 23	91 ± 7
Styrene	185 ± 12	90 ± 10
Benzyl chloride	250 ± 15	72 ± 6
Chloroform	128 ± 8	107 ± 10
Methylchloroform	100 ± 12	88 ± 6
Tetrachloroethane	31 ± 9	82 ± 13
Trichloroethylene	217 ± 15	67 ± 4
Tetrachloroethylene	114 ± 21	103 ± 5

Among the rest of the aromatic compounds, all showed marked potentiation of the mechanical response, while only benzyl chloride had a slight inhibiting effect on the NA uptake. The rest of the halogenated hydrocarbons showed various results. The most remarkable observation was the marked difference between trichloroethylene and methylchloroform. While methylchloroform was more or less without an effect, trichloroethylene strongly potentiated the mechanical response and significantly inhibited the NA uptake. Furthermore tetrachloroethylene behaved more or less like methylchloroform.

It is thus obvious that the industrial solvents tested in these experiments behave quite differently and that their effect is not related to their lipid water partition properties. It is thus possible that other solvents than those tested might have even stronger effects, which has to be ruled out before any final conclusion can be drawn about these specific effects of industrial solvents.

In order to elucidate the reason for these effects, more detailed studies were performed with three of the most potent solvents in the first screening tests. The solvents chosen for these detailed studies are trichloroethylene, toluene, and benzyl chloride.

FURTHER STUDIES WITH TRICHLOROETHYLENE, TOLUENE, AND BENZYL CHLORIDE

As pointed out above, the screening experiments were insufficient in explaining more in detail how the industrial solvents interfere with the adrenergic transmission. In order to rule out that and to get more information about dose response, further studies were performed.

The concentration of the organic solvents in the organbath was lowered and the responses from the lower concentration of trichloroethylene and benzyl chloride can be seen in Figs. 1 and 8. Both trichloroethylene and benzyl chloride in concentrations down to 3 ppm have an obvious effect on the mechanical response. This is a concentration, which can be obtained in blood of human beings during industrial exposure. Therefore it seems reasonable to assume that the observed potentiating effect of organic solvents observed *in vitro* also might occur *in vivo*. However, further studies have to be done in order to elucidate the quantitative aspects.

As has been discussed above, the effect of the organic solvents can be related to one or several steps in the adrenergic transmission. In order to elucidate the sensitivity of the effector cells, the adrenergic nerves were removed by 6-OH-DA, injected the day before to the animals (see Malmfors and Sachs, 1968), and the mechanical response of vas deferens was elicited by exogenous NA added to the organbath. It is a well-known phenomenon that removing the adrenergic nerves markedly increases the sensitivity of the smooth muscle cells to exogenous NA because the inactivating function of the adrenergic nerves has been lost. This increased sensitivity is called the presynaptic supersensitivity (Trendelenburg, 1963). This effect was obtained in this preparation (Figs. 2 and 3). Addition of trichloroethylene (10–100 ppm) increased the mechanical response in the innervated preparation in about the same degree as the denervation. It is thus obvious that trichloroethylene in this situation exerts an effect, which must be considered of important significance. It can be seen that the potentiating effect of 100 ppm trichloroethylene is of the same order of magnitude as that of a three times higher concentration of NA. It can thus be concluded that trichloroethylene at that concentration increases the sensitivity of mouse vas deferens to exogenous NA by about three times.

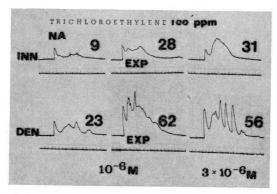

FIG. 2. The mechanical response to exogenous NA in an intact (INN) and a previously denervated (DEN) mouse vas deferens. NA was added to a final concentration of 10^{-6} M and 3×10^{-6} M respectively; exposure time 60 s. At the middle tracing (EXP) trichloroethylene (100 ppm) was present.

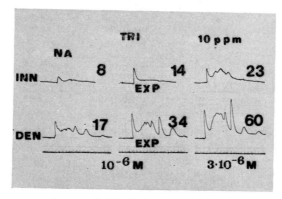

FIG. 3. The same experiment as in Fig. 2, but 10 ppm of trichloroethylene was used.

This might at least partially be explained by the inhibiting effect of trichloroethylene on the NA uptake by the adrenergic nerves as seen in the screening experiment (see above). However, when trichloroethylene was added together with NA to the denervated mouse vas deferens, it was noticed that the potentiating effect of trichloroethylene was present even when the adrenergic nerves were absent. The potentiating effect of trichloroethylene in the denervated mouse vas deferens was of about the same order of magnitude as in the innervated. This is similar to what is obtained about 1 week after decentralizing a sympathetically innervated organ; the postsynaptic supersensitivity (Trendelenburg, 1963).

This effect of trichloroethylene must significantly contribute to the potentiation of the adrenergic transmission. The nature of this postsynaptic supersensitivity is unclear and has to be studied further. However, an effect on the irritability of the smooth muscle cells might be suspected, as trichloroethylene also potentiates the response to acetylcholine in denervated mouse vas deferens (Fig. 4). As this also is the case for the postsynaptic supersensitivity, obtained after decentralization, there is a reason to believe that the nature of the acute postsynaptic supersensitivity, produced by trichloroethylene, is similar to that. As it has been shown (Fleming, personal communication) that the resting membrane potential of the smooth muscle cells at the postsynaptic supersensitivity is reduced, trichloroethylene

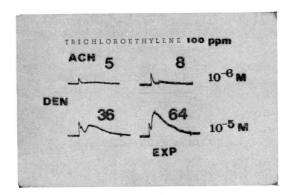

FIG. 4. The mechanical response of previously denervated mouse vas deferens to acetylcholin (10^{-5} and 10^{-6} M). At the two right tracings (EXP) 100 ppm of trichloroethylene was present.

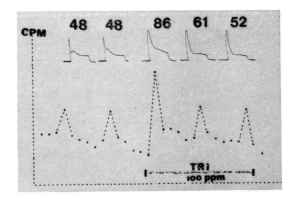

FIG. 5. The mechanical response (upper tracings) and the overflow of the total radioactivity (CPM) (lower tracings) from a mouse vas deferens preincubated in ^{3}H-NA. At the three last tracings trichloroethylene (100 ppm) was present in the superfusion medium.

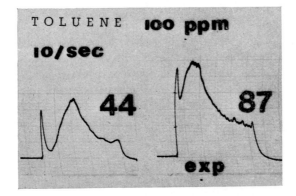

FIG. 6. The mechanical response to electric stimulation (10 per s) before and during exposure to toluene (100 ppm). Stimulation time 30 s.

might in some way or another acutely produce a change of the resting membrane potential of the smooth muscle cells producing the observed hypersensitivity.

Similar experiments using toluene have revealed about the same results (Figs. 6 and 7), thus indicating the same mode of action for toluene as for trichloroethylene. However, as there is little structural resemblance between toluene and trichloroethylene, it is difficult to understand any common mode of action on the molecular level. Further work is needed to rule out the structural effect relationship.

Benzyl chloride has a marked potentiating effect similar to that of toluene and trichloroethylene after nerve stimulation (Fig. 8). However, the effect on nerve response to exogenous NA is different (Fig. 9). There was a slight potentiating effect in the innervated mouse vas deferens, while 100 ppm of benzyl chloride rather had a slight opposite effect in the denervated mouse vas deferens. This indicates that the inhibiting effect on the NA uptake of benzyl chloride might have some importance in the innervated mouse vas deferens, while the absence of postsynaptic supersensitivity in the denervated mouse vas deferens makes the potentiating effect after electric stimulation more difficult to explain. However, unpublished results indicate that 100 ppm of benzyl chloride *in vitro* has a degenerative effect on the smooth muscle cells and thus leading to an irreversible damage of the smooth muscle cells at that concentration. The potentiating effect of benzyl chloride at electric stimulation must therefore be explained by an excessive release of the transmitter by the nerve impulses (see below).

The amount of transmitter released by a nerve impulse is not constant (Farnebo and Malmfors, 1971), but can be varied by different mechanisms. The mechanism regulating the amount of transmitter being released by the nerve impulses is unclear. However, it is obvious that this mechanism might be affected by organic solvents. In order to elucidate this further, a superfusion experiment was performed in mouse vas deferens, where the radioactivity released by nerve stimulation was measured. The mouse vas deferens had been preincubated in ^{3}H-NA. As can be seen in Fig. 5, two pre-exposure stimulations gave about the same mechanical response and radioactive overflow. When trichloroethylene 100 ppm was added, there was a marked potentiation of the mechanical response, as observed earlier, and at the same time the overflow of radioactive material was markedly increased. The second and third stimulation period did not reveal that much overflow, but there was still some potentiation of the mechanical response. From this experiment it is obvious that industrial solvents as trichloroethylene can increase the release of transmitter by nerve impulses. However, in the experiments performed there is a marked tachyphylaxis, which was observed with toluene and benzyl chloride too. The reason for this tachyphylaxis is difficult to assess, but unpublished observations indicate an increased leakage of radioactive material between the stimulation periods, and at some instances a tendency to breakdown of the transmission. It is thus possible that the increased release is a predegeneration sign and of minor importance compared to the postsynaptic supersensitivity.

In conclusion it can be safely stated that the industrial solvents affect the adrenergic transmission, probably both on the nerve and the effector side. The relative importance of the different effects observed has to be further elucidated, but some of the results go along very well with the earlier observations of the increased sensitivity of the heart to catecholamines at exposure to trichloroethylene. The practical significance of the results can not be stated until further *in vivo* experiments have been performed.

In order to elucidate if these effects of some of the industrial solvents were valid also for the central nervous system, a few preliminary studies have been performed. The NA turn-

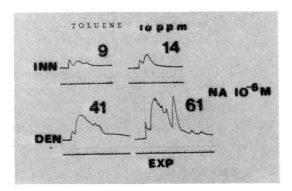

FIG. 7. The mechanical response to NA (10^{-6} M) of an intact mouse vas deferens (INN) and a previously denervated mouse vas deferens (DEN) before and during exposure to toluene (10 ppm).

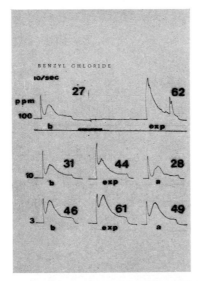

FIG. 8. The mechanical response to electric stimulation (10 per s) before (b), during (exp), and after (a) the exposure to benzyl chloride at different final concentrations (3, 10, and 100 ppm).

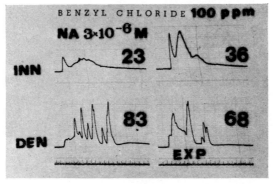

FIG. 9. The mechanical response to NA (3×10^{-6} M) of an intact mouse vas deferens (INN) and a previously denervated mouse vas deferens (DEN) before and during the exposure to benzyl chloride (100 ppm).

over in the whole brain has been estimated by using NA synthesis inhibition by H44/68 (the methylester of α-methyl-*para*-tyrosine). This experiment revealed (Table 2) that trichloroethylene and toluene but not methylchloroform affect the NA in the central nervous system. This is of particular interest, as the two former compounds have been reported being among the most effective and popular solvents for sniffing misuse. They thus have a stimulating effect on the central nervous system and cause addiction. It would be very valuable if this type of animal experiment could be used to test the stimulating effect on the central nervous system of various solvents and mixtures of solvents.

TABLE 2

	NA content (% of controls)
Methylchloroform	98 ± 4
Trichloroethylene	82 ± 5
Tetrachloroethylene	81 ± 6

REFERENCES

FARNEBO, L. O., and MALMFORS, T. (1971) *Acta physiol. scand.*, Suppl. 371, 1–18.
JONSSON, G., HAMBERGER, B., MALMFORS, T., and SACHS, CH. (1969) *Eur. J. Pharmac.* **8**, 58–72.
MALMFORS, T., (1965) *Acta physiol. scand.* **64**, Suppl. 248, 1–93.
MALMFORS, T., and SACHS, CH. (1968) *Eur. J. Pharmac.* **3**, 89–92.
TRENDELENBURG, V. (1963) *Pharmac. Rev.* **15**, 225–276.

AXOPLASMIC TRANSPORT AS A MECHANISM FOR AXONAL SUPPORT AND GROWTH

SESSION I

Chairman: O. ERÄNKÖ

DYNAMICS AND MECHANICS OF NEUROPLASMIC FLOW

PAUL A. WEISS

The Rockefeller University, New York, NY, USA

SUMMARY

In the frame of a condensed review of the relevant features of axonal flow, studied by the author and his coworkers in the last three decades, recent progress in the elucidation of the underlying motile mechanism is described, with indications of its possible relation to a general principle of cell surface pulsation, based on circling intracellular pH rhythms.

Some 30 years ago, when I first stumbled on the phenomenon of neuroplasmic flow (Weiss, 1943; Weiss and Davis, 1943), most of the premises taken for granted at the present day were nonexistent. In fact, I did not even observe the very fact of flow in the nerve fiber directly, but inferred it merely indirectly from observations on accidentally constricted nerves. My conclusion that the axon, far from being the stationary fixture as which it presented itself under the microscope, was in reality a steady stream of substance, moving peripherad from its source in the neuronal cell body to a presumed fate of dissipation *en route* and of dissolution and extrusion at the end, was deduced solely from the "damming up" of axonal content at the proximal side of tight sleeves of live artery around nerves, with concomitant size deficits developing on the distal side (Weiss, 1944a). Evidently the local constriction by the cuffs, in narrowing the diameters of the axons in the ensheathed segments, had established a partial obstruction to the steady downflow of neuroplasm from the central source. Only the later removal of the sleeve (Weiss and Hiscoe, 1948), even many months up to a year after its application (Weiss and Cavanaugh, 1959), permitted us actually to record the process of flow as the accumulated proximal mass then moved into the widened peripheral channel in the manner of a tidal wave. And the rate of the observed advance of that wave front at roughly 1 mm/day gave us the first concrete measure of the kinetics of the movement—a figure confirmed since as an almost universal constant by order of magnitude.

However, the purely quantitative asymmetry at a "bottleneck", that is proximal amassment with commensurate distal want, was early recognized as giving a wholly inadequate description of the phenomenon, for it neglected the *form* in which the proximal "damming" occurred—not as a simple bag-like bulge but as a distortion of the cylindrical shape of the axon into various configurations (convolutions, corkscrews, telescopic inversions, beading, etc.) (Weiss, 1944b; Weiss and Hiscoe, 1948), denoting technologically the wrenching that a solid bar in forward thrust undergoes when it meets a sudden resistance. A quantitative study of these deformations (Weiss and Hiscoe, 1948; Weiss, 1972a), as well as the fact that electron microscopically all the fine-structural intraaxonal features, such as neurotubules and neuro-filaments, showed patterns exactly conformant to the surface configurations of the axon (Weiss, 1969), has unequivocally identified the "axis cylinder" of the neuron as a structur-ally cohesive semisolid-state system and not a column of liquid consistency. Unfortunately, this fact has been and still is widely ignored in the sheer bulk determinations of transfer of mass from nerve cell body into the periphery. It has been clear from the beginning, and firmly substantiated since, that the axonal column moves proximodistally in a state of high structural consistency, though not rigidity, notwithstanding its content of between 80% and 85% of water (see later). Moreover, the neurotubules and mitochondria have also been shown to be carried along by the axonal flow at its standard rate (Weiss and Pillai, 1965), evidently embodied in its substance, much like steel wires in reinforced concrete, merely allowing short-range local excursions of mitochondria through their own wormlike loco-motor activities.

It should be mentioned that Ramon y Cajal (Cajal, 1928) had already noted and illust-rated the deformities of regenerating axons at constrictions, but misinterpreted them as residues of "growth cones", which he considered to be battering rams across dense tissue. In order to avoid further confusion, I would propose not to deal promiscuously with two clearly separable, though interrelated processes, namely, *neuroplasmic flow*, on the one hand, and *regeneration*, on the other, but confine our considerations in the following to the *intact mature nerve fiber* only. Even though axonal flow had happened to come to my notice from observations on regenerating fibers, the basic phenomenon was soon corrobor-ated to occur identically in undisrupted fibers, so that all deviations found in regenerating neurons should be ascribed to peculiarities of the latter. Of course, the close correspondence between the rates of axonal flow and of the fastest advance of the free tips of regenerating axonal sprouts (a few millimeters per day) is hardly sheer coincidence, but, as I shall indicate below, this seems related to a common conveyor mechanism in both, regardless of the marked disparity of the consistency of the conveyed content, which is solid in the former while distinctly more fluid in the latter.

In view of the relative solidity of the mature axoplasm, one might question the approp-riateness of the designation of the translatory motion of the axonal column as "flow." Yet, since the term has come into general use, it might as well be retained, but with the clear understanding that it signifies a strictly non-Newtonian convection, comparable to the flow of lava or even of glaciers. At any rate, the terms "neuroplasmic flow" or "axonal flow" should remain reserved for this steady proximo-distal advance of the axonal column *as a whole*. It actually should be regarded as a process of *growth* in which newly synthesized material is added at the growing point, i.e. in the cell body, much as hair grows from its follicle.

By implication, this view denies to the axon itself, from the hillock down, any intrinsic capacity for growth, but rather marks it as primarily a shipping line for products synthesized and assembled in the perikaryon and a transmission line for excitation, without excluding additional uptake of accessory products along its course. Even though at that early time the instrumental linkage between genes and protein reproduction, so dramatically clarified by the more recent discoveries in molecular biology, had not yet been revealed, I had the temerity of conjecturing, on rather tenuous grounds, that the nucleated territory of the perikaryon was the sole source of all the proteinacious products of the neurons, both structural and enzymatic, and even a major source for nonproteinacious macromolecules assembled with the enzymatic help of the former. My argument in favor of this conjecture was as follows (Weiss and Hiscoe, 1948). Numerous reports in the older literature had pointed to the fact that living nerve gave off far higher amounts of ammonia than did other tissues (Gerard, 1932). In judging this to indicate that split products of stepwise proteolysis in the axon could not be as readily recycled to the far-off synthetic center near the neuronal nucleus as they might over the much shorter distances in all other cell types, and, therefore, considering the ammonia output as terminal de-amination sign, I calculated from the reported output data the amount of daily protein replacement that would have to be shipped down from the cell body in order to maintain a steady supply, and found it to require a proximo-distal supply stream moving at a rate of the order of 1 mm per day, which coincided with the rate we had observed microscopically in fibers released from a damming constriction.

Evidently, the infinitely finer resolution of the mechanism of protein synthesis and degradation, accomplished in the 30 years since, might stamp that early deduction as naive and truly based on coincidence. Yet even if it were, it had a most propitious effect in that it engendered the trend of applying the novel techniques of tracing the vagaries of protein-acious compounds in living cells by radioactive amino acid markers incorporated in proteins. Our own use of various radioactive tracers of substance shifts in nerve dates back to 1944, when we obtained some highly active isotopes from the Atomic Project at the University of Chicago; they revealed a proximo-distal movement of fluid in the endoneurial spaces between peripheral fibers at a rate of several millimeters per hour (Weiss et al., 1945), i.e. about 30 times faster than the axonal flow inside the fibers. Later experiments with radioactive phosphorus in our own and a neighboring laboratory, as well as many subse-quent ones, suffered from the insufficient discriminatory power of the labeling compounds used and from the fact that the conclusions were derived from measurements on "nerve" taken as a whole without distinction between neuronal and sundry nonneuronal contents.

While the latter weakness of resolving power still attaches to many recent investigations, the former inadequacy has been drastically reduced by methodical progress, especially in the last decade. Labeling of amino acids with ^{14}C made possible the singling-out of protein metabolism and confirmed directly the close connection between cellulifugal shift of protein and axonal flow, which had originally been sheer deduction. Yet the most significant technical advance came from the introduction of ^3H-labeled amino acids in 1963 by Droz and Leblond, followed by radioautography of microscopic (Droz and Leblond, 1963) (later, electronmicroscopic) sections. Since even then the isotope was administered by injection to whole animals, thus yielding a stationary background of ubiquitous cells in the process of protein synthesis, the signal-to-noise ratio of the characteristic advance of protein in nerve over the stationary background of labeled surrounding tissue was not yet optimally high. In order to attain more strictly confined localization of the isotope labeling to more sharply circumscribed sites of neuronal cell bodies, we chose with success, firstly, the ganglion cells of the retina as sources of the optic nerve, accessible through injections into the vitreous humor (Taylor and Weiss, 1965), a method thenceforth widely adopted; secondly, the cells of origin of the olfactory nerve in the nasal mucosa by inserting a gelatin pellet soaked in labeling fluid into the nostril (Weiss and Holland, 1967); and, finally, somatic sensory neurons by transient immersion of the excised spinal ganglion into the labeling solution, leaving the nerve attached, but guarded against seepage (Weiss, 1967). Partial localization has also been obtained by topical injections into the spinal cord (Ochs and Burger, 1958; Miani, 1964) or brain parts directly.

Regardless of the growing diversity and refinement of methods and objects, a number of our original conclusions have, in the main, stood the test of time, as listed briefly in the following. (1) The content of the axon is in steady cellulifugal motion. (2) It moves ("grows") as a coherent semisolid column from its base in the perikaryon and succumbs to dissolution at the ending. (3) This translatory advance proceeds at an average rate of the order of 1 μm/min. (4) The primary source of the protein constituents and inclusions of the axonal column lies in the perikaryon. (5) This sharp spatial division into a reproductive and nonreproductive portion, combined with the far excentric position of the former, makes the neuron a uniquely favorable object for the study of cell-biological phenomena. The process described in points (1) to (4) is the only one to which the term "neuroplasmic (or axonal) flow" proper should be reserved. All other movements, especially convections of substance *within* the axon, should be characterized as "intraneuronal (or endoaxonal) transport", regardless of speed and orientation. Before turning to the latter a few supplementary remarks, which have emerged from more recent work, need to be added. The rationale for some of them will be presented further below.

(1) and (2) The axonal content as such possesses no motile power but is driven by a peristaltic pulse wave in the axonal surface, the energy for which is presumably furnished by the Schwann cell. The passivity of the content is attested to by two facts: (a) the direct observation in motion pictures of blockage of the column by obstructions despite the continuing peristaltic activity of the surface drive (Weiss, 1972b); and (b) the accumulation at a block of arrested mitochondria that have been swept along in the stream, revealed electron microscopically (Weiss and Pillai, 1965), as well as biochemically by the local piling up of mitochondrial enzymes (Friede, 1959) in front of the obstruction, while the surface drive keeps on. The neurotubules, whose protein subunits can be marked by their selective affinity to colchicine (Karlsson and Sjöstrand, 1969; Grafstein *et al.*, 1970), are likewise structurally incorporated in the moving mass (Weiss and Mayr, 1971b). Taken together, all these facts militate against interpreting the proximodistal shift of the protein markers as signs of a "transport", much less a "migration" of protein as if they were free molecules in solution. Quite to the contrary, they must be viewed as indicators of the proteinacious constituents of the moving axonal fabric. To designate the movement as "transport", would be no more logical than if one were to describe the moving of a passenger train, built of steel, as transport of steel, even though it might also carry steel on board as freight. Awareness of this misnomer is all the more important as actual "transport" of substances *within* the moving nerve fiber is also a reality (see below).

(3) The custom initiated by our original crude measurements, stating the rate of axonal flow in terms of its linear advance, ignores the fact that normally the rate of linear advance of a unit of mass in a given channel varies in inverse ratio to the square of the lumen. Applied to nerve, this would mean that in fibers of smaller caliber progress in the longitudinal direction would be faster than in larger fibers, if the amount of inflow per unit of time were the same for both. This is a point to be taken into account in comparing different axons in the same nerve, and even more so, between nerves of different size spectra or, due to caliber increase with nerve length during growth, also of different ages. Yet, the case is

not that simple. Firstly, the diameter of an axon and the size of its cell body are positively related, so that a larger axon might be expected to be fed a larger *amount* of neuroplasm per unit of time than a thinner one, which would result in similar rates of advance in both. Secondly, as will be explained presently, the surface drive of the axonal flow proper seems to proceed at a standard rate in all fibers, thus setting the maximum attainable traffic speed for all of them, to which the fiber caliber would adaptively yield, insuring some degree of synchronization among the fiber population. As there are no concrete data on any of these points, it would seem quite appropriate for the time being to abide by the linear dimension for measuring or estimating rates of axonal flow.

(4) Our original supposition of the perikaryon being the sole site of protein reproduction had to be reviewed when it was reported that some protein synthesis occurs at nerve terminals as well. I believe that we have succeeded in clarifying this apparent ambiguity as follows. We had observed that mitochondria arrested in regions of blocked axonal flow accumulate at the block and break down within a few days (Weiss and Pillai, 1965). The same fate meets the mitochondria which are brought daily by the hundreds to a stop at the blind ending of an axon, spilling their content into the "synaptosomal" medium (Weiss and Mayr, 1971a). Considering the fact that mitochondria possess the whole machinery of DNA→RNA→protein reproduction, we compared amino-acid incorporation into protein in continuous series of small nerve samples between those rich and those poor in mitochondrial content, found the rate of protein synthesis in the former about twice as high as in the latter, but also established unequivocally that this difference was abolished by prior brief immersion of both kinds of fragments in chloramphenicol, a specific inhibitor of the synthesis of mitochondrial protein (Weiss and Mayr, 1971a). The protein production at nerve terminals would therefore seem to be attributable to the constantly replenished graveyard of mitochondria, which themselves have originated in the perikaryon, although a more direct chemical identification of the terminal protein would still be desirable.

None of the general statements made up to here about axonal flow in the strict sense can be extended as such by extrapolation to the processes of endoaxonal transport. We shall return to this distinction later, but it seems to be based essentially on the different services the two mechanisms have to perform in the household of the organism. It has become clear by now that neurons operate like the specialized industrial and commercial systems of human design: the perikaryon is the factory, the axon is the shipping line, and the synaptic ending is a site of consumption, transaction, and trans-shipment. While both the production end and the synaptic marketing end have in the last decade received mounting and remarkably successful study, especially as regards the biochemical transactions and the storage and export involved, the shipping mechanism itself has attracted little study. I shall, therefore, briefly sketch whatever beginning we have been able to make in its description and understanding.

We started with a program of phase-contrast, microscopic time-lapse cinemicrography of living neurons from postnatal animals in rigorously controlled *in vitro* conditions, using mostly freshly explanted spinal ganglia of young mice, attached to their sensory nerves, whose fibers were then gently teased apart for visual recording. The results were so concordant that they can readily be summarized as follows (Weiss, 1972b).

(1) The driving mechanism of the axonal flow is clearly visible as a continuous succession of peristaltic pulses, i.e. steadily propagated contraction–relaxation waves which sweep cellulifugally over the axonal surface at intervals of between 15 and 30 min, proceeding at rates of close to 1 μm/min.

(2) The morphological expression of these waves is, *in vitro*, a circumferential indentation of the contour of the axon (including the myelin sheath in medullated fibers), proceeding smoothly without interruptions from the cell body downwards. The size of the traveling ring-like zone of constriction measures a few micra; in its wake the axonal surface returns to its standard diameter until after 15 to 30 min the next wave arrives, and so forth.

(3) As said earlier, the axonal content itself behaves purely passively, driven forward by the "massaging" effect of the surface pulse. This distinction between active drive and passive convection is most marked in fibers in early stages of Wallerian degeneration, when the axonal content has already become fragmented into separate oblong boluses (Cajal's "ovoids"), while its complex envelope (myelin sheath and axolemma) is still continuous over longer stretches; in those cases, one sees the surface wave move smoothly over the whole length of still continuous sheath enclosing the string of discontinuous fragments, each of which is passively shoved forward during the passing of a wave, rebounding afterwards to its prior place.

(4) Since the driving force of the axonal flow thus resides solely in the axonal surface, the speed of this drive, ascertained now directly from the motion picture recordings as close to 1 μm/min, must also be accepted as the upper speed limit at which the semisolid axonal content can advance, much as the speed of a conveyor belt delimits the fastest rate at which its load can be conveyed. Slower advances, down to full arrest, are attributable to local obstructions that impair the *passive displacement* of the content, but not the unhindered *active propagation* of the surface drive. In such instances, the content gets compressed lengthwise and commensurably bloated in width, as shown by the "damming" effect in front of bottlenecks. On the other hand, the far more liquid state of an embryonic or re-generating axon sprout would, as in Newtonian flow in general, permit the fluid to accommodate to an increase of the pressure of the drive by an increase in flow rate in inverse proportion to any reduction in the diameter of the flow channel.

(5) Motion pictures of the mobility of the content of *mature* fibers, forced artificially into more rapid flow than that of the normal axon by gradual compression applied above or below the microscopic field, have in general confirmed and expanded our earlier conclusions regarding the consistency of neuroplasm, its cohesiveness, rheology, shearing properties, etc.

(6) In all of this, neither the nature nor the specific carrier of the peristaltic surface activity has been specified, and I have deliberately refrained from hypothetical predictions beyond the range of our actual knowledge, which is still very meager. As for the dynamics involved, there has, however, a promising clue turned up recently, which will be dealt with farther below. Regarding the identification of the "active surface," the nearest guess would be a cooperative interaction between axolemma and Schwann cell membrane, particularly as the Schwann cell, with its great abundance of mitochondria, could readily supply the necessary energy for the drive, which the axon with its notorious dearth of mitochondria along its course could not. Yet all such questions had better be left to further disciplined research than to premature and perhaps prejudicial speculations.

I have presented these points merely by way of samples of how the purely descriptive term of "axonal flow" can be brought nearer to realistic understanding of the dynamics underlying the process. Encouraged by the insight gained from the cinemicrographic analysis, combined with electron microscopic studies (not to be dealt with in this paper), we then proceeded with some temerity to developing technological models of the peristaltic drive with the aim of not just simulating the phenomenon but of having it conform to strict mathematical formulations by which the pertinence of the model and the validity of its premises could be tested, thereby to furnish guidelines for deeper understanding and further detailed investigations. This work was undertaken at my laboratory as a doctor's thesis in "bioengineering" under the joint supervision of an authority in fluid mechanics, Professor Martin J. Levy, of the Newark College of Engineering, and myself (Biondi et al., 1972).

The candidate, Robert Biondi, who after his master's degree had spent several years in engineering practice, first established by delicate micromethods the apparent viscosity of microsamples of neuroplasm extruded from single axons. The measured value of 2.5×10^6 cP, which is several hundred thousand times that of watery solutions, quantified further our earlier evidence of the semisolid state of the axis cylinder. However, the vast number of unknowns in the field of nonNewtonian rheology of such highly gelated masses, particularly in the microscopic dimensions at issue, was so staggering that it is surprising that we succeeded to come out from our lengthy trial-and-error procedure over the years with a solution in which the behavior of the mechanical model, the underlying theoretical premises, and the records obtained from the living nerve fiber itself, were in essential accordance over the testing range of variables explored in the model (e.g. viscosity of test substances, speed of drive, frequency of pulses, shear forces, etc.) and despite the necessary introduction of many simplifying assumptions to make the model suitable for rigorous mathematical treatment. Even then, recourse to computer handling became crucial.

The details of these studies are far too complicated to be recounted in this brief report. Let me give simply a very sketchy summary of the salient features relevant to the understanding of the dynamics of the axonal drive. The final working model (Biondi et al., 1972) consisted of a planar flow channel, with two Plexiglass plates as bottom and top, several millimeters apart, and the sides made of elastic rubber sheeting with inflow and outflow tubes on the front and rear sides. On each of the two flanks, a series of equidistant horizontal disk-shaped rollers, mounted on a symmetrical pair of moving "caterpillar-tractor" belts, protruded into the lateral rubber walls. The two chains of opposite rollers, traveling continuously and abreast down the channel sides, thus produced periodic transitory symmetrical indentations of the sides of the channel, hence series of rhythmic changes of its lumen in simulation of a peristaltic wave. The device was built to permit deliberate adjustments of wavespeed, wavelength, and wave amplitude. Pressure gauges, dipping into the channel and fixed on the frame, were connected with oscillographs for the recording of local pressure changes in the medium during the passing of a pair of rollers. They registered as a rhythmic pressure diagram, and with the aid of already established theoretical formulations (Shapiro et al., 1969; Yin and Fung, 1969) yielded reliable values for the pressure developed by a peristaltic wave in the axial direction of flow as a function of the flow rate for any particular wave geometry and test fluid viscosity.

Extensive experimentation with this device has made it very likely that it can be considered as a truly representative, though simplified, model of the major features of the dynamics of axonal flow. It has corroborated the theoretical prediction of rheologists that traveling constrictions of a tube, even if of small amplitude far short of total occlusion of the lumen, can set and keep the tube content in translatory motion provided the consecutive waves are adequately spaced in time. The passive convection of the content results from the just mentioned different rates in the rise and fall of pressure in front and in back of the advancing constriction. Finally, and most encouragingly, a comparison between the experimental data of the model with the actual parameters of the axonal flow has led to the conclusion that quantitative predictions from the model, with speed being a function of peristaltic wave geometry and the flow properties of the conveyed material, yield a theoretical mean value for the possible rate of flow of 0.45 mm/day, which is of the same order as that empirically observed in the living nerve fiber.

After these brief remarks about the physical mechanism of the surface drive of the axonal column, let me pass on cursorily to recent observations apt to place that peristaltic wave into a much more general class of cell surface properties. They intimate that the linear advance of the constriction pulse of the axonal surface is simply the linear expression of a cell surface activity which in a spherical cell would manifest itself as three-dimensional pulsation. The occurrence of pulsation, i.e. contraction–relaxation waves sweeping over cell surfaces, has been noted in a wide array of organisms; for instance, in the yolk of fish eggs and embryos, the plasmodial slime molds, and most appropriately in our context, Schwann cells *in vitro* (Pomerat, 1961). Some time ago (Weiss, 1961) I noticed in motion pictures of monkey kidney cells cultured *in vitro* that some of the cells, flattened out to disk shape along the cover slip, displayed a rotatory movement circling along the fringe of the ruffled membrane. I interpreted this as the planar configuration which a spherical pulse wave would assume when constrained into a planar surface; if constrained further into a linear course it would appear as a peristaltic wave as in the nerve fiber.

Alerted by this conjecture, I have recently subjected the respective films to quantitative measurements of the time characteristics of the phenomenon. The apparent circular revolution of the fringe was identified as a circling wave of expansion (adhesion) and retraction (detachment) of the cell fringe (to the substratum) proceeding in a regular rhythm. The time for completing a full turn was between 15 and 30 min, corresponding to a rate of circumferential movement of the order of 1 μm/min. Both periodicity and speed of travel of this wave thus turned out to be surprisingly close to the corresponding values established for the axonal drive. As a test of whether or not this was sheer coincidence, we then investigated other cell types. There we found similar surface rhythms wherever we looked. Macrophages from various sources showed regular pulsations or shuttle movements with periodicities varying, depending on type, size, and state, between 5 and 15 min/cycle, faster than the larger cells but still within the same order of magnitude. Thus rhythmic sequences of contraction–relaxation waves sweeping over cell surfaces seem to be a common cell-biological phenomenon that has escaped general notice only because of its comparatively slow rate, which requires time-lapse accelerations of about 100 times the actual speed to be recognized visually.

Let me now briefly comment on a possible physicochemical explanation of the observed rhythmicity. A. C. Taylor in my laboratory had observed that single cultured cells, well spread out *in vitro* in a balanced salt solution at pH 7.3, would contract and assume spherical shape when the pH of the medium was raised to about 8, which change proved fully reversible as soon as the pH of the medium was returned to normal: the rounded cells would then reattach and spread out flat as before (Taylor, 1962). Going on, we placed bipolar spindle cells, whose motile ruffles are confined to the two opposite poles, between two micropipettes, dispensing the basic medium, one at pH 7.3 and the other buffered to pH 8 (Weiss and Scott, 1963). Only the cell end exposed to the high pH did retract, while the other end continued to spread on. This result unmistakably revealed a highly sensitive *local* reaction of the cell membrane to changes in the local inside–outside pH gradient across the surface. In short, any increase in the local slope of that gradient generates a local contraction. And, accordingly, one can interpret the contraction–expansion wave circling around the fringe of flattened cells in a homogeneous medium (see the first described experiments above) as a wave of lowered intrinsic local pH, signaling a wave of chemical changes in or beneath the cell membrane. In other words, the observed cycling of the pH wave might be just an index of a corresponding sweep around the cell of underlying chemical dynamics.

In contrast to the growing understanding of the axonal flow proper, however, the dynamics of *endoaxonal transport* is still quite obscure. Aside from the abundantly demonstrated fact that transport from center to periphery (and possibly also in reverse) at rates of 1 μm/s and higher exists, neither its routes nor its mechanism have been ascertained. In part, the search has been beclouded by the fact that data for whole nerve (including—besides neurons—blood vessels, endoneural tissue, and interstitial lymph spaces) were lumped with the scanty data on individual axons. Also the data cover the whole range of dimensions from molecules and macromolecules through larger particles (e.g. catecholamine storage granules up to 0.1 μm) up to the pigment granules of chromatophores (of about 0.5 μm in diameter), which latter race equally fast toward the center of the cell under the influence of adrenalin. Elementary physical and rheological considerations would seem to discount explanations in terms of hydrodynamic flow, although peristalsis in submicroscopic dimensions cannot be entirely ruled out (Weiss, 1970). Faster transport of molecules and particles carrying an electric surface charge and being passed on in saltatory fashion along properly spaced "stepladders" of correspondingly charged sites has been observed (Weiss, 1961; Grover, 1966) and might be borne in mind. Neurotubules have also been implicated, mostly because of the blockage of fast transport by colchicine (Kreutzberg, 1969), a drug noted for its interaction with tubular protein; yet, here again, the drug might also have affected coincidentally the real, but unknown, conveyor mechanism other than the tubule. So, it might be wise to defer, for the present, sheer conjecture pending the disclosure of further more concrete information.

There are some suggestive reports on bidirectional fast transport. Those based on the observation of transitory accumulations of axonal content (mitochondria, catecholamines, enzymes) at the proximal end of the distal stump of a transected nerve can be dismissed for having failed to take account of the powerful extraneous effects which the degenerative processes at the site of such a traumatic lesion exert on the adjacent area of live tissue (Schlote, 1970). But those based on distoproximal movement of tracers in intact tissue are creditable (Kristensson *et al.*, 1971). Yet even they need not imply that a given single neuron has shipping lines that can operate in both directions at the same time, such as has been described for the fluid pseudopodia of single-celled organisms. On the other hand, the familiar retrograde "influence" extending from the periphery to the central nerve cell bodies via their nerve fibers makes some centripetal communication device a postulate. But again, it is unwarranted to presume that this process need involve any centripetal convection of *matter* any more than does the propagation of an afferent nerve impulse. In our state of ignorance it would be preferable not to limit our guesses to the narrow range of answers and considerations already at our disposal as of today.

ACKNOWLEDGEMENT

The recent work of the laboratory has been partially supported by the National Science Foundation. Assistance by Mrs. Yvonne Holland is gratefully acknowledged.

REFERENCES

BIONDI, R. J., LEVY, M. J., and WEISS, P. A. (1972) An engineering study of the peristaltic drive of axona flow. *Proc. Natn. Acad. Sci. USA* **69**, 1732–1736.

CAJAL, S. RAMON Y. (1928) *Degeneration and Regeneration of the Nervous System* (translated and ed. by R. M. May), Oxford Univ. Press.

DROZ, B., and LEBLOND, C. P. (1963) Axonal migration of proteins in the central nervous system and peripheral nerves as shown by radioautography. *J. Comp. Neurol.* **121**, 325–346.

FRIEDE, R. L. (1959) Transport of oxydative enzymes in nerve fibers; a histochemical investigation of the regenerative cycle in neurons. *Expl. Neurol.* **1**, 441–466.

GERARD, R. W. (1932) Nerve metabolism. *Physiol. Rev.* **12**, 469–592.

GRAFSTEIN, B., McEWEN, B. S., and SHELANSKI, M. L. (1970) Axonal transport of neurotubule protein. *Nature* **227**, 289–290.

GROVER, N. (1966) Anisodiametric transport of ions and particles in anisotropic tissue spaces. *Biophys. J.* **6**, 71–85.

KARLSSON, J.-O., and SJÖSTRAND, J. (1969) The effect of colchicine on the axonal transport of protein in the optic nerve and tract of the rabbit. *Brain Res.* **13**, 617–619.

KREUTZBERG, G. (1969) Neuronal dynamics and axonal flow: IV, Blockage of intraaxonal enzyme transport by colchicine. *Proc. Natn. Acad. Sci. USA* **62**, 722–728.

KRISTENSSON, K., OLSSON, Y., and SJÖSTRAND, J. (1971) Axonal uptake and retrograde transport of exogenous proteins in the hypoglossal nerve. *Brain Res.* **32**, 399–406.

MIANI, N. (1964) Proximo-distal movement of phospholipid in the axoplasm of the intact and regenerating neurons. In: *Mechanisms of Neural Regeneration* (*Progress in Brain Research*, vol. 13) (Singer, M. and Schadé, J. P., eds.) Elsevier, Amsterdam. pp. 115–126.

OCHS, S., and BURGER, E. (1958) Movement of substance proximo-distally in nerve axons as studied with spinal cord injections of radioactive phosphorus. *Am. J. Physiol.* **194**, 499–506.

POMERAT, C. M. (1961) Cinematology, indispensable tool for cytology. *Int. Rev. Cytol.* **11**, 307–339.

SCHLOTE, W. (1970) Nervus opticus und experimentelles trauma. *Monogr. Gesamtgeb. Neurol. Psychiatrie* **131**, 156 pp.

SHAPIRO, A. H., JAFFRIN, M. Y., and WEINBERG, S. L. (1969) *J. Fluid Mech.* **37**, 799–825.

TAYLOR, A. C. (1962) Responses of cells to pH changes in the medium. *J. Cell Biol.* **15**, (2) 201–209.

TAYLOR, A. C., and WEISS, P. A. (1965) Demonstration of axonal flow by the movement of tritium-labelled protein in mature optic nerve fibers. *Proc. Natn. Acad. Sci. USA* **54**, 1521–1527.

WEISS, P. A. (1943) Endoneurial edema in constricted nerve. *Anat. Rec.* **86**, 491–522.

WEISS, P. A. (1944a) Evidence of perpetual proximo-distal growth of nerve fibers. *Biol. Bull.* **87**, 160.

WEISS, P. A. (1944b) The technology of nerve regeneration: a review: sutureless tubulation and related methods of nerve repair. *J. Neurosurg.* **1**, 400–450.

WEISS, P. A. (1961) Structure as the coordinating principle in the life of a cell. *Proc. of the Robert A. Welch Foundation Conferences on Chemical Research* **5**, 5–31.

WEISS, P. A. (1967) Neuronal dynamics and axonal flow: III, Cellulifugal transport of labelled neuroplasm in isolated nerve preparations. *Proc. Natn. Acad. Sci. USA* **57**, 1239–1245.

WEISS, P. A. (1969) Neuronal dynamics and neuroplasmic ("axonal") flow. In: *Cellular Dynamics of the Neuron* (S. H. Barondes, ed.) Symposium of International Society for Cell Biology, Academic Press, New York **8**, 3–34.

WEISS, P. A. (1970) Neuronal dynamics and neuroplasmic flow. In *The Neurosciences: Second Study Program* (editor-in-chief F. O. Schmitt), The Rockefeller University Press, New York, pp. 840–850.

WEISS, P. A. (1972a) Neuronal dynamics and axonal flow: V, The semisolid state of the moving axonal column. *Proc. Natn. Acad. Sci. USA* **69**, 620–623.

WEISS, P. A. (1972b) Neuronal dynamics and axonal flow: axonal peristalsis. *Proc. Natn. Acad. Sci. USA.* **69**, 1309–1312.

WEISS, P. A., and CAVANAUGH, M. W. (1959) Further evidence of perpetual growth of nerve fibers: recovery of fiber diameter after the release of prolonged constrictions. *J. Exp. Zool.* **142**, 461–473.

WEISS, P. A., and DAVIS, H. (1943) Pressure block in nerves provided with arterial sleeves. *J. Neurophysiol.* **6**, 269–286.

WEISS, P. A., and HISCOE, H. B. (1948) Experiments on the mechanism of nerve growth. *J. Exp. Zool.* **107**, 315–395.

WEISS, P. A., and HOLLAND, Y. (1967) Neuronal dynamics and axonal flow: II, The olfactory nerve as model test object. *Proc. Natn. Acad. Sci. USA* **57**, 258–264.

WEISS, P. A., and MAYR, R. (1971a) Neuronal organelles in neuroplasmic ("axonal") flow: I, Mitochondria. *Acta neuropath. Berl.* Suppl. V, 187–197.

WEISS, P. A., and MAYR, R. (1971b) Neuronal organelles in neuroplasmic ("axonal") flow: II, Neurotubules. *Acta neuropath. Berl.*, Suppl. V, 198–205.

WEISS, P. A., and PILLAI, P. A. (1965) Convection and fate of mitochondria in nerve fibers: axonal flow as vehicle. *Proc. Natn. Acad. Sci. USA* **54**, 48–56.

WEISS, P. A., and SCOTT, B. I. H. (1963) Polarization of cell locomotion *in vitro*. *Proc. Natn. Acad. Sci. USA* **50**, 330–336.

WEISS, P. A., WANG, H., TAYLOR, A. C., and EDDS, M. V. Jr. (1945) Proximo-distal fluid convection in the endoneurial spaces of peripheral nerves demonstrated by colored and radioactive (isotope) tracers. *Am. J. Physiol.* **143**, 521–540.

YIN, F., and FUNG, Y. C. (1969) *J. Appl. Mech.* **36**, 579–587.

EFFECTS OF DEGENERATION AND AXOPLASMIC TRANSPORT BLOCKADE ON SYNAPTIC ULTRASTRUCTURE, FUNCTION, AND PROTEIN COMPOSITION

M. Cuénod, P. Marko,* E. Niederer, C. Sandri, and K. Akert

Brain Research Institute, University of Zürich, Zürich, Switzerland and
*Friedrich Miescher Institute, Basel, Switzerland

SUMMARY

Nerve endings of the pigeon optic fibers present an early enlargement of the vesicles after retinal ablation and intraocular injection of colchicine, suggesting that this ultrastructural alteration might be related to a deficit in material migrating with the fast axoplasmic flow. The blockade of axoplasmic transport by colchicine or vinblastine seems to interfere reversibly with synaptic transmission without affecting the nerve impulse conduction. During the degeneration of the optic nerve, one protein subunit disappears, which seems specific for the pigeon retinal projections. It can be found in the soluble and in one particulate fraction. It is probably a glycoprotein renewed by material transported with the fast flow. Its molecular weight is in the order of 140 000–150 000.

INTRODUCTION

The dependence of the axon and its terminals upon the nerve cell body for the maintenance of their normal structure and function is well established (Grafstein, 1969; Droz, 1973; Weiss, this symposium). The axoplasmic migration of a great variety of molecules provides a mechanism by which the soma supplies axon and terminals with necessary elements. When severed from the perikaryon, the axon and the nerve endings undergo degenerative changes which have been long recognized by the anatomists (Guillery, 1970). This paper presents a review of data concerned (1) with the early ultrastructural changes in degenerating terminals and their relation to axoplasmic transport, and (2) with the disappearance of a protein during the degenerating process and some of its characteristics.

Most of this work has been performed on the visual system of the pigeon, using the ganglion cells of the retina, their axons in the optic nerve and contralateral optic tract, and their terminals in the contralateral optic tectum as a model. The avian retino-tectal system has the advantage of being completely crossed so that one side can be used as control for the

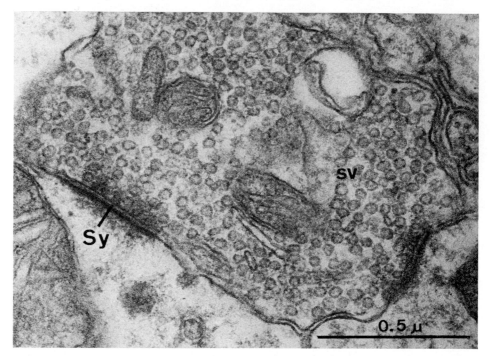

FIG. 1. Normal optic nerve terminal in the optic tectum of the pigeon. sv = synaptic vesicles, Sy = synapse, f = fibrils. Paraformaldehyde perfusion, followed by glutaraldehyde immersion fixation. Osmic acid post fixation; uranylacetate and lead hydroxide contrast. (×40,000.)

other in the same animal. It has been extensively used to study axoplasmic transport because it is easy to apply a radioactive precursor via vitreous humor to the retinal ganglion cells (Taylor and Weiss, 1965; Grafstein, 1967; McEwen and Grafstein, 1968; Karlsson and Sjöstrand, 1971; Elam and Agranoff, 1971; Cuénod et al., 1972a).

EARLY ULTRASTRUCTURAL CHANGES IN DEGENERATING NERVE TERMINALS

After surgical ablation of the retina the optic nerve terminals present ultrastructural changes which appear much earlier than the fibrillar and electron dense boutons. The diameter of the vesicular profiles is larger than that of normal synaptic vesicles (Figs. 1 and 2). This change can be detected 12–24 h after the destruction of the ganglion cell bodies. Then there is a progressive increase in the vesicular diameter and a decrease in vesicular numbers until the classical stage of homogeneous opacity of terminals is reached. These observations were made on material fixed with paraformaldehyde, glutaraldehyde, and acrolein as well as on freeze-etched preparations (Cuénod et al., 1970; Akert et al., 1971). Thus the presence of enlarged vesicles in the presynaptic boutons appear as an early sign of terminal degeneration. Similar observations have been made by Angaut (personal communication) and confirmed in other systems (Kawana et al., 1971; Pecci Saavedra et al., 1973).

The time course of early degenerative changes is nearly identical with the arrival in the nerve endings of proteins transported by fast axoplasmic migration under normal con-

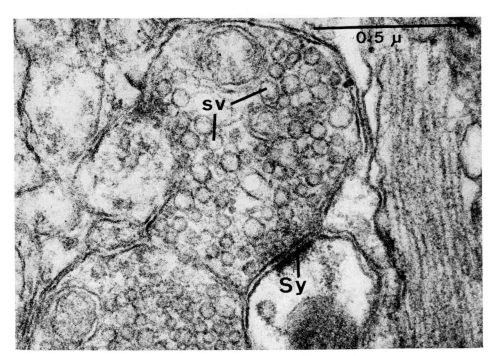

FIG. 2. Optic nerve terminal in the left optic tectum of the pigeon 7 days after ablation of the right retina. Note the enlarged vesicles. Method of fixation and impregnation same as in Fig. 1.

ditions. When a radioactive amino acid is injected into the pigeon vitreous humor, labeled proteins appear within a few hours in the tectal optic nerve terminals and synaptosomes and reach a first peak 12–24 h later (Fig. 4) (Schonbach and Cuénod, 1971; Schonbach et al., 1971; Cuénod and Schonbach, 1971).

INTERFERENCE WITH AXOPLASMIC TRANSPORT

The similar time course of the two events suggested that the early degenerative vesicular changes could be related to a deficit in some material normally provided by the fast axoplasmic transport and missing after destruction of the ganglion cell body. In order to test this hypothesis, colchicine, which has been shown to interfere with the axoplasmic transport (Dahlström, 1968; Kreutzberg, 1968), has been injected intraocularly in doses of 10, 100, or 500 μg at various times before intraocular injection of radioactive amino acid. The animals were sacrificed 24 h later, that is at the peak of fast flowing activity. Colchicine induced a strong depression of the transported radioactivity, which is at a maximum 3 days after injection and completely reversible within a few weeks (Boesch et al., 1972). Similarly, intraocular injection of colchicine in the same doses induces the appearance of large vesicular profiles sometimes associated with a fibrillar proliferation in the tectal optic nerve terminals (Figs. 1 and 3). This phenomenon which can be detected 3–4 days after colchicine application, reaches a peak after 8–14 days, and is completely reversible within a few weeks without the appearance of dark boutons (Cuénod et al., 1972b). Thus it seems likely that the vesicular changes observed during the early stage of degeneration in the pigeon visual system is related to the lack of some factor normally supplied by the fast

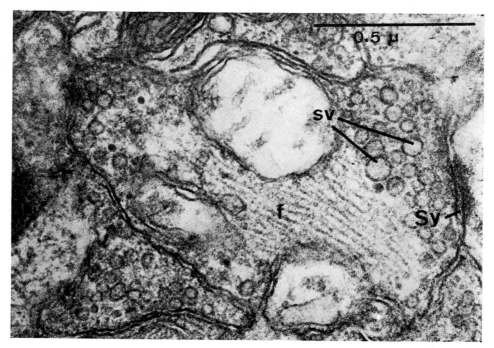

FIG. 3. Optic nerve terminal of the left optic tectum of the pigeon 7 days after injection of 500 μg colchicine in the right vitreous humor. Note the enlarged vesicles and the fibrillar profiles. Method of fixation and impregnation same as in Fig. 1.

axoplasmic flow. Nothing is known about the mechanism responsible for these changes. It could be due to a passive effect of a change in concentration of synaptoplasmic elements or to the lack of a factor implicated in the vesicle formation or renewal.

Furthermore, the ultrastructural changes induced in the nerve terminals by the colchicine blockage of axoplasmic flow correlate well with alterations of the synaptic transmission. Electrical stimulation applied at various times after intraocular injection of colchicine to the optic nerve elicits normal action potentials indicating that the impulse conduction is not affected, while the responses recorded in the middle and deep layers of the optic tectum are strongly depressed, suggesting a deficit in the synaptic transmission. This depression is most conspicuous after 1 week and completely reversible within a few weeks (Perisic and Cuénod, 1972). Recently, similar results have been obtained after intraocular injection of 10–100 μg of Vinblastine (Felder, in preparation), which also blocks very effectively the axoplasmic transport of proteins in the pigeon visual system (Cuénod, unpublished observations).

The results reviewed above show that interference with the supply of material coming from the perikaryon and renewing the axon and its terminals induces early changes in the nerve ending ultrastructure and function. This is consistent with the suggestion that the rapid axoplasmic flow is particularly destined to the nerve ending (McEwen and Grafstein, 1968; Cuénod and Schonbach, 1971; Schonbach et al., 1971; Cuénod et al., 1972a; Droz, 1973) and that a part at least of the material transported rapidly has a half-life of a few days only (Cuénod and Schonbach, 1971; Schonbach and Cuénod, 1971; Marko and Cuénod, 1973). Good agreement exists also with the anatomical observation that after destruction of

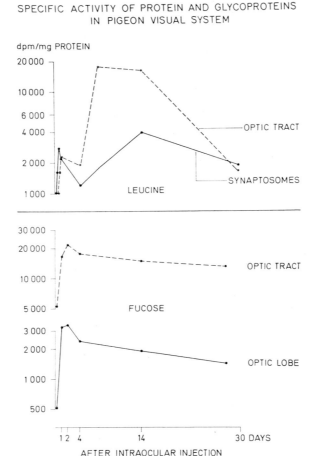

FIG. 4. Time course of the specific activity of proteins and glycoproteins in optic tract homogenate, synaptosomal fraction of optic lobe, or optic lobe homogenate.

afferent fibres to some nuclei investigated in the cat and rat the degenerative changes demonstrated with the aid of suppressive silver technique seem to appear first in the terminals and then in the axon (Grant, personal communication). As the early degenerative changes seem to be related to the lack of material transported by fast axoplasmic flow, one could speculate that the later changes might involve a deficit in slowly migrating material.

CHANGES IN PROTEIN COMPOSITION DURING DEGENERATION

In view of the critical importance of the material supplied by the perikaryon to the axon and terminals, the protein composition of the pigeon optic nerve and tectum was studied at various time intervals after surgical ablation of the retina. The samples were homogenized in 0.32 M sucrose and separated by differential centrifugation in crude mitochondrial, microsomal, and soluble fractions. The crude mitochondrial fraction was placed on a discontinuous sucrose gradient and centrifuged at 250,000 g for 60 min. "Fraction X"

EFFECT OF RETINAL ABLATION ON
SDS ACRYLAMIDE GEL PATTERNS OF
FRACTION X FROM PIGEON OPTIC
TECTUM

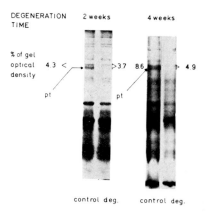

FIG. 5. SDS polyacrylamide gels of fraction X from pigeon optic tectum 2 and 4 weeks after ablation of the retina on one side. The pattern of bands on the degenerating side (deg.) compared with the control side, reveals the progressive disappearance of one band, called pt.

SUBCELLULAR DISTRIBUTION OF PT BAND
IN OPTIC NERVE AND TECTUM

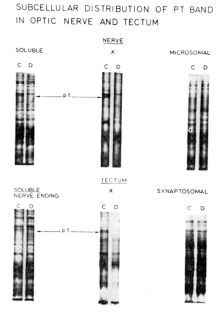

FIG. 6. Subcellular distribution of pt band in pigeon optic nerve and tectum degeneration induced by ablation of the retina 4 weeks earlier. Note the presence of pt band on the control (C) side and its absence on the degenerating (D) side in the soluble and X fraction of nerve and the soluble nerve ending fraction (O) and X fraction of tectum. This band cannot be detected in other fractions, e.g. in the microsomal fraction of nerve or the synaptosomal fraction of tectum on the normal side.

was collected at the interphase between 1.4 and 1.6 M. In other experiments the crude mito-chondrial fraction was submitted to an osmotic shock and fractionated according to Whittaker *et al.* (1964). The soluble and the O fraction were precipitated with 10% TCA, then all fractions were solubilized in 1% SDS, 8 M urea, 0.01 M dithiothreitol, and 0.05 M K_2CO_3. They were separated on SDS polyacrylamide gel electrophoresis according to Grossfeld and Shooter (1971) as modified by Marko *et al.* (1971) (see Cuénod *et al.*, 1973, for technical details).

Although a diffuse diminution of the bands was noticed on the degenerating side in comparison with the intact side, the most striking observation was the strong decrease and disparition of at least one band, 2–4 weeks after operation (Fig. 5). This band, called "pt", is present in fractions of optic fibers and of optic tectum. In the optic nerve and tract, two

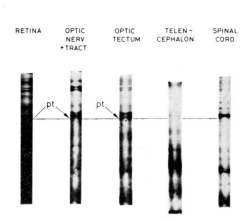

FIG. 7. Anatomical distribution of pt band in intact pigeon nervous system. Note the presence of pt band in X fractions of retina, optic tract, and nerve and optic tectum; but in telencephalon and spinal cord, the band cannot be detected.

fractions are particularly rich in pt band material—the soluble protein fraction and the particulate fraction X. In other membraneous nerve fractions, the pt band cannot be detected. In the optic tectum this band can be found in the X fraction and in the soluble protein fraction obtained from synaptosomes after osmotic shock (O), but not in other fractions (Fig. 6). The pt band has been detected in the retina, but could not be observed either in soluble or X fraction prepared from pigeon telencephalon or spinal cord (Fig. 7). These observations suggest that this protein subunit might be specific for the retinal pro-jections to the mesodiencephalon of the pigeon. Its migration in SDS gel electrophoresis suggest a molecular weight between 140 000–150 000. Labeling the fast and slow migrating proteins by an intraocular injection of [14]C- and ^{3}H-proline respectively reveals that the pt band is renewed mainly by fast moving material (Cuénod *et al.*, 1973). When ^{3}H-fucose is injected intraocularly, the pt band contains about 5% of the total gel radioactivity, although the density of the band is much smaller, suggesting that it is a glycoprotein.

It would be important to know more about the turnover characteristics of this protein. The only data available concern the total fractions (Fig. 4). After intraocular injection of ^{3}H-fucose, the specific activity of the proteins decay in two phases with half-life times of 7 and 57 days in the optic tract, 5 and 30 days in the tectal crude mitochondrial fraction, and 7 and 120 days in the O fraction, all fractions containing the pt band (Marko and Cuénod, 1973; Marko *et al.* in preparation). At the moment, the functional significance of this protein subunit is unknown.

ACKNOWLEDGEMENTS

We thank Dr. Allan Smith for reading the manuscript and the Misses L. Decoppet, R. Emch, E. Schneider, and Mr. A. Fäh for their excellent technical assistance.

Work supported by grants No. 3.329.70 and 3.133.69 from the Swiss National Foundation for Scientific Research and by the Dr. Eric Slack-Gyr Foundation.

REFERENCES

AKERT, K., CUÉNOD, M., and MOOR, H. (1971) Further observations on the enlargement of synaptic vesicles in degenerating optic nerve terminals of the avian tectum. *Brain Res.* **25,** 255–263.

BOESCH, J., MARKO, P., and CUÉNOD, M. (1972) Effects of colchicine on axonal transport of proteins in the pigeon visual pathways. *Neurobiology* **2,** 123–132.

CUÉNOD, M., and SCHONBACH, J. (1971) Synaptic proteins and axonal flow in the pigeon visual pathway. *J. Neurochem.* **18,** 809–816.

CUÉNOD, M., SANDRI, C., and AKERT, K. (1970) Enlarged synaptic vesicles as an early sign of secondary degeneration in the optic nerve terminals of the pigeon. *J. Cell Sci.* **6,** 605–613.

CUÉNOD, M., BOESCH, J., MARKO, P., PERISIC, M., SANDRI, C., and SCHONBACH, J. (1972a) Contribution of axoplasmic transport to synaptic structures and functions. *Int. J. Neurosci.* **4,** 77–87.

CUÉNOD, M., SANDRI, C., and AKERT, K. (1972b) Enlarged synaptic vesicles in optic nerve terminals induced by intraocular injection of colchicine. *Brain Res.* **39,** 285–296.

CUÉNOD, M., MARKO, P., and NIEDERER, E. (1973) Disappearance of particulate tectal protein during optic nerve degeneration in the pigeon. *Brain Res.* **49,** 422–426.

DAHLSTRÖM, A. (1968) Effect of colchicine on transport of amine storage granules in sympathetic nerves of rat. *Eur. J. Pharmac.* **5,** 111–113.

DROZ, B. (1973) Renewal of synaptic proteins. *Brain Res.* **62,** 383–394.

ELAM, J. S., and AGRANOFF, B. W. (1971) Transport of proteins and sulfated mucopolysaccharides in the goldfish visual system. *J. Neurobiol.* **2,** 379–390.

GRAFSTEIN, B. (1967) Transport of protein by goldfish optic nerve fibers. *Science* **157,** 196–198.

GRAFSTEIN, B. (1969) Axonal transport: communication between soma and synapse. In *Advances in Biochemical Psychopharmacology*, vol. 1 (E. Costa and P. Greengard, eds.), Raven Press, New York, pp. 11–25.

GROSSFELD, R. M., and SHOOTER, E. M. (1971) A study of the changes in protein composition of mouse brain during ontogenic development. *J. Neurochem.* **18,** 2265–2277.

GUILLERY, R. W. (1970) Light and electron-microscopical studies of normal and degenerating axons. In *Contemporary Research Methods in Neuroanatomy* (W. J. H. Nauta and S. O. E. Ebbesson, eds.), Springer-Verlag, New York, pp. 77–105.

KARLSSON, J.-O., and SJÖSTRAND, J. (1971) Synthesis, migration and turnover of protein in retinal ganglion cells. *J. Neurochem.* **18,** 749–767.

KAWANA, E., AKERT, K., and BRUPPACHER, H. (1971) Enlargement of synaptic vesicles as an early sign of terminal degeneration in the rat caudate nucleus. *J. Comp. Neurol.* **142,** 297–308.

KREUTZBERG, G. W. (1968) Histochemical demonstration of a colchicine-induced blockage of enzyme transport in axons of peripheral nerves. *Third. Int. Congr. Histochem. Cytochem.*, p. 133.

MARKO, P., and CUÉNOD, M. (1973) Contribution of the nerve cell body to renewal of axonal and synaptic glycoproteins in the pigeon visual system. *Brain Res.* **62,** 419–423.

MARKO, P., SUSZ, J.-P., CUÉNOD, M. (1971) Synaptosomal proteins and axoplasmic flow: Fractionation by SDS polyacrylamide gel electrophoresis. *FEBS Letters* **17,** 261–264.

McEWEN, B. S., and GRAFSTEIN, B. (1968) Fast and slow components in axonal transport of protein. *J. Cell Biol.* **38,** 494–508.

PECCI SAAVEDRA, J., MASCITTI, T. A., and PEREZ LLORET, I. L. (1973) Increased rate of anterograde degeneration in the visual pathway of kittens. *Brain Res.* **50,** 265–274.

PERISIC, M., and CUÉNOD, M. (1972) Synaptic transmission depressed by colchicine blockade of axoplasmic flow. *Science* **175,** 1140–1142.

SCHONBACH, J., and CUÉNOD, M. (1971) Axoplasmic migration of protein: a light microscopic autoradiographic study in the avian retino-tectal pathway. *Exp. Brain Res.* **12,** 275–282.

SCHONBACH, J., SCHONBACH, C., and CUÉNOD, M. (1971) Rapid phase of axoplasmic flow and synaptic proteins: an electron microscopical autoradiographic study. *J. Comp. Neurol.* **141**, 485–498.

TAYLOR, A., and WEISS, C. (1965) Demonstration of axonal flow by the movement of tritium-labeled protein in mature optic nerve fibers. *Proc. Natn. Acad. Sci. USA* **54**, 1521–1527.

WHITTAKER, V. P., MICHAELSON, I. A., and KIRKLAND, R. J. A. (1964) The separation of synaptic vesicles from nerve-ending particles ("synaptosomes"). *Biochem. J.* **90**, 293–303.

AXONAL TRANSPORT OF PROTEINS IN GROWING AND REGENERATING NEURONS

J. Sjöstrand and M. Frizell

Institute of Neurobiology, University of Göteborg, Göteborg, Sweden

SUMMARY

Axonal transport in chick embryonic retinal neurons was studied after intraocular injection of ^{3}H-proline or ^{3}H-fucose. Rapid transport to the contralateral optic tectum could be demonstrated from the seventh day of incubation and the rate of rapid transport increased with age. A relatively larger proportion of retinal fucose-labeled glycoproteins was transported to the tectum throughout development, and the highest percentage of transported glycoprotein radioactivity was observed at 18 days. SDS gel electrophoresis of labeled tectal proteins revealed that a large number of relatively high mol.wt-polypeptides reached the nerve terminals by a rapid phase of axonal transport throughout development.

In other experiments the transport of choline-O-acetyltransferase (ChAc, EC 2.3.1.6), acetylcholinesterase (AChE, EC 3.1.1.7), and rapidly migrating proteins and glycoproteins was studied in normal and regenerating hypoglossal nerves of the adult rabbit, using ligature technique. The accumulation of ChAc and AChE in double ligature experiments on the hypoglossal and vagus nerves suggested that only 5–20% of the enzymes were mobile within an isolated nerve segment, and this mobile fraction was transported with the fast or intermediate rate of axonal flow. The study of ChAc in the perikarya, axons, and terminals of normal hypoglossal neurons revealed that only 2% of the enzyme activity was localized to the nerve cell bodies, whereas 42% was derived from the main hypoglossal nerve trunk and 56% from the preterminal axons and terminals in the tongue. From the transport rate of ChAc in the hypoglossal nerve and its distribution, the half-life of the enzyme in the terminal axons of the hypoglossal nerve was calculated to 16 days.

In regenerating nerves the accumulation of rapidly migrating ^{3}H-leucine labeled proteins, ChAc and AChE, proximal to a single ligature was reduced 1 week after a nerve crush as compared to the contralateral nerve, whereas the accumulation of rapidly migrating ^{3}H-fucose-labeled glycoproteins was markedly increased in the regenerating nerve. These changes were slowly normalized during the following 4–6 weeks of regeneration.

The result indicates an initial depression of the axonal transport of the bulk of rapidly migrating proteins including ChAc and AChE in the chromatolytic hypoglossal neurons, whereas the transport of rapidly migrating glycoproteins is increased. These initial changes were slowly normalized during the subsequent regeneration period.

INTRODUCTION

In the mature nerve cell it is likely that the soma and axon has reached a steady state where the amount of material synthesized and transported is equivalent with that which is catabolized or secreted. In growing nerve cells this steady state has not yet been attained, and the elongation of axons is assumed to involve continuous transport of newly formed material toward the growing tips. After axotomy the neuronal equilibrium is deranged in the regenerating axon with changed demands for maintenance of axonal structures and increased demands for growth. Our studies were carried out to obtain information about axonal transport in embryonic and regenerating neurons.

The axonal transport of proteins and glycoproteins during development was studied in the optic pathway of chick embryos during the period when the formation of retino-tectal connections occur from the seventh day up to the eighteenth day (for review see Cowan, 1971). Labeled precursor (^{3}H-leucine, ^{3}H-proline, and ^{3}H-fucose) was injected into the right eyeball of chick embryos of the White Leghorn strain. In chicks the chiasmal crossing is virtually complete, and in the main experimental series the recovery of protein-bound radioactivity was followed in the contralateral optic tectum using liquid scintillation technique (Marchisio et al., 1973). In another series the axonal transport of proteins from the retina to the contralateral tectum was studied by radioautography according to techniques previously described (Marchisio and Sjöstrand, 1972).

The characteristics of axonal transport in normal and regenerating cholinergic nerves were studied in adult rabbits (Fonnum et al., in preparation; Frizell and Sjöstrand, in preparation) by following the flow of proteins and glycoproteins including the enzymes choline-O-acetyltransferase (ChAc, EC 2.3.1.6) and acetylcholinesterase (AChE, EC 3.1.1.7).

METHODS

EMBRYONIC OPTIC PATHWAY

Chick embryos of the White Leghorn strain were used. Labeled precursor was injected into the right eyeball with a Hamilton syringe as described previously (Marchisio and Sjöstrand, 1971). (^{3}H) fucose (L-(1-^{3}H)-fucose, specific activity 950 mCi/mmol) and (^{3}H) proline (L-(5-^{3}H)-proline, specific activity 6.8 Ci/mmol) were injected at a dose of 2 μCi for 7 day embryos (stage 31) and 5 μCi for 13- and 18-day embryos (stage 39 and 44 respectively).

At various time intervals after the injection the animals were decapitated. After fixation of the embryo head in ice-cold 5% TCA overnight, the relevant parts of the optic system were dissected free. The samples in the ^{3}H-proline series and ^{3}H-fucose series were homogenized in ice-cold 5% (w/v) TCA and 6% TCA-0.5% phosphotungstic acid (PTA) respectively, and treated as earlier described (Karlsson and Sjöstrand, 1971).

In a smaller series of animals, optic tecta were taken 6 h following intraocular isotope injection for gel electrophoresis. The samples were homogenized in 0.25–1 ml of a solution of 3% sodium dodecyl sulphate (SDS), 3% β-mercaptoethanol in 10 mM phosphate buffer (pH 7.0). Polyacrylamide electrophoresis in SDS was carried out as previously described (Karlsson and Sjöstrand, 1971) in the system of Shapiro et al. (1967).

NORMAL AND REGENERATING CHOLINERGIC NERVE

The vagus and hypoglossus nerves of adult albino rabbits were carefully exposed under pentobarbital anesthesia. Ligatures were made with thin silk thread. The distances between the ligatures were 30–35 mm for the vagus nerve and 15–20 mm for the hypoglossus nerve. In the regeneration experiments the right hypoglossal nerve was crushed 5 mm proximal to its entry to the tongue base with a silk thread.

The nerve segments used for enzyme determination were dissected free of adhering tissue and cut into 2.5–5 mm pieces.

The pieces of nerves and hypoglossal nucleus were homogenized in 10 mM-EDTA (pH 7.4) using a glass–glass homogenizer. The tongue was homogenized in an Ultra-Turrax rotating at maximum speed. The homogenates were treated with 0.1 % Triton (final conc.) before assay. ChAc and AChE were assayed as described by Fonnum (1969). The incubation mixture for ChAc consisted of (final concs.): 0.2 mM-(1-^{14}C) acetylCoA, 10 mM-EDTA, 12 mM-choline, 250 mM-NaCl, 50 mM-sodium phosphate buffer (pH 7.4), and 0.1 mM-eserine salicylate. The incubation mixture for AChE contained: 0.7 mM-(1-^{14}C) ACh, 20 mM-sodium phosphate buffer (pH 7.4), and 0.1 mM-ethopropazine (buturylcholinesterase inhibitor).

In the labeling experiments (^{3}H)-leucine or (^{3}H)-fucose (L-(4,5-^{3}H) leucine, specific activity 38 Ci/mmol, conc. 1 mCi/ml and L-(1-^{3}H) fucose, specific activity 2.82 Ci/mmol, conc. 5–10 mCi/ml, Radiochemical Centre, Amersham, England) was applied to the calamus scriptorius according to Miani (1963) (for experimental details, see Frizell and Sjöstrand, in preparation).

The animals were killed from 5 to 20 h after the administration of the isotope and the relevant tissue samples were dissected out. Following homogenization in TCA, the samples were treated as previously described (Karlsson and Sjöstrand, 1971). The radioactivity was measured by liquid scintillation and the values were corrected for quenching. The activity was expressed as disintegrations per minute (dpm) per 2.5 mm nerve tissue.

RESULTS AND DISCUSSION

AXONAL TRANSPORT IN THE OPTIC PATHWAY OF CHICK EMBRYOS

Labeled precursor was incorporated into retinal proteins at all embryonic stages studied. The turnover in the retina of both proteins and glycoproteins was exceedingly high in the 7-day embryos compared to that of later stages.

In the 10-day embryos, labeled proteins and glycoproteins reached the contralateral optic tectum at 2 h after intraocular injection of precursor. Since the length of the optic pathway is 5.3 mm at the 10-day stage (Marchisio and Sjöstrand, 1972), a transport rate of at least 60 mm/day can be calculated. Also, at day 13 and day 18 a phase of rapidly transported protein was detected in the contralateral optic tectum at 2 h following intraocular injection. Since at these stages the length of the optic pathway is 7.9 and 9.3 mm respectively, transport rates of at least 95 and 110 mm/day can be estimated. The velocity of rapid transport thus almost doubles between day 10 and day 18. If the changes in the rate of rapid axonal transport are considered as a function of the embryonic age, a continuous increase in the rate of rapid flow may be observed in the optic pathway (Fig. 1). The changes in the rate of rapid axonal transport observed during development in the present study are in agreement with those reported for the developing optic pathway of newborn rabbits (Hendrickson and Cowan, 1971).

In 7-day embryos the protein-bound radioactivity following intraocular injection was only slightly elevated in the left tectum at 4 h for ^{3}H-proline and at 12 h for ^{3}H-fucose, and no significant difference between the left and the right tectum could be demonstrated by liquid scintillation technique. At this stage, however, radioautography could reveal axonal transport in the still relatively few axons spreading to the surface of the optic tectum. Both rapid and slow axonal transport of protein and glycoprotein could be demonstrated by

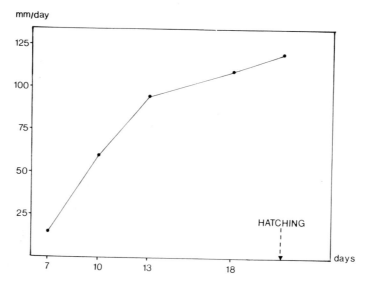

Fig. 1. Transport velocity of the rapid phase of axonal transport during development. The rates are calculated from data obtained from studies using scintillation counting (Marchisio *et al.*, 1973; Marchisio and Gremo, in preparation) or radioautography (Marchisio and Sjöstrand, 1972; Marchisio and Sjöstrand, in preparation).

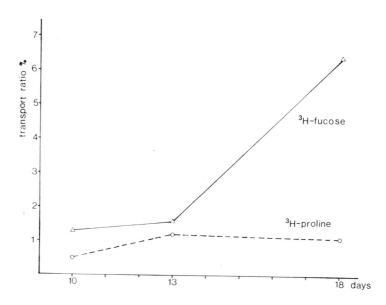

Fig. 2. The amount of protein-bound radioactivity transported to the tectum is expressed as the percentage of protein bound radioactivity recovered in the contralateral retina after injection of ³H-proline (dashed line) and ³H-fucose (solid line). The percentage transport ratio was calculated 6 h after precursor injection when a large portion of rapidly transported proteins could be recovered in the contralateral tectum. (From Marchisio *et al.*, 1973.)

radioautography in the 7-day embryos (Marchisio and Sjöstrand, 1972; Marchisio and Sjöstrand, in preparation). Our results therefore indicate that axonal transport is efficiently working already early in embryogenesis before synaptic contacts have been formed.

In order to study the polypeptide constituents of the rapid transport phase, SDS gel electrophoresis was carried out. The electrophoresis of leucine- or fucose-labeled tectal proteins showed that a large number of relatively high mol.wt.-polypeptides reached the optic tectum by a rapid phase of axonal transport in 13-day and 18-day chick embryos. The labeling pattern of the polypeptides was similar in 13-day and 18-day embryos and no obvious differences were seen when either fucose or leucine was used as precursor.

In the 18-day embryo 6 h after precursor injection a large amount of protein-bound radioactivity transported by the rapid phase may be recovered in the tectum. At this time interval the amount of radioactivity transported to the tectum compared to the level of retinal incorporation was approximately 1.1 % for proline and 6.4% for fucose. When the variations of this "transport index" for fucose and proline 6 h after injection are considered as a function of embryonic age (Fig. 2), it is evident that the relative proportion of fucose radioactivity transported from the retina is consistently higher throughout the development and that a relatively larger proportion of retinal glycoproteins is aimed for rapid axonal transport at 18 days when compared to earlier stages.

DISTRIBUTION AND TRANSPORT OF ChAc AND AChE IN MATURE CHOLINERGIC NEURONS

The hypoglossal nerve fibers originate from the two hypoglossal nuclei and the nerve axons project their terminals to the ipsilateral part of the tongue (Barnard, 1940; Sax, 1969). As ChAc is assumed to be exclusively an intraneuronal enzyme (Kasa, 1971), it is a good marker for cholinergic neurons. This prerequisite makes it possible to determine the ChAc activity of the hypoglossal neurons. The ChAc confined to the hypoglossal nerve cell bodies was calculated to be 43 nmol/h per nucleus. The enzyme activity of the hypoglossal nerve from the nucleus of origin to the entrance into the tongue was found to be 1.16 μmol/h and the enzyme activity of the axon terminals of the tongue was estimated to be 3.10 μmol/h. Taking into account that there are two hypoglossal nuclei, two hypoglossal nerves, and one tongue, the total ChAc activity within the hypoglossal neurons was 5.50 μmol/h. Therefore 2% of the ChAc activity was present in the cell bodies, 42% in the axons of the hypoglossal nerve, and 56% in fine axons and axon terminals within the tongue.

Using single ligatures we found that AChE and ChAc accumulated in a linear way above the ligature during the first 24 h (Frizell et al., 1970), indicating an axonal transport of these constituents. Assuming that all enzyme in the nerve was available for transport, the calculated rates from the accumulation data will be 15 mm/day for vagus and 5 mm/day in the hypoglossal nerve for both enzymes.

If only a small proportion of enzyme is transportable, the calculation will give considerably higher velocity values. Lubińska, using isolated segments of the dog peroneal nerve, showed that only 15% AChE of the activity of the nerve was rapidly moving, while the rest was stationary or slowly migrating (Lubińska and Niemierko, 1971). It was also shown that the terminal accumulation of AChE was dependent on the length of the segment and time. Double ligatures in our system showed that there was a large accumulation proximal to the first ligature, but only a smaller accumulation of AChE and ChAc proximal to the second ligature (Fig. 3).

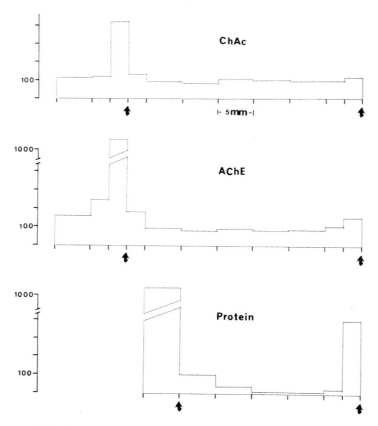

FIG. 3. The distribution of the activity of ChAc-, AChE-, and ³H-labeled proteins in doubly ligated vagus nerve. Ligatures were applied 20–22 h before sacrifice. In the labeling experiments 30 μl of L-(³H) leucine was administered continuously to the fourth ventricle during 30 min, 5 h before the ligation. The activities are expressed as a percentage of the average enzyme or labeled protein activity of the nerve segment between the ligatures. Arrows indicate sites of ligatures. (From Fonnum *et al.*, in preparation.)

These results suggest that only 5–20% of the total enzyme activities were transported in the isolated segment (Table 1). This part was transported with a fast or intermediate rate of axonal flow. The transport rate derived for ChAc and AChE in the table shows that the enzymes are transported from the cell bodies and to the nerve terminals in less than 2 days. The proportion of ChAc transported down the hypoglossal nerve in 22 h was 45.2 nmol/h as calculated from single ligature experiments (Fig. 4a). Since the ChAc activity present in the hypoglossal nucleus was 43 nmol/h, this means that the turnover of ChAc in the peri-karya is very fast and that the enzyme activity may be replaced in less than 1 day. The ChAc activity of the hypoglossal terminals and preterminal axons of the tongue was esti-mated to 3.10 μmol/h, and the half-life of the ChAc in this compartment was calculated to 16 days.

The effect of colchicine on axonal transport was examined by injecting 100 μg of col-chicine into the cisterna cerebello-medullaris. The accumulation of cholinergic enzymes (Fig. 4) and rapidly migrating proteins proximal to a single ligature in the vagus nerve was inhibited.

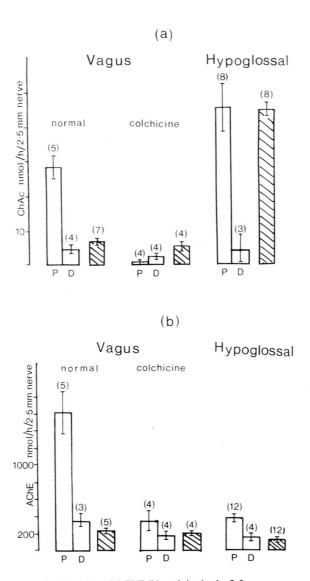

FIG. 4. The increment of ChAc (a) and AChE (b) activity in the 2.5 mm nerve segment proximal (P) and distal (D) to a single ligature applied to the vagus or hypoglossal nerve 22 h before sacrifice. In some experiments of the vagus nerve colchicine (100 μg in 100 μl aqua dest.) was injected intracisternally 28 h before ligation and 48 h before sacrifice. The hatched columns represent the average enzyme activity of the nerves calculated from the enzyme activity of a 5 mm nerve segment 5–15 mm proximal to the ligature. Values are the mean ± SEM, and the number of experiments is indicated within parentheses. The increment of enzyme activity was calculated as the difference between the enzyme activity of the 2.5 mm nerve segment proximal or distal to the ligature and the average enzyme activity. (Data from Fonnum et al., in preparation.)

TABLE 1. THE TRANSPORT OF ChAc AND AChE IN AN ISOLATED NERVE SEGMENT OF THE VAGUS AND HYPO-
GLOSSAL NERVES; CALCULATED TRANSPORT RATES
(From Fonnum et al., in preparation)

Enzyme	Average activity of the segment (nmol/h per 2.5 mm)	Percent mobile enzyme of the segment		Calculated transport rate mm per 24 h	
		Prox.-dist	Retrograde	Prox.-dist.	Retrograde
Vagus nerve					
ChAc	7.5 ± 0.5 (4)	6.7 ± 1.7 (7)	3.3 ± 0.8 (6)	191	64
AChE	209 ± 29 (4)	4.7 ± 0.9 (4)	3.8 ± 1.3 (4)	425	123
Hypoglossal nerve					
ChAc	39.1 ± 1.1 (4)	5.8 ± 1.7 (4)	3.5 ± 1.0 (4)	47	53
AChE	137 ± 14 (9)	11.2 ± 1.5 (9)	4.9 ± 1.0 (9)	73	73

The values are mean $\pm$ SEM. Number of experiments is given in parentheses. The average activity of
the segment is the mean of the total enzyme activity of the isolated nerve segment between double ligatures
as determined from continuous 2.5–5 mm nerve pieces cut out 22 h after ligation.

Percent of mobile enzyme: $\dfrac{\text{(increase of enzyme activity/2.5 mm nerve) at the end of the segment} \times 100}{\text{the total enzyme activity of the segment}}$

Transport rate from double ligature: $\dfrac{\text{transport rate as calculated from single ligature} \times 100}{\text{percentage of mobile enzyme}}$.

AXONAL TRANSPORT DURING REGENERATION

The axonal transport of labeled proteins and cholinergic enzymes was studied during regeneration by following the accumulation above a nerve ligature. The linear accumulation
of various axonal compounds proximal to a nerve ligature for at least 20 h (Dahlström
and Häggendal, 1966; Frizell et al., 1970; Jarrott and Geffen, 1972) and the intact fast
axonal transport in isolated nerve segments (Lubińska and Niemierko, 1971; Bray, Kow
and Breckenridge, 1971) strongly suggest an undisturbed axonal transport in ligated nerves
during this time. The axonal transport of rapidly migrating glycoproteins was also studied
during nerve regeneration, since glycoproteins are membrane-associated (Karlsson and
Sjöstrand, 1971) and might participate specifically in the regenerative process of the neuron.

The accumulation of ChAc and AChE in the 2.5 mm segment proximal to a ligature on
the crushed side was reduced to about 50 and 60% respectively of the enzyme accumulation
on the contralateral side 1 week following crush of the right hypoglossal nerve (Fig. 5).
After 4 weeks of regeneration, however, the accumulation on the regenerating side was
increased to 130 and 100% of the contralateral for ChAc and AChE respectively, and after
2 weeks of further regeneration the corresponding figures decreased slightly to about 80%
for both enzymes (Fig. 5).

Rapidly migrating proteins and glycoproteins accumulated proximal to a ligature both in
regenerating and control nerves (Fig. 6). After 1 week of regeneration, the accumulation of
^{3}H-labeled proteins on the regenerating side was reduced to 60% of that of the control side,

whereas the accumulation of ^{3}H-fucose-labeled proteins was markedly increased to 240% of the control side (Figs. 6 and 7). Four weeks after nerve crush the accumulation of ^{3}H-leucine-labeled proteins showed a somewhat increased percentage as compared to that found after 1 week of regeneration, whereas the accumulation of ^{3}H-fucose-labeled proteins was slightly decreased. After 6 weeks of regeneration the accumulation was about 120 and 160% of the contralateral for ^{3}H-leucine- and ^{3}H-fucose-labeled proteins respectively.

The decreased accumulation of rapidly migrating proteins, ChAc, and AChE after 1 week of regeneration, is in accordance with the reports of decreased protein synthesis and activity of ChAc and AChE in neurons during this period (Kung, 1971; Engh et al., 1971; Schwarzacher, 1958; Hebb and Silver, 1965). Since the accumulation proximal to a nerve ligature is a function of several factors, many changes in the chromatolytic neuron could be responsible for this decrease.

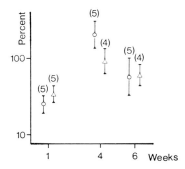

FIG. 5. The accumulation of ChAc (○) and AChE (△) activity in the 2.5 mm segment proximal to a ligature of the right hypoglossal nerve in percentage of the accumulation in the 2.5 mm segment proximal to a ligature of the left hypoglossal nerve applied simultaneously. The mean activity of the nerve segment on the control side was 64.6 ± 7.3 nmol/h per 2.5 mm nerve for ChAc and 525.3 ± 121.3 nmol/h per 2.5 mm nerve for AChE. The right hypoglossal nerve was crushed 1, 4, or 6 weeks before the ligation. The animals were killed 21–23 h after ligature. The values are the mean ± SEM and the number of experiments is indicated within parentheses.

A decreased axonal transport of rapidly migrating proteins (Carlsson et al., 1971) and of noradrenaline (Boyle and Gillespie, 1970) has been found in regenerating nerves and might be responsible for the decreased accumulation proximal to a ligature. The decreased axonal flow could be due to a decreased rate of flow (Carlsson et al., 1971) or a decreased amount of material transported by the flow as a consequence of changed peripheral demands after a nerve crush. A possible correlate to a decreased axonal flow is the reduction of axon diameters noted proximal to a nerve crush during the first weeks of regeneration (Kreutzberg and Schubert, 1971).

Several authors have suggested a shift of the protein synthesis of the neuron during the first period of regeneration from synthesis of rapidly migrating secretory "transmitter" proteins to structural "matrix" proteins (Engh et al., 1971; Matthews and Raisman, 1971; Price and Porter, 1972), and this is in line with the present finding of decreased accumulation of transmitter enzymes. Since the lysosomal activity seems to be increased during chromatolysis (Bodian and Mellors, 1945; Holtzman et al., 1967; Matthews and Raisman, 1971), an increased breakdown of both perikaryal and axonal protein might contribute to the decreased accumulation of rapidly migrating proteins and ChAc and AChE during regeneration.

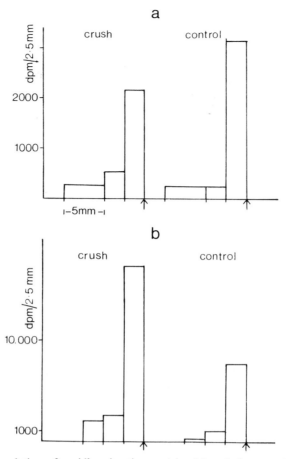

FIG. 6. The accumulation of rapidly migrating proteins (a) and glycoproteins (b) proximal to a ligature applied to both hypoglossal nerves in two representative experiments. The hypoglossal nucleus was labeled with 30 μl of (^{3}H) leucine (1 μCi/μl) (a) or 30 μl of (^{3}H) fucose (10 μCi/μl) (b) 21 h (a) and 19 h (b) before sacrifice. Both hypoglossal nerves were ligated 1 h before the administration of isotope. The right hypoglossal nerve was untreated until ligation (control). The activity of ^{3}H-leucine-labeled proteins in the 2.5 mm nerve segment proximal to the ligature ranged from 250–2000 dpm per 2.5 mm nerve tissue on the crushed side as compared to 400–3000 dpm per 2.5 mm on the control side, in a series of four experiments and the corresponding figures for the ^{3}H-fucose-labeled proteins were 6000–17,000 dpm per 2.5 mm on the crush side and 2000–8000 dpm per 2.5 mm on the control side. Arrows indicate site of ligature. (From Frizell and Sjöstrand, in preparation.)

In sharp contrast to the decreased accumulation of ChAc, AChE, and rapidly migrating (^{3}H)-leucine-labeled proteins, the accumulation of glycoproteins is markedly increased 1 week after regeneration. During the outgrowth period of the regenerating neuron there ought to be an increased demand for membraneous precursors to supply the tips of sprouting axons. Since (^{3}H)-fucose-labeled glycoproteins are associated with the axonal membrane fractions (Karlsson and Sjöstrand, 1971), it is not surprising with an increased accumulation of these compounds during the outgrowth period. The increase in size of the Golgi-complex of the regenerating neuron (Bodian, 1964; Price and Porter, 1972) is interesting, considering that the incorporation of ^{3}H-fucose into glycoproteins mainly takes place at this site

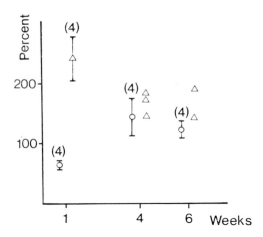

FIG. 7. The accumulation of rapidly migrating proteins(○)and glycoproteins(△)in the 2.5 mm segment proximal to a ligature applied to the right hypoglossal nerve in percentage of the corresponding accumulation proximal to a ligature applied to the hypoglossal nerve. The right hypoglossal nerve was crushed 1, 4, or 6 weeks before the ligation. The hypoglossal nucleus was labeled with (^{3}H) leucine (30 μl, 1 μCi/μl) or (^{3}H) fucose (20–30 μl, 5–10 μCi/μl) 19–21 h before sacrifice, 1–2 h after the ligation. The values are mean ± SEM or single and the number of experiments is indicated within parentheses. (From Frizell and Sjöstrand, in preparation.)

(Winterburn and Phelps, 1972). After 4 weeks of regeneration the accumulation of glyco-proteins is less increased. This coincides with the end of the outgrowth period and beginning of the maturation period. At this time, however, there is a rise in the accumulation of ChAc, AChE, and rapidly migrating ^{3}H-leucine-labeled proteins. After 6 weeks of regenera-tion the accumulation of ChAc and AChE is somewhat decreased as compared to the accumulation at 4 weeks, whereas the accumulation of rapidly migrating proteins and glycoproteins is still elevated at this time. Increased proteins synthesis has been demon-strated in the nerve cell body at the start of the maturation period (Brattgård et al., 1957; Engh et al., 1971). It has been proposed that this increase is due to a trophic signal from the effector organ when the neuromuscular contact is established (Engh et al., 1971). This hypothesis is supported by the increased retrograde transport found in regenerating hypo-glossal neurons 5 weeks after a nerve crush (Kristensson and Sjöstrand, 1972).

REFERENCES

BARNARD, J. W. (1940) The hypoglossal complex of vertebrates. J. Comp. Neurol. **72**, 489–524.
BODIAN, D. (1964) An electron microscopic study of the monkey spinal cord: II, Effects of retrograde chromatolysis. Bull. Johns Hopkins Hosp. **114**, 13–119.
BODIAN, D., and MELLORS, R. C. (1945) The regenerative cycle of motoneurons, with special reference to phosphatase activity. J. Exp. Med. **81**, 469–488.
BOYLE, F. C., and GILLESPIE, J. S. (1970) Accumulation and loss of noradrenaline central to a constriction on adrenergic nerves. Eur. J. Pharmac. **12**, 77–84.
BRATTGÅRD, S. O., EDSTRÖM, J. E., and HYDÉN, H. (1957) The chemical changes in regenerating neurons. J. Neurochem. **1**, 316–325.
BRAY, J. J., KOW, C. M., and BRECKENRIDGE, B. M. (1971) Reversed polarity of rapid axonal transport in chicken motoneurons. Brain Res. **33**, 560–564.
CARLSSON, C.-A., BOLANDER, P., and SJÖSTRAND, J. (1971) Changes in axonal transport during regeneration of feline ventral roots. J. Neurol. Sci. **14**, 75–105.
COWAN, W. M. (1971) Studies on the development of the avian visual system. In Cellular Aspects of Neural Growth and Differentiation (D. C. Pease, ed.), UCLA University Press, Berkeley, pp. 177–222.

DAHLSTRÖM, A., and HÄGGENDAL, J. (1966) Studies on the transport and life-span of amine storage granules in a peripheral adrenergic neuron system. *Acta physiol. scand.* **67**, 278–288.

ENGH, C. A., SCHOFIELD, B. H., DOTY, S. B., and ROBINSON, R. A. (1971) Perikaryal synthetic function following reversible and irreversible peripheral axon injuries as shown by radioautography. *J. Comp. Neurol.* **142**, 465–480.

FONNUM, F. (1969) Radiochemical microassays for the determinations of choline acetyltransferase and acetylcholinesterase activities. *Biochem. J.* **115**, 465–472.

FONNUM, F., FRIZELL, M., and SJÖSTRAND, J. (1973) Transport, turnover and distribution of choline acetyltransferase and acetylcholinesterase in the vagus and hypoglossal nerves of the rabbit. *J. Neurochem.* (In preparation).

FRIZELL, M., and SJÖSTRAND, J. (1973) Transport of proteins, glycoproteins and cholinergic enzymes in regenerating hypoglossal neurons. (In preparation.)

FRIZELL, M., HASSELGREN, P. O., and SJÖSTRAND, J. (1970) Axoplasmic transport of acetylcholinesterase and choline acetyltransferase in the vagus and hypoglossal nerves of the rabbit. *Expl. Brain Res.* **10**, 526–531.

HEBB, C., and SILVER, A. (1965) Axoplasmic flow of protein. In *Protides of the Biological Fluids* (H. Peeters, ed.), Elsevier, Amsterdam.

HENDRICKSON, A. E., and COWAN, W. M. (1971) Changes in the rate of axoplasmic transport during postnatal development of the rabbit's optic nerve and tract. *Expl. Neurol.* **30**, 403–422.

HOLTZMAN, E., NOVINOFF, A. B., and VILLAVERO E. H. (1967) Lysosomes and GERL in normal and chromatolytic neurons of the rat ganglion *J. Cell Biol.* **33**, 419–435.

JARROTT, B., and GEFFEN, L. B. (1972) Rapid axoplasmic transport of tyrosine hydroxylase and other cytoplasmic constituents. *Proc. Natn. Acad. Sci. USA* **69**, 3440–3442.

KARLSSON, J. O., and SJÖSTRAND, J. (1971) Axonal transport of proteins in retinal ganglion cells: amino acid incorporation into rapidly transported proteins and distribution of radioactivity to the lateral geniculate body and the superior colliculus. *Brain Res.* **37**, 279–285.

KASA, P. (1971) Ultrastructural localization of choline acetyltransferase and acetylcholinesterase in central and peripheral nervous tissue. In *Progress in Brain Research* (O. Eränkö, ed.), Elsevier, Amsterdam, pp. 337–344.

KREUTZBERG, G. W., and SCHUBERT, P. (1971) Volume changes in the axon during regeneration. *Acta neuropath. Berlin* **17**, 220–266.

KRISTENSSON, K., and SJÖSTRAND, J. (1972) Retrograde transport of protein tracer in the rabbit hypoglossal nerve during regeneration. *Brain Res.* **45**, 175–181.

KUNG, S. H. (1971) Incorporation of tritiated precursors in the cytoplasm of normal and chromatolytic sensory neurons as shown by radioautography. *Brain Res.* **25**, 656–660.

LUBINSKA, L., and NIEMIERKO, S. (1971) Velocity and intensity of bidirectional migration of acetylcholinesterase in transected nerves. **27**, 329–342.

MARCHISIO, P. C., and SJÖSTRAND, J. (1971) Axonal transport in avian optic pathway during development. *Brain Res.* **26**, 204–211.

MARCHISIO, P. C., and SJÖSTRAND, J. (1972) Radioautographic evidence for protein transport along the optic pathway of early chick embryos. *J. Neurocytol.* **1**, 101–108.

MARCHISIO, P. C., SJÖSTRAND, J., AGLIETTA, M., and KARLSSON, J.-O. (1973) The development of axonal transport of proteins and glycoproteins in the optic pathway of chick embryos. *Brain Res.* (In press.)

MATTHEWS, M. R., and RAISMAN, G. (1971) A light and electron microscopic study of the cellular response to axonal injury in the superior cervical ganglion of the rat. *Proc. R. Soc. Lond.* B, **181**, 43–79.

MIANI, N. (1963) Analyses of the somato-axonal movement of phospholipids in the vagus and hypoglossal nerves. *J. Neurochem.* **10**, 859–874.

PRICE, D. L., and PORTER, K. R. (1972) The response of ventral horn neurons to axonal transection. *J. Cell Biol.* **53**, 24–37.

SAX, D. S. (1969) Anatomy of lingual movement. In: *Psychotropic Drugs and Dysfunctions of the Basal ganglia* (G. Crane and R. Gardnei Jr., eds.), Public Health Service Publication No. 1938, pp. 75–85.

SCHWARZACHER, H. G. (1958) Der Cholinesterasegehalt motorischer Nervenzellen während der axonalen Reaktion. *Acta anat.* **32**, 51–65.

SHAPIRO, A. L., VINUELA, E., and MAIZEL, J. V. (1967) Molecular weight estimation of polypeptide chains by electrophoresis in SDS-polyacrylamide gels. *Biophys. Res. Commun.* **28**, 815–820.

WINTERBURN, P. J., and PHELPS, C. F. (1972) The significance of glycosylated proteins. *Nature* **236**, 147–151.

THE ROLE OF AXOPLASMIC FLOW IN TROPHISM OF SKELETAL MUSCLE

S. Thesleff

Department of Pharmacology, University of Lund, Lund, Sweden

SUMMARY

In mammalian skeletal muscle, denervation causes the appearance of extrajunctional cholinergic receptors and of action potentials resistant to the blocking effect of tetrodotoxin. Reinnervation reverses these changes. The alterations in membrane excitability that are observed after denervation are prevented by the administration of actinomycin D to the animal, suggesting that they are the result of genetically induced synthesis of new proteins.

Denervation changes appear earlier in muscles with a short nerve stump distal to the site of neurectomy, i.e. the length of the nerve distal to the site of sectioning influences the time course of the appearance of the excitability changes.

The application of colchicine or vinblastine to motor nerve axons induces denervation changes in the muscle without affecting nerve impulse conduction, transmitter release, or neuromuscular transmission.

Blockade of transmitter release from motor nerve terminals by botulinum toxin produces the same effects as surgical denervation.

It is concluded that substances carried by axoplasmic transport are released from motor nerve terminals, presumably by the same mechanism as the transmitter, and that these substances exert a repressive influence on that part of the muscle genome which controls the synthesis of the proteins necessary for the development of extrajunctional cholinergic receptors and of tetrodotoxin resistant action potentials.

Following denervation, the chemical and electrical excitability of mammalian skeletal muscle changes in a characteristic way. In innervated muscles, cholinergic receptors are present only in the limited area of the subsynaptic region, occupying a small fraction of the muscle membrane. After denervation, receptors develop on the entire muscle surface, the cell acquiring a high and uniform sensitivity to applied acetylcholine (ACh) as shown by Fig. 1 (Axelsson and Thesleff, 1959). The action potential is also altered by denervation (Fig. 2). In innervated muscles, tetrodotoxin (TTX) blocks the inward sodium current of the action potential thereby completely blocking spike generation. After denervation the action potential becomes resistant to the blocking effect of TTX (Redfern and Thesleff, 1971). Reinnervation completely reverses both of these changes in membrane excitability.

The appearance in denervated muscles of extrajunctional cholinergic receptors and of

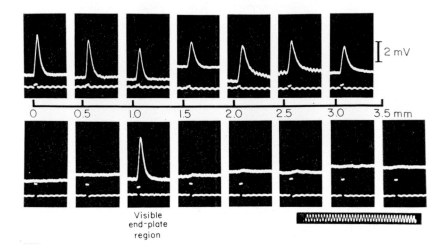

FIG. 1. The sensitivity of a muscle fiber of the cat tenuissimus muscle to microiontophoretically applied ACh. The membrane potential is recorded in the upper tracing and the current passing through the pipette in the lower tracing of each record. In an innervated fiber (lower records) only the visible end plate region responded to the drug. In a 14-day denervated fiber a constant pulse of ACh produced at each point of the membrane depolarization (upper records). Time marker 100 Hz. (Axelsson and Thesleff, 1959.)

TTX resistant action potentials is prevented by the administration of actinomycin D to the animal. Since this drug, in the dosages used, blocks DNA-dependent RNA synthesis, it appears that the aforementioned denervation changes result from the synthesis of new muscle proteins and that the motor nerve normally exerts a regulatory influence on the genome of the muscle cell (Grampp *et al.*, 1972).

This conference is devoted to the dynamics of neurons and therefore it seems appropriate to ask to what an extent is the nervous control of muscle protein synthesis secondary to synaptically induced muscle activity or the consequence of the actions of regulatory or "trophic" substances being released from the nerve. To differentiate between these two possibilities we have studied the effect of the peripheral nerve stump length on the time course of the appearance of TTX resistant action potentials in denervated muscles (Harris and Thesleff, 1972). The experiments were made on the extensor digitorum longus (EDL) muscle of adult Wistar rats. The muscles were denervated "close" by cutting the deep peroneal nerve at the knee or "distant" by cutting the sciatic nerve in the sciatic foramen. In most cases a bilateral denervation was made—"close" on one side and "distant" on the other, mechanical inactivity resulting in both muscles at the moment of sectioning of the nerve. The difference in the peripherel nerve stump length achieved by the cutting at the two levels was approximately 3 cm. The muscles were removed between 24 and 72 h after denervation at intervals of 6 h and examined with intracellular electrodes for their capability of producing action potentials in the presence of TTX 10^{-6} M. As shown by Fig. 3, TTX resistant action potentials were recorded about 6 h earlier in "close" denervated muscles than in "distant" denervated ones. Since inactivity resulted in both muscles at the same moment, the results offer evidence against the concept that the denervation changes of skeletal muscle are primarily the result of mechanical inactivity. The results indicate that denervation changes are delayed by 1 h for each 5 mm of nerve stump remaining. This time

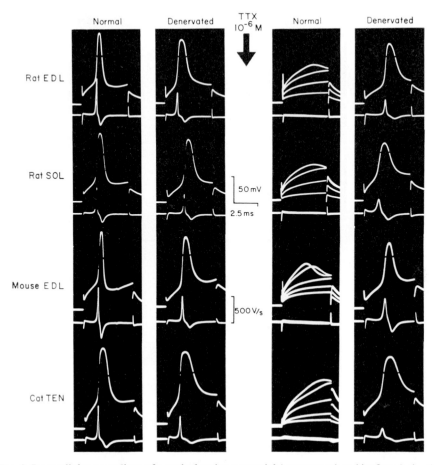

FIG. 2. Intracellular recordings of a typical action potential (upper trace) and its first derivative (lower trace) in innervated and in 6–7-day denervated rat EDL, soleus (SOL), mouse EDL, and cat tenuissimus (TEN) muscles. The records in the left-hand panel were obtained in the absence of TTX, and those in the right-hand panel in the presence of 10^{-6} M TTX. The break in the action potential tracing indicates the zero potential level of the cell.

is within the range of quoted rates of axonal transport and is thus indicative of trophic substances being released from the nerve.

To study this possibility we applied colchicine to the sciatic nerve of adult rats (Hofmann and Thesleff, 1972). Colchicine is a drug which, when applied to neurons, destroys the organization of microtubules in axons and in dendrites. As shown by Kreutzberg (1969) and Dahlström (1968), the injection of the drug (5–10 μl of a 135–250 mM solution) under the perineurium of the sciatic nerve interrupts the proximo-distal flow of macromolecules and organelles at the site of application. The values presented in Table 1 show that colchicine failed to affect the twitch as well as the tetanic tension of the EDL muscle in response to indirect stimulation proximal to the site of colchicine application. Neither did the rats show any sign of paralysis of the hindleg, spontaneous movements being normal. Spontaneous transmitter release of normal frequency and amplitude, recorded as miniature endplate potentials (mepps), were, as shown in Table 2, present in all superficial muscle fibers.

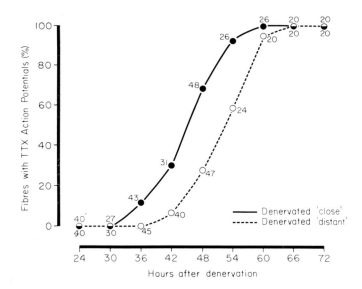

FIG. 3. Percentage of muscle fibers with TTX resistant action potentials in rat EDL muscles at various times after denervation. The muscles were denervated "close" (closed circles) or "distant" (open circles). Pooled results from 48 muscles; the figures indicate the number of fibers examined. (Harris and Thesleff, 1972.)

TABLE 1. TWITCH AND TETANIC TENSIONS OF INDIRECTLY STIMULATED RAT EDL MUSCLES

Colchicine 0.25 M was applied to the sciatic nerve distal to the site of nerve stimulation and the EDL muscle of the contralateral untreated leg was used as control

	Time after colchicine (days)	Mean twitch tension (g)	Mean tetanic (100 Hz) tension (g)
1	Colchicine treated	18.5	48.3
	Control	20.5	49.0
2	Colchicine treated	21.2	49.5
	Control	20.7	46.8
3	Colchicine treated	19.5	50.2
	Control	20.3	47.8

It is therefore unlikely that the drug caused degeneration even of a portion of the motor nerve axons or of their terminals. When the extrajunctional cholinergic sensitivity of the muscles was examined it was observed that by the fourth day after colchicine application practically all the fibers were sensitive to microiontophoretically applied ACh (Table 2). The range of extrajunctional ACh sensitivity varied between the fibers from 2 to 129 mV/nC passed through the ACh pipette and was therefore not as uniform as that observed in surgically denervated muscles. The average sensitivity of 36 units was, however, of about the same magnitude as that following denervation. The action potentials were resistant to the blocking effect of TTX as shown in Table 2. With a single application of colchicine the appearance of extrajunctional ACh sensitivity and of TTX resistant action potentials was transient and the muscle properties returned towards normal 5–6 days after the drug

TABLE 2. EFFECTS OF LOCAL APPLICATION OF COLCHICINE TO THE SCIATIC NERVE ON THE FREQUENCY AND THE AMPLITUDE OF SPONTANEOUS MEPPS AND ON THE PRESENCE OF EXTRAJUNCTIONAL ACh SENSITIVITY AND TTX RESISTANT ACTION POTENTIALS IN THE EDL MUSCLE

In each fiber 50 mepps were measured. The table includes, for comparison, values obtained from normal, untreated animals and from surgically denervated ones

Time and type of treatment	Frequency of mepps (per s) (mean ± SEM)	Amplitude of mepps (mV) (mean ± SEM)	Presence of ACh sensitivity (>2 mV/nC)	Presence of action potentials in TTX (10^{-6} M)
Control untreated	3.1 ± 0.24 (26)[b]	0.50 ± 0.04 (26)[b]	0/26[a]	0/26[a]
1 day after colchicine	5.7 ± 0.60 (14)	0.41 ± 0.04 (14)	0/12	0/10
1 day after denervation	—	—	0/10	0/10
2 days after colchicine	4.0 ± 0.45 (18)	0.42 ± 0.03 (18)	0/18	0/10
2 days after denervation	—	—	0/11	8/12
3 days after denervation	—	—	12/12	12/12
4 days after colchicine	3.1 ± 0.60 (8)	0.52 ± 0.07 (8)	15.16	13/14
5 days after colchicine	5.4 ± 0.51 (21)	0.35 ± 0.22 (20)	6/20	0/14
5 days after denervation	—	—	12/12	12/12
6 days after colchicine	1.5 ± 0.56 (6)	0.42 ± 0.02 (6)	8/15	2/10
7 days after denervation	—	—	12/12	12/12

Number of fibers responding/number of fibers examined. [b] Number of fibers examined.

treatment. Recently, Albuquerque et al. (1972) have reported similar results following chronic application to the sciatic nerve of colchicine or vinblastine.

From these studies it appears that materials carried by axoplasmic transport are important for the prevention of the development of the membrane changes generally referred to as resulting from denervation.

Botulinum toxin blocks neuromuscular transmission by selectively interfering with the release of the transmitter from cholinergic nerve terminals, nerves releasing other transmitters being unaffected. This toxin effect is achieved without apparent degenerative changes in the nerve and its terminals, nor is impulse transmission in nerve nor in muscle interfered with (Lamanna, 1959). Present evidence indicates that the toxin is irreversibly bound to cholinergic nerve terminals, and that this binding interferes with the mechanism by which ACh is released from the nerve (Thesleff, 1960; Zacks et al., 1962).

When botulinum toxin is applied to a mammalian skeletal muscle in a dose sufficient to block neuromuscular transmission, the chemical and electrical excitability of muscle fibers is altered qualitatively and quantitatively in the same way as after surgical denervation (Thesleff, 1960; Josefsson and Thesleff, 1961). It therefore appears that the release of a trophic factor or factors from nerve terminals is coupled to the release of ACh or that, alternatively, the release occurs by a mechanism equally sensitive to the toxin as that of ACh liberation.

In conclusion the results presented indicate that trophic substances, carried by axoplasmic transport, are released, presumably by the same mechanism as the transmitter, from motor nerve terminals and that these substances exert a repressive influence on that part of the muscle genome which controls the synthesis of the proteins necessary for the development of extrajunctional ACh receptors and of TTX resistant action potentials. The studies show that muscle inactivity cannot alone be responsible for the denervation changes, but they do not exclude that activity–inactivity influence the process.

ACKNOWLEDGEMENT

The researches reported on here were supported by grants from the Swedish Medical Research Council.

REFERENCES

ALBUQUERQUE, E. X., WARNICK, J. E., TASSE, J. R., and SANSONE, F. M. (1972) Effects of vinblastine and colchicine on neural regulation of the fast and slow skeletal muscles of the rat. *Exptl. Neurol.* **37**, 607–634.

AXELSSON, J., and THESLEFF, S. (1959) A study of supersensitivity in denervated mammalian skeletal muscle. *J. Physiol. Lond.* **149**, 178–193.

DAHLSTRÖM, A. (1968) Effect of colchicine on transport of amine storage granules in sympathetic nerves of rat. *Eur. J. Pharmac.* **5**, 111–113.

GRAMPP, W., HARRIS, J. B., and THESLEFF, S. (1972) Inhibition of denervation changes in skeletal muscle by blockers of protein synthesis. *J. Physiol. Lond.* **221**, 743–754.

HARRIS, J. B., and THESLEFF, S. (1972) Nerve stump length and membrane changes in denervated skeletal muscle. *Nature New Biol.* **236**, 60–61.

HOFMANN, W. W., and THESLEFF, S. (1972) Studies on the trophic influence of nerve on skeletal muscle. *Eur. J. Pharmac.* **20**, 256–260.

JOSEFSSON, J.-O., and THESLEFF, S. (1961) Electromyographic findings in experimental botulinum intoxication. *Acta physiol. scand.* **51**, 163–168.

KREUTZBERG, G. W. (1969) Neuronal dynamics and axonal flow: IV, Blockage of intra-axonal enzyme transport by colchicine. *Proc. Natn. Acad. Sci. USA* **62**, 722–728.

LAMANNA, C. (1959) The most poisonous poison. *Science* **130**, 763–772.

REDFERN, P., and THESLEFF, S. (1971) Action potential generation in denervated rat skeletal muscle: II, The action of tetrodotoxin. *Acta physiol. scand.* **82**, 70–78.

THESLEFF, S. (1960) Supersensitivity of skeletal muscle produced by botulinum toxin. *J. Physiol. Lond.* **151**, 598–607.

ZACKS, S. I., METZGER, J. F., SMITH, C. W., and BLUMBERG, J. M. (1962) Localization of ferritin labelled botulinum toxin in the neuromuscular junction of the mouse. *J. Neuropath. Exp. Neurol.* **21**, 610–633

AXOPLASMIC TRANSPORT AS A MECHANISM FOR AXONAL SUPPORT AND GROWTH

SESSION II

Chairman: U. S. VON EULER

DIFFERENTIAL ACCUMULATION OF ENZYMES IN CONSTRICTED NERVES ACCORDING TO THEIR SUBCELLULAR LOCALIZATION

PIERRE LADURON

Department of Neurobiochemistry, Janssen Pharmaceutica, Research Laboratoria, B-2340 Beerse, Belgium

SUMMARY

The axonal flow of enzymes can provide a suitable tool for the study of the intracellular localization of enzymes, namely by specifying whether two or several different enzymes are contained within the same subcellular structure. For this, kinetics of accumulation for each given component must be performed in order to obtain a possible dissociation of different classes of enzymes. Various examples, reported throughout the present paper, illustrate this statement. Thus the accumulation and the disappearance of enzymes of the catecholamine biosynthesis, in the proximal and distal segments of constricted sympathetic nerves, have brought further evidence for a double intracellular localization. Indeed, the rate of transport of tyrosine hydroxylase and dopa decarboxylase is much lower than that of dopamine β-hydroxylase, which is in agreement with an extragranular localization for the first two steps and an intragranular for the last enzyme.

In this field, however, one should proceed with caution when interpreting certain results, e.g. when tyrosine hydroxylase is measured in sciatic nerves. Therefore, for this particular problem, it seems much more appropriate to work on more specifically sympathetic neurons like splenic or hypogastric nerves.

The axonal flow of enzymes, namely of dopamine β-hydroxylase, may afford a new approach in the study of the turnover of vesicles or other subcellular organelles characterized by marker enzymes.

Various enzymes belonging to different subcellular entities, like mitochondrial, lysosomal, and microsomal, as well as pinocytic vesicles characterized by exogenous peroxidase, have also been reported to move along an axon. For these enzymes the accumulation rate was found to be generally lower than for dopamine β-hydroxylase. By means of double ligature experiments or of graded determination of the enzyme activity near a single ligature, it has been possible to find a differential accumulation for marker enzymes of lysosomes and microsomes for which a transport rate was nearly identical (0.3 mm/h).

Finally, a possible digestive phenomenon attributed partly to lysosomes transported along the axon, must be taken into consideration to explain certain dynamic aspects of neurotransmission.

INTRODUCTION

The fact that in all the iiving cells many biological processes are confined to different subcellular compartments, implies the occurrence of intracellular transport mechanisms. Thus the secretion of proteins in addition to catecholamines from chromaffin cells requires a movement of granules from the Golgi apparatus where the proteins are packaged, to the plasma membrane where an exocytic release occurs. In the same way, organelles synthesized in the cell body of a neuron must be transported along the axon to reach the nerve terminal in order to be secreted outside. However, in the neuron, this transport mechanism, currently named axonal flow, is much longer both in space and in duration.

The purpose of the present paper is not to give a complete review of the axonal flow of all kinds of enzymes in myelinated and unmyelinated nerves (Dahlström, 1971), but rather to emphasize some properties of the transport of certain enzymes as related to their subcellular localization.

In other words, the axonal flow, in a way, performs a kind of "physiological fractionation" of enzymes (Laduron, 1970a) which can be estimated by the rate of accumulation above a constriction, for instance. Therefore when two given enzymes flow down along an axon at a different rate they have most probably a different subcellular localization. The activity of various enzymes can easily be measured in several segments near the site of construction at different times after ligature of the nerve. However, the data provided by this method possess some important limitations in connection with the origin of the observed enzyme activity, which can originate from the axon itself but also from surrounding cells, such as Schwann cells.

METHODOLOGICAL REMARKS

Various techniques have been introduced to study the axonal flow of neurotransmitters or proteins in the nerves. One among those is based on the use of labeled tracers and has the great advantage of being carried out on intact rather than interrupted nerves. Nevertheless, an important limitation of this method is the lack of specificity, with regard to the identification of labeled compounds which are really transported, as well as the nature of the subcellular particles carrying the radioactive tracer. For this latter, however, autoradiography can sometimes solve certain problems without providing certainty, however, whether the labeling is really contained in a given organelle or only linked to the outside of the membrane.

Another method widely used and suggesting a flow along the axon is based on the accumulation of different components, which can be observed on one or even both sides of a constricted nerve. In this regard it is, however, necessary to interpret the obtained data with some caution.

As a one-way movement is characterized by an accumulation of a given enzyme, for instance above a constriction, and at the same time, by a disappearance of this enzyme in the distal part of the neuron, it can be interpreted quite easily since such a phenomenon cannot originate otherwise than from the axon itself. Indeed, it is not possible for the enzyme activity to increase in the surrounding cells only above and not below the constriction. On the other hand, a bidirectional movement raises difficulties in forwarding a valid interpretation of this phenomenon. Nevertheless, a combined biochemical and morphological approach as described in a remarkable paper for the mitochondriae in cat hypogastric nerves (Banks et al., 1969) allows us to assess the axonal nature of this movement However, for the myelinated nerves, the problem remains often very complex. For instance, in sciatic nerves which possess both sensory and motor neurons, a bidirectional movement could result either from a unidirectional axonal flow in each type of neuron or from a bidirectional one in both.

Moreover, a biochemical analysis of an enzyme on both sides of a ligature does not in itself allow to ascertain whether increased enzyme activity originates from the axon, since it could reflect a stimulation of injured Schwann cells. Therefore, in order to furnish a valid interpretation of such an observation, further investigation is needed using cytochemical and morphological methods or including additional experiments, like double ligatures, local drug applications or kinetic studies.

Before presenting some examples of enzyme accumulation in constricted nerves, I would like to make two remarks concerning the methodology commonly used.

In several studies bearing on the axonal transport of enzymes, the activities were generally expressed in micromoles of the formed product per hour or minute and per centimeter of nerve. In our opinion, this kind of presentation can raise difficulties for the interpretation of results more especially as the accumulation rate is lower.

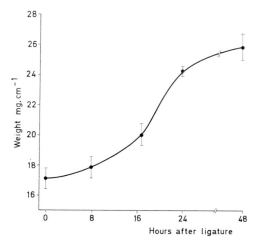

FIG. 1. Wet weight of a 1 cm proximal segment of rat sciatic nerve at different times after ligature.

For the synaptic vesicles which flow down very rapidly, the problem is less critical, but for enzymes which are transported at a lower rate, an increased enzyme activity can partly result from the increase in protein concentration or even in the tissue weight in the nerve. This point is illustrated in Fig. 1 which shows an increase in the wet weight in a 1 cm proximal segment of rat sciatic nerve at different times after ligature. Therefore, it seems very important to express the observed results in a manner commonly used in biochemistry i.e. μmoles h^{-1} or min^{-1} g^{-1} tissue or mg^{-1} protein. Without considering this limitation when interpreting their results, Jarrot and Geffen (1972) apparently found a rapid accumulation for tyrosine hydroxylase in sciatic nerves. In this case, the enzyme activity referred to 1 cm of chicken nerve, which was inadequate for measuring a kinetic of accumulation. For an unbiased observer, it appears as evident that a proximal part of a constricted nerve is seriously swollen, which therefore produces a modification of its weight or its protein concentration.

A second methodological remark is concerned with the homogenization and fractionation of nerves before analysis by enzymatic assays. It is well known in cellular biochemistry that excessive homogenization or the use of very high shearing forces as produced, for instance by an Ultraturrax, may cause considerable damage so that particle-bound enzymes can be made soluble or soluble enzymes can bind upon unspecific structures. Therefore, the estimation of the total amount of a given enzyme contained in a tissue needs to be carried out from a total homogenate. But, if this determination is performed from a supernatant yielded by a first centrifugation run, as reported in recent studies (Thoenen et al., 1971; Coyle and Wooten, 1972), a certain amount of enzyme which can vary according to the experimental conditions, i.e. time after ligation, effect of drug, centrifugation time, etc., is lost in the discarded pellet in such a way that a complete recovery of total enzyme activity is never reached, and this activity even becomes an uncontrolled variable. This remark is of particularly great importance for tyrosine hydroxylase which is known to bind unspecifically upon various structures namely in homogenizing in media containing sucrose or Ca^{++} (Laduron and Belpaire, 1968a). It is rather surprising that, in the same study (Coyle and Wooten, 1972), dopamine β-hydroxylase was measured from a total homogenate and tyrosine hydroxylase from a supernatant. In such conditions one must not be surprised if results are interpreted erroneously.

ENZYMES OF THE CATECHOLAMINE BIOSYNTHESIS

The three enzymes involved in the biosynthesis of noradrenaline have been studied for their ability to be transported along the axon of sympathetic neurons. In the first report dealing with this group of enzymes, Laduron and Belpaire (1968c) showed that dopamine β-hydroxylase which, for the first time, was measured enzymatically in a sympathetic nerve, accumulated on the proximal side but not on the distal side of a ligature applied to dog splenic nerves (Table 1). Three main features characterized this observation; the high rate of transport (3 mm/h), the structure-linked latency of the dopamine β-hydroxylase in splenic nerves as well as its equilibration properties in a density gradient (Laduron, 1969), and, finally, the unidirectional nature (proximo-distal) of this movement assessed by the accumulation above the ligature and a disappearance below the ligature. These results strongly suggested the existence of an axonal flow of granules containing dopamine β-hydroxylase at a rate which is very similar to that previously found for noradrenaline (Dahlström, 1971).

Ever since then this finding has been confirmed in different sympathetic nerves using biochemical methods (Smith et al., 1970; de Potter and Chubb, 1971; Lamprecht et al.,

TABLE 1. ACTIVITY OF ENZYMES INVOLVED IN THE BIOSYNTHESIS OF CATECHOLAMINES AND NORADRENALINE CONTENT IN CONSTRICTED SYMPATHETIC NERVES, 48 HOURS AFTER LIGATURE

		Control	Proximal segment		Distal segment	
			Units/g	% of control	Units/g	% of control
Tyrosine hydroxylase	μmoles $h^{-1} g^{-1}$	0.39 ± 0.09	0.21 ± 0.09	54	0.12 ± 0.07	31
Dopa decarboxylase	μmoles $h^{-1} g^{-1}$	0.254 ± 0.016	0.57 ± 0.03	224	0.094 ± 0.025	37
Dopamine-β-hydroxylase	μmoles $h^{-1} g^{-1}$	0.79 ± 0.59	15.1 ± 6.8	1910	0.39 ± 0.35	49
Noradrenaline	μg g^{-1}	9.3 ± 2.8	63.0 ± 148	677		

1972; Brimijoin, 1972; Coyle and Wooten, 1972; Jarrot and Geffen, 1972) and immuno-histochemical techniques (Livett *et al.*, 1969).

In contrast to the rapid transport of dopamine β-hydroxylase, the accumulation of tyrosine hydroxylase and dopa decarboxylase has been interpreted in different ways, sometimes even contradictory. Tyrosine hydroxylase was first reported to be unchanged and even slightly decreased in the proximal segment of canine splenic nerves 48 h after ligature (Laduron and Belpaire, 1968c). In the distal part, the decreased activity was still more pronounced (Table 1). From this observation it was concluded that tyrosine hydroxylase was certainly not contained in the granule containing catecholamines and dopamine β-hydroxylase owing to the complete dissociation of the accumulation rates for the two enzymes. This was quite in agreement with the extragranular localization of tyrosine hydroxylase in the adrenal medulla (Laduron and Belpaire, 1968a) and in splenic nerves (de Potter *et al.*, 1970).

Recently results, apparently quite opposite, were obtained in other laboratories. Lamprecht *et al.* (1972) (see also Kopin and Silberstein, 1972) have shown an obvious dissociation of the accumulation of dopamine β-hydroxylase and that of tyrosine hydroxylase in ligated sciatic nerves, the former accumulating more rapidly than the latter. In contrast, Coyle and Wooten (1972) using the same experimental system in the same laboratory, observed a rapid accumulation for both enzymes. About this latter study, a problem of methodology has already been discussed which highly restricts the implications of these data. Finally, another paper is rather surprising (Jarrot and Geffen, 1972). Although these authors reported an accumulation of tyrosine hydroxylase significantly lower than that of dopamine β-hydroxylase in constricted sciatic nerves of chickens, they concluded astonishingly that the increase in calculated transport rates of dopamine β-hydroxylase and tyrosine hydroxylase was parallel. In addition to this contradiction, I have already called the attention for a methodological point concerning the increase of weight of the proximal segment as illustrated in Fig. 1. Owing to the complex nature of its framework and to the difficulty in performing a good homogenization, the sciatic nerve does not represent an appropriate tool for the study of the axonal transport of tyrosine hydroxylase, an enzyme known to form aggregates and to absorb to particulate fraction (Wurzburger and Musacchio, 1971). In this regard, pure sympathetic nerves, like splenic or hypogastric nerves, are much more appropriate.

Another "soluble" enzyme, dopa decarboxylase has been firstly described to accumulate above a ligature at a rate of 1 to 2 mm/h corresponding approximately to that of noradrenaline (Dahlström and Jonason, 1968). However, it must be emphasized that the onset of such an accumulation was delayed up to 24 h after ligature. More recently it has been shown by means of a more sensitive assay for dopa decarboxylase that the activity of this enzyme increased gradually above the ligature up to the second day after ligature while it decreased below the ligature (Laduron, 1970b; see also Table 1). From this study the rate was estimated to be only 0.27 mm/h. As shown in Fig. 2, the distribution pattern is typical of a phenomenon occurring in the axon rather than in other surrounding cells, since an accumulation corresponds to the disappearance of enzyme on the other side of the ligature. The results of Dahlström and Jonason (1968) are somewhat surprising, namely with regard to the rapid accumulation rate occurring only between 24 and 48 h after the ligature. This must be attributed most probably to the lack of sensitivity in the determination of dopa decarboxylase.

Therefore, as a general conclusion, one may say that tyrosine hydroxylase and dopa decarboxylase flow down along the axon at a much lower rate than dopamine β-hydroxylase, depending on their own intracellular localization—one extragranular, the other intra-granular.

Furthermore, this kind of study can afford new possibilities for the determination of turnover of organelles and enzymes linked to these structures. By measuring the dopamine β-hydroxylase above the ligature in dog splenic nerves, it has been possible to calculate the life-span of the vesicle running up to 1.5 days (de Potter and Chubb, 1971) which is certainly much more consistent with the turnover of noradrenaline than the 3–5 weeks previously postulated (Dahlström, 1971).

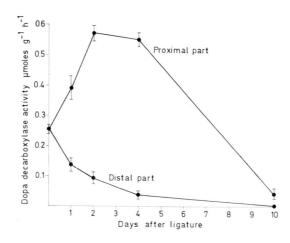

FIG. 2. Dopa decarboxylase activity above (proximal part) and below (distal part) a ligature in sciatic nerves. The enzyme activities were measured from a total homogenate and the result expressed in micromoles of dopamine formed per h and per gram of tissue (mean of at least five experiments $\pm$ SEM).

MITOCHONDRIAL ENZYME

Owing to a bidirectional accumulation, the movement of mitochondria in nerves raises difficulties in forwarding a valid interpretation of the phenomenon. In the sympathetic nerves, Banks *et al.* (1969) have shown by means of a combined biochemical and morphological approach that the accumulation of cytochrome oxidase occurred above as well as below a ligature at an approximate rate of 0.6 mm/h. Although a morphological examination and biochemical determination, namely on both sides of two constrictions indicated a bidirectional movement of mitochondria in constricted and therefore damaged nerves, these authors carefully noted that these results must not be applied to normal nerves without some reservations.

Similar results were obtained in myelinated nerves (see Zelena, 1969). More recently, MAO activities were also studied in constricted sciatic nerves (Dahlström *et al.*, 1969). The enzyme was found to accumulate slowly above a ligature and to reach a maximum value after 7 days before returning toward a normal value. It is noteworthy that sympathectomy only delayed this maximum activity to the fourteenth day, suggesting that only the axons of sympathetic nerves participated to a small extent in this phenomenon.

LYSOSOMAL AND MICROSOMAL ENZYME

Another example of a double accumulation in the proximal as well as in the distal part of crushed nerves was given by the behavior of lysosomal enzymes like acid phosphatase, acid desoxyribonuclease, or glucuronidase (Laduron, 1970a, b; Johnson, 1970). Again a valid interpretation in this regard was rendered difficult by the existence of a possible double origin either from the axon or from surrounding cells like the Schwann cells. Relying on his observations, Johnson (1970) suggested that there should most likely be a marked increase in the formation of acid phosphatase and glucuronidase in the sciatic nerve next to the region of the crush. Cytochemical data pointed to this view (Holtzman, 1969). On the other hand, our own interpretation suggested a possible double origin for this lysosomal accumulation (Laduron, 1970b). This problem was further studied by comparing the accumulation

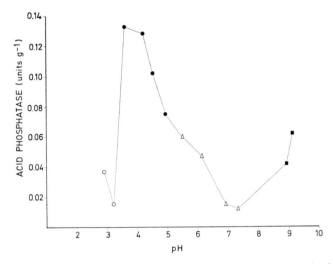

Fig. 3. pH curve for acid phosphatase from a proximal part of constricted sciatic nerves.

of acid phosphatase and inosine diphosphatase in constricted sciatic nerves under various experimental conditions. Various biochemical data provided evidence of the lysosomal nature of acid phosphatase. Firstly, it has the typical pH curve of acid hydrolases with an optimum pH between 3.4 and 4.2 (Fig. 3). Moreover, experiments bearing on the structure-linked latency indicated that this enzyme belongs to subcellular particles. By measuring the acid phosphatase and the inosine disphosphatase in 2-mm pieces on both sides of a constriction, a completely different distribution pattern was obtained for each enzyme as illustrated in Fig. 4. For acid phosphatase, a graded accumulation with the highest activity near the ligature can be seen on both sides of the constriction, while for inosine diphosphatase equally increased activities were found in all the segments, in the proximal as well as in distal part. Such a distribution pattern for inosine diphosphatase is more compatible with an axonal origin than with an injury-stimulated reaction in the Schwann cells, whilst a graded accumulation of acid phosphatase on both sides of the ligature remained consistent with both concepts. Nevertheless, by means of double ligature experiments it has been possible to distinguish the two possible origins. Figure 5 shows such an experiment where acid phosphatase was measured in various segments 4, 7, and 10 days after a double ligature

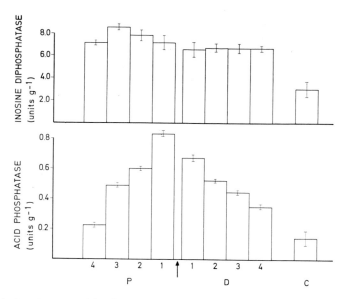

FIG. 4. Acid phosphatase and inosine diphosphatase activity in 2-mm segments of rat sciatic nerve above (P) and below (D) a ligature (↑) after 7 days, as compared with control values (C) (nerve of the unoperated side).

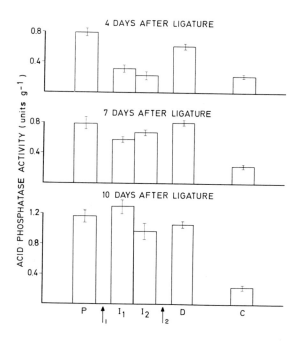

FIG. 5. Acid phosphatase activities in several segments of rat sciatic nerve at different times after two ligatures; proximal part (P) above the first ligature (↑¹), distal (D) part below the second ligature (↑²), two intermediary (I₁I₂) segments and control (C) nerves from the unoperated side (mean of at least six experiments ± SEM).

applied on rat sciatic nerves. After 4 days the activity was only found to increase in the proximal and distal segment, whereas the intermediary parts were found almost unchanged as compared with the controls. However, after a longer time, 7 or 10 days, the increase of acid phosphatase activity became progressively identical in all the segments. Similar experiments performed by estimating acid desoxyribonuclease activities gave identical results, whereas alkaline phosphatase was found unaltered when compared to controls.

The foregoing data seem to be consistent with a possible double origin of this increase of lysosomal activity on both sides of a ligature. As no change was observed between the two ligatures during the first days, one may assume that the accumulation of acid hydrolases above the first and below the second constriction could originate from a flow of lysosomes along the axon. Thereafter the increased activity observed between the two ligatures should be due to an injury-induced reaction of Schwann cells or other surrounding cells. Consequently it is likely that the lysosomes, like other subcellular organelles, can flow down in axons. Moreover, it is not unlikely that the accumulation of granules or vesicles containing catecholamines and mitochondriae reached a maximum level after 2 or 3 days owing to the digestive process of lysosomal enzymes. Whether an axonal flow occurs in normal nerves remains, however, is a question to be elucidated. As for the inosine diphosphatase, the transport rate of lysosomes in constricted nerves should be approximately 0.3 mm/h. It is noteworthy that this microsomal enzyme migrates much more slowly than acetylcholinesterase which has been reported to flow down at about 11 mm/h in the proximo-distal and at 5.6 mm/h in the disto-proximal direction (Lubinska and Niemerko, 1971).

Finally, it must be stressed that the increase of inosine diphosphatase along a relatively long part of the proximal and distal segment does not support the view of a local axonal reaction (Pellegrino de Iraldi and de Robertis, 1970). These data are, however, much more in agreement with an increased activity in elongated structures like membranes, in contrast to the graded accumulation of hydrolytic enzymes which is more compatible with an axonal flow of lysosomes.

EXOGENOUS ENZYME

Until now, attention has only been focused on the axonal flow of enzymes occurring either in one direction, but only centrifugal, or in both directions. Recently, another kind of unidirectional movement, centripetal this time, also called retrograde, has been reported to occur in the neurons.

When the granules or vesicles containing noradrenaline have reached the terminals by a rapid proximo-distal flow along the axon, it is beyond doubt that the neurotransmitters cannot be released otherwise than by exocytosis (Smith and Winkler, 1972). This process implies that the granular membrane can be incorporated in the membrane of nerve endings. Consequently, if this exocytosis phenomenon was not followed by an endocytosis phenomenon directly related to the first one, one might expect a nearly unlimited growth of the nerve endings, which is certainly not in agreement with reality (Fig. 6). Such an endocytic process has already been demonstrated in several types of neurons (Holtzman and Peterson, 1969; Zacks and Sait, 1969; Kristenson et al., 1971; Guidetta et al., 1971) in neurosecretory terminals of posterior pituitary glands (Douglas et al., 1971) and more recently also in the adrenal medulla (Abraham and Holtzman, 1973). For this, the uptake of horseradish peroxidase previously injected into the animal can be visualized to occur in the nerve endings by means of a specific histochemical procedure. This technique has also allowed to

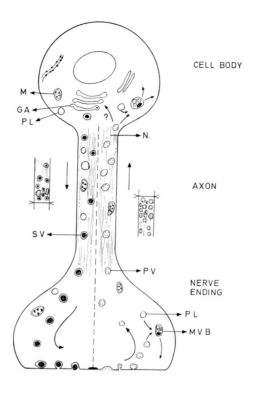

CELL BODY

AXON

NERVE
ENDING

FIG. 6. Diagram illustrating the dynamic aspects of the neurotransmission occurring at the subcellular level of adrenergic neurones and involving namely process of biosynthesis, axonal flow,
exocytosis, endocytosis and degradation. M, mitochondria; GA, Golgi apparatus; PL, primary
lysosome; SV, synaptic vesicle; PV, pinocytic vesicle; MVB, multivesicular body; N, neurotubule.

demonstrate the accumulation of this exogenous protein below a ligature (Kristensson *et
al.*, 1971; Kristensson and Olson, 1971; Lavail and Lavail, 1972). This finding suggests the
occurrence of a retrograde flow of pinocytic vesicles originated most probably from the
nerve endings. The finding of such a centripetal movement represents an important step in
neuronal dynamics and will allow to explain the role of these long-time enigmatic structures,
the agranular vesicles, or empty "synaptic vesicles".

That endocytosis is closely related to exocytosis is supported by a recent experiment
showing that the uptake of peroxidase into small vesicles within nerve endings in lobster
stretcher muscles can be enhanced by electric stimulation of transmitter release by the
endings (Holtzman *et al.*, 1971). One should hope that this new concept of endocytosis in
the neuron may lead to new studies on the uptake of labeled exogenous noradrenaline which
most likely should also be performed by the same endocytic process. In this regard we have
shown that labeled noradrenaline was taken up by the lysosomes in the spleen of dogs and
in the kidney of rats (Laduron *et al.*, 1966; Laduron, 1969). At that time we wrote: "It is
too early to know whether this storage (of labeled noradrenaline in the lysosomes) occurs by
endocytosis. . . . It appears however clearly that radioactive perfused noradrenaline cannot
be used to characterize the specific storage site of endogenous catecholamine containing
particles." This early finding, which was in complete disagreement with the common concept

according to which labeled noradrenaline is taken up by vesicles containing endogenous catecholamines (Axelrod, 1971), appears today as much more compatible with the phenomenon of endocytosis recently described.

REFERENCES

ABRAHAM, S. J., and HOLTZMAN, E. (1973) Secretion and endocytosis in insulin-stimulated rat adrenal medulla cells. *J. Cell Biol.* **56**, 540–558.

AXELROD, J. (1971) Noradrenaline: fate and control of its biosynthesis. *Science* **173**, 598–606.

BANKS, P., MANGNALL, D., and MAYOR, D. (1969) The re-distribution of cytochrome oxidase, noradrenaline and adenosine triphosphate in adrenergic nerves constricted at two points. *J. Physiol.* **200**, 745–762.

BRIMIJOIN, S. (1972) Transport and turnover of dopamine β-hydroxylase (EC 1.14.2.1) in sympathetic nerves of the rat. *J. Neurochem.* **19**, 2182–2193.

COYLE, J. T., and WOOTEN, G. F. (1972) Rapid axonal transport of tyrosine hydroxylase and dopamine β-hydroxylase. *Brain Res.* **44**, 701–704.

DAHLSTRÖM, A. (1971) Axoplasmic transport (with particular respect to adrenergic neurons). *Phil. Trans. R. Soc. Lond.* **B, 261**, 325–358.

DAHLSTRÖM, A., and JONASON, J. (1968) Dopa decarboxylase activity in sciatic nerves of the rat after constriction. *Eur. J. Pharmac.* **4**, 377–383.

DAHLSTRÖM, A., JONASON, J., and NORBERG, K. A. (1969) Monoamine oxidase activity in rat sciatic nerves after constriction. *Eur. J. Pharmac.* **6**, 248–254.

DE POTTER, W. P., and CHUBB, I. W. (1971) The turnover rate of noradrenergic vesicles. *Biochem. J.* **125**, 375–376.

DE POTTER, W. P., SMITH, A. D., and DE SCHAEPDRYVER, A. F. (1970) Subcellular fractionation of splenic nerves: ATP, chromogranin A and dopamine β-hydroxylase in noradrenergic vesicles. *Tissue & Cell* **2**, 529–546.

DOUGLAS, W. W., NAGASAWA, J., and SCHULZ, R. A. (1971) Coated microvesicles in neurosecretory terminals of posterior pituitary glands shed their coats to become smooth "synaptic" vesicles. *Nature* **232**, 340–341.

GUIDETTA, A., D'UDINE, B., and PEPE, M. (1971) Uptake of protein by the giant axon of the squid. *Nature* **229**, 29–30.

HOLTZMAN, E. (1969) Lysosomes in the physiology and pathology of neurons. In: *Lysosomes in Biology and Pathology*. (J. T. Dingle and H. B. Fell, eds.) North-Holland, Amsterdam, p. 192.

HOLTZMAN, E., and PETERSON, E. R. (1969) Uptake of protein by mammalian neurons. *J. Cell Biol.* **40**, 863–869.

HOLTZMAN, E., FREEMAN, A. R., and KASHMER, L. A. (1971) Stimulation-dependent alterations in peroxidase uptake at lobster neuromuscular junctions. *Science* **173**, 733–736.

JARROT, B., and GEFFEN, L. B. (1972) Rapid axoplasmic transport of tyrosine hydroxylase in relation to other cytoplasmic constituents. *Proc. Natn. Acad. Sci. USA* **69**, 3440–3442.

JOHNSON, J. L. (1970) Changes in acetylcholinesterase, acid phosphatase and betaglucuronidase proximal to a nerve crush. *Brain Res.* **18**, 427–440.

KOPIN, I. J., and SILBERSTEIN, S. D. (1972) Axons of sympathetic neurons: transport of enzymes *in vivo* and properties of axonal sprouts *in vitro*. *Pharmac. Rev* **24**, 245–254.

KRISTENSSON, K., and OLSSON, Y. (1971) Retrograde axonal transport of protein. *Brain Res.* **29**, 363–365.

KRISTENSSON, K., OLSSON, Y., and SJÖSTRAND (1971) Axonal uptake and retrograde transport of exogenous proteins in the hypoglossal nerve. *Brain Res.* **32**, 399–406.

LADURON, P. (1969) Biosynthèse, localisation intracellulaire et transport des catécholamines. Thesis, Vander, Louvain.

LADURON, P. (1970a) Axonal flow of enzymes involved in the biosynthesis of catecholamines. *Acta physiol. scand.*, Suppl. **357**, 15.

LADURON, P. (1970b) Differential accumulation of various enzymes in constricted sciatic nerves. *Archs. int. Pharmacodyn. Thér.* **185**, 200–203.

LADURON, P., and BELPAIRE, F. (1968a) Tissue fractionation and catecholamines: 2, Intracellular distribution patterns of tyrosine hydroxylase, dopa decarboxylase, dopamine β-hydroxylase, phenylethanolamine *N*-methyltransferase and monoamine oxidase in adrenal medulla. *Biochem. Pharmac.* **17**, 1127–1140.

LADURON, P., and BELPAIRE, F. (1968b) Transport of noradrenaline and dopamine β-hydroxylase in sympathetic nerves. *Life Sci.* **7**, 1–7.

LADURON, P., and BELPAIRE, F. (1968c) Evidence for an extragranular localization of tyrosine hydroxylase. *Nature* **217**, 1155–1156.

Laduron, P., de Potter, W., and Belpaire, F. (1966) Storage of labeled noradrenaline in lysosomes. *Life Sci.* **5,** 2085–2094.

Lamprecht, F., Weise, V. K., and Kopin, I. J. (1972) Effect of colchicine and vinblastine on the tyrosine hydroxylase and dopamine β-hydroxylase content of the rat superior cervical ganglion and salivary gland. *Fed. Proc.* **31,** 544.

Lavail, J. H., and Lavail, M. M. (1972) Retrograde axonal transport in the central nervous system. *Science* **176,** 1416–1417.

Livett, B. G., Geffen, L. B., and Rush, R. A. (1969) Immunohistochemical evidence for dopamine β-hydroxylase and a catecholamine binding protein in sympathetic nerves. *Biochem. Pharmac.* **18,** 923–924.

Lubinska, L., and Niemerko, S. (1971) Velocity and intensity of bidirectional migration of acetylcholinesterase in transected nerves. *Brain Res.* **27,** 329–342.

Pellegrino de Iraldi, A., and de Robertis, E. (1970) Studies on the origin of the granulated and non-granulated vesicles. In *Bayer Symposium II* (H. J. Schümann and H. Kroneberg, eds.), Springer-Verlag, Berlin, pp. 4–17.

Smith, A. D., and Winkler, H. (1972) Fundamental mechanisms in the release of catecholamines. In: *Catecholamines* (H. Blaschko and E. Muscholl, eds.) Springer-Verlag, Berlin, pp. 538–617.

Smith, A. D., Mayor, D., and Banks, P. (1970) Unpublished results cited by P. Banks and K. B. Helle (1971) *Phil. Trans. R. Soc. Lond.* B, **261,** 305–310.

Thoenen, H., Mueller, R., and Axelrod, J. (1971) Phase difference with induction of tyrosine hydroxylase in cell body and nerve terminals of sympathetic neurones. *Proc. Natn. Acad. Sci. USA* **65,** 58–72.

Wurzburger, R. J., and Musacchio, J. M. (1971) Subcellular distribution and aggregation of bovine adrenal tyrosine hydroxylase. *J. Pharmac.* **177,** 155–168.

Zacks, S. I., and Sait, A. (1969) Uptake of exogenous horseradish peroxidase by coated vesicles in mouse neuromuscular junctions. *J. Histochem. Cytochem.* **17,** 161–170.

Zelena, J. (1969) Bidirectional shift of mitochondria in axons after injury. In *Cellular Dynamics of the Neuron* (S. H. Barondes ed.), Academic Press, New York, p. 73–94.

IMPORTANCE OF AXOPLASMIC TRANSPORT FOR TRANSMITTER LEVELS IN NERVE TERMINALS

J. Häggendal, A. Dahlström, S. Bareggi, and P.-A. Larsson

Department of Pharmacology and Institute of Neurobiology, University of Göteborg, Göteborg, Sweden

SUMMARY

The disappearance of transmitter content in rat adrenergic and cholinergic nerve terminals following axotomy at different levels of the axons has been studied. The transmitter disappearance was considered to reflect degenerative changes of the nerve terminals. The length of attached axonal stump after axotomy could influence the course of transmitter decrease and degeneration; with a longer stump attached the course of degeneration was delayed. This delay was interpreted to be due to the centrifugal axonal transport of some factor(s) essential for the maintenance of the nerve terminal integrity. The rate of transport of this factor was calculated and compared with the fast rate of intra-axonal transport of transmitter, presumably particle bound, which occurs in both adrenergic and cholinergic neurons.

In peripheral adrenergic nerves the rate of transport of amine storage granules was reconsidered and calculated after investigating certain factors of importance for the calculations, such as (a) the noradrenaline (NA) loading of granules accumulated above a crush, which seem to increase somewhat during the accumulation period; (b) the fraction of NA in normal sciatic nerve which is transportable at fast rates. Only part of the NA was transportable; the same was found also for the acetylcholine in cholinergic neurons.

In all three systems investigated the transmitter particles and the factor(s) essential for nerve terminal integrity was found to be transported at approximately similar rates; this rate was in peripheral adrenergic neurons about 8 mm/h; in central adrenergic neurons much slower, about 0.5 mm/h; and in peripheral autonomic cholinergic neurons about 4–5 mm/h. The transport of both substances is blocked by vinblastine. This could suggest that the two substances were connected with each other. However, some results from experiments using reserpine indicate that this is probably not the case.

INTRODUCTION

The neuron has a high metabolic activity in which different compounds are continuously formed in the cell body and by different mechanisms transported towards the nerve terminals. Studies of these problems were initiated and highly stimulated by the works of Weiss and coworkers (Weiss and Hiscoe, 1948; Weiss, 1961, 1963). The transport seems to occur at different rates. While the rate of the axonal flow is slow, a few millimeters per day,

257

such organelles like amine storage granules are transported intra axonally at a fast rate at the order of millimeters per hour (e.g. Dahlström, 1965; Dahlström and Häggendal, 1966; Banks et al., 1969). The mechanism for the fast transport appears to be connected to the neurotubules. It can thus be blocked by such drugs as colchicine and vinblastine (VIN), which disrupt the neurotubules (for details and references, see, e.g. Dahlström, 1970, 1971). The fast transport of proteins (Ochs and Ranish, 1969) and amine storage granules (Dahlström, 1967; Häggendal et al., 1974), is functioning with the normal rate also in axons distal to a cut or crush. The nerve terminals will thus after an axotomy be supplied with compounds present in the axonal stump and transported distally at a fast rate until the stores in the stump are used up. The longer the attached stump, the longer is the time until the stores are used up.

After a period of latency following axotomy a number of "degeneration phenomena" occur at the nerve terminal-effector cell level, e.g. transmission failure, disappearance of the transmitter from the nerve terminals, destruction of the nerve terminal membrane, increased sensitivity of the effector cell to the transmitter, and leakage of the transmitter from the degenerating nerve terminals which may cause activation of the effector cells, noticeable as, e.g., contraction of the periorbital smooth muscle some hours after removal of the superior cervical ganglion (cf. Lundberg, 1969). (For a recent review of degeneration activity after parasympathetic and sympathetic denervation, see Emmelin and Trendelenburg, 1972.)

Several studies have shown that degenerative changes occur later after "distant" axotomy, when the attached nerve stump is long, than when the stump is short (e.g. Birks et al., 1960; Emmelin, 1967; Harris and Thesleff, 1972). Also the appearance of morphological changes in the nerve terminals is delayed by increasing the length of the attached nerve stump (Miledi and Slater, 1970). These studies indicate that some factor of importance for the maintenance of the functional and the structural integrity of the nerve terminals is transported distally in the axons. These factors will in the following be referred to as nerve terminal factors (NTF). Based on the differences in the nerve stump lengths and the delay in the appearance of degeneration phenomena the transport rate of NTF can be calculated. The rate was found to be 2–10 mm/h in parasympathetic fibers to the cat parotid gland (Emmelin, 1968), 5 mm/h in the rat extensor digitorum longus nerve (Harris and Thesleff, 1972) and 13 mm/h in the rat phrenic nerve (Miledi and Slater, 1970).

This rate of transport in cholinergic neurons is thus of the same order of magnitude as the fast rate found for the transport of amine storage granules in peripheral adrenergic neurons (about 5–10 mm/h) in the rat sciatic nerve (Dahlström and Häggendal, 1966). Also it is similar to the rate of transport of acetylcholine (ACh) in motor and preganglionic nerves (for references, see Dahlström et al., this volume).

In a series of experiments we have compared the transport rates of NTF and the fast transport rates of NA and ACh in adrenergic and cholinergic neurons respectively. The transmitter levels in different tissues have been followed after axotomy with different lengths of the remaining stump. The decrease of transmitter levels in the tissue during denervation reflects a loss of transmitter stored in the nerve terminals. However, the decreased levels at a certain time after axotomy reflect the condition of the nerve terminals as a mean. As pointed out by Malmfors and Sachs (1965), the adrenergic nerve terminal branches of one individual neuron in the iris lose their NA content within 1–2 h when they start to degenerate. At the same time nerve terminals from other adrenergic neurons in the same tissue appear to be completely unaffected. Sachs and Jonsson (1973) also found that the transmitter storage mechanism of the granules is affected before the nerve membrane. It may thus be that the early, small changes in transmitter levels primarily reflect degenerative changes of the nerve terminal storage granules.

In this study three different types of neurons have been studied in the rat with respect to degenerative changes in nerve terminals following axotomy:

(1) peripheral NA containing neurons of the long type;
(2) central NA containing neurons (bulbospinal neurons);
(3) peripheral ACh containing neurons (preganglionic fibers to the superior cervical ganglion).

1. PERIPHERAL NA-CONTAINING NEURONS

Almost all the NA in the skeletal muscle is present in the nerve terminals of adrenergic vasoconstrictors (Fuxe and Sedvall, 1965). The axons to more than 90% of these nerve terminals in the rat gastrocnemic muscle are running in the sciatic nerve. The NA levels

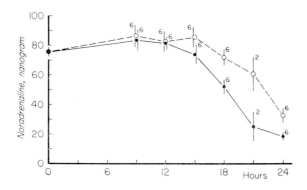

FIG. 1. The amounts of NA (ng/muscle) in rat gastrocnemic muscles at different times after cutting the sciatic nerves. ●——● shows the values after cutting the nerve close to the muscle on one side; ○ – – –○ indicates the values after cutting about 3 cm proximal to the level on the contralateral side. Mean ± SEM are given. Small numerals indicate number of observations. (From Häggendal and Dahlström, *Acta Neuropath.*, Suppl. V, 238–248 (1971).) Springer-Verlag, Berlin, Heidelberg, New York.

were followed in the gastrocnemic muscle after cutting the sciatic nerve close to the muscle unilaterally, and on the contralateral side at about 3 cm distance.

On the "close" side the NA levels started to decrease about 12 h after the axotomy (Fig. 1). The levels had declined to 50% at about 18 h after the operation and to 20% after 24 h. On the "distal" side, the decrease followed the same pattern, but was delayed for about 3 h (Häggendal and Dahlström, 1971). The difference of 3 cm in nerve stump length thus delayed onset of degeneration by about 3 h. The transport of NTF therefore corresponds to a transport rate of about 10 mm/h.

This is a fast rate of transport of the same order of magnitude as the fast transport of amine storage granules earlier calculated to be about 5 mm/h (Dahlström and Häggendal, 1966). In a recent paper, Lundberg (1972) has calculated the rate of transport for the "axotomy information" to be 4 mm/h in the adrenergic neurons to the eye using colchicine as a tool. However, our figures for the rate of transport of NTF and amine storage granules obviously differ by a factor of about 2. Both these figures have therefore been re-estimated.

A.   TRANSPORT RATE OF NTF

When the difference between "distal" and "close" axotomy of sciatic nerve was 3.3 cm, as a mean, the delay in the NA disappearance was found to be 4 h, as a mean (Fig. 2) (Bareggi *et al.*, 1974). The transport rate of NTF can thus be calculated to be about 8 mm/h.

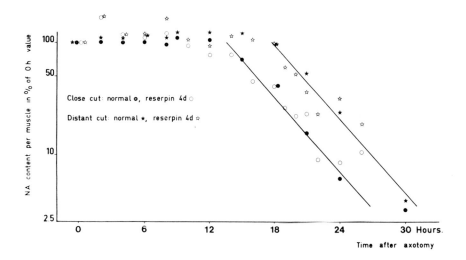

FIG. 2. The amounts of NA in rat gastrocnemic muscle at different times after cutting the sciatic nerve either close to the muscle (circles) or 3.3 cm proximal to it (stars). Normal rats, filled symbols; reserpine treated rats (10 mg/kg i.p., 4 days prior to operation), open symbols. The NA is expressed on a logarithmic scale in percent of the 0 h values, i.e. at the time of operation.

B.   TRANSPORT RATE OF AMINE STORAGE GRANULES

The transport rate of about 5 mm/h in the sciatic nerve was calculated from the amount of NA that accumulated per hour above a constriction, related to the amount of NA found per unit of length of uncrushed nerve. The endogenous NA was in these experiments considered to be a marker of the amine storage granules. The assumption was made that the granules did not markedly increase their NA content during the experiments. Control experiments with simultaneous double ligations indicated that this probably was not the case (Dahlström and Häggendal, 1966). However, even if the assumptions were valid for discussing the order of magnitude of the fast transport, a more exact figure was needed, and we therefore have considered in detail some factors of importance for the calculations.

(a) The endogenous NA in amine storage particles above a nerve crush seems to increase somewhat with time during the accumulation period (Dahlström and Häggendal, 1970, 1972; Dahlström *et al.*, in preparation). In the sciatic nerve segment between simultaneous or "delayed" double crushes the NA amounts were followed at different time intervals. When "delayed" double crushes were performed, amine granules were first allowed to accumulate above a distal crush for 6 h; therafter a second crush was made about 1.5 cm proximal to the first one. The increase of NA content within the isolated segment of the nerve may be interpreted as an increased NA loading of the amine granules present in the segment. It is unlikely that the increase was due to an increased amount of *granules*, since these probably must be provided by the cell body via the axons, a connection which is interrupted by the second high crush. The increase seemed not to be very high, but is of importance when calculating the rate of transport. The increase by 9 h after the high crush corresponded to about 35% of the NA amount found above the low 6 h crush prior to the second crush. These and other experiments may indicate that the amine granules at a high level of uncrushed nerve might have the capacity to increase their NA loading by about 100%

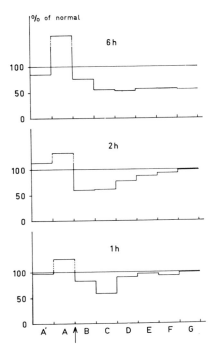

FIG. 3. The NA content in 5 mm segments of rat sciatic nerve distal to a crush which was made 1, 2, or 6 h before dissection. The ordinate shows the NA values expressed as percent of the NA content in the respective 5 mm segments of control nerve, crushed just prior to dissection (0 h crush). The abscissa indicates the different 5 mm segment from the level of the foramen infrapiriformis and distally along the nerve. The arrow indicates the site of the crush.

while transported distally in the axons. Correction for this increased loading will give a somewhat reduced figure of about 3 mm/h for the rate of transport of amine storage granules. However, correction for a second factor will yet again *increase* the rate of transport.

   (b) Not all the NA in the uncrushed sciatic nerve seems to be transportable at a fast rate. As discussed in an earlier paper by Dahlström (1967), some of the NA must be present in the adrenergic vasoconstrictors of the blood vessels in the sciatic nerve.

   In order to estimate the NA fraction that is transportable at a fast rate in the sciatic nerve, the NA amounts were followed in 0.5 cm long consecutive segments distal to a crush 1–12 h after operation (Häggendal *et al.*). As mentioned above, the mechanism for fast transport is functioning in spite of the ligation. Thus a fraction of the NA disappeared first in the segments near the crush and with increasing time also in the more distal segments (Fig. 3). The rate of distal transport of this mobile NA fraction could be estimated and found to be about 8 mm/h. The transportable NA fraction was 45% of the total NA content per unit of length. To some extent the stable (or less mobile) NA fraction may represent the NA present in the adrenergic vasoconstrictor nerves to the blood vessels in the sciatic nerve. However, it cannot at present be excluded that it is also present in other tissues in the nerve, and it can even be situated within adrenergic axons. Thus, e.g., Tranzer (1972) discusses the tubular reticulum in association with amines.

We can thus assume that the accumulation of NA above a crush is due to transport of only 45% of the NA in uncrushed nerve. When this factor is also included in the corrections, the rate of transport for amine storage granules was estimated to be 8 mm/h. This figure is in good agreement with the observed rate of transport *distal* to a crush being about 8 mm/h.

There are also some other factors that may be of importance for the calculation of the normal rate of transport.

(c) The axotomy may affect the cell bodies, influencing the production and down-transport of granules (Dahlström and Häggendal, 1972). Under normal environmental temperature conditions, this effect, however, seems to be of minor importance at least up to 12 h after crushing.

(d) At some conditions a possible retrograde accumulation of NA (Dahlström, 1965) may disturb the calculations. Thus there were signs of retrograde accumulation of NA in the 0.5 cm segment just distal to the crush. The nature and importance of this accumulation must be further investigated, but its role for these calculations probably is small.

Granular constituents other than NA can be used for the calculation of the fast transport of amine granules, e.g. dopamine-β-hydroxylase (DBH, EC 1.14.2.1) (for references, see Geffen and Livett, 1971). When measuring the transportable fraction distal to a constriction of the rat sciatic nerve in the mode just discussed for NA, the rapidly transportable DBH fraction was found to correspond to less than 50% of the DBH in unligated nerve (Dahlström and Häggendal, in preparation). Wooten and Coyle (1973) have found the transportable fraction of the DBH in unligated nerve to be about 30% and the rate of proximo-distal transport to be 6.3 mm/h. In a recent paper Brimijoin (1972) reports the rate to be 4.3 mm/h. However, this figure was based only on estimates of the accumulation of DBH above a crush, and no correction for the nonmobile fraction of DBH was made. This means that the figure of 4.3 mm/h in all probability must be increased, perhaps doubled, yielding a figure of about 9 mm/h.

To conclude: the rate of transport of amine storage granules in rat long adrenergic neurons appears to be about 8 mm/h, estimated with different techniques. This fast rate was also found for the transport of NTF.

2.   BULBOSPINAL NA-CONTAINING NEURONS

The cell bodies of these neurons are located in the lower brain stem, the axons descend in the spinal cord, and a rich nerve terminal net innervates the gray matter of the spinal cord, as demonstrated both biochemically and histochemically (e.g. Magnusson and Rosengren, 1963; Andén et al., 1964; Carlsson et al., 1964; Dahlström and Fuxe, 1965). When comparing the rates of transport for amine storage granules and for NTF, these neurons are of particular interest since the transport rate of amine storage granules, estimated by the accumulation of endogenous NA above a transection, is very low. The rate was found to be about 0.7 mm/h (Häggendal and Dahlström, 1969). This transport rate is thus approximately one-tenth of the corresponding rate in the peripheral adrenergic neuron, but must still be looked upon as a relative fast rate, more rapid than the axonal flow of 1–2 mm/day.

NA was followed both biochemically and histochemically in three consecutive 1 cm segments distal to a transection of the rat spinal cord in the midthoracic region (Häggendal and Dahlström, 1973). The nerve terminals present within a particular 1 cm length of the spinal cord will, as a mean, have 1 cm shorter axons than the nerve terminals in the more distal 1 cm segment. The onset and the course of the NA decrease in three consecutive sections were found to be delayed with increasing length of the axons (Fig. 4). Based on the delay in onset observed between the different 1 cm segments, the rate of transport of NTF

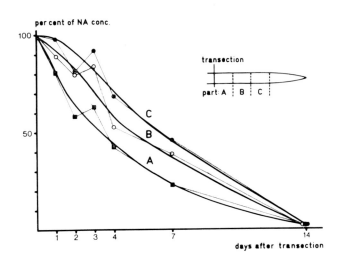

FIG. 4. The NA content in the caudal part of rat spinal cord after transection. The values are given in percent of the NA concentration in parts A, B, and C (see inlet figure) in 0 h transected rats. Part A (■——■), part B (○——○), and part C (●——●). Mean values are indicated. For SEM and number of estimations see Table 1 in Häggendal and Dahlström (1973). (From Häggendal and Dahlström, *Neuropharmacology*, **12**, 349–354 (1973) Pergamon Press.)

could be calculated to be about 0.3–0.4 mm/h. This rate is thus also markedly slower than the rate for NTF in peripheral adrenergic neurons and comparable with the estimated rather slow rate for the transport of NA granules within these central neurons.

It may be mentioned in this connection that the same type of slow rate is found for the transport of serotonin in bulbospinal neurons (about 0.5 mm/h; Dahlström et al., 1973a), and for the NTF transport in these neurons as judged by histochemical observations (Häggendal and Dahlström, 1973).

3. ACH-CONTAINING PREGANGLIONIC NEURONS

Part of the ACh present in the sciatic nerve appears to be transported at a fast rate of 3–5 mm/h (Häggendal et al., 1971; Dahlström et al., 1974), which is in agreement with the findings of rapid axonal transport of labeled ACh in *Aplysia* (Koike et al., 1972) (see also Dahlström et al., this volume). Based on the amount of ACh accumulating per hour proximal to a cut of the preganglionic nerve fibers to the rat superior cervical ganglion and the fraction of transportable ACh per unit of length of normal nerve, the rate of transport of ACh was found to be about 4 mm/h.

After cutting the preganglionic cholinergic nerves, the general course of ACh decrease in the ganglia was similar after a cut close to the ganglion and after a cut 10–14 mm caudal, (distant cut) to the ganglion on the contralateral side (Fig. 5). However, after a distant cut there was a time-lag in the ACh decrease of about 4 h as compared to after a close cut (Fig. 5). This corresponds to a transport rate of NTF of 3–4 mm/h. Thus it was also here a good correlation between the fast transport of the transmitter vehicles and NTF.

As mentioned in the introduction, different degeneration phenomena have been followed in motor nerves with increasing length of the nerve stump. Following the development of tetrodotoxin resistant action potentials in rat extensor digitorum longus muscles, Harris

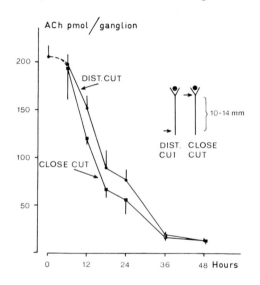

FIG. 5. The ACh content of rat superior cervical ganglia at different times after preganglionic denervation either close to the ganglion (■——■) or at a distance of 10–14 mm (●——●). Means ± SEM are indicated. $N = 4$ except where indicated. Paired operations were done except at 0 and 6 h. On a paired t-test the mean differences at 12 h and 24 h were significantly different ($p < 0.05$). (From Häggendal et al., 1973.)

and Thesleff (1972) reported the protecting effect of the longer axonal stump to correspond to a transport rate of 5 mm/h. This rate is in agreement with the rate of ACh transport in the sciatic nerve of 4–5 mm/h (see above).

In the different neurons studied, both aminergic and cholinergic, it seems as if the transport rates for transmitter (-particles) and for NTF are the same, also in neurons with a relatively slow rate of "fast" transport, like the bulbospinal neurons.

The mechanism for transport of NA and ACh may possibly be connected to the microtubules since local treatmentwith colchicine or VIN will interrupt the transport of both NA (e.g. Dahlström, 1968, 1970) and ACh (see Dahlström et al., this volume), probably by destroying the neurotubules (for references, see Mayor and Banks, this volume). Also the relatively slow rate of NA transport in bulbospinal neurons is arrested by VIN (Dahlström, 1971). The transportable NA is in all probability bound to amine storage granules. The fast transport mechanism (probably connected with microtubules) appears, so far, to be used mainly by particle bound substances. This is likely to be the case also for the rapidly transportable ACh. After local treatment of the superior cervical ganglion, with high concentrations of VIN, 5–10 mM, signs of degeneration, such as disappearance of NA from the nerve terminals and degeneration release, occur in the same manner as if the ganglion had been removed (Dahlström, 1970; Lundberg, 1972; Dahlström *et al.*, 1973b). VIN can thus produce a chemical axotomy, but interestingly enough the propagation of pre- and postganglionic nerve impulses appears not to be affected for several hours in this system. The results indicate that the NTF may be using microtubules for the transport and that it may be particle bound.

The fast transport of transmitters and of NTF show many features in common:

(1) the rate of transport seems to be the same within different types of neurons;
(2) the transport system may be connected with the neurotubules, which indicates that also NTF is particle bound.

It may then be asked if the transmitters and NTF are transported within the same particles, e.g. amine storage granules in adrenergic neurons? Several possibilities may exist, e.g.:

(1) NTF is a normal component of the transmitter granules, implying that the granules protect the nerve terminals from degeneration.
(2) NTF is connected with the granules during the transport, but the two may or mat not be produced separately in the cell bodies.
(3) NTF is produced in the cell bodies and transported distally, probably particle bound, but separate from amine granules.
(4) NTF is not preventing degeneration. It is formed at the place for the axonal damage and then by axonal transport mechanisms reaching the nerve terminals, where it after a period of latency produces the signs of degeneration. The necessity of considering also this possibility has been discussed by, e.g. Lundberg (1972).

However, even if this last possibility is difficult to exclude, it appears at present less likely than the other three possibilities, where NTF is considered to prevent degeneration. As mentioned in the introduction the peripheral parts of the neuron are supplied, via transport mechanisms, with compounds formed in the cell bodies. For the fast transport of some compounds an apparently highly developed mechanism is available. If this transport is arrested by axotomy or treatment with such drug as colchicine or VIN, it seems likely that a lack of one or several factors of importance for the maintenance of the nerve terminals will occur when (a) the stores in the remaining axonal stump are empty (explaining the importance of increased length of the axonal stump), and (b) the stores in the nerve terminals have been consumed (explaining the fact that onset of degeneration signs occurs with a delay of several hours following arrest of the axonal contribution).

If possibility (1) (the transmitter granules contain the NTF) is true it could be expected that ACh-containing particles would protect the cholinergic nerve terminals and NA-containing particles the adrenergic terminals. In order to investigate if this is the case for the adrenergic neuron a nerve degeneration study was performed in reserpine pretreated rats. Reserpine, even in a large dose, does not *per se* induce nerve terminal degeneration (ref. Malmfors, 1965). After a large dose of reserpine a supranormal amount of new amine storage granules is probably transported to the terminals between day 3 and day 6 (Dahlström and Häggendal, 1969). This is in food agreement with the enzyme induction found in the ganglion cell bodies after reserpine (Thoenen *et al.*, 1969; Molinoff *et al.*, 1970), where enzymes dealing with the monoamine metabolism, including DBH, are increased. On the fourth day after reserpine the nerve terminals may therefore contain a supranormal amount of recently downtransported amine storage granules, which may be the cause of e.g. a supranormal capacity for uptake–storage of small amounts of ^{3}H-NA (Häggendal and Dahlström, 1972). If the newly downtransported granules contained the factor of importance for maintaining the nerve terminal membrane, the time course for the degeneration phenomena following axotomy, e.g. NA disappearance, would be expected to be delayed in reserpine treated rats (where an increased amount of granules are transported distally) as compared to normal rats. This was not the case. After close and distal axotomy of the sciatic nerve the NA disappearance in gastrocnemic muscle followed the same course as in normal rats (Fig. 2).

The observations by Hofmann and Thesleff (1972) also support the view that a trophic factor can be separated from transmitter particles. In rat extensor digitorum longus muscles denervation-like changes occurred some days after the injection of colchicine into the nerve. Since impulse conduction and ACh release at nerve stimulation were unaffected, it was concluded that no nerve terminal degeneration had occurred. The colchicine injection had obviously arrested the intraaxonal transport of a "trophic factor" without interfering notably with transmission, indicating that the "trophic factor" was not directly connected with ACH releasing vesicles.

It therefore seems most likely that if NTF has any connection with the transmitter particles, this connection may be the utilization of a common transport mechanism at an approximately similar rate of transport rather than a localization within the same organelle.

ACKNOWLEDGEMENTS

The work has been supported by the Swedish Medical Research Council (grants Nos. 10X-166, 14X-2207, and 04P–4173) and by Wilhelm och Martina Lundgrens's Foundation. Dr. Silvio Bareggi from Istituto di Ricerche Farmacologiche "Mario Negri", Italy, was a trainee at the Department of Pharmacology, University of Göteborg, under the European Program in Brain and Behavior Research.

REFERENCES

ANDÉN, N.-E., HÄGGENDAL, J., MAGNUSSON, T., and ROSENGREN, E. (1964) The time course of the disappearance of noradrenaline and 5-hydroxytryptamine in the spinal cord after transection. *Acta physiol. scand.* **62**, 115–118.

BANKS, P., MANGNALL, D., and MAYOR, D. (1969) The redistribution of cytochrome oxidase, noradrenaline and adenosine triphosphate in adrenergic nerves constricted at two points. *J. Physiol. Lond.* **200**, 745–762.

BAREGGI, S., DAHLSTRÖM, A., and HÄGGENDAL. J. (1974) Intra-axonal transport and degeneration of adrenergic nerve terminals after axotomy with a long or short nerve stump. *Med. Biol.* (in press).

BIRKS, R., KATZ, B., and MILEDI, R. (1960) Physiological and structural changes at the amphibian myoneural junction, in the course of nerve degeneration. *J. Physiol. Lond.* **150**, 145–168.

BRIMIJOIN, S. (1972) Transport and turnover of dopamine-β-hydroxylase in sympathetic nerves of the rat. *J. Neurochem.* **19**, 2183–2193.

CARLSSON, A., FALCK, B., FUXE, K., and HILLARP, N.-Å. (1964) Cellular localization of monoamines in the spinal cord. *Acta physiol. scand.* **60**, 112–119.

DAHLSTRÖM, A. (1965) Observations on the accumulation of noradrenaline in the proximal and distal parts of peripheral adrenergic nerves after compression. *J. Anat. Lond.* **99**, 677–689.

DAHLSTRÖM, A. (1967) The transport of noradrenaline between two simultaneously performed ligations of the sciatic nerves of rat and cat. *Acta physiol. scand.* **69**, 158–166.

DAHLSTRÖM, A. (1968) Effect of colchicine on transport of amine storage granules in sympathetic nerves of rat. *Eur. J. Pharmac.* **5**, 111–113.

DAHLSTRÖM, A. (1970) The effects of drugs on axonal transport of amine storage granules. *Bayer-Symposium II*, Springer-Verlag, pp. 20–36.

DAHLSTRÖM, A. (1971) Effects of vinblastine and colchicine on monoamine containing neurons of the rat, with special regard to the axoplasmic transport of amine granules. *Acta neuropath. Berlin*, Suppl. V, 226–237.

DAHLSTRÖM, A., and FUXE, K. (1965) Evidence for the existence of monoamine-containing neurons in the central nervous system: II, Experimentally induced changes in the intraneuronal amine levels of bulbo-spinal neuron systems. *Acta physiol. scand.* **64**, Suppl. 247, 1–35.

DAHLSTRÖM, A., and HÄGGENDAL, J. (1966) Some quantitative studies on the noradrenaline content in the cell bodies and terminals of a sympathetic adrenergic neuron system. *Acta physiol. scand.* **67**, 271–277.

DAHLSTRÖM, A., and HÄGGENDAL, J. (1969) Recovery of noradrenaline in adrenergic axons of rat sciatic nerves after reserpine treatment. *J. Pharm. Pharmac.* **21**, 633–638.

DAHLSTRÖM, A., and HÄGGENDAL, J. (1970) Transport of life-span of amine storage granules studied by histochemical and biochemical methods. *Acta physiol. scand.*, Suppl. 357, p. 7.

DAHLSTRÖM, A., and HÄGGENDAL, J. (1972) Effect of axotomy on synthesis and transport of amine granules in sympathetic neurons. *Abstract to Fifth Internat. Congr. of Pharmacol.*, p. 50.

DAHLSTRÖM, A., HÄGGENDAL, J., and ATACK, C. (1973a) Localization and transport of serotonin. In *Serotonin and Behaviour* (E. D. Barchas and E. Usdin, eds.), Academic Press, New York, 87–96.

DAHLSTRÖM, A., HÄGGENDAL, J., and LINDER, A. (1973b) Degeneration contraction after local vinblastine treatment of superior cervical ganglia in the rat. *Eur. J. Pharmac.* **21**, 41–45.

DAHLSTRÖM, A., EVANS, C. A. N., HÄGGENDAL, J., HEIWALL, P.-O., and SAUNDERS, N. (1974) Rapid transport of acetylcholine in rat sciatic nerve proximal and distal to a lesion. *J. Neural Transm.* (in press).

EMMELIN, N. (1967) Parotid secretion after cutting the auriculotemporal nerve at different levels. *J. Physiol. Lond.* **188**, 44–45 P.

EMMELIN, N. (1968) Degeneration secretion from parotid glands after section of the auriculotemporal nerves at different levels. *J. Physiol. Lond.* **195**, 407–418.

EMMELIN, E., and TRENDELENBURG, U. (1972) Degeneration activity after parasympathetic or sympathetic denervation. *Rev. Physiol.* **66**, 147–211.

FUXE, K., and SEDVALL, G. (1965) The distribution of adrenergic nerve fibres to the blood vessels in skeletal muscle. *Acta physiol. scand.* **64**, 75–86.

GEFFEN, L. B., and LIVETT, B. G. (1971). Synaptic vesicles in sympathetic neurons. *Physiol. Rev.* **51**, 98–157.

HÄGGENDAL, J., and DAHLSTRÖM, A. (1969) The transport and life-span of amine storage granules in bulbo-spinal noradrenaline neurons of the rat. *J. Pharm. Pharmac.* **21**, 55–57.

HÄGGENDAL, J., and DAHLSTRÖM, A. (1971) The importance of the axoplasmic transport of amine granules for the functions of adrenergic neurons. *Acta neuropath.*, Suppl. V, 238–248.

HÄGGENDAL, J., and DAHLSTRÖM, A. (1972) The recovery of the capacity for uptake-retention of ^{3}H-nor-adrenaline in rat adrenergic nerves after reserpine. *J. Pharm. Pharmac.* **24**, 565–574.

HÄGGENDAL, J., and DAHLSTRÖM, A. (1973) The time course of noradrenaline decrease in rat spinal cord following transection. *Neuropharm.* **12**, 349–354.

HÄGGENDAL, J., SAUNDERS, N., and DAHLSTRÖM, A. (1971) Rapid accumulation of acetylcholine in nerve above a crush. *J. Pharm. Pharmac.* **23**, 552–555.

HÄGGENDAL, J., DAHLSTRÖM, A., and SAUNDERS, N. (1973) Axonal transport and acetylcholine in rat pre-ganglionic neurons. *Brain Res.* **58**, 494–499.

HÄGGENDAL, J., DAHLSTRÖM, A., and LARSSON, P.-A. (1974) Rapid transport of noradrenaline in rat sciatic nerve distal to a crush. *Acta physiol. Scand.* (submitted).

HARRIS, J. B., and THESLEFF, S. (1972) Nerve stump length and membrane changes in denervated skeletal muscle. *Nature, Lond.* **236**, 60–61.

HOFMANN, W. W., and THESLEFF, S. (1972) Studies on the trophic influence of nerve on skeletal muscle. *Eur. J. Pharmac.* **20**, 256–260.

KOIKE, H., EISENSTADT, M., and SCHWARTZ, J. H. (1972) Axonal transport of newly synthesized acetyl-choline in an identified neuron of *Aplysia*. *Brain Res.* **37**, 152–159.

LUNDBERG, D. (1969) Adrenergic-neuron blockers and transmitter release after sympathetic denervation studied in the conscious rat. *Acta physiol. scand.* **75**, 415–426.

LUNDBERG, D. (1972) Effects of colchicine, vinblastine and vincristine on degeneration transmitter release after sympathetic denervation studied in the conscious rat. *Acta physiol. scand.* **85**, 91–98.

MAGNUSSON, T., and ROSENGREN, E. (1963) Catecholamines of the spinal cord, normally and after tran-section. *Experentia* **19**, 229.

MALMFORS, T. (1965) Studies on adrenergic nerves: the use of rat and mouse iris for direct observations on their physiology and pharmacology at cellular and subcellular levels. *Acta physiol. scand.* **64**, Suppl. 248, 1–93.

MALMFORS, T., and SACHS, C. (1965) Direct studies on the disappearance of the transmitter and changes in the uptake-storage mechanisms of degenerating adrenergic nerves. *Acta physiol. scand.* **64**, 211–223.

MILEDI, R., and SLATER, C. R. (1970) On the degeneration of rat neuro-muscular functions after nerve section. *J. Physiol. Lond.* **207**, 507–528.

MOLINOFF, P., BRIMIJOIN, S., WEINSHILBOUM, R., and AXELROD, J. (1970) Neuronally mediated increase in dopamine-β-hydroxylase activity. *Proc. Natn. Acad. Sci. USA* **66**, 453–458.

OCHS, S., and RANISH, N. (1969). Characteristics of the fast transport system in mammalian nerve fibres. *J. Neurobiol.* **2**, 247–261.

SACHS, CH., and JONSSON, G. (1973) Quantitative microfluorimetric and neurochemical studies on degenerating adrenergic nerves. *J. Histochem. Cytochem.* **21**, 902–911.

THOENEN, H., MUELLER, R. A., and AXELROD, J. (1969) Increased tyrosine hydroxylase activity after drug-induced alteration of sympathetic transmission. *Nature* **221**, 1264.

TRANZER, J. P. (1972) A new amine storing compartment in adrenergic neurons. *Nature, New Biol.* **237**, 57–58.

WEISS, P. (1961) The concept of perpetual neuronal growth and proximo-distal substance convection. *Regional Neurochemistry* (S. S. Kety and J. Elkes, eds.), Pergamon, London, pp. 220–242.

WEISS, P. (1963) Self-renewal and proximo-distal convection in nerve fibres. *The Effect of Use and Disuse of Neuromuscular Functions.* (E. Gutmann and P. Hnik, eds.), Elsevier, Amsterdam, pp. 171–183.

WEISS, P., and HISCOE, H. B. (1948) Experiments on the mechanism of nerve growth, *J. Exp. Zool.* **107**, 315–395.

WOOTEN, F., and COYLE, J. (1973) Axonal transport of catecholamine synthesizing and metabolizing enzymes. *J. Neurochem.* **20**, 1361–1371.

INTRA-AXONAL TRANSPORT MECHANISMS IN THE NORADRENERGIC NEURON

P. Banks and D. Mayor

Department of Biochemistry and Department of Human Biology and Anatomy, The University, Sheffield S10 2TN, United Kingdom

THE dense-cored or granular vesicles which store noradrenaline in noradrenergic neurons are synthesized in the cell body and subsequently move proximo-distally along the axon towards the sites of transmitter release (Dahlström, 1971; Banks and Mayor, 1972). While the production of these vesicles is dependent upon the continued synthesis of protein, their movement along the axon is not (Banks *et al.*, 1973a). Furthermore, it has been shown that the movement of dense-cored vesicles does not depend upon continuity of the axon with its cell body but appears to be generated by processes occurring within the axon (Dahlström, 1967; Mayor and Kapeller, 1967; Banks *et al.*, 1969).

In this paper an attempt will be made to suggest avenues of investigation which might tell us more about the mechanisms underlying the movement of dense-cored vesicles. This movement can be conceived either as a consequence of displacement by random Brownian motion or as a vectorial process driven by an input of energy derived from metabolism.

The rate of granule displacement along the axon is reported to be in the range of 2.8 to 0.3 μ/s (Dahlström, 1971). These rates of displacement encompass the root-mean-square displacement suffered by particles of the size of dense-cored vesicles (Shea and Karnovsky, 1966), when suspended in a medium with a viscosity equal to that reported for lobster nerve, namely 0.06 poise (Heilbrünn, 1956). These data indicate that diffusion merits serious consideration as a possible mechanism for the translocation of dense-cored vesicles in non-myelinated axons. However, recent determinations of the viscosity of axoplasm from frog sciatic nerves have given values of about 10^4 poise (Biondi *et al.*, 1972). The root-mean-square displacement of dense-cored vesicles in a medium with that viscosity would be only 3.7 mμ/s. On this basis the observed rate of movement of noradrenaline storage vesicles along the axon is about 100 to 1000 times greater than could be accounted for by displacement resulting from Brownian motion. The recent determinations of the viscosity of axoplasm would thus seem to rule out diffusion as an adequate explanation of vesicle movement, especially as they reject the possibility that axoplasm has any significant time-dependent thixotropic properties (Biondi *et al.*, 1972).

The view that Brownian movement is unable to account for vesicle displacement receives support from experiments in which a segment of nerve is isolated by means of two ligatures *in vivo*. Proximo-distal movement of dense-cored vesicles continues within such an isolated length of nerve trunk and they accumulate proximal to the lower ligature but not distal to the upper one (Dahlström, 1967; Mayor and Kapeller, 1967; Banks *et al.*, 1969). Since diffusion would bring about a uniform distribution of the vesicles within the isolated axonal segments rather than a concentration of vesicles at one point, it alone could not account for the above-mentioned observations. Alternatively, it could be argued that the accumulation of vesicles proximal to the lower ligature might be a result of microelectrophoresis sustained by the flow of injury currents (Friede, 1964). However, this fails to account for the lack of vesicle accumulation distal to the upper ligature where similar injury currents would be expected to exist.

It is, of course, possible that injury to the axon causes changes that allow vesicles to become tightly bound to other cell structures near to the point of damage and that their accumulation reflects diffusion followed by binding. There is no evidence to support this view which fails to explain why similar binding sites are not produced distal to the upper ligature and which neglects the low rate of vesicle diffusion occurring in axoplasm of high viscosity.

Thus it would appear that simple diffusion is not able to account adequately for the translocation of dense-cored vesicles in sympathetic axons. Therefore attention must be focused on the more complicated of the two original hypotheses, namely that vesicle translocation is dependent upon a supply of energy derived from metabolism. If this is the case, it immediately raises questions concerning the molecular mechanisms by which metabolic energy is transduced into mechanical work.

Experiments with colchicine and vinblastine have suggested that the intra-axonal movement of dense-cored vesicles is dependent upon the integrity of the axonal system of microtubules (Dahlström, 1968; Banks *et al.*, 1971a, b). There are many other situations in which the movement of subcellular particles or cell processes depends upon an organized system of microtubules, for example in cilia (Warner and Satir, 1973), mitotic spindles (Wilson, 1969; Hepler *et al.*, 1970) and melanophores (Bickle *et al.*, 1966; Green, 1968).

In cilia each A tubule in the circle of 9 doublet microtubules carries, as arm-like projections, an enzyme called dynein. This is considered to be a mechano-enzyme which, by interacting with the B tubules of the adjacent doublet, may be responsible for generating ciliary movement (Mooseker and Tilney, 1973).

Chromosomes possess a structure, the kinetochore, which is apparently necessary for their attachment to the microtubules of the mitotic spindle prior to their migration during mitosis (Hepler *et al.*, 1970).

In the central axons of the lamprey spinal cord discrete bridges of electron-dense material have been seen connecting presumptive synaptic vesicles to axonal microtubules (Smith, 1971).

These various observations can be used to build an hypothesis concerning the movement of dense-cored vesicles within non-myelinated noradrenergic axons; namely, that vesicles are attached to microtubules via cross-bridges consisting of a mechano-enzyme similar to dynein.

On hydrolysing ATP, the mechano-enzyme undergoes a conformational change such that the vesicle moves relative to the stationary microtubule in a manner analogous to the movement of thin filaments relative to thick ones during the contraction of striped muscle. When, during this type of "cross-bridge" movement, the linkage is broken at one point, it is immediately replaced by a new "cross-bridge" further along the microtubule. This cycle can be repeated with the net result that the vesicle moves along the tubule. In principle it does not matter whether the mechano-enzyme is an appendage of the vesicle or the microtubule, but it is necessary for the microtubule to possess a definite polarity to ensure unidirectional movement of the vesicle.

How then can this working hypothesis be tested?

If the vesicle movement is ATP-dependent, it should be prevented by inhibiting energy supplying pathways; this has indeed been found to be the case (Kirpekar et al., 1973; Banks et al., 1973a). However, as ATP is a widely required metabolite and since the resolving power of such experiments is extremely low, nothing very useful concerning the fundamental mechanism of vesicle translocation within axons can be obtained from this type of approach.

Another approach is to examine the sensitivity of vesicle movement to drugs or treatments known to inhibit certain forms of intracellular motility, especially if they are also believed to interfere with some well-defined intracellular or axonal structure.

Experiments using colchicine and vinblastine fall into this category and their use has led to the intra-axonal microtubules being implicated in the movement of noradrenaline containing dense-cored vesicles (Banks et al., 1971a, b). However, the microtubule hypothesis would be destroyed if a drug or treatment was discovered which dispersed microtubules but did not prevent vesicle movement.

Recently it has been shown that cooling ganglion/sympathetic nerve preparations to 0°C for 4 h causes an almost complete loss of axonal microtubules, but that on rewarming to 37°C the microtubules reappear and vesicle movement proceeds unimpaired (Banks et al., unpublished observations). Thus by using physical means it has not been possible to separate the transport of dense-cored vesicles from the integrity of axonal microtubules.

Certain forms of cell motility, which are sensitive to low concentrations (about 1 μg/ml) of cytochalasin B, are believed to depend upon a system of microfilaments (Wessells et al., 1971). These structures have been implicated in the formation and movement of axonal growth cones in developing neurones in vitro (Yamada et al., 1970). However, even at concentrations of 10 μg/ml, this drug fails to inhibit vesicle movement in noradrenergic nerves and it has no effect on the abundance of microtubules (Banks et al., 1973b). Therefore, axonal transport of the type under consideration does not seem to be related to a cytochalasin sensitive mechanism.

If microtubules or some other fibrous protein system are involved in vesicle transport, further experiments of the type considered above may help to clarify their role in this process. However, it is also necessary to know more about the structural organization of microtubules and other components within the axon before further progress can be made. To obtain this information considerable thought must be given to methods of fixation for electron microscopy that will preserve the protein fibres in their natural arrangement. The effect of temperature on the numbers of microtubules apparent per axon in nerves maintained in vitro has been mentioned previously. From these observations it might be expected that the temperature of fixation would affect the preservation of microtubules. It has recently been shown that fixing samples of normal hypogastric nerves at 0°C in phosphate buffered glutaraldehyde yields only 16.1 $\pm$ 0.3 SEM microtubules per axonal cross-section compared with 36.6 $\pm$ 0.3 SEM when fixation is carried out at 20°C (Banks et al., unpublished observations). The possibility that fixation at higher temperatures, such as 37°C, may permit even better preservation and retention of microtubules and other fibrous structures for more detailed electron-microscopic study is being examined. Further improvements may be obtained by fixation at different values of pH or ionic strength than those currently in use.

As well as improving techniques for electron microscopy, another way to tackle the problem of vesicle movement is to isolate proteins from nerves that might be involved in the generation of the movement and to examine their properties and interactions. Several possibilities immediately spring to mind, such as the isolation and characterization of tubulin (the microtubule subunit) followed by a study of its possible interactions with other axonal proteins and organelles, in particular with dense-cored vesicles. The possibility exists that the axon contains a dynein-like ATP-ase; if so is it able to associate with tubulin or with dense-cored vesicles? Experiments to investigate these possibilities are currently in progress in our laboratory.

Filarin, the protein subunit of neurofilaments, has been isolated from squid axons (Huneeus and Davison, 1970). However, little is known about its properties and functions. An actomyosin-like protein has been isolated from brain (Puszkin *et al.*, 1968) where it has been implicated in the release of neurotransmitters (Berl *et al.*, 1973). A similar protein has recently been found in noradrenergic nerves (Banks, unpublished observations) but its precise location and possible functional role remain to be discovered.

Clearly much remains to be learned about the protein components of axoplasm and the structure of dense-cored vesicles.

There is considerable evidence to suggest that axonal microtubules are labile structures; the speed with which they disappear on cooling and reappear on rewarming illustrates this clearly. Observations of this type invite questions concerning the mechanisms by which the fibrous systems found within axons are assembled. The growth of mitotic spindles from centrioles and the continuity between the basal bodies and microtubules of cilia and flagellae raises the possibility that microtubule assembly within axons occurs by a process of crystal growth emanating from some (centriole-like) structure within the cell body. However, this does not necessarily seem to be the case in mature neurones since, after cooling and re-warming isolated lengths of nerve, microtubules reappear in axons separated from their neuronal cell bodies and centrioles (Banks *et al.*, unpublished observations). Reassembly and alignment with the axonal axis can thus occur locally within the axon.

Little further progress will be made in understanding the mechanisms of vesicle translocation and the cell biology of axoplasm until much more basic information concerning the molecular architecture and dynamics of the axon has been obtained. The easy work has been done. From now on progress will be uphill.

REFERENCES

BANKS, P., and MAYOR, D. (1972) Intra-axonal transport in noradrenergic neurones in the sympathetic nervous system. *Biochem. Soc. Symp.* **36**, 133–149.

BANKS, P., MANGNALL, D., and MAYOR, D. (1969) The redistribution of cytochrome oxidase, noradrenaline and adenosine triphosphate in adrenergic nerves constricted at two points. *J. Physiol.* **200**, 745–762.

BANKS, P., MAYOR, D., MITCHELL, M., and TOMLINSON, D. (1971a) Studies on the translocation of noradrenaline-containing vesicles in post-ganglionic sympathetic neurones *in vitro*: inhibition of movement by colchicine and vinblastine and evidence for the involvement of axonal microtubules. *J. Physiol.* **216**, 625–639.

BANKS, P., MAYOR, D., and TOMLINSON, D. R. (1971b) Further evidence for the involvement of microtubules in the intra-axonal movement of noradrenaline storage vesicles. *J. Physiol.* **219**, 755–761.

BANKS, P., MAYOR, D., and MRAZ, P. (1973a) Metabolic aspects of the synthesis and intra-axonal transport of noradrenaline storage vesicles. *J. Physiol.* **229**, 383–394.

BANKS, P., MAYOR, D., and MRAZ, P. (1973b) Cytochalasin B and the intra-axonal movement of noradrenaline storage vesicles. *Brain Res.* **49**, 417–421.

BERL, S., PUSZKIN, S., and NICKLAS, W. J. (1973) Actomyosinlike protein in brain. *Science* **179**, 441–446.

BICKLE, D., TILNEY, L. G., and PORTER, K. R. (1966) A mechanism for pigment granule migration in the melanophores of *Fundulus heteroclitus. Protoplasma* **61**, 323.

BIONDI, R. J., LEVY, M. J., and WEISS, P. A. (1972) An engineering study of the peristaltic drive of axonal flow. *Proc. Natn. Acad. Sci. USA* **69**, 1732–1736.

DAHLSTRÖM, A. (1967) The transport of noradrenaline between two simultaneously performed ligations of the sciatic nerves of the rat and cat. *Acta physiol. scand.* **69**, 158–166.

DAHLSTRÖM, A. (1968) Effect of colchicine on transport of amine storage granules in sympathetic nerves of rat. *Eur. J. Pharmac.* **5**, 111–113.

DAHLSTRÖM, A. (1971) Axoplasmic transport (with particular reference to adrenergic neurones). *Phil. Trans. R. Soc. Lond.* B, **261**, 325–358.

FRIEDE, R. L. (1964) Electrophoretic production of "reactive" axon swellings *in vitro* and their histochemical properties. *Acta neuropath.* **3**, 217–228.

GREEN, L. (1968) Mechanism of movements of granules in melanocytes of *Fundulus Heteroclitus. Proc. Natn. Acad. Sci. USA* **59**, 1179–1186.

HEILBRÜNN, L. V. (1956) *The Dynamics of Living Protoplasm*, Academic Press, New York.

HEPLER, P. K., McINTOSH, J. P., and CLELAND, S. (1970) Intermicrotubule bridges in mitotic spindle apparatus. *J. Cell Biol.* **45**, 438–444.

HUNEEUS, F. C., and DAVISON, P. F. (1970) Fibrillar proteins from squid axons: I, Neurofilament protein. *J. Molec. Biol.* **52**, 415–428.

KIRPEKAR, S. M., PRATT, J. C., and WAKADE, A. R. (1973) Metabolic and ionic requirements for the intra-axonal transport of noradrenaline in the cat hypogastric nerve. *J. Physiol.* **228**, 173–180.

MAYOR, D., and KAPELLER, K. (1967) Fluorescence microscopy and electron microscopy of adrenergic nerves after constriction at two points. *J.R. Microsc. Soc.* **87**, 277–294.

MOOSEKER, M. S., and TILNEY, L. G. (1973) Isolation and reactivation of the axostyle: Evidence for a dynein-like ATP-ase in the axostyle. *J. Cell Biol.* **56**, 13–26.

PUSZKIN, S., BERL, S., PUSZKIN, E., and CLARKE, D. D. (1968) Actomyosin-like protein isolated from mammalian brain. *Science* **161**, 170–171.

SHEA, S. M., and KARNOVSKY, M. J. (1966) Brownian motion: a theoretical explanation for the movement of vesicles across the endothelium. *Nature* **212**, 353–355.

SMITH, D. S. (1971) On the significance of cross-bridges between microtubules and synaptic vesicles. *Phil. Trans. R. Soc. Lond.* B, **261**, 395–405.

WARNER, F. D., and SATIR, P. (1973) The substructure of ciliary microtubules. *J. Cell Sci.* **12**, 313–326.

WESSELS, N., SPOONER, B. S., ASH, J. F., BRADLEY, M. O., LUDNENA, M. A., TAYLOR, E. L., WRENN, J. J., and YAMADA, K. M. (1971) Microfilaments in cellular and developmental processes. *Science* **171**, 135–143.

WILSON, H. J. (1969) Arms and bridges on microtubules in the mitotic apparatus. *J. Cell Biol.* **40**, 854–589.

YAMADA, K. M., SPOONER, B. S., and WESSELS N. K. (1970) Axonal growth; roles of microfilaments and microtubules. *Proc. Natn. Acad. Sci. USA* **66**, 1206.

PROXIMODISTAL TRANSPORT OF ACETYLCHOLINE IN PERIPHERAL CHOLINERGIC NEURONS

A. Dahlström, J. Häggendal, E. Heilbronn, P.-O. Heiwall, and N. R. Saunders

Departments of Neurobiology and Pharmacology, University of Göteborg, Fack, S-400 33 Göteborg, Sweden, Research Institute of the National Defence, Dept I, 17204 Sundbyberg, Sweden, and Department of Physiology, University College London, Gower Street, London WC1, England

SUMMARY

The intra-axonal transport of acetylcholine (ACh) and choline acetyltransferase (ChAc) in peripheral cholinergic neurons has been studied during the past 3 years. A brief review of the results is given.

In both motor nerves (the rat sciatic nerve) and a preganglionic sympathetic nerve (the preganglionic cervical trunk) ACh accumulated on the proximal side of a crush or cut. Some local synthesis of ACh due to the axonal trauma also occurred. In rat sciatic nerve ChAc accumulated above the crush much more slowly than ACh. In nerve distal to the axotomy a decrease of ACh, but not of ChAc, was observed. This decrease indicates that a proximo-distal transport of a certain fraction of the axonal ACh continues in distal segments, and thus that the transport mechanism is localized within the axon. The decrease in the distal parts of short-term crushed nerves gave information about the fraction of ACh which is rapidly transportable in the axons. In rat sciatic and preganglionic nerves this fraction was 20–25% and 5% respectively of the total ACh content. Since the accumulation characteristics of ChAc were very different from those of ACh, it is possible that the rapid increase of ACh above a crush was due to a rapid proximo-distal transport of ACh and not merely to accumulation of the synthesizing enzyme. When local crush-induced synthesis and transportable fractions were taken into account, the rate of transport of ACh appeared to be 4–5 mm/h in rat sciatic nerve and 4 mm/h in rat preganglionic nerve. ChAc appeared in rat sciatic nerve to move distally at a slow rate, but it cannot be excluded that a small fraction moves rapidly.

Subcellular fractionation studies may indicate that accumulated ACh is bound to a particle which is denser than "synaptic vesicles." Since large dense core vesicles have been observed in myelinated and preganglionic fibres proximal to a crush, it is suggested that these particles may possibly constitute the transport organelle for ACh.

INTRODUCTION

The axons of cholinergic neurons contain acetylcholine (ACh). But the significance of its presence there is not clear, in contrast to its well-known and much studied involvement in impulse transmission at axon terminals (Katz, 1966). The hypothesis of Nachmansohn (1959) that ACh is involved in impulse transmission in the axon appears untenable on the basis of evidence so far advanced (Hebb, 1963). Another explanation for the presence of ACh in axons is that some or all of the components of the ACh-synthesizing system are formed in the perikaryon and are transported to the terminals within the axon. This idea was put forward by Feldberg and Vogt (1948) in agreement with the hypothesis of axonal flow (Weiss and Hiscoe, 1948). Some support for it came from studies of Hebb and Waites (1956) on redistribution of choline acetyltransferase (ChAc) in transected nerves. However, the time periods studied were rather long, and it is difficult to know how much of the changes were due to interruption of axonal transport and how much were due to early regeneration phenomena. Until recently the problem has not been studied very much. In contrast, there have been many investigations of adrenergic neurons; these have led to the hypothesis that noradrenaline (NA) storage particles are formed in the perikaryon and are transported distally to the nerve terminals at a rate of several millimeters per hour, thus suggesting an explanation for the presence of transmitter (NA) in the axons as well as in their terminals (Dahlström and Häggendal, 1966, 1970; Banks et al., 1969). The functional significance of this transport has been suggested to be the supply of storage-release organelles to the nerve terminals rather than of transmitter itself (Dahlström and Häggendal, 1966; Geffen and Rush, 1968; Häggendal and Dahlström, 1971).

Investigations similar to those on adrenergic neurons are now being carried out on cholinergic neurons. This brief review is a summary of the findings so far. The main experimental approach has been to investigate the redistribution of ACh and ChAc in peripheral nerves at various times after axotomy (Häggendal et al., 1971, 1973; Dahlström et al., 1974; Heiwall et al., 1974; Saunders et al., 1973). If axonal transport continues in axons subjected to a localized lesion, then substances which are transported would be expected to accumulate proximal to the lesion and decline distal to it. On the other hand, any local effect would be expected to produce a similar change on both sides of the lesion. The subcellular distribution of ACh and ChAc in normal and crushed nerves is also being investigated by subcellular fractionation (Heilbronn et al., 1974). Also, some effects on axonal transport of ACh and ChAc of drugs which interfere with microtubules, (vinblastin VIN and colchicine COL) are being investigated in an attempt to study the mechanism of transport of these substances.

METHODS

Rats were used in most experiments (Sprague–Dawley, 180–250 g, males). For subcellular fractionation studies, cats were used because larger amounts of material could be obtained per animal. The sciatic nerve was exposed under ether (rats) or nembutal (cats) anesthesia and crushed with a fine silk thread (Lubińska, 1959). In some rats the nerve, instead of being crushed, was cut or ligated with a silk thread which was left around the nerve. All operations were bilateral. In some cases two crushes were made 15 mm apart. At different times after operation the rats were made unconscious with a blow on the head, the nerves rapidly dissected out, put on ice-cooled glass plates, and divided into 5 mm lengths (Figs. 1 and 4), and put immediately into ice-cooled 10% trichloroacetic acid (TCA). Two to eight pieces were pooled for each determination. Uncrushed nerves, or nerves crushed just prior to dissection (0 h crush), were used as controls. The cervical preganglionic nerves of rats were exposed under an operation microscope and cut with scissors either close to the ganglion or at a distance of 10–14 mm, just above the clavicle. Six to forty-eight hours later the rats were reanesthetized with ether, the nerve parts removed, placed on an ice-cooled plate, and cut into 3–4 mm segments. Eight to twenty-four segments were usually pooled for each determination and homogenized in cold TCA. Zero hour cut nerves were used as controls.

Assay of ACh. The ACh was extracted from the nerves according to MacIntosh and Perry (1950) and assayed on a guinea-pig ileum preparation (Blaber and Cuthbert, 1961) using Schild's (1942) four-point assay technique. An antihistamine (Mepyramine®) was added to the Krebs solution used. The activity in the samples was identified as ACh by inactivation with purified AChE and by either complete or parallel inhibition by atropine of the response of the gut to standard and sample. The activity measured was thus ACh-like, but will be referred to as ACh.

Injection of VIN and COL. The sciatic nerves of rats were injected with 5 μl of COL (10^{-2}, 10^{-1} M) or VIN (10^{-4}–10^{-2}) dissolved in saline. Two hours later the sciatic nerves were crushed as described above about 15 mm distal to the site of injection. After a further 6 h the sciatic nerves were removed, divided as shown in Fig. 6, and extracted for ACh. In some experiments VIN or COL was injected into the lumbar region of the spinal cord (4 $\times$ 5 μl; see Fig. 7) 6 h before crushing the sciatic nerves. Twelve hours later the 5 mm part of nerve above the crush was removed and extracted for ACh.

Subcellular fractionation studies. Fifteen to eighteen hours after operation the cats were reanesthetized with nembutal and 1 cm just above the crush was dissected out and kept cold. In some experiments the nerves were initially dropped into liquid nitrogen. Ten to fourteen nerves were pooled together and gently homogenized in an ultraturrax, followed by homogenization in a teflon–teflon homogenizer in isotonic sucrose (12 strokes up and down, 840 r.p.m., recooling after 6 strokes), with or without eserine (conc. 3 $\times$ 10^{-5} M). The homogenate was then diluted 1:1 with isotonic sucrose and centrifuged at 9500 g for 30 min in an SS 34 head. The supernatant was carefully layered on discontinuous sucrose gradients (0.6–1.8 M sucrose) and centrifuged in an SW 25:2 ultracentrifuge head at 170,000 g for 2 h. The fractions obtained were separated and analyzed for ACh content and enzyme activities (AChE, ChAc, lactate-dehydrogenase, acid phosphatase, glucose-6-phosphatase, thiamine-pyrophosphatase, cytochrome-oxidase, and dopamine-β-hydroxylase). After spinning down pellets at 39,000 r.p.m., 1 h (SW 41 T:), electron microscopy was carried out on the pellets (Heilbronn *et al.*, 1974).

RESULTS AND DISCUSSION

I. CRUSH EXPERIMENTS

1. *Sciatic Nerves*

The distribution of ACh in cat sciatic nerves at different times after crushing has been investigated by Häggendal *et al.* (1971) and Dahlström *et al.* (1974). The main changes (Fig. 1) were (1) with increasing time after crushing the nerve there was a progressive accumulation of ACh in part A, just proximal to the crush (Fig. 2), (2) a smaller accumulation of ACh was observed in part B just distal to the crush, and (3) in the nerve segments distal to part B (segments D–F) there was a fall below control of 16 % (at 6 h) and 21 % (at 12 h).

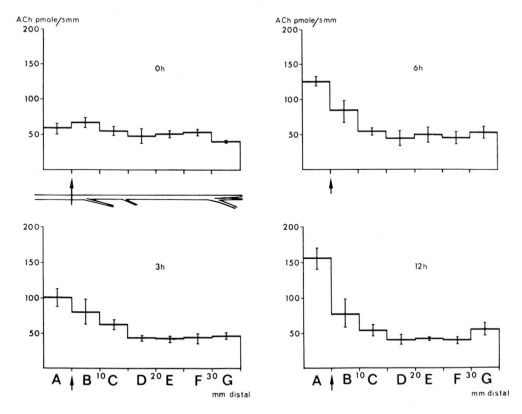

FIG. 1. The ACh content (pmol/5 mm segment) of rat sciatic nerve up to 12 h after crushing. Mean ± SEM are indicated in 5 mm segments of nerve from a level just above the foramen infrapiriformis and distally. The arrows indicate the site of the crush performed 0, 3, 6, or 12 h before dissection. (From Dahlström et al., 1974.)

The cause of the accumulation of ACh proximal to the crush could be (a) local synthesis induced by the crush procedure, (b) increased local synthesis of ACh due to an accumulation of ChAc or precursors of ACh proximal to the crush, (c) the proximo-distal transport and accumulation of ACh itself, or a combination of these. Now local synthesis induced by the crush procedure would be expected to affect both part A and B to a similar extent. This was the case immediately after axotomy and up to 3 h afterwards. However, this symmetrical increase was only about 60% more than control and by 6 h after crushing the accumulations on either side of the crush were markedly asymmetrical; by 12 h piece A contained nearly 3× control, whereas no further increase was seen in part B. It is known that injury to a cholinergic nerve may stimulate local synthesis of ACh (Feldberg, 1943; Evans and Saunders, 1967). This could account for the initial rise in ACh on both sides of the crush and would be expected to affect both sides equally. Dahlström et al. (1974) have used the increase in B as a maximum estimate of the rise in ACh due to local synthesis. When this amount was subtracted from the content of the A piece the net increase in part A followed a straight line with time (Fig. 2, II) up to 12 h after crushing.

Of the ACh precursors choline is probably present in nervous tissues in excess (cf. Ansell and Spanner, 1970). Acetyl-Co-A appears to be produced by mitochondria (Tuček,

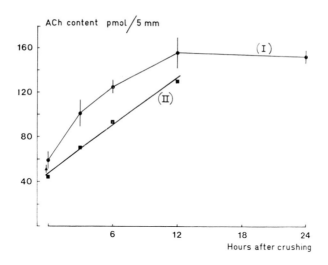

FIG. 2. The increase in ACh in rat sciatic nerve in the 5 mm segment just above a crush at different times after operation I. Curve II was obtained when correction for local crush-induced ACh synthesis was performed (for explanation see text). (From Dahlström *et al.*, 1974.)

1970) which seem to be transported at too slow a rate (6–14 mm/day; Banks *et al.*, 1969; Karlsson and Sjöstrand, 1971) to account for the rapid accumulation of ACh. The amount of accumulation of ChAc proximal to a crush in sciatic nerves has been found (Saunders *et al.*, 1973) to be much smaller than that of ACh (cf. Figs. 2 and 3A). At first sight this might appear to indicate that the ChAc accumulation could not account for the ACh accumulation. However, the kinetic factors which set the level of ACh in an axon are unknown, and it is possible that even a small increase in ChAc could result in a large increase in ACh concentration. Calculation of the rate of transport for ACh and ChAc is another way of considering the possible relation between the two.

When attempting to calculate a rate of transport it is necessary to have information about (1) the normal content of the transported material in the nerve, (2) the net accumulation of the material not due to crush induced local synthesis (in the case of ACh), and (3) the fraction of the material which is transported at a rate faster than the bulk flow of axoplasm. Information about the transportable fraction can be obtained by studying the level of the transported material in the distal segments of the nerve after crushing.

(a) *Rate of transport of ACh.* Information on points 1 and 2 can be obtained from Figs. 1 and 2. Information about the transportable fraction can be obtained by studying the ACh content in distal segments of the nerve soon after crushing. It has been shown that fast transport of material in axons is not interrupted by axotomy, but continues in a proximo-distal direction in the nerve distal to the crush (cf. Ochs and Ranish, 1969). If part of the ACh were transportable at a fast rate, this fraction would be expected to have moved from distal segments D–F into segments further distally by 3–6 h after crushing. The remaining fraction would thus be stationary or transported at a very slow rate. From Fig. 1 it can be seen that there is a significant fall in ACh content in segments D–F at 6 and 12 h after crushing which amounts to 16 and 21 % respectively. In a separate experiment where 15 mm of nerve distal to a 6 h crush (corresponding to segments C–E) was compared to normal nerve the fall was 25% ($p < 0.025$) (Dahlström *et al.*, 1974). The rapidly transportable

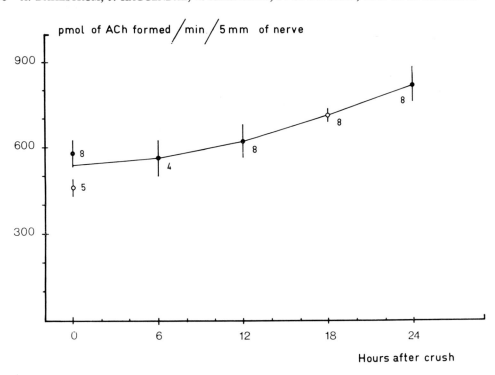

FIG. 3A. Accumulation of ChAc activity in the 5 mm above a crush in rat sciatic nerve at different times after crushing. Mean values $\pm$ SEM are shown. Numbers indicate the number of observations. The line drawn joins the mean values. At 0 h a weighed mean has been calculated taking into account the different n values for two control series. (From Saunders *et al.*, 1973.)

fraction of ACh in rat sciatic nerve would thus amount to 20–25%, the rest being stationary or transported slowly. When performing such experiments to estimate the transportable fraction of ACh it is of course necessary that the postoperative time chosen is as short as possible, and certainly less than the time when degenerative changes begin to occur.

Based on this knowledge, the rate of transport of the transportable fraction of ACh in rat sciatic nerve can be calculated: the normal content of 5 mm nerve was 46 ± 1.9 pmol ($n = 47$); the total rise in a 5 mm piece just above a 6 h crush was 130% above normal or, when correction for local synthesis had been made, about 120% above control; the transportable fraction was 20–25% of total. This means that the transportable fraction in 24 mm $\left(\dfrac{1.2 \times 5 \text{ mm}}{25\%}\right)$ to 30 mm $\left(\dfrac{1.2 \times 5 \text{ mm}}{20\%}\right)$ of nerve was moved into the A piece in 6 h, indicat-

ing a rate of transport of 4–5 mm/h. This estimate may be regarded as a minimum figure; in the 5 mm segment central to piece A a rise of about 65% above control was observed at 6 h in some experiments. This indicates that the transport rate may be somewhat faster than 4–5 mm/hr.

(b) *Rates of transport of ChAc.* Saunders *et al.* (1973) found no detectable decline in ChAc activity distal to a single lesion and no redistribution in ChAc activity between two crushes (Fig. 3B). This was in contrast to ACh for which there was a decline of 20–25%

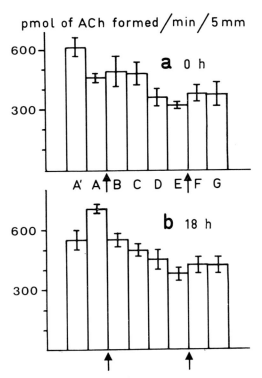

FIG. 3B. Distribution of ChAc activity in rat sciatic nerves which were crushed twice simulta-neously (double-crushed nerves). Arrows indicate the positions of the crushes. Means ± SEM are shown. $n = 4$–5 at 0 h and 7–8 at 18 h. (From Saunders *et al.*, 1973.)

distal to a lesion (see above) and a marked redistribution between crushes (Fig. 4, B, from Häggendal *et al.*, 1971). Because of these differences it was suggested that all of the ChAc moved at the same slow rate and that on this basis the transport of ChAc and ACh was separated. However, as was pointed out by Saunders *et al.* (1973), these experiments do not exclude the possibility that a very small fraction of the ChAc could be moving rapidly. The accumulation of ChAc in Fig. 3A could be accounted for by rapid transport of 5% of the total ChAc at a rate of about 3 mm/h. If the transportable fraction was really as small as this, neither a decline in ChAc distal to a single crush nor a redistribution between two crushes 20 mm apart (Fig. 3B) would have been detectable. The problem can be resolved by repeating the experiments in longer nerves and placing the crushes further apart. Fonnum (1970) has presented evidence that ChAc is present in axoplasm as a soluble enzyme. But his experiments would not exclude the possibility that a very small fraction of the ChAc activity is particle bound. Thus at present it remains uncertain whether or not the rate of transport of ChAc and ACh are different. Even if they are similar, because of the difference in size of the transportable fraction for ACh and for ChAc as estimated above, it will still not be clear if the ACh accumulation is independent of the smaller accumulation of ChAc until experiments using ChAc inhibition are performed. As will be discussed below, a rapid rate of intra-axonal transport probably means that the transported material is associated with some subcellular particle. If the rates of transport of the transportable fraction of ACh and ChAc are in fact similar, it may well be that the same transport particle is involved for both.

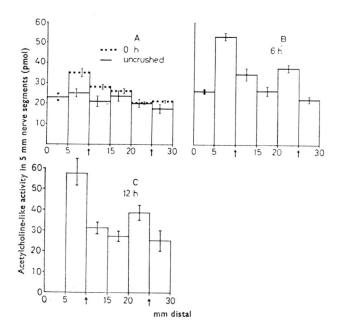

FIG. 4. The amount of ACh in 5 mm nerve segments of rat sciatic nerves which were crushed at two points simultaneously (double-crushed nerves). Means ± SEM are given. $n = 4–6$. Where $n = 2$ the individual values are given. The ordinate shows the amount of ACh in pmol per 5 mm segments (uncorrected for losses). The abscissa indicates the distance along the nerve from the highest level 8–9 mm above foramen infrapiriformis. The arrows show the sites of nerve crush made 0, 6, or 12 h before dissection. In A the solid lines are uncrushed nerves. In A–C the total amount of ACh between the crushes is: A, 0 h crush 73.1; uncrushed 63.2; B, 98.0; C, 96.1 pmol. (From Häggendal *et al.*, 1971.)

2. *Cervical preganglionic nerve*

On the proximal side of the cut (part A, Fig. 5) the ACh content increased to 40 % above normal in 12 h. Some rise was also observed in the 4 mm further proximal to A (Fig. 5, from Häggendal *et al.*, 1973). Distal to the cut a progressive decrease was seen in part B as well as further distally. This is in contrast to the rise in B seen in the crushed sciatic nerve experiments (see above). However, in experiments in which the sciatic nerves were cut rather than crushed, Dahlström *et al.* (1974) found that there was also no increase in ACh content in part B. This difference from the crushed nerves might have been due to some loss of axoplasm from the cut ends of the nerves; or it may be that there is less local synthesis in the nerves which are cut rather than crushed. We do not yet have any measurements of ChAc in cervical preganglionic nerve, but a rate of transport of ACh itself which could account for the experimental findings can be calculated from the rise in ACh proximal to the cut and from an estimate of the transportable fraction of ACh.

In order to estimate the transportable fraction of ACh in this nerve, four consecutive segments of 3 mm each were taken between the cut and the ganglion and were assayed for ACh 6 h after axotomy; they were compared to the ACh content of control nerves. A decrease in ACh content of 5 % was observed in the 6 h cut nerves (p < 0.01). If the transportable fraction of ACh is as small as 5 %, which is indicated by these experiments, then

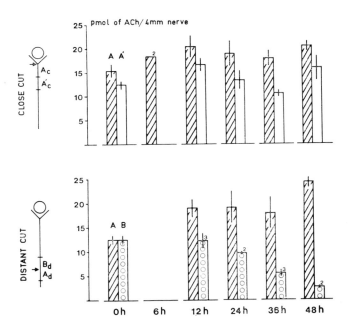

FIG. 5. The ACh content in different 4 mm sections of the cervical preganglionic nerve at different times after cutting either close to the ganglion or at a distance of 10–14 mm. Upper = the ACh content in parts A and A' at different times after cutting close to the ganglion. Lower = the ACh content in parts A and B after a distant cut. Mean ± SEM is indicated. $n = 4$ except where indicated. (From Häggendal et al., 1973.)

the rate of transport of ACh or ACh storage factor would be approximately 4 mm/h, i.e. similar to that in the sciatic nerve (see Section I, 1).

The low values for the transportable fraction of ACh (20–25% in sciatic nerve and 5% in preganglionic nerve) are consistent with observations suggesting that most axonal ACh is free in the axoplasm (Carlini and Green, 1963; Evans and Saunders, 1974) and would therefore not be expected to move rapidly.

II. MECHANISM OF TRANSPORT

If the early decrease in ACh content in the more distal parts of the nerve is due to continued transport of ACh, it means that axonal transport of ACh is independent of continuity with the nerve cell body. This is also suggested by the redistribution of ACh which occurs in double-crushed nerves (Häggendal et al., 1971). In these nerves there was an accumulation of ACh above both a proximal and a distal lesion.

Several drugs, including some local anesthetics and the mitotic inhibitors COL and VIN, disrupt microtubules and appear to have effects upon transport of various materials in different types of axons (Edström and Mattson, 1972), e.g. NA in adrenergic nerves (Dahlström, 1968, 1971; Banks et al., 1971). It has therefore been suggested that microtubules are involved in the mechanism of rapid transport. However, the reported effects of these drugs seem to be quite numerous and variable; it may be that they depend upon the dose and preparation used. Some of the effects do not seem likely to be directly related to disruption of microtubules. For example, high concentrations of VIN (10^{-2} M) injected sub-

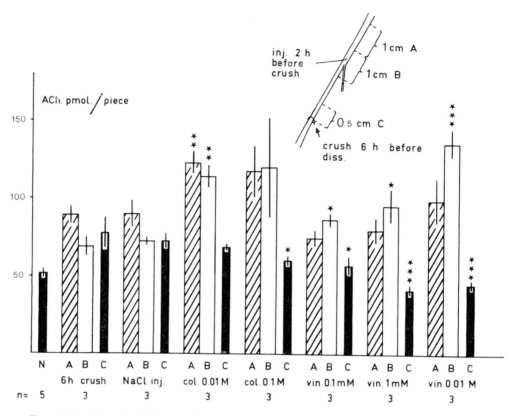

FIG. 6. The effect of colchicine and vinblastine on ACh-transport in rat sciatic nerve. Mean ± SEM are given. *n* indicates number of observations. The ordinate shows the amount of ACh in pmol per 5 or 100 mm piece of nerve after different treatments which are indicated along the abscissa. The injections to the upper right of the figure 2 h before a low crush was made. The stars indicate levels of significance in differences against control nerves, injected with saline or only crushed 6 h prior to dissection.

epineurally (5 µl) produced rapid block of axonal conduction in rat sciatic nerve (Dahlström *et al.*, unpublished observations), while the same concentration when soaked on the efferent part of the cervical superior ganglion did not notably affect impulse conduction for several hours after VIN application (Dahlström. 1971; Dahlström *et al.*, 1973). Also Byers *et al.* (1973) have found that the local anesthetic lidocaine can have effects upon rapid axonal transport of labeled protein at concentrations which are without apparent effects upon the morphology of microtubules. Thus in attempting to use drugs as a tool for investigating possible mechanisms for axonal transport, it is important to study a range of possible effects of these drugs at different dose levels.

A start has been made in cholinergic neurons to investigate the effects of COL and VIN on transport of ACh and ChAc, on impulse conduction, and upon axonal morphology. Some of the preliminary results are presented here.

COL and VIN injected either under the epineurium of the nerve (application to the axons) or injected into the lumbar part of the spinal cord (application to the cell bodies) have been found to depress the accumulation of ACh above a crush (Figs. 6 and 7). In the nerve experiments 5 µl of saline (control), COL (10^{-2}, 10^{-1} M) or VIN (10^{-4}–10^{-2} M)

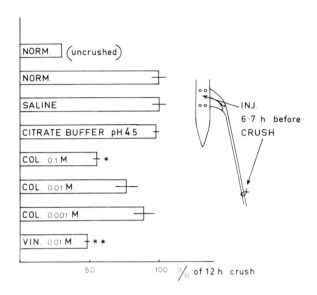

FIG. 7. The effect of colchicine and vinblastine injections into the lumbar part of the rat spinal cord on the accumulation of ACh in the sciatic nerve above bilateral 12 h crushes. Mean ± SEM are indicated. $n = 3–5$. Four injections of 5 μl each were made as indicated in the figure to the right (o) 6–7 h before crushing the nerve. Five millimeters of the nerves just above the crush were dissected out 12 h after the crush operation. The top bar shows the ACh content in 5 mm of normal, uncrushed nerve. ACh is expressed in percent of the amounts in 12 h crushed nerves of normal rats.

dissolved in saline, was injected carefully subepineurally into the nerve at its central end (Fig. 6). Two hours later a crush was made 15–20 mm distal to the site of injection 6 h before killing the animal. The segments above the injection (A), around the site of injection (B), and just above the crush (C), were extracted and assayed for ACh. These results are shown in Fig. 6. In the area of injection (B) and above it (A), COL and VIN caused an increase in ACh, which was not due to the injection trauma *per se* since saline-injected nerves did not produce any increase. The increase in ACh was proportional to the concentration of the mitotic inhibitor used (Fig. 6). Above the crush (part C) there was an inverse relationship between concentration of the test substance and the accumulation of ACh. In saline-injected nerves a usual amount of ACh accumulated in part C (Fig. 6). The results suggest that VIN and COL block the proximo-distal transport of ACh, in a dose-dependent manner. The increase in parts A and B following COL or VIN may be due to accumulation of ACh which was arrested by the injection. It could also be due to an altered reaction of the guinea-pig ileum used in the ACh estimation caused by VIN or COL remaining in the nerve samples. However, VIN or COL when added to ACh containing samples did not affect the contractions of the gut to ACh. Another possibility is that the test substances caused a pronounced local synthesis of ACh; this is difficult to test at present since no good inhibitors of ACh synthesis are available. The decreased accumulation in part C is likely to be due to an inhibition of ACh transport through the injected segment to the part above the crush. It is interesting to observe that the C segments of the nerves injected with the two highest concentrations of VIN are about 15% lower than the content of a normal, uncrushed 5 mm segment. This fraction may well correspond to the transportable fraction of ACh which at the time of crushing could have already passed into more distal parts of the nerve (Fig. 6).

When VIN or COL was injected into the lumbar part of the spinal cord 5–6 h before the sciatic nerves were crushed, a marked decrease in ACh accumulation above the crush was observed (Fig. 7). Injections of saline or citrate buffer (pH 4.5, which is the pH of the highest concentration of VIN used) did not cause any detectable decrease in ACh accumulation as compared to un-injected rats with 12 h crushes (Fig. 7). This indicates that if these test substances are applied close to the cell bodies of motor neurons, an inhibitory effect on ACh transport and accumulation may also occur. (For further details on the VIN–COL experiments, see Heiwall *et al.*, 1974.)

Previous investigators have reported that COL interrupts transport of AChE in rat sciatic nerves (Kreutzberg, 1969) and both AChE and ChAc in rabbit vagus and hypoglossal nerves (Sjöstrand *et al.*, 1971). Our own experiments are incomplete, but did show that VIN (10^{-4}–10^{-2} M) and COL (10^{-2} M) blocked accumulation of ChAc in rat sciatic nerves. As already mentioned, high concentrations of VIN (10^{-2} M) when injected into the sciatic nerve (5 μl) block axonal impulse conduction, possibly by disruption of axonal membrane proteins (cf. Wilson *et al.*, 1970). Lower concentrations (10^{-3} M) produce impulse conduction block only after 18–20 h when degenerative changes could also be seen histologically (Dahlström *et al.*, unpublished). Still lower concentrations (10^{-4}–10^{-5} M) were without effect on impulse conduction, but did block both ACh and ChAc accumulation, thus suggesting a more selective effect at lower concentrations. These results with mitotic inhibitors suggest that microtubules may be involved in the proximo-distal transport of various materials in cholinergic axons, but further work is needed to elucidate the mechanism of transport.

III. TRANSPORT COMPARTMENT FOR ACETYLCHOLINE

Our experiments show that materials important for the ACh transmitter system are transported rapidly in cholinergic neurons. It is not yet quite certain that the material transported is ACh itself, or the enzyme ChAc or both of these, as discussed above. However, whatever it is, the question arises as to the subaxonal compartment in which this transport occurs. Rapid transport is generally thought to involve organelles such as vesicles or tubular structures (e.g. ER), whereas substances located freely in the axoplasm are considered to be transported with the slow phase (1–2 mm/day) of axonal flow (see discussion in Skrangiel-Kramska *et al.*, 1969). Therefore it is likely that the transportable fraction of ACh (and ChAc?) is situated in some particulate compartment. In nerve terminals ACh is considered to be stored in synaptic vesicles (e.g. Whittaker, 1969). However, synaptic vesicles have rarely been seen in axons, and usually only in association with axon damage (e.g. Wettstein and Sotelo, 1963). The fractionation studies on cat crushed sciatic nerves which have been carried out (Heilbronn *et al.*, 1974) have demonstrated that a considerable part of the accumulated ACh in this nerve was sedimentable (Fig. 8) and equilibrated in the interphase between 1.2 and 1.4 M sucrose. This indicates a density which is larger than that of the typical synaptic vesicles of 400 Å (e.g. Whittaker, 1969). So far this denser ACh particle has not been identified electronmicroscopically, and it can therefore not yet be excluded that this sedimentable ACh is due to some artefact induced by the homogenization.

The paucity of clear 400 Å synaptic vesicles in normal cholinergic axons and the observation of the comparatively dense ACh particles present in crushed sciatic nerves of the cat might indicate that the transport organelle for ACh is not identical with the synaptic vesicle of 400 Å. Recent electron microscopical observatipns have demonstrated the accumulation in

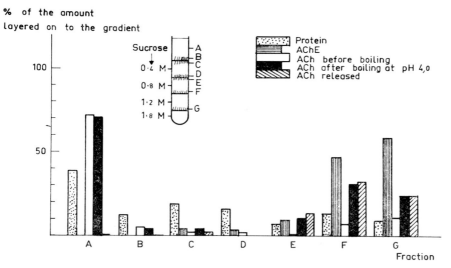

Fig. 8. Total amounts of protein, acetylcholinesterase (AChE), and free and "bound" ACh, found in subcellular fractions from 1 cm pieces of the proximal part of crushed (18 h) sciatic nerves from the cat. The part nearest to the crush was taken from altogether 8 nerves (2 from each of 4 cats).

crushed cholinergic preganglionic nerves of large dense core vesicles in glutaraldehyde-OsO_4-fixed material. These accumulations were observed proximal to the crush but not distal to it (Woog and Bennett, 1972). Similar accumulations of dense core vesicles (> 700 Å in diameter) have been seen also in myelinated nerves of rat sciatic nerve (Woog and Bennett, 1972; Liebermann et al., 1974; Mayor, personal commun.) Large dense core vesicles are usually connected with adrenergic axons but are also present in adrenergic nerve terminals together with the typical small dense core vesicles (seen preferentially in $KMnO_4$-fixed material, e.g. Hökfelt, 1969). The presence of a dense core in glutaraldehyde-OsO_4-fixed material does not necessarily represent a catecholamine but may indicate the presence of a matrix protein in the organelles (cf. Bloom and Aghajanian, 1968). In cholinergic axons such large dense core vesicles have been observed during regeneration (Lentz, 1967; Pellegrino de Iraldi and de Robertis, 1968). In motor terminals they have been observed both in normal (Miledi and Slater, 1970) and in regenerated endplates (Lüllmann-Rauch, 1971), and their significance has been suggested to be related to some trophic nerve influence.

In adrenergic neurons the typical small dense core vesicles appear to be present mainly in nerve terminals, whereas the large vesicles are more frequent in axons, particularly on the proximal side of a crush (e.g. Geffen and Ostberg, 1969). An increasing amount of evidence indicates that the large dense core vesicles in adrenergic neurons represent (a) the transport organelle for NA, supplying the nerve terminals with the essential storage-release granules, and (b) the precursor of the typical small dense core vesicles (for reviews see Geffen and Livett, 1971; Häggendal and Dahlström, 1971; Smith, 1971). The large NA-containing dense core vesicle in adrenergic neurons may thus be considered as a young, or early, type of NA storage particle (e.g. Dahlström and Häggendal, 1972). It may be that the large dense core vesicles in crushed cholinergic nerves are the transport organelle for ACh and a precursor of the small clear synaptic vesicles of cholinergic nerve terminals.

ACKNOWLEDGEMENTS

This work was supported by the Swedish Medical Research Council (grants Nos. 14X-2207, 14X-166, and 04P-4173), by Wilhelm and Martina Lundgren's Foundation, and by the Wellcome Trust, London.

REFERENCES

ANSELL, G. B., and SPANNER, S. (1970) The origin and turn-over of choline in the brain. In *Drugs and Cholinergic Mechanisms in the CNS*. (E. Heilbronn and A. Winter, eds.), Almqvist & Wiksell, Stockholm, pp. 143–159.

BANKS, P., MANGNALL, D., and MAYOR, D. (1969) The redistribution of cytochrome oxidase, noradrenaline and adenosine triphosphate in adrenergic nerves constricted at two points. *J. Physiol.* **200**, 745–762.

BANKS, P., MAYOR, D., MITCHELL, M., and TOMLINSON, D. (1971) Studies on the translocation of noradrenaline-containing vesicles in post-ganglionic sympathetic neurones *in vitro*: inhibition of movement by colchicine and vinblastine and evidence for the involvement of axonal microtubules. *J. Physiol.* **216**, 625–639.

BLABER, L. C., and CUTHBERT, A. W. (1961) A sensitive method for the assay of acetylcholine. *J. Pharm. Pharmac.* **13**, 445–446.

BLOOM, F. E., and AGHAJANIAN, G. K. (1968) An electron microscopic analysis of large granular synaptic vesicles of the brain in relation to monoamine content. *J. Pharmac. Exp. Ther.* **159**, 261–273.

BYERS, M. R., FINK, B. R., KENNEDY, R. D., MIDDAUGH, M. E., and HENDRICKSON, A. E. (1973) Effects of Lidocaine on axonal morphology, microtubules and rapid transport in rabbit vagus nerve *in vitro*. *J. Neurobiol.* **4**, 125–143.

CARLINI, E. A., and GREEN, J. P. (1963) Acetylcholine activity in the sciatic nerve. *Biochem. Pharmac.* **12**, 1367–1376.

DAHLSTRÖM, A. (1968) Effect of colchicine on transport of amine storage granules in sympathetic nerves of rat. *Eur. J. Pharmac.* **5**, 111–113.

DAHLSTRÖM, A. (1971) Effects of vinblastine and colchicine on monoamine-containing neurons of the rat, with special regard to the axoplasmic transport of amine granules. *Acta neuropath. Berlin*, Suppl. V, 226–237.

DAHLSTRÖM, A., and HÄGGENDAL, J. (1966) Studies on the transport and life-span of amine storage granules in a peripheral adrenergic neuron system. *Acta physiol. scand.* **67**, 278–288.

DAHLSTRÖM, A., and HÄGGENDAL, J. (1970) Axonal transport of amine storage granules in sympathetic adrenergic neurons. In: *Biochemistry of Simple Neuronal Models* (E. Costa and C. Giacobini, eds.), *Adv. Biochem. Psychopharmacol.* **2**, 65–93.

DAHLSTRÖM, A., and HÄGGENDAL, J. (1972) On the possible relation between different pools of adrenergic transmitter and heterogeneity or amine storage granules in nerve terminals. *Acta physiol. Pol.* XXIII, Suppl. 4, 67–69.

DAHLSTRÖM, A., HÄGGENDAL, J., and LINDER, A. (1973) Degeneration contraction after local vinblastine treatment of superior cervical ganglia in the rat. *Eur. J. Pharmac.* **21**, 41–45.

DAHLSTRÖM, A., EVANS, C. A. N., HÄGGENDAL, C. J., HEIWALL, P. O., and SAUNDERS, N. R. (1974) Rapid transport of acetylcholine in rat sciatic nerve proximal and distal to a lesion. *J. Neur. Transm.* (in press).

EDSTRÖM, A., and MATTSON, H. (1972) Fast axonal transport *in vitro* in the sciatic system of the frog. *J. Neurochem.* **19**, 205–221.

EVANS, C. A. N., and SAUNDERS, N. R. (1967) The distribution of acetylcholine in normal and in regenerating nerves. *J. Physiol.* **192**, 79–92.

EVANS, C. A. N., and SAUNDERS, N. R. (1974). An outflow of acetylcholine from normal and regenerating ventral roots of the cat. *J. Physiol.* (In press.)

FELDBERG, W. (1943). Synthesis of acetylcholine in sympathetic ganglia and cholinergic nerves. *J. Physiol.* **101**, 432–445.

FELDBERG, W., and VOGT, M. (1948). Acetylcholine synthesis in different regions of the central nervous system. *J. Physiol.* **107**, 372–381.

FONNUM, F. (1970). Surface charge of choline acetyltransferase from different species. *J. Neurochem.* **17**, 1905–1910.

GEFFEN, L. B., and RUSH, R. A. (1968). Transport of noradrenaline in sympathetic nerves and the effect of nerve impulses on its contribution to transmitter stores. *J. Neurochem.* **15**, 925–930.

GEFFEN, L. B., and OSTBERG, A. (1969) Distribution of granular vesicles in normal and constricted sympathetic neurones. *J. Physiol.* **204**, 583–592.

GEFFEN, L. B., and LIVETT, B. G. (1971) Synaptic vesicles in sympathetic neurons. *Physiol. Rev.* **51**, 98–157.

HÄGGENDAL, J., and DAHLSTRÖM, A. (1971) The functional role of the amine storage granules of the sympatho-adrenal system. *Mem. Soc. Endocrinol.* **19**, 651–669.

HÄGGENDAL, J., SAUNDERS, N. R., and DAHLSTRÖM, A. (1971) Rapid accumulation of acetylcholine in nerve above a crush. *J. Pharm. Pharmacol.* **23**, 552–555.

HÄGGENDAL, J., DAHLSTRÖM, A., and SAUNDERS, N. R. (1973) Axonal transport and acetylcholine in rat preganglionic neurons *Brain Res.* **58**, 494–499.

HEBB, C. (1963) Formation, storage and liberation of acetylcholine. In: *Handbuch der Experimentellen Pharmacologie.* Eds. Eichler, O. and Farah, A., Springer Verlag, Berlin. **15**, 56–88.

HEBB, C., and WAITES, G. M. (1956). Choline acetyltransferase in antero- and retrograde degeneration of a cholinergic neuron. *J. Physiol.* **132**, 667–671.

HEILBRONN, E., WIDLUND, L., HÄGGENDAL, J., SAUNDERS, N. R., and DAHLSTRÖM, A. (1974) The subcellular localization of accumulated acetylcholine in crushed sciatic nerves of cat (in preparation.)

HEIWALL, P.-O., DAHLSTRÖM, A., SAUNDERS, N. R., and HÄGGENDAL, J. (1974) Effect of mitotic inhibitors on the transport of acetylcholine in rat sciatic nerve (in preparation).

HÖKFELT, T. (1969) Distribution of noradrenaline storing particles in peripheral adrenergic neurons as revealed by electronmicroscopy. *Acta physiol. scand.* **76**, 427–440.

KARLSSON, J. O., and SJÖSTRAND, J. (1971) Synthesis, migration and turnover of the protein in retinal ganglion cells. *J. Neurochem.* **18**, 749–767.

KATZ, B. (1966) *Nerve, Muscle and Synapse*, McGraw-Hill, New York.

KREUTZBERG, G. W. (1969) Neuronal dynamics and axonal flow: IV, Blockage of intra-axonal enzyme transport by colchicine. *Proc. Natn. Acad. Sci. USA* **62** (3) 722–728.

LENTZ, T. L. (1967) Fine structure of nerves in the regenerating limb of the newt *Triturus. Am. J. Anat.* **121**, 647–670.

LIEBERMAN, A. R., SAUNDERS, N. R., HEILBRONN, E., HÄGGENDAL, J., and DAHLSTRÖM, A. (1974) (in preparation.)

LUBIŃSKA, L. (1959) Region of transition between preserved and regenerating parts of myelinated nerve fibres. *J. Comp. Neurol.* **113**, 315–335.

LÜLLMANN-RAUCH, R. (1971) The regeneration of neuromuscular junctions during spontaneous re-innervation of the rat diaphragm. *Z. Zellforsch.* **113**, 315–335.

MACINTOSH, F. C., and PERRY, W. L. M. (1950) Biological estimation of acetylcholine. *Meth. Med. Res.* **3**, 78–92.

MILEDI, R., and SLATER, C. R. (1970) On the degeneration of rat neuromuscular junctions after nerve sectioning. *J. Physiol.* **207**, 507–528.

NACHMANSOHN, D. (1959) *Chemical and Molecular Basis of Nerve Activity*, Academic Press, New York.

OCHS, S., and RANISH, N. (1969) Characteristics of the fast transport systems in mammalian nerve fibres. *J. Neurobiol.* **1**, 247–261.

PELLEGRINO DE IRALDI, A., and DE ROBERTIS, E. (1968) The neurotubular system of the axon and the origin of granulated and non-granulated vesicles in regenerating nerves. *Z. Zellforsch.* **87**, 330–344.

SAUNDERS, N. R., DZIEGIELEWSKA, K., HÄGGENDAL, J., and DAHLSTRÖM, A. (1973) Slow accumulation of choline acetyltransferase in crushed sciatic nerves of the rat. *J. Neurobiol.* **4**, 95–103.

SCHILD, H. O. (1942) A method of conducting a biological assay on a preparation giving repeated graded responses illustrated by the estimation of histamine. *J. Physiol.* **101**, 115–130.

SJÖSTRAND, J., FRIZELL, M., and HASSELGREN, P.-O. (1971) Effects of colchicine on axonal transport in peripheral nerves. *J. Neurochem.* **17**, 1563–1570.

SKRANGIEL-KRAMSKA, J., NIEMIERKO, S., and LUBIŃSKA, L. (1969). Comparison of the behaviour of a soluble and a membrane-bound enzyme in transected peripheral nerves. *J. Neurochem.* **16**, 921–926.

SMITH, A. D. (1971) Secretion of proteins (chromogranin A and dopamine-β-hydroxylase) from a sympathetic neuron. *Phil. Trans. R. Soc. Lond.* B, **261**, 363–370.

TUČEK, S. (1970) Subcellular localization of enzymes generating acetyl-CoA and their possible relation to the biosynthesis of acetylcholine. In *Drugs and Cholinergic Mechanisms in the CNS* (E. Heilbronn and A. Winter, eds.), Almqvist & Wiksell, Stockholm, pp. 117–131.

WEISS, P. A., and HISCOE, H. (1948). Experiments on the mechanism of nerve growth. *J. Exp. Zool.* **107**, 315–396.

WETTSTEIN, R., and SOLETO, J. R. (1963) Electron microscope study on the regenerative process of peripheral nerves of mice. *Z. Zellforsch.* **59**, 708–730.

WHITTAKER, V. P. (1969) The nature of acetylcholine pools in brain tissue. *Progr. Brain Res.* **31**, 211–222.

WILSON, L., BRYAN, J., RUBY, A., and MAZIA, D. (1970) Precipitation of proteins by vinblastine and calcium ions. *Proc. Natn. Acad. Sci. USA* **66**, 807–814.

WOOG, R. H., and BENNETT, M. R. (1972) Vesicle types in injured nerve fibres. *Proc. Austr. Physiol. Pharmac. Soc.* **3**, 89–90.

AXONAL TRANSPORT OF DOPAMINE-β-HYDROXYLASE BY ABNORMAL HUMAN SURAL NERVES

STEPHEN BRIMIJOIN AND PETER JAMES DYCK

Departments of Pharmacology and Neurology, Mayo Medical School, Rochester, Minnesota 55901, USA

SUMMARY

Axoplasmic transport of dopamine-β-hydroxylase was measured in normal human sural nerves and in sural nerves from twelve patients with various peripheral neuropathies. As compared to the normals, most nerves from patients exhibiting loss of sensation or of autonomic function showed decreased transport of dopamine-β-hydroxylase. In general this decrease was greater than was the associated reduction of enzyme activity.

Dopamine-β-hydroxylase (DBH), which catalyzes the final stage in biosynthesis of norepinephrine, is an enzyme of particular interest on account of its localization to catecholamine storage vesicles in adrenergic nerves (Hörtnagl *et al.*, 1969). Immunofluorescence experiments have shown that DBH accumulates proximal to a constriction of adrenergic axons (Geffen *et al.*, 1969). Quantitative measurements of the rate of accumulation of DBH activity above a ligature on the rat sciatic nerve (Brimijoin, 1972; Coyle and Wooten, 1972) indicate that DBH is transported proximodistally with a high velocity comparable to that for axonal transport of norepinephrine (Dahlström and Häggendal, 1966).

Although the problem of the mechanism of rapid axoplasmic transport has attracted much attention, little is presently known about the role of transport in maintaining neuronal integrity. It seemed to us that some light might be shed on this question by comparing axonal transport of DBH in normal human nerves with transport in nerves from patients with peripheral neuropathies.

The sural nerve was chosen for these studies as a superficial cutaneous nerve which contains autonomic fibers (Mitchell, 1953) and which can be conveniently biopsied without leading to substantial functional impairment (Dyck and Lofgren, 1968). Fascicular samples, 3–5 cm in length, were obtained at ankle level under local anesthesia with informed consent from healthy human volunteers, ages 21–28. Similar samples were obtained as a part of biopsies performed for diagnostic reasons on patients with peripheral neuropathies. The nerves were incubated in 200 ml of bicarbonate-buffered physiological salt solution, pH 7.4 (for composition see Brimijoin *et al.*, 1973). This solution was maintained at 37°C and continuously gassed with 95 % O_2, 5 % CO_2. After 15 min of incubation *in vitro*, ligatures of silk thread were applied to the nerve. After a further incubation for a variable period of time, the nerve was cut into 3 mm segments which were individually homogenized in glass homogenizers containing 0.6 ml of ice-cold buffer (0.005 M Tris, pH 7.4; bovine serum albumin, 0.2 %; and Triton X-100, 0.1 %). Homogenates were centrifuged at 15,000 × g for 10 min, and the supernatant fractions were assayed for DBH activity as previously described (Molinoff *et al.*, 1971). Partially purified bovine adrenal DBH was added to duplicate samples as an internal standard to correct for any variation of activators or inhibitors of DBH.

The results obtained with normal sural nerves have been reported in detail elsewhere (Brimijoin *et al.*, 1973). The main feature was a progressive increase in DBH activity in the segment immediately above the ligature placed near the distal end of the nerve. This increase could be seen in nerves incubated for 1.5 h *in vitro* and was substantial in nerves incubated for 3–5 h. Elsewhere along the nerve, changes in DBH activity were inconsistent, although after several hours of incubation there was a suggestion of DBH accumulation distal to a ligature placed on the proximal end of the nerve.

Total DBH activity did not change during incubation. The mean DBH activity, per 3 mm segment, between the proximal and distal ligatures was taken as a baseline against which to measure accumulation. This baseline was subtracted from the DBH activity in the segment above the distal ligature; the result was assumed to represent DBH which had been transported into the segment above the ligature during the incubation. Accumulated DBH activity was then divided by the baseline activity to obtain a relative measure of transport. This measure increased linearly with time of incubation ($r = 0.944$). The rate of increase corresponded to proximodistal transport of DBH at a velocity of 2 mm/h (or greater, if part of the DBH in the nerve had been stationary).

Sural nerves from patients with diseases of peripheral nerve were incubated *in vitro* for 3 h after application of ligatures. The relative rate of accumulation of DBH activity was calculated just as for the normal nerves. Table 1 presents this measure as a percentage of the mean rate of accumulation in normal nerves, estimated from a least squares fit of the normal data (Brimijoin *et al.*, 1973). It is apparent that, in patients who had only motor symptoms (cases 1 and 2), both the levels of DBH activity and the rate of transport of DBH were normal. In all except one patient so far examined who had sensory symptoms or both motor and sensory symptoms, however, the transport of DBH was significantly lower than control. Some of this group of patients had subnormal levels of DBH activity, possibly as a result of degeneration of adrenergic fibers. Others, who had equally little transport, had normal levels of enzyme activity. Further investigation is necessary to determine if normal enzyme levels are associated with reduced enzyme transport during the earlier stages of degenerative nerve diseases.

One exception to the correlation of sensory symptoms with loss of transport was observed in a case of inflammatory neuropathy, probably of allergic origin (case 9). This patient had normal transport and normal levels of DBH. It is unfortunate that we have at present no good clinical measure of adrenergic function in these patients, since this case of inflammatory neuropathy points up the coincidental nature of the correlation between sensory loss and loss of transport. In all probability, this correlation depends on a tendency of the diseases we have studied to involve sensory fibers and autonomic fibers at the same time. Apparently the autonomic fibers were not involved in the inflammatory neuropathy of case 9. Case 12 shows the opposite picture in which there were no observable defects in motor or

TABLE 1. TRANSPORT OF DBH IN ABNORMAL HUMAN SURAL NERVES

Case	Origin	Diagnosis	Sympto-matology	DBH activity per mg (percent of control)	DBH transport (percent of control)
1		Motor neuropathy	Motor	96	151
2		Charcot-Marie-tooth (progressive muscular atrophy)	Motor	82	124
3		Charcot-Marie-tooth (neuronal)	Motor and sensory	100	10[a]
4	Hereditary	Charcot-Marie-tooth (hypertrophic)	Motor and sensory	42	16[a]
5		Dejerine–Sottas	Motor and sensory	125	0[a]
6		Olivo-ponto-cerebellar degeneration, plus	Motor and sensory	110	31[a]
7		Sensory neuropathy	Sensory	24[a]	39[a]
8		Sensory neuropathy	Sensory	17[a]	0[a]
9		Uremia	None	170[a]	56
10	Acquired	Uremia	Motor and sensory	100	6[a]
11		Inflammatory neuropathy	Motor and sensory	50	100
12	Unknown	Undiagnosed neuropathy	Loss of sweating	37	18[a]

[a] Signifies more than two standard deviations from the control mean. Control DBH activity was 96 ± 12 (SEM) pmole octopamine formed per hour of incubation per milligram wet weight. Control transport corresponded to an increase in DBH activity in the segment just above the distal ligature to 2.6 times the baseline activity.

sensory function but in which there was an abnormality in sweating, a function controlled by cholinergic sympathetic fibers. Transport of DBH was grossly abnormal in this patient, but even in this case we lack evidence of an association of this finding with a deficit in adrenergic function.

Much work remains to be done before we understand whether loss of DBH transport is an incidental feature of these neuropathies or whether a defect in rapid axonal transport is actually an early link in the chain of events leading to loss of nerve function and, ultimately, degeneration of the neuron. In any case, studies of axonal transport offer the possibility of new insights into the mechanism of peripheral nerve diseases in man.

ACKNOWLEDGEMENTS

Supported in part by NIMH grant MH-21413, NIH grants NS05811 and NS0741, and by the Gallmeyer Miller, and Upton funds.

REFERENCES

BRIMIJOIN, S. (1972) Transport and turnover of dopamine-β-hydroxylase (EC 1.14.2.1) in sympathetic nerves of the rat. *J. Neurochem.* **19**, 2183–2193.

BRIMIJOIN, S., CAPEK, P., and DYCK, P. (1973) Axonal transport of dopamine-β-hydroxylase by human sural nerves *in vitro*. *Science* **180**, 1295–1297.

COYLE, J., and WOOTEN, F. (1972) Rapid axonal transport of tyrosine hydroxylase and dopamine-β-hydroxylase. *Brain Res.* **44**, 701–704.

DAHLSTRÖM, A. and HÄGGENDAL, J. (1966) Studies on the transport and life span of amine storage granules in a peripheral adrenergic neuron system. *Acta physiol. scand.* **67**, 278–288.

DYCK, P. J., and LOFGREN, E. P. (1968) Nerve biopsy: choice of nerve, method, symptoms, and usefulness. *Med. Clinc. N. Am.* **52**, 885–893.

GEFFEN, L. B., LIVETT, B. G., and RUSH, R. A. (1969) Immunohistochemical localization of protein components of catecholamine storage vesicles. *J. Physiol. Lond.* **204**, 593–606.

HÖRTNAGL, H., HÖRTNAGL, H., and WINKLER, H. (1969) Bovine splenic nerve: characterization of noradrenaline-containing vesicles and other cell organelles by density gradient centrifugation. *J. Physiol. Lond.* **205**, 103–114.

MITCHELL, G. A. G. (1953) *Anatomy of the Autonomic Nervous System*, Livingstone, Edinburgh, p. 207.

MOLINOFF, P. B., WEINSHILBOUM, R., and AXELROD, J. (1971) A sensitive enzymatic assay for dopamine-β-hydroxylase. *J. Pharmac. Exp. Ther.* **178**, 425–432.

GROWTH

SESSION I

Chairman: U. S. VON EULER

CONTROL MECHANISMS OF THE ADRENERGIC NEURON

RITA LEVI-MONTALCINI

Laboratorio di Biologia Cellulare (CNR), Rome, Italy
and Department of Biology, Washington University, St. Louis, Missouri, USA

SUMMARY

The discovery that sympathetic neurons are highly receptive to a nerve growth factor (NGF) which is normally present in tissues and body fluids and plays a vital role in the life of these cells, was the starting point of an investigation on growth regulatory mechanisms of these cells. Daily injections of NGF in newborn rodents call forth a dramatic increase in size and number of these neurons, where as injections of a specific antiserum to the NGF result in death of sympathetic nerve cells. The process is known as immunosympathectomy. It was subsequently found that two pharmacological agents, 6-hydroxydopamine (6-OH-DA) and guanethidine, when injected in newborn mice or rats, produce destruction of sympathetic neurons comparable to that elicited by an antiserum to the NGF. Ultra-structural studies showed, however, that the sequence and localization of degenerative events in the cell compartments differ markedly from those produced by the antiserum, and also differ from each other. It seemed, therefore, of considerable interest to see whether the simultaneous administration of NGF would mitigate or prevent the toxic effects produced by 6-OH-DA or guanethidine. To this aim, littermate newborn rats were divided into four groups and injected daily from the day of birth with NGF, NGF and guanethidine, guanethidine, or saline. In a second experimental series, 6-OH-DA instead of guanethidine was used alone or in combination with NGF. The destructive effects of guanethidine are apparent earlier than those of 6-OH-DA. Ganglia of guanethidine-injected rats consist of satellite cells and only a few atrophic sympathetic neurons at 8 days; ganglia of 6-OH-DA-treated rats show a similar picture at the end of the third week. Simultaneous injections of NGF prevent the destructive effects of guanethidine or 6-OH-DA, but marked differences are apparent at stereo-, optic, and electron microscopic inspection in ganglia of the two series. Ganglia of NGF and guanethidine-treated rats compare in size to those treated with NGF alone; both are about three times larger than controls at 8 days. Ganglia of 6-OH-DA- and NGF-treated rats are three to four times larger than those treated with NGF at the end of the third week. The massive volume increase is due to an extraordinary increase in number and size of postganglionic axons and moderate increase in glial and satellite cells.

INTRODUCTION

In biological sciences, perhaps more than in all other experimental sciences, progress has depended upon the fortunate choice of the system which was to play a leading role in the understanding of other systems of more elaborate, but basically similar, design.

Thus in the fields of molecular biology, microbiology and genetics, bacteriophage, *Escherichia coli*, and fruit fly, to mention only some of the most celebrated models, provided ideal objects to explore the molecular basis of organization of a virus, a simple bacterial cell, and of the genetic material stored in the nuclear compartment of cells of pluricellular organisms. Even more important, however, than the knowledge gained in each given sector is the impact that these investigations exerted in the general field of biology. All of a sudden, in fact, the gates of what was to become known as "the golden age" stood wide open in front of the biologist, who is still dazzled by the light which poured in.

Of all areas, that of neurobiology is the one which has benefited least from the coming to existence of the golden age; the obvious and all too well known reason is the tremendous complexity of a system which consists of an immense population of different cells interconnected by even more complex wiring circuits. While these cells obey the same basic rules which hold for all animal cells, they also obey rules which are unique to this system and cannot be uncovered unless the same cells are explored in their natural surroundings. Of all cells which build the nervous system, one suggests itself as a possible candidate for such a role: the adrenergic sympathetic neuron.

Long before the opening of the new area of biology, this cell had already played a key role in unveiling some of the basic principles which operate in the nervous system. Without it, the discovery of the chemical nature of neurotransmitters and the subsequent identification of some of them would perhaps never have been achieved. And yet even if it was soon proved that intercentral neurons communicate by releasing humoral agents in the same way as the sympathetic neuron, still the concept prevailed that this nerve cell population forms a class apart from that of other neurons, being—as it is—excluded from the main stream and endowed with what seemed to be only a sort of auxiliary role to that of the centrally located neurons. Hence only a decade ago the neurobiologist would have been reluctant to accept this cell as a valid model of neurons responsible for higher brain functions.

The discovery by Swedish workers (Dahlström and Fuxe, 1964a, b; Falck *et al.*, 1962; Fuxe *et al.*, 1970) that nerve cells lodged in the central nervous system share many properties in common with the sympathetic adrenergic neuron and at the same time play a fundamental role in the structural and functional organization of the brain, opened what can be defined as the golden era in neurobiological sciences. Thus the sympathetic adrenergic neuron acquired full status as a first class citizen and all of a sudden came to the forefront of research in this field. The heavy investment of this past decade in the study of adrenergic central neurons and of the role that they play in manifold brain activities, gives impressive evidence for this new development which, in turn, reflects on the peripheral adrenergic neuron for the vicarious and most serviceable function that it can play as a model of the central, much less approachable, adrenergic nerve cell.

Our interest in the sympathetic neuron did not stem, however, from these considerations nor, until recently, did we make any attempt to explore the adrenergic central neuron. Ever since we started this line of investigation more than two decades ago, the object has been the sympathetic nerve cell as such, with its structural and functional properties which, at that time, seemed to share few if any properties in common with those of neurons lodged in the CNS.

The objective of this research was, in fact, entirely confined to the realm of neuro-embryology, the science which analyzes the role of extrinsic factors in neurogenesis. Nor did we even conceive of the sympathetic neuron as a most suitable cell for these studies. The sensory and motor embryonic nerve cells were, in fact, far more in favor than the sympathetic neuron, and it was the latter which imposed itself on our attention, snatching the role held by somatic neurons ever since the beginning of the century as the favorite object of the neuroembryologist.

The history of this investigation and of the tortuous way in which it shifted from the analysis of the effects of the periphery on the growth and differentiation of associated nerve centers to that of a protein molecule which plays a key role in the life of the adrenergic neuron has been reported many times and need not be repeated here. By way of introduction we shall, however, summarize in a most condensed fashion the early steps of this investigation which is at present still in full development, although its objective has little if anything in common with that which promoted this search.

HISTORICAL BACKGROUND

Neuroembryological studies in the first four decades of the century gave unequivocal evidence for the role played by peripheral tissues and end organs in the development and growth of associated nerve structures. The experiments performed in amphibian larvae and avian embryos showed that ablation of a limb bud at early developmental stages would result in severe atrophy of sensory and motor nerve centers which innervate the limb, whereas implantation of an additional limb will produce the opposite effect, namely a size increase of the same nerve centers. In order to explore the mechanism of action of peripheral tissues, Bueker, conceived the idea of grafting a rapidly growing tissue into the flank of 3-day chick embryos. To this aim he implanted three different types of mouse tumors. One of these, sarcoma 180, became established, and in a few days covered an area considerably larger than that of the adjacent limb bud. Five days later the embryos were sacrificed and serially sectioned. The finding that sensory nerve fibers growing out from adjacent spinal ganglia had branched into the neoplastic tissue and that the same ganglia were larger than those of the contralateral side, seemed to give support to the hypothesis that the size of a given primary nerve center depends upon the extent of the peripheral areas which it innervates (Bueker, 1948). A more extensive analysis of the phenomenon in our laboratory,[†] however, showed other facets of this stimulus–response effect which called for a different interpretation of the growth response elicited by the tumor from the adjacent sensory ganglia of the host. In three ways the effect produced by the neoplastic tissue differed from that of a normal limb bud or other embryonic tissues: (a) the sympathetic ganglia of the host appeared to be much more enlarged than the spinal ganglia, (b) the effect was not restricted to ganglia which innervated the tumor but was clearly apparent on the entire sympathetic chain ganglia of the host, and (c) sympathetic nerve fibers produced by the hypertrophic and hyperplastic ganglia in embryos bearing transplants of mouse sarcomas 180 or 37 (the second tumor produced the same effect as sarcoma 180) massively invaded the viscera and even forced their way into the blood vessels. The hypothesis that the tumor elicited these dramatic effects by releasing a growth promoting agent into the circulation of the host received confirmation from experiments of tumor implantation onto the chorio-allantoic membrane of 4- to 6-day chick embryos. In this position, the tumor and the embryo shared the circulation but no direct contact was established between embryonic and neoplastic tissues. The effects elicited by the tumor on sympathetic ganglia of the host

† This and subsequent experiments were performed in the laboratory directed by the eminent neuro-embryologist V. Hamburger. The author wishes to express her gratitude to him for the hospitality and invaluable help received during the many years of their association and everlasting friendship.

were, however, of the same nature and nearly the same magnitude as those elicited by intraembryonic transplants (Levi-Montalcini, 1952).

These findings, while giving support to the hypothesis of the release by neoplastic tissues of a humoral growth promoting agent, also suggested a different experimental approach. The chick embryo was replaced by an *in vitro* technique which permitted a more immediate exploration of the effects elicited by the tumor on the target sensory and sympathetic ganglia. To this aim, these ganglia from 8-day chick embryos were explanted in a semisolid medium consisting of chicken plasma and embryonic extract in proximity to fragments of the tumors under investigation. In control experiments, the same ganglia were combined *in vitro* with embryonic tissue or with tumors which did not produce any growth promoting effect upon their transplantation into the chick embryo. The results of these experiments gave even more impressive evidence than the *in vivo* experiments for the release of a humoral growth promoting factor from mouse sarcomas 180 and 37. Sensory and sympathetic ganglia facing explants of these tumors produced a dense fibrillar halo in a 6–8 h period, while in control experiments the same ganglia produced few or no nerve fibers in the first 24 h of culture. The discovery of this effect (Levi-Montalcini *et al.*, 1954) signaled the turning point of the investigation. The magnitude of the effect elicited by the two sarcomas in the target sensory and sympathetic nerve cells, as well as the rapidity of the growth response which materializes in a few hours, set, in fact, the stage for the next step—the characterization of the growth factor. At that time this seemed a fairly straightforward project to us as well as to the outstanding biochemist, S. Cohen, who joined us. How far off it really was is best documented by the fact that the nerve growth factor (NGF), as this factor was to become known, was characterized only 16 years later, in spite of the full-time investment in this project by our team. And this would perhaps never have been achieved were it not for some extraordinary chance discoveries which provided a short cut and made possible the identification of the NGF and of the full range of the growth response of the target cells.

THE NERVE GROWTH FACTOR: ITS MAIN SOURCES AND ITS DISTRIBUTION IN TISSUES AND BODY FLUIDS

A first successful attempt to elucidate the chemical nature of the humoral factor released by mouse sarcomas 180 and 37 was made in 1954, soon after the discovery of the *in vitro* effect of both tumors on sensory and sympathetic ganglia. Addition to the culture medium of the tumor extract calls forth the formation of the typical fibrillar halo. A nucleoprotein particle isolated from the extract and named "nerve growth promoting factor" proved to be endowed with this growth promoting activity (Cohen *et al.*, 1954). In an attempt to further purify this factor, Cohen made use of phosphodiesterase obtained from snake venom. These experiments gave an unexpected and unforeseeable result: the snake venom itself was found to possess a nerve-growth-promoting activity far more pronounced than that of the tumors under investigation (Cohen and Levi-Montalcini, 1956). In 1958 a third and even more potent source of the NGF was discovered in mouse submaxillary salivary glands (Cohen, 1958; Levi-Montalcini, 1958). Here it may suffice to mention that these glands remain up to the present time the richest source of the NGF; in extracts of adult male submaxillary salivary glands, its concentration reaches about 1% of the soluble proteins. Extensive studies performed ever since the discovery of the NGF activity of these glands have given evidence for (a) the localization of the NGF in the tubular portion of the gland, (b) its *in situ* production, and (c) its control by the male hormone, testosterone (Levi-

Montalcini and Angeletti, 1968). The NGF is in fact absent from the same gland of pre-puberal mice, in which the tubular portion is still not differentiated, and increases in parallel with the differentiation of these tubules from puberty to full maturity. In females the NGF is present at a concentration ten times lower than in males, but upon testosterone injection it reaches the same level as in males. As in males, the injection of the hormone brings about a marked increase in the tubular portion. While evidence was also obtained that the NGF is not released in a hormonal fashion from these glands and does not compare in many other respects with hormones (Levi-Montalcini, 1966), still no satisfactory explanation can be offered for the potent nerve growth activity elicited by snake venom and mouse salivary glands on the embryonic sensory and embryonic and fully differentiated sympathetic neurons.

Perhaps more important than the finding of very large amounts of this factor in snake venom and mouse salivary glands, at least in connection with the problem of the role which it plays in the life of the target cells, is the finding that the NGF is present in trace amounts in all tissues and body fluids, also in organisms where it cannot be detected in the salivary glands, and these are, indeed, the great majority. A systematic screening for its presence revealed in fact its widespread distribution in embryonic (Bueker et al., 1960) as well as in fully differentiated tissues (Levi-Montalcini and Angeletti, 1961). Recent studies with homogenates of heart and spleen from mice and rats, upon further purification of various fractions by differential centrifugation, gave evidence for its localization in a fraction sedimented at $100,000\ g$. The presence of the NGF in this fraction was also confirmed immunochemically by microcomplement fixation, using the antiserum to the salivary NGF (P. U. Angeletti et al., 1972b). The possibility that the NGF activity could somehow be associated with adrenergic terminals in peripheral tissues and play a role in the maintenance and function of the sympathetic adrenergic neurons is at present under investigation.

Finally, it is of interest to mention that the NGF is also detectable in the serum of all species investigated, man included, in saliva, milk, and urine. These findings give support to the hypothesis that the NGF plays a functional role in the life of the target nerve cells. More crucial evidence for such a role came from other work to be considered in a following section.

CHEMICAL PROPERTIES AND STRUCTURE OF THE SALIVARY NGF SUBUNIT

It was mentioned on p. 300 that first attempts to identify the chemical nature of the growth factor indicated that the activity was bound to a nucleoprotein fraction. The subsequent discovery that the venom itself is a most potent source of this factor brought new and most important information on the chemical nature of the NGF. The factor was identified by Cohen in a protein, rather than nucleoprotein, fraction (Cohen, 1959). Since the growth-promoting activity of the tumor extract persisted also after inactivation of the nucleic acid present in the active fraction, the conclusion was reached that the tumor NGF is a protein, rather than a nucleoprotein, molecule. However, since the discovery that both snake venom and salivary glands are far richer sources of NGF than the tumor, no further attempts were made to purify and characterize the tumor molecule endowed with this growth-promoting activity. In view of the marked similarity of effects elicited by the active fractions isolated from snake venom and from mouse salivary glands and of the more extensive work invested in the characterization of the latter, we shall consider here only the salivary NGF. It suffices to mention that biochemical and immunological studies performed first by Cohen (1960) and then extended by Zanini et al. (1968) and R. H. Angeletti (1969) gave evidence for the striking similarity of the venom and salivary NGF. In fact the results obtained from immunological studies show that the NGFs isolated from these two different animal sources belong to a family of closely related proteins whose mechanism of action on the responsive nerve cells must be essentially the same.

Studies first initiated by Cohen and pursued then in our laboratory (Salvi et al., 1965) as well as others (Pérez-Polo et al., 1972; Varon et al., 1967) showed that the NGF possesses a marked tendency to aggregate both with itself and with other active molecules. Cohen, who first purified the mouse salivary NGF, reported a molecular weight of 44,000, whereas later work (Bocchini and Angeletti, 1969) indicated a molecular weight of 30,000. Zanini et al. (1968) have reported the isolation of a fully active protein of only 14,000 mol. wt. The immunochemical properties of this smaller species were indistinguishable from those of the 28,000 mol. wt. form when judged by immunoelectrophoresis and complement fixation tests. More recent work by R. H. Angeletti et al. (1971) gave evidence that the NGF molecule represents a dimer of two identical subunits bound together by noncovalent bonds alone in a tight complex which is difficult to dissociate. These studies were climaxed by the elucidation of the complete primary and secondary structure of the fundamental subunit of 2.5 S mouse NGF (R. H. Angeletti and Bradshaw, 1971). It contains 118 amino acids with amino terminal serine and carboxyl terminal arginine and has a molecular weight of 13,259. Studies now in progress are probing the structure–function relationship of this factor.

THE TARGET CELLS

Of the extensive work performed ever since the discovery of the growth response elicited by mouse sarcomas 180 and 37 in the sensory and sympathetic ganglia of the chick embryo, we shall here consider only the most relevant features of this response at the structural, ultrastructural, metabolic, and enzymatic levels. Since there is definite evidence for the identity of the growth effect called forth by the NGFs isolated from mouse sarcomas, snake venom, and mouse salivary glands, only the latter, as the most thoroughly investigated, will be considered here.

CHARACTERISTICS OF THE *IN VITRO* AND *IN VIVO* GROWTH RESPONSE AT THE STRUCTURAL AND ULTRASTRUCTURAL LEVELS

Studies *in vitro* with the highly purified NGF show that the typical fibrillar halo illustrated in Fig. 1a, b is elicited by the addition to the culture medium of 0.01 μg of NGF per ml of culture medium. This is defined as one biological unit (BU). Ten biological units call forth the formation of a shorter and denser fibrillar halo, while the addition of 100 BU results in the total suppression of the radial nerve fiber outgrowth from the ganglia. Histological studies, reported in detail elsewhere (Levi-Montalcini et al., 1972), indicate that the NGF excess does not, however, prevent the excessive production of nerve fibers from sensory or sympathetic ganglia but calls forth a different pattern of nerve fiber outgrowth: the fibers do not grow out radially but in a circular fashion around the ganglion and form a dense fibrillar capsule which increases in width in parallel with the increase in NGF content in the medium.

Studies with sensory and sympathetic nerve cells dissociated respectively from ganglia of 8- and 12-day chick embryos showed that both nerve cell types survive indefinitely and build

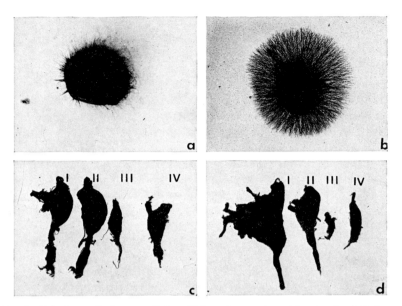

FIG. 1.a, b: Spinal ganglia from an 8-day chick embryo cultured *in vitro* for 24 h in control medium (a) and in a medium containing 1 BU of salivary NGF (b). Silver stain. ×45. c: Whole mounts of superior cervical ganglia from 13-day-old littermate rats injected daily since birth with NGF and guanethidine (I), NGF (II), guanethidine (III), and saline solution (IV). ×10. d: Whole mounts of superior cervical ganglia from 19-day-old littermate rats injected daily since birth with 6-OH-DA and NGF (I), NGF (II), 6-OH-DA (III), and saline (IV). ×10.

a dense fibrillar network in a minimum essential medium in the presence of 1–10 NGF BU. In its absence, nerve cells undergo rapid deterioration and die in the first 24–48 h of culture. These findings are taken as indicative of the essential role played by NGF in the life of both nerve cell types (Levi-Montalcini and Angeletti, 1963).

Daily injections of NGF in newborn mice and rats in the amount of 10–50 $\mu g/g$ body weight bring about increase in size of sympathetic ganglia up to ten-fold their normal size in a 10-day period, while sensory ganglia are not affected by the treatment. The volume increase of sympathetic ganglia is due to an increase in cell number and size of individual neurons. Evidence that the adrenergic sympathetic nerve cells remain receptive throughout life to the effect of the NGF was obtained by injection of this protein molecule in adult mice and rats. In both instances, sympathetic ganglia underwent a marked volume increase. Histological studies showed that this effect is due to hypertrophy of individual neurons, while their number did not increase (Levi-Montalcini, 1966).

Detailed studies performed by Olson (1967) with the Falck–Hillarp fluorescent technique gave an impressive demonstration of the increased density of the adrenergic fibrillar network in peripheral organs of baby mice injected with the NGF.

A recent most interesting development, which may open a new area of exploration, is the report that the adrenergic neurons in the CNS are also receptive to the action of the NGF, provided the factor is administered by intracisternal injection. A marked increase of adrenergic nerve fibers is suggested from photographic documentation by Björklund and Stenevi (1972) and Berger *et al.* (1973).

Studies of the NGF response at the EM, performed at short time intervals after addition of the NGF to the culture medium or injection of this factor in newborn mice, showed that the earliest effect consists of a massive increase in neurofibrillar material and in a marked enlargement of the Golgi complex (Levi-Montalcini *et al.*, 1968). The question whether the NGF increase in neurotubules and consequent excessive formation *in vivo* and *in vitro* of nerve fibers is due to a polymerization and assembly effect of the basic neurotubular structure or to *de novo* synthesis of the primary protofibril units was studied by incorporating into the tissue culture medium 0.1 μM of vincristine, an alkaloid which suppresses nerve fiber extension by disrupting the microtubule structures of neurotubules and neurofilaments. Under these conditions, the ganglia failed to produce the fibrillar halo when treated with the NGF, but EM studies showed that the nerve cell perikarya were filled with masses of protofilaments. The conclusion was reached that the NGF calls forth the extraordinary increase in neurofibers by stimulating *de novo* synthesis of the protofilaments (Levi-Montalcini and Angeletti, 1970). Recent biochemical experiments directed to exploring the mechanism of action of the NGF at the biochemical level corroborated these findings (Hier *et al.*, 1972).

NGF-INDUCED METABOLIC CHANGES IN SENSORY AND SYMPATHETIC GANGLIA

The growth response elicited by NGF is accompanied by several metabolic changes such as increase in RNA, protein and lipid synthesis, and carbohydrate utilization. The latter occurs through activation of the pentose-phosphate pathway (P. U. Angeletti *et al.*, 1964a, b, 1965).

The primary site of action of NGF is, however, not yet identified. The hypothesis first submitted, that it could be at the level of DNA transcription (Levi-Montalcini, 1966), was not supported by subsequent investigations with actinomycin-D. The addition of this specific inhibitor to the culture medium at doses which block RNA synthesis does not completely prevent the production of a neurofibrillar halo around the ganglia cultured in presence of NGF (Larrabee, 1969, 1972; Levi-Montalcini and Angeletti, 1971).

More revealing than the demonstration of widespread metabolic changes called forth by NGF in sensory and sympathetic embryonic ganglia *in vitro* were subsequent studies on the biosynthesis of noradrenaline in the sympathetic adrenergic neuron. At variance with previous experiments, the latter were performed on ganglia dissected out from infant rats sacrificed immediately after NGF treatment. It was, in fact, rightly objected (Larrabee, 1969) that the activation of various metabolic pathways in ganglia incubated in presence of NGF could be due not so much, or at least not only, to a growth-stimulating effect by this factor as to a "maintenance effect" elicited by NGF; control ganglia undergo progressive deterioration, as already mentioned. This criticism obviously does not apply to *in vivo* experiments where NGF-treated and littermate rats are in comparably healthy condition.

The results showed that the NGF produces a selective fifteen- to twenty-fold increase in the activity of tyrosine hydroxylase and dopamine-β-hydroxylase, the two key enzymes exclusively located in the adrenergic neuron and involved in noradrenaline synthesis. In contrast, the activity of other nonspecific enzymes which operate in the synthesis and degradation of the neurotransmitter, dopa decarboxylase and monoaminoxidase, rose only in proportion to the increase in volume of sympathetic ganglia and to the four-fold increase in their protein content. It is of considerable interest to note that a similar increase in the two key enzymes of noradrenaline biosynthesis occurs also upon physiological stimulation (cold exposure) or reserpine induced depletion of noradrenaline (Thoenen *et al.*, 1971). The similarities and differences in the regulative processes called forth by NGF and functional activity in the synthesis of noradrenaline are at present under study.

GROWTH INHIBITION OF SYMPATHETIC NERVE CELLS BY ANTIBODIES TO THE NGF

The key role played by NGF in growth and differentiative processes of the adrenergic sympathetic neuron, as well as in its maintenance upon reaching maturity, came sharply into focus from immunological studies. In 1960 Cohen produced a specific antiserum to the NGF by the usual procedure of injecting the purified protein molecule into rabbits (Cohen, 1960). Addition of the antiserum to the culture medium entirely prevented the formation of the fibrillar halo by the NGF, thus indicating the presence of specific antibodies to this molecule. The antiserum was then injected in newborn mice and rats for a 1-week period. A month later, the treated animals were sacrificed. At inspection under the stereomicroscope, the ganglia appeared reduced to exceedingly small nodules. Histological studies performed on all para- and prevertebral chain ganglia showed that sympathetic neurons had been reduced to a vanishingly small population consisting of 2–5% that of controls. Glial cells, still in rather large numbers 3–4 weeks after discontinuation of the treatment, underwent atrophy and disappeared in turn in subsequent months (Levi-Montalcini and Booker, 1960). In 1961 this process became known as "immunosympathectomy". The procedure of selectively destroying the sympathetic chain ganglia by injecting a specific antiserum to the NGF has been used ever since to produce colonies of immunosympathectomized mice and rats for experimental purposes. The same treatment was also applied to larger animals, cats, and rabbits, and proved to be effective. However, for reasons of convenience and also in view of the fact that the effects are more consistent in mice and rats, the latter remained the objects of choice. Here we shall not consider the latitude of the destructive effects called forth by antibodies to the NGF, which may differ from case to case and also in the same animal from ganglion to ganglion: the extent of the degenerative effects is always more pronounced in the para- than in the prevertebral ganglia. The reasons for these differences have been discussed in other articles and tentatively explained as due to difference in the maturation of the adrenergic cell population in different ganglia at birth. The paravertebral ganglia are less differentiated at birth than the prevertebral ganglia, and this may account for their higher vulnerability to antibodies to the NGF. A less complete degree of immunosympathectomy obtained in some laboratories is instead easily explained as due to the use of a less potent antiserum (Vogt, 1964; Zaimis, 1964; Klingman and Klingman, 1972). In all instances it became apparent that sympathetic ganglia innervating the sex organs, the vas deferens in males and the uterus in females, are not affected either by the NGF or by the antiserum, thus giving evidence for some biochemical differences which are at present under investigation.

The treatment with the antiserum to the NGF (AS-NGF) in adult animals results in a marked, but reversible, size decrease of sympathetic adrenergic neurons, which are adversely affected by antibodies to the NGF but recover upon discontinuation of the treatment (P. U. Angeletti et al., 1971).

Ultrastructural studies performed during the first 24 h after injection of the AS in newborn animals gave evidence for the sequence and localization of degenerative events produced by antibodies to the NGF in the different cell compartments in sympathetic immature neurons. These effects are already apparent 2 h after the first injection of the antiserum and consist of marked changes in the fine structure of the nucleoli. In proximity to the altered nucleolus, the chromatin clumps in large areas and appears considerably denser than in controls. In immediately subsequent stages, between 4 and 12 h after injection, the nuclear material becomes intermixed. Vacuolization, pyknosis, rupture of the plasma membrane, and other signs of cytolysis are seen in most neurons surrounded by macrophages and histiocytes (Levi-Montalcini *et al.*, 1969).

THE NEW APPROACH TO THE STUDY OF CONTROL MECHANISMS IN THE ADRENERGIC NEURONS

While the studies on the mechanism of action of the NGF and of the AS-NGF were in progress, a new and most revealing facet of growth control mechanisms in the sympathetic nervous system came to light with the discovery that the same neurons in newborn mice and rats are also destroyed by an entirely different procedure, namely by treatment with some adrenergic blocking agents. The discovery in 1969 (P. U. Angeletti and Levi-Montalcini, 1970a; P. U. Angeletti, 1972) that injections of the dopamine analog, 6-hydroxy-dopamine (6-OH-DA), in newborn mice and rats produce the destruction of para- and prevertebral sympathetic ganglia and no adverse effects in other organs or structures, opened an entirely new field of investigation and, at the same time, quite unexpectedly provided a new and most valuable tool to explore the effects of the NGF and its possible mechanism of action.

Previous investigations (Porter *et al.*, 1963) had shown that this dopamine analog produces a long-lasting depletion of norepinephrine storage in sympathetically innervated organs. Subsequent electronmicroscopic studies showed that this effect is due to the selective destruction of adrenergic synaptic vesicles by this agent (Thoenen and Tranzer, 1968; Tranzer and Thoenen, 1968; Malmfors and Thoenen, 1971). No lesions were detected in the cell perikarya. A time sequence study gave evidence for the reversibility of the damages inflicted by 6-OH-DA in the synaptic vesicles. Regeneration of these organelles takes place after discontinuation of the treatment and parallels the gradual and progressive restoration of function. Upon daily injection of 6-OH-DA in newborn mice and rats in the amount of 50 μg/g body weight for the first week of life, the immature sympathetic nerve cells in para- and prevertebral ganglia undergo progressive deterioration, clearly apparent at the light microscope 3 days after initiation of the treatment. In subsequent days, the degenerative processes extend to all nerve cells until, toward the end of the first week, practically all neurons show marked signs of alterations, whereas glial cells appear normal. Electron microscope studies of sympathetic ganglia at different time intervals during the first days after the beginning of treatment showed the precocity of cytoplasmic alterations called forth by 6-OH-DA. They consist of shrinking of mitochondria, appearance of large and numerous lacunar spaces, and disorganization of the endoplasmic reticulum. The cytoplasmic lesions precede the alterations in the fine structure in the nuclear compartment. The latter become apparent at later stages. At 7 days only few atrophic neurons and normal glial and connective cells are seen in most sections (P. U. Angeletti and Levi-Montalcini, 1970b). As in the case of immunosympathectomy, the process is irreversible and results in the production of animals entirely deprived of sympathetic function but otherwise comparable to controls in somatic development and vitality.

These results promoted an intensive search for possible noxious effects elicited by other adrenergic blocking agents. Almost at the same time, similar results were reported with another drug, guanethidine, from three laboratories (Burnstock *et al.*, 1971; L. Eränkö and O. Eränkö, 1971; O. Eränkö and L. Eränkö, 1971; P. U. Angeletti and Levi-Montalcini, 1972; P. U. Angeletti *et al.*, 1972a; Heath *et al.*, 1972). In newborn mice and rats, injections of guanethidine at doses of 20–30 μg/g of body weight call forth massive destruction of immature sympathetic neurons; the effects are of the same range and severity as those induced by AS-NGF and 6-OH-DA, but the intracellular localization of lesions produced by guanethidine are markedly different from those elicited by AS-NGF and 6-OH-DA. They are apparent at the EM toward the third day and increase progressively in severity and range in subsequent days. Dilation and rupture of mitochondria and widespread lesions of the endoplasmic reticulum are evident in almost all immature neurons between the third and fourth day of treatment. At 8 days practically no intact nerve cells are seen in any section, and the residual nerve cell population amounts to less than one-tenth that of controls. Dissection of ganglia at the end of the first month show that the ganglia are reduced to extremely small nodules comparable in size to those described in AS-NGF and 6-OH-DA-treated mice. At variance with the other treatments, guanethidine is much more effective in rats than in mice. Evidence was given by Burnstock *et al.* (1971) and L. Eränkö and O. Eränkö (1971) that guanethidine causes destruction not only of the immature, but also of fully differentiated, adrenergic neurons in adult rats.

A third drug, bretylium tosylate, tested in our laboratory, was also found to elicit selective degenerative effects in sympathetic adrenergic neurons, but, at variance with those elicited by AS-NGF, 6-OH-DA, and guanethidine, the lesions produced by this adrenergic neuron

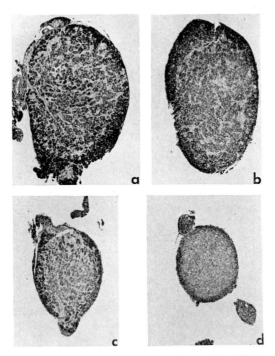

FIG. 2. Transverse sections through stellate sympathetic ganglia of 8-day-old littermate rats injected daily since birth with (a) NGF, (b) NGF and guanethidine, (c) saline, and (d) guanethidine. Note that no nerve cells are present in ganglion treated with guanethidine. All sections at ×80. (Unpublished photos by L. Aloe.)

blocking agent are retricted to the mitochondria and are, at least in part, reversible. The adrenergic cell population is only moderately reduced, and there is evidence for restoration to normality of surviving cells months after treatment (Caramia *et al.*, 1972).

INTERACTION BETWEEN NGF, GUANETHIDINE, AND 6-OH-DA

It was of interest to see whether NGF could prevent the toxic effects called forth by the two drugs guanethidine and 6-OH-DA. Preliminary experiments *in vitro* showed that the addition to the culture medium of 100–150 μg/ml of 6-OH-DA does not prevent the formation of the fibrillar halo from ganglia cultured in presence of 1–10 NGF BU. The same halo failed, however, to form if guanethidine was added to the culture medium at the concentration of 10 μg/ml. In spite of lack of nerve fiber outgrowth from ganglia cultured in presence of guanethidine and NGF, clearcut evidence for a "protective effect" exerted by NGF against the ganglion-blocking agent became apparent from histological studies of the same ganglia. While, in fact, nerve cells in ganglia cultured in a medium containing guanethidine undergo massive degeneration at the end of the first day of culture, the same cells in ganglia cultured in presence of guanethidine and 100 NGF BU are perfectly preserved and compare to those of NGF-treated ganglia.

These results suggested an investigation of the combined guanethidine and NGF treat-

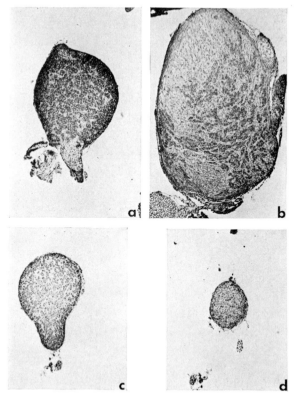

FIG. 3. Transverse sections through stellate sympathetic ganglia of 19-day-old littermate rats injected daily since birth with (a) NGF, (b) NGF and 6-OH-DA, (c) saline, and (d) 6-OH-DA. Axons surrounded by glial cells in upper and lower sections of ganglion (b). All sections at ×60. (Unpublished photos by L. Aloe.)

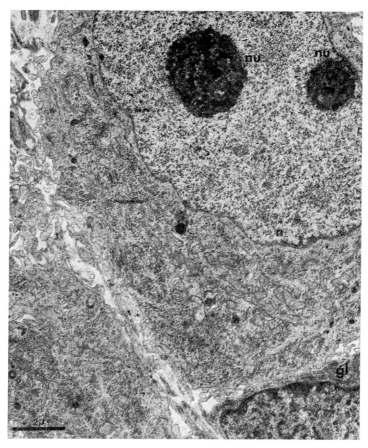

FIG. 4. Electron microscope of segment of a sympathetic neuron from superior cervical ganglion of 8-day-old rat injected since birth with NGF and guanethidine. All cell compartments are perfectly preserved. n, Nucleus, nu, nucleoli; gl, glial cell. (Unpublished photo by L. Aloe.)

ment and 6-OH-DA and NGF. The results are reported in detail in another publication Johnson and Aloe, submitted). Here we shall only mention that in both experimental series, sympathetic nerve cells were not only spared from destruction but underwent hypertrophy and hyperplastic effects. Figures 1c and 2 illustrate the results of these experiments.

A paradoxic effect was obtained with the combined NGF and 6-OH-DA treatment. As illustrated in Figs. 1d and 3, ganglia of rats injected with this drug and NGF and fixed at 20 days reach a size which is about three times larger than that of ganglia treated only with NGF. Observations at the dissecting microscope on specimens sacrificed at 6, 8, 12, and 19 days, show that the size difference between ganglia treated with NGF and NGF + 6-OH-DA increases progressively between the eighth and the nineteenth day. Histological studies provided the answer for such a paradoxic effect. It was, in fact, found that nerve cells in the combined treatment undergo hypertrophy of the same range, although more cells are present in the ganglia of the NGF-treated than in those of rats submitted to the combined treatment. The size difference, which is strikingly in favor of animals injected with NGF and 6-OH-DA, is due to an extraordinary increase in number and cross-section of postganglionic

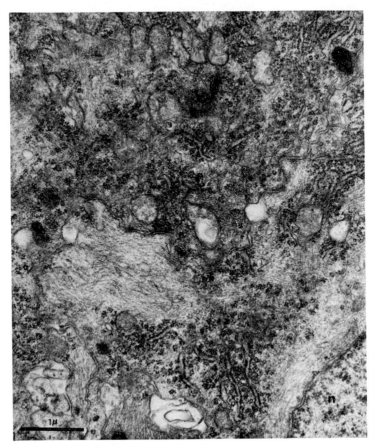

Fig. 5. Electron microscope of a sympathetic neuron from superior cervical ganglion of 19-day-old rat injected daily since birth with NGF and 6-OH-DA. Large neurofilament bundles are seen in the cell perikaryon. The endoplasmic reticulum is well preserved. n, Nucleus.

axons which force apart the nerve cells and fill all available space among neurons (Fig. 3b). Glial and satellite cells are also more numerous than in controls. No such increase in axons or in the glial cell population is instead apparent in sympathetic ganglia of guanethidine treated rats. No increase in glial cells occurs, however, in sympathetic ganglia of guanethidine treated rats (Fig. 2b). The hypertrophic and hyperplastic nerve cell population compares in size to that of NGF-treated littermates and appears even more densely packed than in the latter ganglia (Fig. 2a). One gets the impression that a normal or perhaps a subnormal quota of glial and satellite cells surrounds the neurons.

It is tempting to correlate these findings with the different mechanism of action of the two drugs. The dopamine analog accumulates in the storage vesicles of the adrenergic nerves and causes selective destruction of the end terminals of these fibers (Tranzer and Richards, 1971; Thoenen, 1971, 1972); guanethidine, although also gaining access into the synaptic adrenergic vesicles (Mitchell and Oates, 1970), does not produce such degenerative effects. Upon combined 6-OH-DA and NGF treatment, two opposite and conflicting processes set in. The growth-promoting factor enhances all metabolic processes and calls forth a tremendous increase in neurofibrillar material, as documented by their accumulation in the cell perikarya and in the increased axon diameter; 6-OH-DA, by destroying the adrenergic end terminals, blocks the efflux and influx processes related to the release and uptake of the neurotransmitter. The remarkable increase in number and size of post-ganglionic axons as well as the increase in glial and satellite cells populations may result from the highly aberrant condition in axonal flow along the adrenergic fibers. Brisk proliferation in perineuronal microgliacytes, has been described by many authors upon nerve fiber transection (Blinzinger and Kreutzberg, 1968; Torvik and Skjörten, 1971).

Ultrastructural studies of ganglia injected with guanethidine and NGF show that the cells at the end of the eighth day of treatment are well preserved and compare to those treated with the NGF alone. Figure 4 shows a segment of one of these cells. Likewise, sympathetic neurons in rats treated with 6-OH-DA and NGF are in excellent condition after 3 weeks of combined treatment, as illustrated in Fig. 5.

CONCLUDING REMARKS

Perhaps the most striking and unusual feature of this long search, which started more than two decades ago and is still in progress, is the continuous shift in the goal as well as in the methodological approach. Each new finding diverted the attention from the old to a new, more fundamental aspect of nerve cell growth and differentiation, and each discovery did not so much provide an answer to the question which promoted this quest as raise new questions which led into new areas of exploration and required a different approach. Thus the microbistoury of the neuroembryologist was discarded when biochemical, rather than morphological, information was of more immediate interest. When, in turn, the biochemical analysis proved to be insufficient, it was supplemented by techniques borrowed from immunological and pharmacological fields. In all phases of these studies, however, the structural and ultrastructural approach remained in the forefront and provided the unifying thread which held together the manifold facets of this everchanging and everbroadening investigation.

Today, as the barriers which prevented access into the central nervous system have broken down, thanks to the invaluable tool provided by histofluorescent techniques, again the structural approach will play a major role in the analysis of growth regulatory mechanisms of the central adrenergic neurons.

ACKNOWLEDGEMENTS

This work was supported in part by grants from the National Institute of Neurological Diseases and Stroke (NS-03777), from the National Science Foundation (GB-16330X), and from the North Atlantic Treaty Organization (449).

REFERENCES

ANGELETTI, P. U. (1972) Chemical sympathectomy in the newborn. In *Immunosympathectomy* (G. Steiner and E. Schönbaum, eds.), Elsevier, Amsterdam, pp. 237–250.

ANGELETTI, P. U., and LEVI-MONTALCINI, R. (1970a) Sympathetic nerve cell destruction in newborn mammals by 6-hydroxydopamine. *Proc. Natn. Acad. Sci. USA* **65**, 114–121.

ANGELETTI, P. U., and LEVI-MONTALCINI, R. (1970b) Specific cytotoxic effect of 6-hydroxydopamine on sympathetic neuroblasts. *Arch. ital. Biol.* **108**, 213–221.

ANGELETTI, P. U., and LEVI-MONTALCINI, R. (1972) Growth inhibition of sympathetic cells by some adrenergic blocking agents. *Proc. Natn. Acad. Sci. USA* **69**, 86–88.

ANGELETTI, P. U., LIUZZI, A., LEVI-MONTALCINI, R., and GANDINI-ATTARDI, D. G. (1964a) Effects of a nerve growth factor on glucose metabolism by sympathetic and sensory nerve cells. *Biochim. biophys. Acta* **90**, 445–450.

ANGELETTI, P. U., LIUZZI, A., and LEVI-MONTALCINI, R. (1964b) Stimulation of lipid biosynthesis in sympathetic and sensory ganglia by a specific nerve growth factor. *Biochim. biophys. Acta* **84**, 778–781.

ANGELETTI, P. U., GANDINI-ATTARDI, D., TOSCHI, G., SALVI, M. L., and LEVI-MONTALCINI, R. (1965) Metabolic aspects of the effect of nerve growth factor on sympathetic and sensory ganglia: protein and ribonucleic acid synthesis. *Biochim. biophys. Acta* **95**, 111–120.

ANGELETTI, P. U., LEVI-MONTALCINI, R., and CARAMIA, F. (1971) Analysis of the effects of the antiserum to the nerve growth factor in adult mice. *Brain Res.* **27**, 343–355.

ANGELETTI, P. U., LEVI-MONTALCINI, R., and CARAMIA, F. (1972a) Structural and ultrastructural changes in developing sympathetic ganglia induced by guanethidine. *Brain Res.* **43**, 515–525.

ANGELETTI, P. U., LEVI-MONTALCINI, R., and VIGNETI, E. (1972b) Localization of the nerve growth factor in subcellular fractions of peripheral tissues. In *Nerve Growth Factor and its Antiserum* (E. Zaimis and J. Knight, eds.), Athlone Press, London, pp. 39–45.

ANGELETTI, R. H. (1969) Nerve growth factor (NGF) from snake venom and mouse submaxillary gland: interaction with serum proteins. *Brain Res.* **12**, 234–237.

ANGELETTI, R. H., and BRADSHAW, R. A. (1971) Nerve growth factor from mouse submaxillary gland: amino acid sequence. *Proc. Natn. Acad. Sci. USA* **68**, 2417–2420.

ANGELETTI, R. H., BRADSHAW, R. A., and WADE, R. D. (1971) Subunit structure and amino acid composition of mouse submaxillary gland nerve growth factor. *Biochemistry* **10**, 463–469.

BERGER, B. D., WISE, C. D., and STEIN, L. (1973) Nerve growth factor: enhanced recovery of feeding after hypothalamic damage. *Science* **180**, 506–508.

BJÖRKLUND, A., and STENEVI, U. (1972) Nerve growth factor: stimulation of regenerative growth of central noradrenergic neurons. *Science* **175**, 1251–1253.

BLINZINGER, K., and KREUTZBERG, G. (1968) Displacement of synaptic terminals from regenerating motoneurons by microglial cells. *Z. Zellforsch.* **85**, 145–157.

BOCCHINI, V., and ANGELETTI, P. U. (1969) The nerve growth factor: purification as a 30,000 molecular weight protein. *Proc. Natn. Acad. Sci. USA* **64**, 787–794.

BUEKER, E. D. (1948) Implantation of tumors in the hind limb field of the embryonic chick and developmental response of the lumbosacral nervous system. *Anat. Record* **102**, 369–390.

BUEKER, E. D., SCHENKEIN, I., and BANE, J. L. (1960) The problem of a nerve growth factor specific for spinal and sympathetic ganglia. *Cancer Res.* **20**, 1220–1228.

BURNSTOCK, G., EVANS, B., GANNON, B. J., HEATH, J. W., and JAMES, V. (1971) A new method of destroying adrenergic nerves in adult animals using guanethidine. *Br. J. Pharmac.* **43**, 295–301.

CARAMIA, F., ANGELETTI, P. U., LEVI-MONTALCINI, R., and CARRATELLI, L. (1972) Mitochondrial lesions of developing sympathetic neurons induced by bretylium tosylate. *Brain Res.* **40**, 237–246.

COHEN, S. (1958) A nerve growth promoting protein. In *A Symposium on the Chemical Basis of Development* (W. D. McElroy and B. Glass, eds.), Johns Hopkins Press, Baltimore, pp. 665–667.

COHEN, S. (1959) Purification and metabolic effects of a nerve growth promoting protein from snake venom. *J. Biol. Chem.* **234**, 1129–1137.

COHEN, S. (1960) Purification of a nerve growth promoting protein from the mouse salivary gland and its neurocytotoxic antiserum. *Proc. Natn. Acad. Sci. USA* **46**, 302–311.

COHEN, S., and LEVI-MONTALCINI, R. (1956) A nerve growth stimulating factor isolated from snake venom. *Proc. Natn. Acad. Sci. USA* **42**, 571–574.

COHEN, S., LEVI-MONTALCINI, R., and HAMBURGER, V. (1954) A nerve growth stimulating factor isolated from sarcomas 37 and 180. *Proc. Natn. Acad. Sci. USA* **40**, 1014–1018.

DAHLSTRÖM, A., and FUXE, K. (1964a) A method for the demonstration of monoamine containing nerve fibres in the central nervous system. *Acta physiol. scand.* **60**, 293–295.

DAHLSTRÖM, A., and FUXE, K. (1964b) Evidence for the existence of monoamine containing neurons in the central nervous system: I, Demonstration of monoamines in the cell bodies of brain stem neurons. *Acta physiol. scand.* **62**, Suppl. 232, 1–55.

ERÄNKÖ, L., and ERÄNKÖ, O. (1971) Effect of guanethidine on nerve cells and small intensely fluorescent cells in sympathetic ganglia of newborn and adult rats. *Acta pharmac. tox.* **30**, 403–416.

ERÄNKÖ, O., and ERÄNKÖ, L. (1971) Histochemical evidence of chemical sympathectomy by guanethidine in newborn rats. *Histochem. J.* **3**, 451–456.

FALCK, B., HILLARP, N.-Å., THIEME, G., and TORP, A. (1962) Fluorescence of catecholamines and related compounds condensed with formaldehyde. *J. Histochem. Cytochem.* **10**, 348–354.

FUXE, K., HÖKFELT, T., JONSSON, G., and UNGERSTEDT, U. (1970) Fluorescence microscopy in neuroanatomy. In *Contemporary Research Methods in Neuroanatomy* (W. Nauta and S. Ebbesson, eds.), Springer, Berlin, pp. 275–314.

HEATH, J. W., EVANS, B. K., GANNON, B. J., BURNSTOCK, G., and JAMES, V. B. (1972) Degeneration of adrenergic neurons following guanethidine treatment: an ultrastructural study. *Virchows Arch.*, Abt. B, Zellpath. **11**, 182–197.

HIER, D. B., ARNASON, G. G. W., and YOUNG, M. (1972) Studies on the mechanism of action of nerve growth factor. *Proc. Natn. Acad. Sci. USA* **69**, 2268–2272.

JOHNSON, E. M., and ALOE, L. (submitted). Suppression of *in vitro* cytotoxic effects by guanethidine in sympathetic adrenergic neurons by the Nerve Growth Factor, *Brain Res.*

KLINGMAN, G. I., and KLINGMAN, J. D. (1972) Immunosympathectomy and biogenic amines. In *Immunosympathectomy* (G. Steiner and E. Schönbaum, eds.), Elsevier, Amsterdam, pp. 111–130.

LARRABEE, M. G. (1969) Metabolic effects of nerve impulses and nerve growth factor in sympathetic ganglia. *Progress in Brain Res.* **31**, 95–110.

LARRABEE, M. G. (1972) Metabolism during development in sympathetic ganglia of chickens: effects of age, nerve growth factor and metabolic inhibitors. In *Nerve Growth Factor and its Antiserum* (E. Zaimis and J. Knight, eds.), Athlone Press, London, pp. 71–88.

LEVI-MONTALCINI, R. (1952) Effects of mouse tumor transplantation on the nervous system. *Ann. N.Y. Acad. Sci.* **55**, 330–343.

LEVI-MONTALCINI, R. (1958) Chemical stimulation of nerve growth. In *A Symposium on the Chemical Basis of Development* (W. D. McElroy and B. Glass, eds.), Johns Hopkins Press, Baltimore, pp. 646–664.

LEVI-MONTALCINI, R. (1966) The nerve growth factor: its mode of action on sensory and sympathetic nerve cells. *Harvey Lect.*, Ser. 60, 217–259.

LEVI-MONTALCINI, R. and ANGELETTI, P. U. (1961) Biological properties of a nerve growth promoting protein and its antiserum. In *Regional Neurochemistry, Proc. 4th Intn. Neurochemical Symp.* (S. S. Kety and J. Elkes, eds.), Pergamon Press, New York, pp. 362–376.

LEVI-MONTALCINI, R., and ANGELETTI, P. U. (1963) Essential role of the nerve growth factor in the survival and maintenance of dissociated sensory and sympathetic nerve cells *in vitro*. *Devel. Biol.* **7**, 653–659.

LEVI-MONTALCINI, R., and ANGELETTI, P. U. (1968) Biological aspects of the nerve growth factor. In *Ciba Fdtn. Symp. on Growth of the Nervous System* (G. E. W. Wolstenholme and M. O'Connor, eds.), J. & A. Churchill, London, pp. 126–142.

LEVI-MONTALCINI, R., and ANGELETTI, P. U. (1970) Action of nerve growth factor on synthesis of neurofilaments and neurotubules in the target nerve cells. (Abstract) *Proc. Natn. Acad. Sci. USA* **67**, 7A.

LEVI-MONTALCINI, R., and ANGELETTI, P. U. (1971) Ultrastructure and metabolic studies on sensory and sympathetic nerve cells treated with the nerve growth factor and its antiserum. In *Hormones in Development* (M. Hamburgh and E. J. W. Barrington, eds.), Appleton–Century–Crofts, New York, pp. 719–730.

LEVI-MONTALCINI, R., and BOOKER, B. (1960) Destruction of the sympathetic ganglia in mammals by an antiserum to the nerve growth promoting factor. *Proc. Natn. Acad. Sci. USA* **42**, 384–391.

LEVI-MONTALCINI, R., MEYER, H., and HAMBURGER, V. (1954) *In-vitro* experiments on the effects of mouse sarcoma 180 and 37 on the spinal and sympathetic ganglia of the chick embryo. *Cancer Res.* **14**, 49–57.

LEVI-MONTALCINI, R., CARAMIA, F., LUSE, S. A., and ANGELETTI, P. U. (1968) *In vitro* effects of the nerve growth factor on the fine structure of the sensory nerve cells. *Brain Res.* **8**, 347–362.

LEVI-MONTALCINI, R., CARAMIA, F., and ANGELETTI, P. U. (1969) Alterations in the fine structure of nucleoli in sympathetic neurons following NGF-antiserum treatment. *Brain Res.* **12**, 54–73.

LEVI-MONTALCINI, R., ANGELETTI, R. H., and ANGELETTI, P. U. (1972) The nerve growth factor. In *Structure and Function of Nervous Tissue*, vol. 5 (G. H. Bourne, ed.), Academic Press, New York, pp. 1–38.

MALMFORS, T., and THOENEN, H., (eds.) (1971) 6-*Hydroxydopamine and Catecholamine Neurons*, North-Holland, Amsterdam, 368 pages.

MITCHELL, J. R. and OATES, J. A. (1970) Guanethidine and related agents. I. Mechanism of the selective blockade of adrenergic neurons and its antagonism by drugs. *J. Pharmac. Exp. Ther.* **172**, 100–107.

OLSON, L. (1967) Outgrowth of sympathetic adrenergic neurons in mice treated with a nerve growth factor. *Z. Zellforsch.* **81**, 155–173.

PÉREZ-POLO, J. R., BAMBURG, J. P., DE JONG, W. W. W., STRAUS, D., BAKER, M., and SHOOTER, E. M. (1972) Nerve growth factors of the mouse submaxillary gland. In *Nerve Growth Factor and its Antiserum* (E. Zaimis and J. Knight, eds.), Athlone Press, London, pp. 19–34.

PORTER, C. C., TOTARO, J. A., and STONE, C. A. (1963) Effect of 6-hydroxydopamine and some other compounds on the concentration of norepinephrine in the hearts of mice. *J. Pharmac. Exp. Ther.* **140**, 308–316.

SALVI, M. L., ANGELETTI, P. U., and FRATI, L. (1965) Frazionamento delle proteine solubili della ghiandola sottomascellare del topo: localizzazione di alcune componenti biologicamente attive. *Il Farmaco* **20**, 12–21.

THOENEN, H. (1971) Biochemical alterations induced by 6-hydroxydopamine in peripheral adrenergic neurons. In *6-Hydroxydopamine and Catecholamine Neurons* (T. Malmfors and H. Thoenen, eds.), North-Holland, Amsterdam, pp. 75–85.

THOENEN, H. (1972) Chemical sympathectomy: a new tool in the investigation of the physiology and pharmacology of peripheral and central adrenergic neurons. In *Perspectives in Neuropharmacology* (S. H. Snyder, ed.), Oxford University Press, New York, pp. 301–338.

THOENEN, H., and TRANZER, J. P. (1968) Chemical sympathectomy by selective destruction of adrenergic nerve endings with 6-hydroxydopamine. *Naunyn-Schmiedeberg's Arch. exp. Path. Pharmak.* **261**, 271–288.

THOENEN, H., ANGELETTI, P. U., LEVI-MONTALCINI, R., and KETTLER, R. (1971) Selective induction by nerve growth factor of tyrosine hydroxylase and dopamine-β-hydroxylase in the rat superior cervical ganglia. *Proc. Natn. Acad. Sci. USA* **68**, 1598–1602.

TORVIK, A., and SKJÖRTEN, F. (1971) Electron microscopic observations on nerve cell regeneration and degeneration after axon lesions: II, Changes in the glial cells. *Acta neuropath. Berl.* **17**, 265–282.

TRANZER, J. P., and RICHARDS, J. G. (1971) Fine structural aspects of the effect of 6-hydroxydopamine on peripheral adrenergic neurons. In *6-Hydroxydopamine and Catecholamine Neurons* (T. Malmfors and H. Thoenen, eds.), North-Holland, Amsterdam, pp. 15–31.

TRANZER, J. P., and THOENEN, H. (1968) An electron microscope study of selective, acute degeneration of sympathetic nerve terminals after administration of 6-hydroxydopamine. *Experientia* **24**, 155–156.

VARON, S., NOMURA, J., and SHOOTER, E. M. (1967) The isolation of the mouse nerve growth factor protein in a high molecular weight form. *Biochemistry* **6**, 2202–2209.

VOGT, M. (1964) Sources of noradrenaline in the "immunosympathectomized" rat. *Nature, Lond.* **204**, 1315–1316.

ZAIMIS, E. (1964) The immunosympathectomized animal: a valuable tool in physiological and pharmacological research. *J. Physiol.* **177**, 35–36.

ZANINI, A., ANGELETTI, P., and LEVI-MONTALCINI, R. (1968) Immunochemical properties of the nerve growth factor. *Proc. Natn. Acad. Sci. USA* **61**, 835–842.

REGULATION OF ENZYME SYNTHESIS BY NEURONAL ACTIVITY AND BY NERVE GROWTH FACTOR

H. Thoenen, I. A. Hendry, K. Stöckel, U. Paravicini, and F. Oesch

Department of Pharmacology, Biocenter of the University, Basel, Switzerland

SUMMARY

The synthesis of specific proteins in the terminal adrenergic neurons of rats and mice is regulated by the activity of the preganglionic cholinergic nerves and by the nerve growth factor (NGF) both during development and adult life. In adult animals an increased activity of the preganglionic cholinergic fibers results in an enhanced synthesis of tyrosine hydroxylase and dopamine-β-hydroxylase, whereas dopa decarboxylase, the third enzyme involved in the synthesis of norepinephrine, remains unchanged. There is good evidence that acetylcholine is the first messenger in this trans-synaptic induction of specific enzymes, whereas the identity of the second messenger, particularly the possible involvement of cyclic nucleotides, is not yet settled. NGF, a protein isolated from mouse salivary glands, produces in the sympathetic ganglia of newborn animals changes in the enzyme pattern which are very similar to those resulting from increased preganglionic activity in adult animals. For normal postnatal development of the terminal adrenergic neurons both the activity of the preganglionic cholinergic fibers and NGF is necessary. NGF is also essential for the maintenance of normal function in adult animals. This can be deduced from the fact that the decay of plasma NGF after removal of the submaxillary glands in mice is followed by a gradual decrease of all the enzymes involved in norepinephrine synthesis in superior cervical and stellate ganglia. However, although the submaxillary glands seem to be the major site of synthesis of NGF under normal physiological conditions, other tissues are also able to synthesize NGF and to take over this function of the salivary glands. Furthermore, it has been shown that NGF is accumulated in sympathetic ganglia and that it is transported retrogradely from the nerve terminals to the cell body. Whether NGF produces its effects essentially by this latter mechanism or rather by a direct action on the cell body, remains to be established.

INTRODUCTION

Until fairly recently the neuron was considered to be a relatively stable entity concerned with generating, transmitting, and modulating electrical impulses. Thus the main interest was focused on the electrical phenomena of neuronal activity and the underlying ionic events. Little attention was paid to the macromolecular cell constituents of the neuron and their investigation generally remained on the static-descriptive level.

However, in the last decade increasing experimental evidence has been accumulated indicating that the neurons, in spite of their nonproliferation and generally poor regeneration capabilities after completed development, have a high rate of protein turnover (cf. Richter,

315

1970) and an efficient transport system for macromolecules from the cell body (cf. Weiss, 1969; Davison, 1970; Ochs, 1971) to the periphery. This transport is essential for the functional integrity of the nerve terminals (Perišić and Cuénod, 1972) where transformation of electrical impulses into chemical messages takes place. Furthermore, it has been shown that the rate of synthesis of specific macromolecules is regulated by the activity of the neuron. This latter aspect is of particular interest, since it has been recognized that such mechanisms are involved in the long-term adaptation to increased transmitter utilization (cf. Molinoff and Axelrod, 1971; Thoenen and Oesch, 1973), in the regulation of ontogenetic processes (cf. Black et al., 1971a, b; Thoenen, 1972a), and possibly also in the long-term storage of information.

Investigations over the last few years have shown that the relatively simply organized peripheral sympathetic nervous system is a favorable object for such studies. An increased activity of the preganglionic cholinergic nerves produces in the adrenergic neurons an enhanced synthesis of specific enzymes involved in the formation of the adrenergic transmitter (cf. Molinoff and Axelrod, 1971; Thoenen, 1972b) while the total protein concentration is not measurably increased (Mueller et al., 1969a). Furthermore, it has been shown that the administration of nerve growth factor (NGF) produces changes in the enzyme pattern of newborn rats which are very similar to those resulting from increased preganglionic nerve activity in adult animals (Thoenen et al., 1971b). Thus the peripheral sympathetic nervous system offers the unique opportunity to study in the same neuron the trophic action of neuronal activity and the effect NGF, which is so far the only well-defined trophic factor (Levi-Montalcini and Angeletti, 1968) specifically influencing a given population of neurons. As a consequence of all these observations, a great number of interesting problems may now become experimentally amenable: specifically, the relationship between the functional state of the neuronal cell membrane and the regulation of the expression of the available genetic information, the question whether neuronally and NGF-mediated regulation of enzyme synthesis involves similar mechanisms, and to what extent NGF and the activity of the preganglionic cholinergic nerves are important for the development of the terminal adrenergic neurons and for the maintenance of their functional properties in adult life.

NEURONALLY MEDIATED INDUCTION OF ENZYMES INVOLVED IN THE SYNTHESIS OF NOREPINEPHRINE

An increased activity of peripheral and central adrenergic neurons resulting from electrical stimulation or increased reflex discharge is followed by an immediate increase in the synthesis of norepinephrine (NE) from tyrosine. This immediate adaptation is not accompanied by an increase in the in vitro activity of the enzymes involved in NE synthesis. The mechanism of this immediate adaptation is not fully elucidated, and various factors may be involved such as decreased endproduct inhibition of tyrosine hydroxylase (TH) and changes in the availability of pteridine cofactor possibly by activation of its reductase (cf. Weiner et al., 1972).

In addition to this immediate adaptation to increased transmitter utilization, a long-term adaptation comes into play after a prolonged increase in the activity of the sympathetic nervous system involving an increased in vitro activity of TH and dopamine-β-hydroxylase (DBH). The activity of the third enzyme engaged in NE synthesis, DOPA decarboxylase

(DDC), does not change indicating that the three enzymes involved in this metabolic pathway are not regulated as an operational unit (cf. Molinoff and Axelrod, 1971; Thoenen, 1972b). It is noteworthy that TH and DBH are exclusively located in adrenergic neurons and adrenal chromaffin cells, whereas DDC has a more ubiquitous distribution.

The increase in TH and DBH activity is neuronally mediated since it can be prevented by transecting the preganglionic cholinergic fibers (Thoenen et al., 1969; Molinoff et al., 1970) and by administration of ganglionic blocking agents (Mueller et al., 1970). The augmented enzyme activity is due to an increase in enzyme protein rather than the formation of activators or diminution of inhibitors, since the activity of enzyme preparations of controls and experimental animals is always additive, the K_m values remain unchanged, and the increase in enzyme activity can be abolished by administration of inhibitors of protein synthesis (Mueller et al., 1969a, b; Molinoff et al., 1972).

Since more than 95% of the NE liberated by nerve impulses from adrenergic neurons is synthesized in the nerve terminals (cf. Geffen and Livett, 1971), an increased amount of enzyme protein in the nerve endings rather than in the perikaryon is essential if the mechanism of trans-synaptic enzyme induction should be relevant as a long-term adaptation to increased transmitter utilization. Indeed, a proximo-distal transport of induced enzyme protein seems to take place since an increase of TH activity in the rat heart after administration of reserpine occurs about 24 h later than the corresponding increase in the stellate ganglia (Thoenen et al., 1970) which supply the heart with adrenergic fibers. Moreover, after administration of reserpine the induction of TH in the rat lumbar ganglia is followed by a gradual proximo-distal increase of enzyme activity in the sciatic nerve (Thoenen et al., 1970), in which a major part of the adrenergic fibers, originating in the lower lumbar ganglia, run to the periphery. In order to obtain an accurate determination of the net rate of transport of the enzymes involved in the synthesis of NE, we studied their rate of accumulation proximal to a ligature of the rat sciatic (Oesch et al., 1973). Since the rate of accumulation for all enzymes studied was linear for 9–12 h and since neither their level nor the degree of their inducibility by administration of reserpine changed within 48 h after ligation, this procedure seems to be reliable, and ligation of the axon does not seem to influence either the rate of axonal transport or the enzyme-synthetic properties of the perikaryon.

Interestingly, a good correlation between the subcellular distribution of the enzymes involved in NE synthesis and their rate of proximo-distal transport became apparent. DBH which is mainly localized in the particulate fraction of the rat sciatic was transported at the fastest rate, whereas DDC, exclusively located in the high speed supernatant, was transported at the slowest rate (Oesch et al., 1973).

FIRST AND SECOND MESSENGER OF TRANS-SYNAPTIC INDUCTION

The fact that trans-synaptic induction of TH can be prevented by administration of ganglionic blocking agents (Mueller et al., 1970) and that high doses of acetylcholine (Patrick and Kirschner, 1971) and carbachol (Guidotti and Costa, 1973) are able to mimic trans-synaptic induction in denervated adrenals, provides good evidence that acetylcholine acts as first messenger rather than another so far unknown trophic factor liberated from the preganglionic cholinergic nerves.

In view of the widespread function of adenosine 3′,5′-monophosphate (cyclic AMP) as a second messenger in many neurohumoral and hormonal systems (cf. Pastan and Perlman,

1971; Rall, 1972), this nucleotide was one of the most obvious candidates to look at as a possible mediator between the functional state of the neuronal membrane and the regulation of the expression of the available genetic information. The fact that dibutyryl cyclic AMP leads to an increased TH activity in mouse superior cervical ganglia in tissue culture (MacKay and Iversen, 1972) speaks in favor of this assumption. Moreover, the increased cyclic AMP levels in rabbit superior cervical ganglia after stimulation of the preganglionic cholinergic fibers (McAfee et al., 1971) could also be taken to indicate that cyclic AMP plays a role in trans-synaptic induction. It seems that the increased cyclic AMP levels are caused by dopamine which is liberated by acetylcholine from interneurons by a muscarinic mechanism and that the liberated dopamine then acts on the adrenergic neurons by an α-adrenergic mechanism (cf. Greengard and McAfee, 1972). That the increase in cyclic AMP takes place in the neuronal and not in the satellite cells has directly been demonstrated very recently by fluorescence immunocytochemical methods (Bloom, personal communication). However, the increased cyclic AMP levels in the rabbit superior cervical ganglion seem to be causally related to the slow inhibitory postsynaptic potential (Greengard and McAfee, 1972) and not to the nicotinic excitatory potential which, at least in rats, seems to be causally related to the *trans*-synaptic induction of TH and DBH (Mueller *et al.*, 1970, Molinoff *et al.*, 1970, 1972). Accordingly, the increase in cyclic AMP in the rabbit superior cervical ganglion can be blocked by atropine and phentolamine but not by hexamethonium (Greengard and McAfee, 1972). On the other hand, the nicotinic blocking agents pempidine and chlorisondamine effectively block the trans-synaptic induction of TH and DBH in the rat superior cervical ganglion, whereas atropine and phentolamine not only fail to block but even potentiate the trans-synaptic induction of TH resulting from swimming stress (Otten, unpublished results). Furthermore, in recent experiments it has been shown that swimming and cold stress, experimental conditions which lead to trans-synaptic induction of TH in the rat superior cervical ganglion, produce no changes in the level of cyclic AMP (Thoenen *et al.*, 1973).

The strongest argument in favor of a role for cyclic AMP as a second messenger in trans-synaptic induction, namely that dibutyryl cyclic AMP leads to an increase in TH activity in superior cervical ganglia kept in tissue culture, is considerably weakened by the recent finding that dibutyryl cyclic GMP also produces an increase in the *in vitro* activity of TH under the same experimental conditions (Goodman *et al.*, to be published). This latter observation, together with the increase in cyclic AMP in decentralized superior cervical ganglia of the rat, is of particular interest in view of the fact that in many systems the direct action of acetylcholine reduces the level of cyclic AMP and increases that of cyclic GMP (Lee *et al.*, 1972; George *et al.*, 1973). However, this increase of cyclic GMP seems to be mediated—according to the information available so far—by a muscarinic mechanism (Lee *et al.*, 1972).

In conclusion, the problem of the second messenger in the trans-synaptic induction of enzymes in the sympathetic ganglia, particularly the possible involvement of cyclic AMP and cyclic GMP is far from being settled and also in the adrenal medulla there is still a series of ambiguities which remain to be elucidated (Thoenen *et al.*, 1973).

RELATIONSHIP BETWEEN DURATION OF INCREASED NEURONAL ACTIVITY AND TIME REQUIREMENT FOR THE SINGLE STEPS OF ENZYME INDUCTION

After injecting rats with a single dose of reserpine, no consistent increase in adrenal and ganglionic TH activity could be observed earlier than 18 h after drug administration (Mueller *et al.*, 1969a). From these experimental data it could not be decided whether an increased neuronal activity over this whole time period was necessary or whether a relatively short period of increased firing would be sufficient with subsequent time consuming changes of enzyme synthesis at the transcription and/or translation level. To obtain more detailed information on these points, we exposed rats to an intense intermittent swimming stress at a water temperature of 15°C (Thoenen *et al.*, 1973). A swimming stress of 1 h (three swimming periods of 5–7 min) consistently produced a small increase in TH activity after 48 h in both sympathetic ganglia and adrenal medulla, although a statistically significant level was not always reached in the ganglia. However, a 2 h swimming stress (six swimming periods) regularly produced a statistically significant ($p < 0.05$) increase in TH activity in sympathetic ganglia and adrenals both after 24 and 48 h.

The increase in TH activity was completely abolished if actinomycin D was given immediately before or after the swimming stress and was very markedly reduced if given 6 h later. However, administration of actinomycin 12 h after the stress reduced the increase of TH by 30% only and had no effect at all if given after 24 h. Similar results were obtained by Patrick and Kirshner (1971) in the rat adrenal after TH induction by administration of insulin.

Thus it seems that the transcription step is terminated after 18–24 h, while the enhanced ribosomal synthesis of TH continues for a further 24–36 h (Otten *et al.*, 1973), indicating that the turnover of messenger RNA—either that of TH itself or that of a specific regulatory protein (Tomkins *et al.*, 1972)—is relatively slow.

EFFECT OF NGF ON THE ENZYMES INVOLVED IN THE SYNTHESIS OF NOREPINEPHRINE

The work of Levi-Montalcini and others has firmly established that the development of the major part of the sympathetic nervous system depends on NGF (cf. Levi-Montalcini and Angeletti, 1968).

If newborn rats and mice are treated with this protein, their sympathetic nervous system shows a very impressive acceleration of growth resulting from hyperplasia and hypertrophy of the adrenergic neurons. The biochemical correlates to these morphological changes revealed a quite impressive parallelism to the changes in the enzyme pattern occurring in adult animals after an increase in the activity of preganglionic cholinergic nerves (Thoenen *et al.*, 1971a, b). Besides the increase in monoamine oxidase and DDC activity which represents a manifestation of the general growth and which remained within the proportions of the increase in the total protein content, there was a very marked increase in the specific activity of TH and DBH. Although it cannot be excluded with certainty that part of the increase in the specific activity of TH and DBH results from an activation of the preganglionic cholinergic nerves (Angeletti *et al.*, 1972a), the majority of the effect arises from the direct action of NGF, since in decentralized ganglia of newborn rats NGF produces a marked increase in the specific activity of TH and DBH (Thoenen *et al.*, 1972b).

The similarity of the changes in the enzyme pattern produced by administration of NGF to newborn animals and the increased activity of the preganglionic cholinergic fibers in adults raises the question as to whether the specific induction of TH and DBH under these two experimental conditions is effected by a common mechanism or at least by mechanisms which converge to a common final step. This problem is under investigation but has not yet been settled.

RELATIVE IMPORTANCE OF NGF AND THE ACTIVITY OF PREGANGLIONIC CHOLINERGIC NERVES FOR THE DEVELOPMENT OF THE TERMINAL ADRENERGIC NEURONS

Black *et al.* (1971a, b) have shown that in the mouse superior cervical ganglion the number of synapses increases in parallel with the activity of choline acetyltransferase (CAT). Thus the level of this enzyme seems to be a reliable biochemical measure for the formation of synapses between the preganglionic cholinergic nerve endings and the terminal adrenergic neuron. Furthermore, it has been shown that in the postnatal development of the mouse superior cervical ganglion the increase in CAT activity precedes that of TH (Black *et al.*, 1971b), suggesting a relationship between the formation of synapses and the development of the rate-limiting enzyme of NE synthesis in the terminal adrenergic neurons.

Such a relationship was much less apparent in the rat superior cervical ganglion (Thoenen *et al.*, 1972a). There the specific activity of TH increased by only 40% and reached its maximum as early as 10–14 days after birth. In contrast, the much larger increase in CAT activity occurred mainly between 8 and 30 days after birth reaching the maximum of a fifteen-fold increase after 30 days (Fig. 1). While the specific activity of DDC did not change at all, the development of DBH showed some parallelism to that of CAT. However, the extent of the increase in specific activity of DBH was much smaller and the maximum activity was reached 10 days later than that of CAT.

From these findings it could be concluded that in the rat the activity of the preganglionic cholinergic nerves is of minor importance for the development of the terminal adrenergic neurons. However, since it cannot be excluded that the formation of a minimal number of synaptic contacts provides a prerequisite for the action of NGF, the effect of decentralization of the superior cervical ganglion was studied. The transection of the preganglionic cholinergic nerves in newborn animals reduced but did not block the developmental increase in TH, DBH, and DDC, whereby the increase in total activity was more impaired than that of the specific activity (Thoenen *et al.*, 1972b). However, the effect of NGF does not seem to depend on an intact preganglionic cholinergic innervation since TH and DBH revealed the same proportional increase in the intact and decentralized sides both with respect to specific and total activity. Thus it seems that both NGF and the activity of preganglionic cholinergic nerves are essential for the development of the terminal adrenergic neuron in the rat.

The formation of synapses and the activity of the preganglionic cholinergic fibers appear to be of greater importance for the postnatal development of terminal adrenergic neurons in mice than in rats (cf. Black *et al.*, 1971; Thoenen, 1972a). Moreover, this difference in the importance of preganglionic activity between the two species seems to hold not only for development but also for maintenance of a normal level of specific enzymes in adult animals. After decentralization of the superior cervical ganglion, the decay in TH activity is more rapid and more marked in mice than in rats (Hendry *et al.*, 1973). On the other

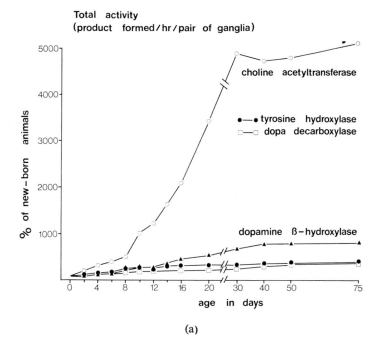

(a)

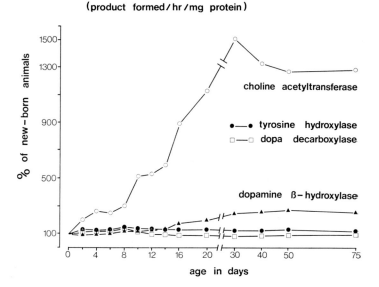

(b)

FIG. 1. Time course of the postnatal development of choline acetyltransferase and the enzymes involved in the synthesis of norepinephrine (according to Thoenen, 1972a). The changes in total (a) and specific (b) activities are expressed in percent of the values of newborn animals. The activity of choline acetyltransferase was determined according to Fonnum (1969), tyrosine hydroxylase according to Mueller *et al.* (1969a), DBH according to Molinoff *et al.* (1971), DOPA decarboxylase according to Håkanson and Owman (1966).

hand, the induction of TH in superior cervical ganglia after administration of reserpine is much smaller—if detectable at all—in mice than in rats (Hendry *et al.*, 1973).

Thus it appears that the normal activity of the preganglionic cholinergic neuron is higher in mice than in rats and that therefore a marked trans-synaptic induction of TH produced by an increase in the preganglionic nerve activity is only possible in rats where the basal level of preganglionic nerve activity is relatively low. Therefore the development of TH during maturation and the maintenance of normal levels of this enzyme in adult animals may depend in mice much more on the activity of the preganglionic cholinergic nerves than in rats.

IMPORTANCE OF NGF FOR THE SYMPATHETIC NERVOUS SYSTEM IN ADULT ANIMALS

PLASMA TURNOVER OF NGF

The removal of the submaxillary glands in adult mice causes a marked reduction in the level of circulating NGF (Hendry and Iversen, 1973). In male mice the plasma concentrations fell to 50% in about 9 days and reached a minimum of 15% of controls by day 33. Thereafter there was a fairly rapid recovery, and normal levels were reached again at 60 days after salivectomy. This rapid recovery took place in spite of any detectable regeneration of the submaxillary glands, indicating that after a certain period of adaptation other tissues become capable of taking over the synthesis of NGF normally accomplished by these glands. The question arises as to whether this initial rate of decay after salivectomy corresponds to the normal plasma turnover of NGF or whether this rate of decay is also influenced by the slowly adapting contribution of other tissues to the plasma NGF level. To answer this question we injected adult male mice with NGF and determined the rate of decay in the plasma. Since it is not clear whether plasma NGF is present in the form of the active β subunit (2.5 S NGF) or in the complex form of the α, β, and γ subunits (7 S NGF), we studied the rate of decay of both forms. As shown in Fig. 2, the half-time is the same for both the 7 S and the 2.5 S NGF. It could be assumed that the difference between the rate of decay of endogenous NGF after removal of the submaxillary glands and the rate of decay of injected NGF could result from a major contribution of the submaxillary gland to the catabolism of plasma NGF. However, preliminary experiments showed that the rate of decay of injected NGF in salivectomized animals did not markedly differ from that in intact controls.

Very recently, Angeletti *et al.*, (1972a) reported on a half-time of radioactive NGF which is considerably longer than that obtained in the present experiments with cold NGF, i.e. 110 versus 25 min. In a few experiments with I^{125} NGF we could confirm the much slower rate of decay of the radioactivity. However, if the determination of the decay rate was confined to the moiety of radioactivity which binds to specific NGF-antiserum bound to a solid phase, the rate of decay was much faster, i.e. very similar to the rate of decay of injected 2.5 or 7 S NGF. Thus it seems that after injection of labeled NGF a considerable part of the radioactivity represents degradation products and not active NGF.

The slow fall in plasma NGF after removal of the submaxillary glands may represent an initial inadequacy of other tissues to replace the synthesis of NGF normally accomplished by the submaxillary gland and to maintain a normal level of circulating NGF. Furthermore, it seems that the submaxillary glands are not only involved in the synthesis of NGF but that they also have a regulatory effect on NGF synthesis in other tissues and that full

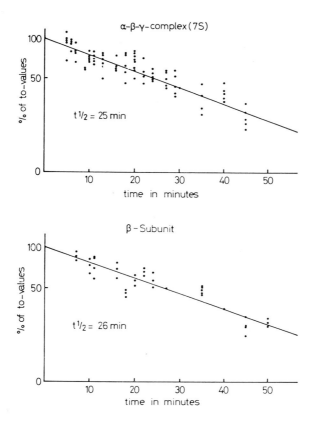

FIG. 2. Plasma half-time of intravenously injected nerve growth factor (NGF). Male albino mice of 30–35 g body weight were injected with 10 μg of 2.5 S (β subunit) or 7 S (complex of α, β, and γ subunit) NGF into the femoral vein. Starting 4 min after injection, blood samples of 10 μl were collected from the tail vein at different time intervals. NGF concentrations were determined by a radioimmunoassay as described by Hendry (1972). For each single animal the regression line was calculated by the method of least squares and the plasma concentration at zero time was determined by extrapolation. The values of the different experiments are expressed in terms of percent of the corresponding zero time values. The correlation coefficient amounts to $r = 0.959$ for 7 S NGF and to $r = 0.957$ for 2.5 S NGF.

compensation by these tissues, independent of the regulatory function of the submaxillary glands, does not occur earlier than 50–60 days after salivectomy.

EFFECT OF NGF ON THE ENZYME PATTERN OF SYMPATHETIC GANGLIA IN ADULT MICE

The fall in plasma NGF after salivectomy is followed with some delay by a fall in the NGF concentration of most tissues, including the sympathetic ganglia (Hendry and Iversen, 1973). This fall in tissue NGF is accompanied by a fall in the activity of TH in both the superior cervical and the stellate ganglia. In order to examine the specificity of this reduction, we determined the other enzymes involved in the synthesis of NE and CAT which is responsible for the synthesis of acetylcholine in the preganglionic cholinergic fibres. As shown in Fig. 3, the removal of the submaxillary glands resulted in a reduction of all the enzymes located in the adrenergic neurons. The fall in enzyme activity was accompanied by a reduction of the total protein content which is reflected by the relatively smaller changes in the specific activity of these enzymes. The effect on the presynaptically located CAT was much smaller and occurred with considerable delay. This delayed reduction of CAT activity may result from a retrograde trans-synaptic regulation which has been shown to occur in neonatal animals after destruction of the adrenergic neurons with 6-hydroxydopamine or NGF-antiserum (Black *et al.*, 1972; Thoenen, 1972a) or after increased growth of the adrenergic neurons by administration of NGF (Thoenen, 1972a).

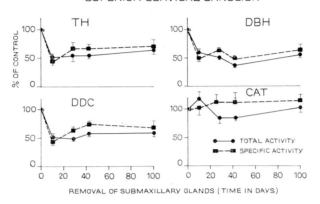

FIG. 3. Effect of salivectomy on the enzymes involved in the synthesis of norepinephrine and acetylcholine in the mouse superior cervical ganglion. In male mice of 30–35 g body weight, both submaxillary glands were removed under ether anesthesia. The animals were killed 10, 28, 42, and 100 days after salivectomy. In the superior cervical ganglion the enzymes involved in the synthesis of norepinephrine and acetylcholine were determined by the methods indicated in Fig. 1. The values of both total (activity/pair ganglia) and specific (activity/mg protein) activities are expressed in percent (mean ± SE) of intact controls.

The reduction of the enzymes involved in the synthesis of NE occurring after removal of the submaxillary glands could be reversed by administration of exogenous NGF (Fig. 4). In intact animals the injection of NGF resulted in an increase of all enzymes involved in NE synthesis above control levels together with an increase in total protein. From these results it can be concluded that NGF has a specific trophic effect on adrenergic neurons not only in neonatal but also in adult animals. Preliminary experiments have shown that removal of the submaxillary glands produces not only a reduction of the enzyme levels in the sympathetic ganglia of mice, but also of rats.

RETROGRADE TRANSPORT OF NGF

In previous experiments, Hendry and Iversen (1973) brought forward evidence that NGF might act on the adrenergic cell body as a retrograde trophic factor conveying information from the nerve terminals to the perikaryon.

The possibility of a retrograde transport of NGF was investigated by injecting I^{125} NGF into the anterior chamber of one eye in adult mice. The rate of accumulation of radio-activity in the superior cervical ganglia of injected and noninjected sides was determined

SUPERIOR CERVICAL GANGLIA

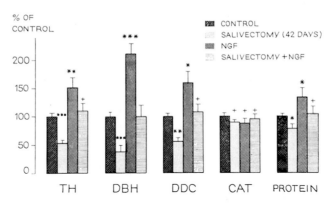

FIG. 4. Effect of nerve growth factor on the superior cervical ganglion of adult salivectomized and intact mice. Male albino mice of 30–35 g body weight were salivectomized under ether anesthesia. After 42 days, salivectomized and intact animals were treated for 4 days with 2.5 S NGF (50 μg/animal s.c.). 24 h after the last injection the animals were killed, the superior cervical ganglia removed and the enzymes involved in the synthesis of norepinephrine and acetylcholine were determined according to the methods indicated in Fig. 1. The values given are expressed in percent (mean $\pm$ SE) of intact untreated controls. *Differs from control $p < 0.05$. **Differs from control $p < 0.005$. ***Differs from control $p < 0.001$. †Does not differ from control $p > 0.1$.

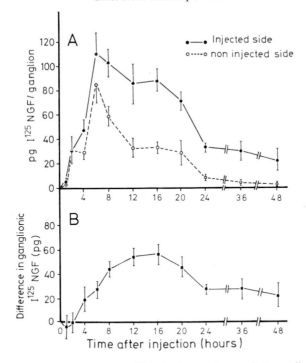

FIG. 5. Time course of accumulation of I^{125} NGF in superior cervical ganglia after unilateral intraocular injection. 0.25 μg of I^{125}-labeled 2.5 S NGF were injected in 2 μl of buffered (pH 7.4) saline into the anterior chamber of the left eye of adult Swiss albino mice weighing 30–35 g. The accumulation of radioactivity in both superior cervical ganglia was determined at different time intervals after injection, using a Packard gamma-counter. The determined radioactivity is expressed in terms of pg (mean $\pm$ SE) I^{125} NGF per ganglion.

and the difference between the two ganglia was taken as a measure of retrograde transport (Fig. 5). A difference between the two ganglia became apparent after 4 h and reached a maximum after 16 h. The distance between the nerve terminals in the iris and the superior cervical ganglion was estimated to be about 1 cm, and thus a retrograde transport of approximately 2.5 mm/h could be assumed. This rate of transport falls within the margins of the so-called rapid axonal transport described in other systems for ortho and retrograde transport (cf. Davison, 1970; Ochs, 1971; Geffen and Livett, 1971; Kristensson et al., 1971; la Vail and la Vail, 1972). The difference in the accumulation of radioactivity between the injected and noninjected sides was abolished by surgical transection of the postganglionic nerve trunk on the injected side. Furthermore, injection of colchicine prior to injection of I^{125} NGF also abolished the difference between injected and noninjected sides, indicating that the retrograde transport depends on intact neurotubules as does the orthograde rapid axonal transport. On the other hand, the destruction of the adrenergic nerve terminals with 6-hydroxydopamine (intraocular or systemic injection) did not impair the retrograde transport of I^{125} NGF, indicating that the resealed stumps or the preterminal parts of the axons are able to take up NGF. This could be of functional importance for the regeneration of adrenergic neurons.

ACKNOWLEDGEMENTS

This work was supported by the Swiss National Foundation for Scientific Research (Grant No. 3.653.71). I. A. Hendry was the recipient of a fellowship from the postgraduent medical foundation of Sydney University.

REFERENCES

ANGELETTI, P. U., LEVI-MONTALCINI, R., KETTLER, R., and THOENEN, H. (1972a) Comparative studies on the effect of nerve growth factor on sympathetic ganglia and adrenal medulla in newborn rats. Brain Res. 44, 197–206.

ANGELETTI, R. H., ANGELETTI, P. U., and LEVI-MONTALCINI, R. (1972b) Selective accumulation of I^{125} labelled nerve growth factor in sympathetic ganglia. Brain Res. 4, 421–425.

BLACK, I. B., BLOOM, F. E., HENDRY, I. A., and IVERSEN, L. L. (1971a) Growth and development of a sympathetic ganglion: maturation of transmitter enzymes and synapses formation in the mouse superior cervical ganglion. J. Physiol. Lond. 215, 24–25P.

BLACK, I. B., HENDRY, I. A., and IVERSEN, L. L. (1971b) Trans-synaptic regulation of growth and development of adrenergic neurons in a mouse sympathetic ganglion. Brain Res. 34, 229–240.

BLACK, I. B., HENDRY, I. A., and IVERSEN, L. L. (1972) The role of post-synaptic neurones in the biochemical maturation of presynaptic cholinergic nerve terminals in the mouse sympathetic ganglion. J. Physiol. 221, 149–159.

DAVISON, P. F. (1970) Axoplasmic transport: physical and chemical aspects. The Neurosciences: Second Study Program (F. O. Schmitt, ed.), The Rockefeller University Press, New York, pp. 851–857.

FONNUM, F. (1969) Radiochemical microassay for the determination of choline acetyltransferase and acetylcholinesterase activities. Biochem. J. 115, 465–472.

GEFFEN, L. B., and LIVETT, B. G. (1971) Synaptic vesicles in sympathetic nerves. Physiol. Rev. 51, 98–157.

GEORGE, W. J., WILKERSON, R. D., and KADOWITZ, PH. J. (1973) Influence of acetylcholine on contractile force and cyclic nucleotide levels in the isolated perfused rat heart. J. Pharmac. Exp. Ther. 184, 228–235.

GREENGARD, P., and McAFEE, D. A. (1972) Adenosine 3':5'-cyclic monophosphate as a mediator in the action of neurohumoral agents. Biochem. Soc. Symp. 36, 87–102.

GUIDOTTI, A., and COSTA, E. (1973) Involvement of adenosine 3',5'-monophosphate in the activation of tyrosine hydroxylase elicited by drugs. Science 179, 902–904.

HÅKANSON, R., and OWMAN, CH. (1966) Pineal dopa decarboxylase and monoamine oxidase activities as related to the monoamine stores. J. Neurochem. 13, 597–605.

HENDRY, I. A. (1972) Developmental changes in tissue and plasma concentrations of the biologically active species of nerve growth factor in the mouse, by using a two-site radioimmunoassay. Biochem. J. 128, 1265–1272.

HENDRY, I. A., and IVERSEN, L. L. (1973) Changes in tissue and plasma concentrations of nerve growth factor following removal of the submaxillary glands in adult mice and their effects on the sympathetic nervous system. Nature 243, 500–504.

HENDRY, I. A., IVERSEN, L. L., and BLACK, I. B. (1973) A comparison of the neural regulation of tyrosine hydroxylase activity in sympathetic ganglia of adult mice and rats. *J. Neurochem.* **20**, 1683–1689.

KRISTENSSON, K., OLSSON, Y., and SJÖSTRAND, J. (1971) Axonal uptake and retrograde transport of exogenous proteins in the hypoglossal nerve. *Brain Res.* **32**, 399–406.

LA VAIL, J. M. and LA VAIL, M. M. (1972) Retrograde axonal transport in the central nervous system. *Science* **176**, 1416–1417.

LEE, T. P., KUO, J. F., and GREENGARD, P. (1972) Role of muscarinic cholinergic receptors in regulation of guanosine 3′:5′-cyclic monophosphate content in mammalian brain, heart muscle and intestinal smooth muscle. *Proc. Natn. Acad. Sci. USA* **69**, 3287–3291.

LEVI-MONTALCINI, R., and ANGELETTI, P. U. (1968) The nerve growth factor. *Physiol. Rev.* **48**, 534–569.

MCAFEE, D. A., and GREENGARD, P. (1972) Adenosine 3′,5′-monophosphate: Electrophysiological evidence for a role in synaptic transmission. *Science* **178**, 310–312.

MCAFEE, D. A., SCHORDERET, M., and GREENGARD, P. (1971) Adenosine 3′,5′-monophosphate in nervous tissue: increase associated with synaptic transmission. *Science* **171**, 1156–1158.

MACKAY, A. V. P., and IVERSEN, L. L. (1972) Increased tyrosine hydroxylase activity of sympathetic ganglia cultured in the presence of dibutyryl cyclic AMP. *Brain Res.* **48**, 424–426.

MOLINOFF, P. B., and AXELROD, J. (1971) Biochemistry of catecholamines. *A. Rev. Biochem.* **40**, 465–500.

MOLINOFF, P. B., BRIMIJOIN, S., WEINSHILBOUM, R., and AXELROD, J. (1970) Neurally mediated increase in dopamine β-hydroxylase activity. *Proc. Natn. Acad. Sci. USA* **66**, 453–458.

MOLINOFF, P. B., WEINSHILBOUM, R., and AXELROD, J. (1971) A sensitive enzyme assay for dopamine β-hydroxylase. *J. Pharmac. Exp. Ther.* **178**, 425–431.

MOLINOFF, P. B., BRIMIJOIN, S., and AXELROD, J. (1972) Induction of dopamine β-hydroxylase in rat hearts and sympathetic ganglia. *J. Pharmac. Exp. Ther.* **182**, 116–129.

MUELLER, R. A., THOENEN, H., and AXELROD, J. (1969a) Increase in tyrosine hydroxylase activity after reserpine administration. *J. Pharmac. Exp. Ther.* **169**, 74–79.

MUELLER, R. A., THOENEN, H., and AXELROD, J. (1969b) Inhibition of trans-synaptically increased tyrosine hydroxylase activity by cycloheximide and actinomycin D. *Molec. Pharmac.* **5**, 463–469.

MUELLER, R. A., THOENEN, H., and AXELROD, J. (1970) Inhibition of neuronally induced tyrosine hydroxylase by nicotinic receptor blockade. *Eur. J. Pharmac.* **10**, 51–56.

OCHS, S. (1971) Characteristics and a model for fast axoplasmic transport in nerve. *J. Neurobiol.* **2**, 331–345.

OESCH, F., OTTEN, U., and THOENEN, H. (1973) Relationship between the rate of axoplasmic transport and subcellular distribution of enzymes involved in the synthesis of norepinephrine. *J. Neurochem.* **20**, 1691–1706.

OTTEN, U., PARAVICINI, U., OESCH, F., and THOENEN, H. (1973) Tyrosine hydroxylase induction: time requirement for completion of transcription. *Experientia* **29**, 765.

PASTAN, I., and PERLMAN, R. L. (1971) Cyclic AMP in metabolism. *Nature,* **229**, 5–9.

PATRICK, R. L., and KIRSHNER, N. (1971) Effect of stimulation on levels of tyrosine hydroxylase, dopamine β-hydroxylase and catecholamine in intact and denervated rat adrenal glands. *Molec. Pharmac.* **7**, 87–96.

PERIŠIĆ, M., and CÚENOD, M. (1972) Synaptic transmission depressed by colchicine blockade of axoplasmic flow. *Science* **175**, 1140–1142.

RALL, TH. W. (1972) Role of adenosine 3′,5′-monophosphate (cyclic AMP) in actions of catecholamines. *Pharmac. Rev.* **24**, 399–409.

RICHTER, D. (1970) Protein metabolism and functional activity. In *Protein Metabolism of the Nervous System* (Lajtha, ed.), Plenum Press, New York and London, pp. 241–258.

THOENEN, H. (1972a) Comparison between the effect of neuronal activity and nerve growth factor on enzymes involved in the synthesis of norepinephrine. *Pharmac. Rev.* **24**, 255–267.

THOENEN, H. (1972b) Neuronally mediated enzyme induction in adrenergic neurons and adrenal chromaffin cells. *Biochem. Soc. Symp.* **36**, 3–15.

THOENEN, H., and OESCH, F. (1973) New enzyme synthesis as a long-term adaptation to increased transmitter utilization. In *New Concepts in Neurotransmitter Regulation* (A. J. Mandell, ed.), Plenum, New York, pp. 33–52.

THOENEN, H., MUELLER, R. A., and AXELROD, J. (1969) Increased tyrosine hydroxylase activity after drug-induced alteration of sympathetic transmission. *Nature* **221**, 1264.

THOENEN, H., MUELLER, R. A., and AXELROD, J. (1970) Phase difference in the induction of tyrosine hydroxylase in cell body and nerve terminals of sympathetic neurons. *Proc. Natn. Acad. Sci. USA* **66**, 58–62.

THOENEN, H., KETTLER, R., BURKARD, W., and SANER, A. (1971a) Neuronally mediated control of enzymes involved in the synthesis of norepinephrine: are they regulated as an operational unit? *Naunyn Schmiedeberg's Arch. exp. Path. Pharmak.* **270**, 146–160.

THOENEN, H., ANGELETTI, P. U., LEVI-MONTALCINI, R., and KETTLER, R. (1971b) Selective induction by nerve growth factor of tyrosine hydroxylase and dopamine β-hydroxylase in the rat superior cervical ganglia. *Proc. Natn. Acad. Sci. USA* **68**, 1598–1602.

THOENEN, H., KETTLER, R. and SANER, A. (1972a) Time course of the development of enzymes involved in the synthesis of norepinephrine in the superior cervical ganglion of the rat from birth to adult life. *Brain Res.* **40**, 459–468.

THOENEN, H., SANER, A., KETTLER, R., and ANGELETTI, P. U. (1972b) Nerve growth factor and preganglionic cholinergic nerves: their relative importance to the development of the terminal adrenergic neuron. *Brain Res.* **44**, 593–602.

THOENEN, H., OTTEN, U., and OESCH, F. (1973) Trans-synaptic regulation of tyrosine hydroxylase. In *Frontiers in Catecholamine Research*, Pergamon Press, in press.

TOMKINS, G. M., LEVINSON, B. B., BAXTER, J. D., and DETTILEFSEN, L. (1972) Further evidence for post-transcriptional control of inducible tyrosine aminotransferase synthesis in cultured hepatoma cells. *Nature*, **239**, 9–14.

WEINER, N., CLOUTIER, G., BJUR, R., and PFEFFER, R. I. (1972) Modification of norepinephrine synthesis in intact tissue by drugs and during short-term adrenergic nerve stimulation. *Pharmac. Rev.* **24**, 203–221.

WEISS, P. A. (1969) Neuronal dynamics and neuroplasmic ("axonal") flow. *Symp. Int. Soc. Cell Biol.* **8**, 3–34.

ASSAY OF NERVE GROWTH FACTOR (NGF) IN MOUSE TISSUE AND THE ROLE OF NGF AND DEPOLARIZING STIMULI IN THE LONG-TERM REGULATION OF TYROSINE HYDROXYLASE ACTIVITY IN ADRENERGIC NEURONS

L. L. Iversen, I. A. Hendry, and A. V. P. Mackay

MRC Neurochemical Pharmacology Unit, Department of Pharmacology, University of Cambridge, Cambridge, England

SUMMARY

A two-site radioimmunoassay for the biologically active β-subunit of mouse salivary gland nerve growth factor (NGF) is described. Using this assay, it has been confirmed that the NGF content of mouse submaxillary glands is under endocrine control, particularly by circulating testosterone. The plasma concentration of NGF is higher in male mice than in females, and the changes in plasma concentrations of NGF during development parallel those occurring in the submaxillary glands in which a sex difference becomes apparent only after puberty. The only other tissue to show a sex difference in NGF content was the superior cervical ganglion. Plasma and tissue concentrations of NGF declined markedly after surgical removal of both submaxillary glands and after castration in male animals. The reduced tissue levels of NGF were accompanied by falls in tyrosine hydroxylase activity of superior cervical and stellate ganglia. After sialectomy there was a gradual recovery in plasma and tissue NGF contents, not accompanied by regeneration of NGF stores in the salivary glands.

Treatment of neonatal mice with NGF caused increases in the size, cell population, and tyrosine hydroxylase activity in superior cervical ganglia. The latter change was reversible if NGF treatment was discontinued. NGF administration could not abolish the inhibition of development of sympathetic ganglia caused by surgical decentralization or by ganglion blocking drugs in neonatal animals. Antisera to NGF caused a dose-dependent decrease in tyrosine hydroxylase activity in sympathetic ganglia, and antisera with high complement-fixing activity were found to be most effective in causing immunosympathectomy.

In superior cervical ganglia maintained in organ culture for up to 48 h there was a loss of approximately 40% of tyrosine hydroxylase activity and approximately 40% of ganglion cells. The cultured ganglia responded to added NGF by increased cell survival and increased tyrosine hydroxylase activity, the effects of NGF being most marked in ganglia from 6-day-old mice and less prominent in ganglia from neonatal rats or from adult mice. Addition of high potassium concentrations (54 mM) to neonatal or adult mice ganglia induced increases of up to 100% in ganglionic tyrosine hydroxylase activity. Another depolarizing stimulus, ouabain (1 mM), also had similar effects. In each case the rise in enzyme activity could be blocked by addition of cycloheximide to the culture medium. The induction of tyrosine hydroxylase by high potassium was not related to concomitant changes in ganglionic noradrenaline content, since enzyme induction occurred to a similar extent with increased, decreased, or unaltered noradrenaline content. The effects of high potassium could be enhanced by the addition of theophylline to the culture medium, and mimicked by dibutyryl cyclic AMP or dibutyryl cyclic GMP, suggesting a possible involvement of cyclic nucleotides in the control of enzyme synthesis. Studies with the antibiotics cycloheximide, actinomycin D, anisomycin, and sparsomycin suggested that tyrosine hydroxylase synthesis may be controlled by a post-transcriptional regulation system similar to that described in other mammalian cells.

I. INTRODUCTION

The discovery of the nerve growth factor (NGF) and the unique activity of this protein in stimulating the growth of adrenergic and sensory neurons has stimulated numerous studies of the possible biological role of NGF in controlling the development and differentiation of such neurons (for review, see Levi-Montalcini and Angeletti, 1968; Angeletti et al., 1968; Zaimis and Knight, 1972; Levi-Montalcini, a preceding chapter). In recent years, interest has also focused on the trans-synaptic control by nerve activity of the synthesis of transmitter-related enzymes in mature adrenergic neurons (for review, see Thoenen, 1972). In our laboratory we have obtained evidence that neural activity may also play a role in the trans-synaptic control of the biochemical specialization of adrenergic neurons during development (Black et al., 1971; Black, this volume). We have also examined the interaction between NGF and trans-synaptic influences in controlling the development and plasticity of adrenergic neurons, both in vivo and in isolated sympathetic ganglia maintained in organ culture, and this work will be reviewed briefly here.

II. ASSAY OF NGF IN MOUSE TISSUES

1. RADIOIMMUNOASSAY PROCEDURE

One of the difficulties in studying the possible biological functions of NGF stems from the problems encountered in assaying the very small amounts of this protein normally present in most animal tissues or body fluids. Most assay methods have hitherto been based on a bioassay, using the fibre outgrowth response of chick sensory ganglia in tissue culture as the test system (Cohen, 1960; Angeletti et al., 1968; Fenton, 1970). Hendry (1972) has accordingly developed a radioimmunoassay procedure for NGF which is both simpler and requires less material for assay than the tissue culture methods.

The immunoassay is designed to measure the biologically active-β-subunit of mouse submaxillary gland NGF; the β-subunit is measured whether present in free form, or in association with α- and γ-subunits in the 7 S molecule (Varon et al., 1967, 1968). The principle of the assay is outlined in Fig. 1. The reaction is carried out in two stages. The first stage involves incubation of the sample containing NGF with an immunoadsorbent paper (containing covalently bound NGF antibodies). Any NGF in the solution will bind to the paper during the 12–16 h incubation, and the paper can then be washed free of contaminating proteins. The paper is incubated, in the second stage of the reaction, with purified ^{125}I-labelled NGF antibodies (prepared by immunoadsorption to an NGF solid phase adsorbent). NGF bound to the paper will bind labelled antibodies to a second antigenic site on the molecule, hence the term "two-site assay" used to describe this type of radioimmunoassay (Addison and Hales, 1971). The amount of bound radioactivity on the papers is determined by liquid scintillation counting, and is linearly related to the amount of NGF in the assay samples in the range 0.25–5.00 ng.

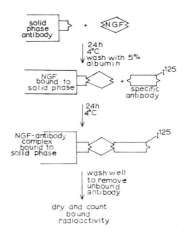

FIG. 1. Outline of protocol for two site immunoassay of β-subunit of NGF.

Values obtained with this assay for NGF content of various adult mouse tissues agreed well with those previously reported (Table 1) (Hendry, 1972). Mouse submaxillary glands have a very high NGF content compared with any other tissues. The concentrations of NGF in submaxillary glands are controlled by circulating sex hormones; there is marked difference in the concentration in adult male and female animals (Table 2). Castration reduces the NGF concentration in both male and female animals to very low levels, which can be restored to near normal male values by testosterone treatment (Lyon *et al.*, 1973). The NGF content of submaxillary glands is very low in infant mice, and there is no sex-related difference; this appears only after puberty (between 21–28 days after birth) (Table 2).

TABLE 1. CONCENTRATIONS OF β-NGF IN VARIOUS ORGANS OF THE ADULT MOUSE

Tissue	β-NGF (ng/mg wet weight)	
	Male	Female
Superior cervical ganglion[a]	0.41 ± 0.07	0.15 ± 0.02
Diaphragm	0.41 ± 0.06	0.42 ± 0.05
Uterus	—	0.27 ± 0.01
Vas deferens	0.36 ± 0.04	—
Adrenal	0.25 ± 0.02	0.37 ± 0.06
Heart	0.28 ± 0.04	0.26 ± 0.06
Kidney	0.17 ± 0.02	0.19 ± 0.01
Spleen	0.18 ± 0.01	0.16 ± 0.02
Liver	0.10 ± 0.02	0.12 ± 0.02
Spinal cord	0.12 ± 0.01	0.13 ± 0.01
Brain	0.09 ± 0.02	0.08 ± 0.01

The results are expressed as the mean values ± SEM for five animals in each group. The assay was performed using a 16 h incubation for the first stage and a 6 h incubation in the second stage.

[a] Values as ng β-NGF per ganglion, four ganglia pooled for each assay. Data from Hendry (1972).

TABLE 2. CHANGES WITH AGE and ENDOCRINE STATE OF β-NGF CONTENT OF MOUSE SUBMAXILLARY GLAND

Age (days)	β-NGF (ng/mg)		
	Male	Both sexes combined	Female
5		1.0 ± 0.14	
10		0.4 ± 0.10	
21	4.8 ± 0.35		2.2 ± 0.17*
28	17.2 ± 1.6		10.8 ± 0.8*
60+	404.0 ± 50.30		51.0 ± 3.30*
60+ after gonadectomy	36.0 ± 1.7 (2)		17.0 ± 5.3 (2)
60+ castrated treated testosterone	335.0 ± 60.1 (2)		—
60+ normal female treated testosterone			544.0 ± 73.5

Values are means ± SEM of 6–8 animals except for some values from groups of 2 animals (indicated with parentheses). Gonadectomy was performed 60 days previously, and testosterone-treated animals received daily injections of 0.5 mg of the hormone for 7 weeks prior to assay. Data from Hendry (1972) and Lyon *et al.* (1973).

* Differs significantly from male ($p < 0.001$).

NGF could be detected in small amounts in the plasma of newborn mice. There was a decrease in plasma NGF concentrations during the first 2 weeks of life followed by a progressive increase to adult values (Fig. 2). The plasma concentrations after 3 weeks paralleled the development of NGF content in submaxillary glands with a marked difference between adult male and female values. The only other tissues to show a sex-related difference in NGF content, however, was the superior cervical ganglion (Table 1), which contained a relatively high concentration in both male and female animals (approximately 1–2 ng/mg) when compared with other tissues (0.08–0.42 ng/mg). The values obtained in our laboratory agree well, with some exceptions, with results reported using a radioimmunoassay which

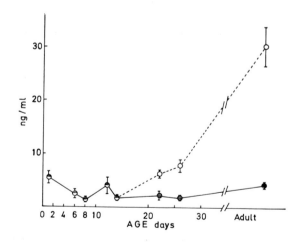

FIG. 2. Changes in the content of β-NGF in mouse plasma with age. Values are means ± SEM for 4–6 determinations; for animals less than 8 days old plasma was pooled to give 250 μl of plasma for each determination. Open circles = male animals; filled circles = female animals; half-filled circles pooled values from male and female animals, which were not significantly different before 20 days of age.

measures the 7 S form of NGF (Johnson *et al.*, 1971) and with results obtained previously using a bioassay procedure (Cohen, 1960). We believe, however, that the two-site radio-immunoassay procedure for NGF has advantages over these and other previously described techniques. Since the present assay is directed against the active β-subunit of NGF there is no possibility of spurious results being obtained by the possible presence of excess amounts of the inactive α- and γ-subunits in plasma or tissues. The requirement for two antigenic sites in this assay also increases the immunochemical specificity of the technique.

2. CHANGES IN TISSUE NGF CONCENTRATION AFTER SUBMAXILLARY GLAND REMOVAL AND CASTRATION

Further experiments were designed in an attempt to determine the sources of NGF in peripheral tissues and plasma. The changes in plasma NGF concentration after puberty appear to parallel those occurring in the salivary glands, suggesting that circulating NGF

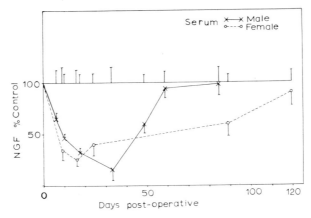

FIG. 3. Effects of removal of both submaxillary glands on the plasma concentrations of β-NGF in adult mice. Results expressed as mean values $\pm$ SEM for groups of 4–6 mice. Control values (100%) were 2.6 $\pm$ 0.63 ng/ml for female animals and 11.5 $\pm$ 0.38 ng/ml for males.

might originate in the latter tissue. At birth, however, the plasma concentrations of NGF are relatively high when compared with the low concentration present in neonatal sub-maxillary glands. The plasma concentration of NGF also decreased during the first 2 weeks after birth. Hendry (1972) thus speculated that circulating NGF in foetal and neonatal animals might represent material derived largely by trans-placental transfer from the maternal circulation. NGF concentrations in the plasma of female animals increase significantly as a consequence of endocrine changes during pregnancy, and preliminary experiments showed that ^{125}I-labelled NGF penetrated readily into the foetus after intravenous administration to pregnant animals. It has proved difficult, so far, however, to test this hypothesis. It was found to be impossible to obtain an adequate survival rate in neonatal mice subjected to bilateral sialectomy. Attempts to examine the effects of lowering the maternal plasma concentrations of NGF by sialectomy (see below) have also proved unsuccessful because this operation produced a temporary infertility in adult female mice.

In adult animals, however, removal of the submaxillary glands did cause a marked reduction in plasma concentrations of NGF (Fig. 3). In male animals plasma NGF fell with a half-time of approximately 9 days to a minimum of 15% of normal values after 33 days. After this there was a fairly rapid recovery to normal plasma concentrations, which were attained by 60 days postoperatively. In adult females, NGF in plasma also fell, with a half-time of about 6.5 days, reaching a minimum value of approximately 25% of normal and again recovering, rather slowly, to reach normal values after 120 days. The return to normal plasma levels of NGF occurred in the absence of any significant regeneration of the NGF stores in the remaining salivary glands or in the scar tissue around the site of removal of the submaxillary glands (Hendry and Iversen, 1973). The source of NGF in plasma during this unexpected recovery phase remains unknown. Whatever the nature of the cellular sites responsible, they are clearly responsive to circulating sex hormones, since in both males and females plasma NGF concentrations returned to values similar to those found in normal animals, with a persistent sex difference. Because of the difference in plasma concentrations

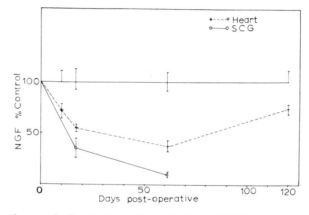

FIG. 4. Effects of removal of both submaxillary glands on β-NGF concentrations in heart and superior cervical ganglia of adult female mice. Values are means ± SEM for groups of 6 animals and are expressed as percentages of control values (0.26 ± 0.09 ng/mg for heart and 0.05 ± 0.012 ng per ganglion).

in normal animals, the absolute values of NGF in plasma at the minima following sialectomy were similar. These results suggest that circulating NGF may derive normally from the submaxillary gland stores, but that under certain conditions other source tissues may take over this role. Alternatively, the submaxillary glands may normally exert a trophic influence on the NGF source tissues from which circulating NGF is derived, a point which is discussed in more detail by Thoenen et al., in this volume.

The fall in plasma concentrations of NGF in both male and female animals after sialectomy was accompanied by a temporary reduction in the concentration of NGF in the heart and in superior cervical ganglia (Fig. 4), suggesting that these in turn may derive some or all of their NGF content from the circulation. The reduced availability of NGF in the tissues and plasma was also accompanied by a reduction in the activity of tyrosine hydroxylase (T-OH) in superior cervical and stellate sympathetic ganglia, this also recovered to normal when plasma and tissue concentrations of NGF were restored (Hendry and Iversen, 1973). This phenomenon is described in more detail in the accompanying article by Thoenen et al.

Castration of adult male mice also led to a marked reduction in plasma and tissue

TABLE 3. EFFECTS OF CASTRATION ON NGF AND TYROSINE HYDROXYLASE IN MOUSE TISSUES

	n	Control	Castrated
NGF concentration:			
Submaxillary glands	4	100 ± 29.9	7.8 ± 0.4**
Plasma	6	100 ± 12.0	40.0 ± 8.0***
Heart	6	100 ± 19.0	5.0 ± 1.0***
Tyrosine hydroxylase activity:			
Superior cervical ganglia	6	100 ± 7.0	67.0 ± 7.1***
Stellate ganglion	6	100 ± 11.0	69.0 ± 7.2*

Animals were killed 30 days after castration, and the tissues assayed for NGF and tyrosine hydroxylase activity as described in text. Values are means $\pm$ SEM for number of animals indicated (n), and are expressed as per cent of control values from similar numbers of unoperated animals (for NGF control values see Fig. 2 and Tables 1 and 2). Mean control values for tyrosine hydroxylase activities of superior cervical and stellate ganglia were 15.8 and 18.6 pmol DOPA h^{-1} per ganglion respectively.
* $= p < 0.05$, ** $= p < 0.01$, *** $= p < 0.005$, when compared with corresponding control values. From Hendry and Iversen (1973).

concentrations of NGF, which was again accompanied by a reduced T-OH activity in sympathetic ganglia (Table 3). These results suggest that there may be a relation between T-OH activity in adrenergic neurons and the presence of NGF in tissues and circulation, even in adult animals. Hendry and Iversen (1973) suggested that NGF in tissues innervated by sympathetic terminals might exert a "retrograde trophic" role in controlling the development and maintenance of adrenergic neurons in the sympathetic nervous system. It was proposed that such neurons may require NGF for their normal development and survival, and that such NGF might be derived from the end-organs with which such neurons make synaptic contact. Evidence has recently been obtained that radioactively labelled NGF can be transported in a retrograde manner from sympathetic terminals in the mouse eye to adrenergic neuron cell bodies in the superior cervical ganglia (Thoenen et al., this symposium).

III. EFFECTS OF NGF AND ANTI-NGF ANTISERA IN VIVO

In confirmation of other reports (Levi-Montalcini and Angeletti, 1968; Thoenen et al., 1971, 1972; Edwards et al., 1972) we have found that treatment of infant mice with NGF causes a significant increase in the volume, number of neurons, and T-OH activity of superior cervical ganglia (Table 4). These effects are dose-related, and lead to approximately a doubling in cell numbers and a fourfold increase in total ganglionic T-OH activity in animals treated with 10 µg NGF (7 S) per gram daily for 10 days from 4 days of age and assayed at age 14 days (Table 4). The increased T-OH activity evoked by such treatment, however, like the increase in ganglion size (Edwards et al., 1972), is reversible if NGF treatment is not continued. In animals similarly treated with NGF for 10 days on days 4–14 and assayed at 60 days, the T-OH activity of superior cervical ganglia had declined to values not significantly different from those in untreated controls (Hendry, 1973). Thus although NGF causes dramatic increases in T-OH and growth of immature ganglionic neurons, these effects do not seem to be permanent. NGF treatment was also found to be insufficient to prevent the failure of normal development of neurons and T-OH activity in mice subjected to unilateral surgical decentralization of the superior cervical ganglion at age 4

TABLE 4. EFFECTS OF NGF ADMINISTRATION ON DEVELOPMENT OF MOUSE SUPERIOR CERVICAL
GANGLIA

	Total ganglion volume ($\mu^3 \times 10^{-6}$)	Total number of cells	Tyrosine hydroxylase activity (pmol DOPA h^{-1} per ganglion)
Untreated control	55.8 ± 7.2 (11)	14,700 ± 770 (11)	12.7 ± 0.9 (6)
NGF treated 3 μg/g	121.7 ± 33.5 (4)	23,900 ± 1370 (4)	26.8 ± 4.1 (6)
NGF treated 10 μg/g	96.9 (1)	23,600 (1)	52.5 ± 7.4 (6)

In separate experiments superior cervical ganglia from untreated control animals, 14 days of age, and from animals treated from days 4 to 14 with 7 S NGF were analysed histologically to determine ganglion size and cell numbers, and biochemically to assay tyrosine hydroxylase activity. Values are means ± SEM for number of experiments indicated in parentheses. Data from Black *et al.* (1972).

days (Black *et al.*, 1972) or in infant animals treated with the ganglion-blocking drug pempidine (Hendry, 1973).

Administration of NGF antisera to infant mice has the well-known effect of causing a destruction of a large proportion of the developing adrenergic neurons in mouse superior cervical ganglia. This is accompanied by a pronounced reduction in T-OH activity. We have found that the extent of reduction in T-OH activity is related to the dose of antiserum used in animals assayed on day 7 after treatment with a single dose of antiserum on day 1 (Hendry and Iversen, 1971). This offers a simple and accurate method for comparing the biological potency of various batches of NGF antisera. Such comparisons, performed in collaboration with Drs. Edwards and Fenton at the Wellcome Research Laboratories, have revealed some interesting clues about the mode of action of NGF antisera in causing immunosympathectomy. The effectiveness of various antisera fractions, taken from a horse at different times during the immunization process, was found to be related to the presence of complement fixing activity in these preparations. Antisera with a high *in vitro* anti-NGF titre but low complement-fixing activity were less effective in causing a reduction in ganglionic T-OH activity than preparations with lower *in vitro* anti-NGF titres but containing high complement fixing ability. This suggests that the NGF antisera may act not by absorbing free NGF in the body, but perhaps by promoting a lysis of adrenergic neurons by reacting in conjunction with complement and membrane-bound antigen (Edwards *et al.*, in preparation).

IV. EFFECTS OF NGF AND DEPOLARIZING STIMULI ON TYROSINE HYDROXYLASE ACTIVITY IN CULTURED ADRENERGIC NEURONS

1. CULTURE SYSTEM

In order to examine the control of T-OH activity in adrenergic neurons in a controlled environment, superior cervical ganglia from rats and mice of various ages have been maintained in an organ culture system. The culture system used is similar to that described by Trowell (1959). The excised ganglia are supported on sterile Millipore filter rafts on a stainless-steel mesh bridge and bathed in culture medium (Eagles Minimum Essential

Medium enriched with 600 mg glucose percent and containing 10% neonatal calf serum and penicillin/streptomycin). The system is incubated for up to 48 h at 37°C in an atmosphere of 95% oxygen/5% carbon dioxide. Ganglia excised from mice of 6 days of age lost approximately 40% of their total tyrosine hydroxylase activity over a 48 h culture period. Ganglia from neonatal and adult rats behaved similarly. In all cases, however, histological examination revealed that a marked reduction in ganglionic cell numbers occurred during the culture period. The 40% loss of tyrosine hydroxylase activity in ganglia from neonatal mice, for example, was associated with a loss of 40% of ganglionic neurons.

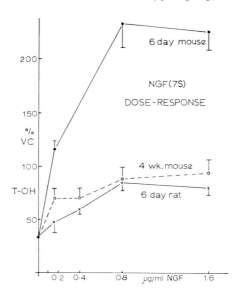

FIG. 5. Effects of various concentrations of added NGF (7 S species from mouse submaxillary glands) on tyrosine hydroxylase activity in superior cervical ganglia of neonatal and adult mice and neonatal rats maintained for 48 h in organ culture. Values are means ± SEM for 6–8 ganglia and are expressed as percentages of enzyme activity per ganglion in ganglia assayed immediately after removal from control animals.

2. EFFECTS OF ADDED NGF

The addition of NGF (7 S species from mouse submaxillary glands) to the culture medium for the 48 h culture period resulted in an increase in total ganglionic T-OH activity which was most marked in ganglia excised from 6-day-old mice (Fig. 5). In contrast, ganglia from adult mice and from 6-day-old rats showed a significantly smaller response to added NGF. The increased T-OH activity in NGF-treated ganglia was accompanied by an increased survival of ganglionic neurons; there was, however, also an increase in T-OH activity per neuron after exposure to NGF. Maximum responses were obtained with a concentration of NGF of 0.8 μg/ml (Fig. 5). The discrepancy observed in the responses of ganglia from neonatal and adult mice is in agreement with many previous studies that have shown NGF to be less effective in adult than in neonatal animals when administered *in vivo*. The increases in T-OH activity evoked by NGF in cultured ganglia were almost completely prevented if cycloheximide (2 μg/ml) was present in the culture medium, suggesting that the rise in enzyme activity was dependent on protein synthesis.

3. DEPOLARIZING STIMULI

It was hoped that sympathetic ganglia maintained in organ culture might provide an *in vitro* model for studies of the mechanisms involved in the trans-synaptic regulation of T-OH activity in adrenergic neurons. *In vivo*, the evidence obtained from previous studies (Patrick and Kirshner, 1971; Thoenen, 1972; Black and Geen, 1973; Hendry, 1973) suggests that an increased release of acetylcholine from preganglionic neurons is responsible for the rises in T-OH activity associated with sustained increases in preganglionic impulse traffic. Addition of acetylcholine with and without an acetylcholinesterase inhibitor, or addition of carbamylcholine, failed to cause any consistent changes in T-OH activity in cultured sympathetic ganglia. Such results, however, are inconclusive since prolonged exposure of ganglionic receptors to cholinergic agonists is known to result in receptor desensitization, and changes in receptor sensitivity are also known to occur after axotomy (Brown and Pascoe, 1954).

We have, therefore, resorted to the use of other more direct means of causing membrane depolarization of ganglionic neurons (Mackay and Iversen, 1972a). For example, increasing the external potassium concentration by addition of potassium chloride to the culture medium or addition to the medium of the cardiac glycoside ouabain. Exposure of ganglia from 6-day-old mice to a range of potassium concentrations for 48 h resulted in a graded increase in T-OH activity which was greatest (more than 200 % of control) after exposure to a tenfold increase in potassium concentration (54 mM). This rise in T-OH activity was blocked by cycloheximide (5 μg/ml) and did not occur when ganglia were exposed to an increase in sodium chloride concentration of the same magnitude. Exposure to the elevated potassium concentration for a period as short as 30 min, with subsequent maintenance in normal medium led to significant increases in T-OH activity at the end of a 48 h culture period (Fig. 6). Maximum responses were obtained after a 3 h exposure to 54 mM potassium, followed by maintenance in normal medium for 45 h (Fig. 6). The presence of cycloheximide during the 3 h exposure to elevated potassium did not significantly alter the rise in T-OH activity unless the drug was also present for the entire period of culture (Fig. 6). This suggests that brief exposure to a depolarizing stimulus is sufficient to activate a long-term regulatory mechanism which subsequently leads to an increased synthesis of the enzyme T-OH. Subsequent studies have shown that the full expression of this activation in terms of increased enzyme synthesis requires at least 24 h.

Addition of ouabain at a concentration of 1 mM to the culture medium resulted in increases in T-OH activity after 48 h in culture similar to those caused by high potassium. These increases could also be prevented by cycloheximide (5 μg/ml).

The increases in T-OH activity evoked by exposure to elevated concentrations of potassium could not be explained by improved cell survival in such media. Histological examination indicated that the number of ganglionic neurons surviving after 48 h in culture was not significantly different after exposure to high potassium or normal media.

Elevated potassium concentrations have also been found to lead to increases in T-OH activity in rat adrenal medullary tissue maintained in culture (Silberstein *et al.*, 1972a) and to increases in dopamine-β-hydroxylase activity in cultured rat superior cervical sympathetic ganglia (Silberstein *et al.*, 1972b).

In further experiments we have examined the interaction between added NGF and elevated potassium concentrations in causing increases in ganglionic T-OH activity. These results indicate that the increased T-OH activity resulting from these two stimuli are not

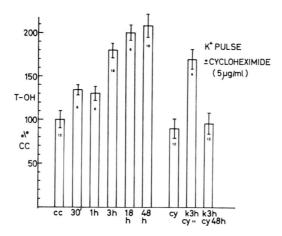

FIG. 6. Effects on ganglionic tyrosine hydroxylase activity of exposure of neonatal mice superior cervical ganglia to elevated potassium concentrations (54 mM KCl) after culture for 48 h. High potassium was present for the first 30 min, 1 h, 3 h, 18 h, or for the entire 48 h culture period. Columns to the right show results obtained with ganglia exposed to high potassium for 3 h in the presence of cycloheximide (5 μg/ml) with subsequent culture for 42 h in the presence or absence of cycloheximide. Results are means ± SEM for numbers of ganglia indicated; tyrosine hydroxylase activity per ganglion is expressed as percentage of values obtained in ganglia cultured for 48 h in normal media (CC).

simply additive. Ganglia exposed to supramaximal concentrations of NGF (1.6 μg/ml) were incapable of further increases in T-OH activity in response to raised potassium. The largest increases in T-OH activity, relative to the culture control, in response to raised potassium, were observed in ganglia cultured in the absence of added NGF. This condition was thus chosen for most subsequent experiments. The non-additive nature of the response elicited by a depolarizing stimulus (raised potassium) and by added NGF suggests that the expression of these two effects may depend upon a common mechanism, although the primary biochemical events involved may be different.

4. LACK OF RELATION BETWEEN GANGLIONIC NORADRENALINE CONTENT AND CHANGES IN T-OH ACTIVITY

The short-term regulation of catecholamine biosynthesis is thought to involve changes in the intracellular concentrations of free catecholamines, operating through an end product inhibition mechanism (see Udenfriend, 1966). It has also been suggested that a similar mechanism might underly the long-term changes in the synthesis of biosynthetic enzymes in response to trans-synaptic control. Silberstein *et al.* (1972a), for example, found that raised potassium concentrations resulted in an increase in T-OH activity in cultured adrenal medullary tissue, and that this was associated with a loss of intracellular catecholamines. We have accordingly examined the relationship between changes in T-OH activity and ganglionic noradrenaline content in cultured sympathetic ganglia. The noradrenaline content of 6-day-old or adult mouse superior cervical ganglia was assayed by an enzymic radiochemical method, utilizing the enzyme phenylethanolamine-*N*-methyl transferase partially purified from bovine adrenals (Jarrott and Iversen, 1971).

Ganglia from neonatal or adult mice showed no significant change in their noradrenaline content during a 48 h culture period under normal conditions. Since such ganglia exhibit marked losses of T-OH activity and neuron numbers, the intracellular noradrenaline of the remaining ganglionic neurons must have increased considerably during the culture period. Exposure of neonatal or adult ganglia to high potassium for 48 h produced a doubling in their noradrenaline content (Fig. 7). Ouabain (1 mM), however, which led to a similar increase in ganglionic T-OH activity, produced an 80% reduction in ganglionic noradrenaline. Simultaneous exposure to high potassium and ouabain resulted in an increase in T-OH activity to 195% of control, a rise which was greater than observed when either stimulus was used alone, but there was no significant difference in ganglionic noradrenaline content when compared with cultured controls. From these results it was already apparent that long-term increases in ganglionic T-OH activity in cultured ganglia could occur independently of changes in noradrenaline content. Further evidence in support of this

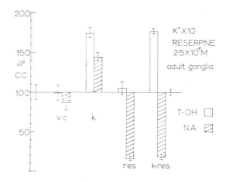

FIG. 7. Effects on ganglionic tyrosine hydroxylase activity (open columns) and noradrenaline content (hatched columns) of exposure of adult mice superior cervical ganglia to elevated potassium (K; 54 mM potassium chloride) and/or reserpine (res; 2.5 × 10⁻⁵ M) for culture periods of 48 h. Values are expressed as percentages of those obtained from ganglia cultured for 48 h in control media, and are means ± SEM for groups of 6–12 ganglia. VC refers to values obtained from ganglia assayed immediately after excision from adult mice, which were not significantly different from culture control values. Similar results were obtained with ganglia from neonatal mice.

conclusion was obtained from studies with drugs that are known to affect the noradrenaline content of adrenergic neurons. Reserpine at a concentration of 2.5×10^{-5} M in the culture medium produced a virtually complete depletion of ganglionic noradrenaline, but was without significant effect on T-OH activity after 48 h culture. Reserpine also failed to influence the increase in T-OH activity evoked by high potassium (Fig. 7), although there was again a severe depletion of ganglionic noradrenaline content. The monoamine oxidase inhibitor clorgyline at a concentration of 10^{-6} M produced a 60% rise in noradrenaline content of cultured ganglia without any concomitant change in T-OH activity. The T-OH inhibitor α-methyl-p-tyrosine at a concentration of 2×10^{-5} M caused a 50% reduction in ganglionic noradrenaline content but had no significant effect on T-OH activity assayed *in vitro* after thorough washing of the cultured ganglia. These results show that ganglionic T-OH activity bears no consistent relationship to long-term changes in the noradrenaline content of the adrenergic neurons. It thus seems unlikely that changes in intraneuronal noradrenaline concentrations are responsible for the long-term changes in T-OH activity observed in response to depolarizing stimuli.

5. POSSIBLE INVOLVEMENT OF CYCLIC AMP IN REGULATION OF GANGLIONIC T-OH ACTIVITY

Previous reports have indicated that depolarization of a variety of nervous tissues, including sympathetic ganglia, leads to a rise in the cyclic adenosine 3′,5′-monophosphate (cAMP) content of these tissues (Kakiuchi *et al.*, 1969; McAfee *et al.*, 1971; Shimizu and Daly, 1972; Rall, 1972). An increased intracellular production of cAMP in response to depolarizing stimuli might provide an alternative mechanism linking membrane depolarization with changes in the synthesis of biosynthetic enzymes.

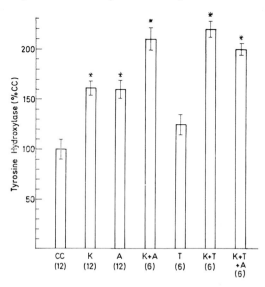

Fig. 8. Effects on ganglionic tyrosine hydroxylase activity and noradrenaline content of increased potassium concentration (K; 54 mM), dibutyryl cyclic AMP (A; 1 mM), and theophylline (T; 5 μM) in neonatal mice superior cervical ganglia cultured for 48 h. Tyrosine hydroxylase and noradrenaline content per ganglion are expressed as percentages of values obtained in ganglia cultured for 48 h in control media (CC) and values are means ± SEM for 6–12 ganglia. Results obtained from ganglia exposed to various combinations of drugs are indicated as KA, KT, and KAT.

The T-OH activity and noradrenaline content of ganglia from neonatal mice cultured for 48 h in the presence of dibutyryl cyclic AMP (dbcAMP) or the phosphodiesterase inhibitor theophylline were observed, and their interaction with the high potassium stimulus investigated (Mackay and Iversen, 1972b). Dibutyryl cAMP (1 mM) when added to the culture medium resulted in a 70% rise in T-OH activity and a 100% rise in noradrenaline content after a 48 h culture period (Fig. 8). Combining dbcAMP with high potassium (54 mM) produced a 110% rise in T-OH activity and a 120% increase in noradrenaline content after 48 h. The increase in T-OH activity evoked by the combined stimulus of dbcAMP and high potassium was significantly greater than that produced by either agent alone. Theophylline at a concentration of 5 μM had no significant effect on either T-OH activity or noradrenaline content but produced a significant enhancement of the responses of both of these parameters to high potassium (Fig. 8). Simultaneous exposure to theophylline, high potassium, and dbcAMP produced no further increase in T-OH activity. As a control, the effects of sodium butyrate (1 mM) were examined, since this substance was reported to effect the T-OH activity of neuroblastoma cells in culture (Waymire *et al.*, 1972; Richelson, 1973). Sodium butyrate had no effect on T-OH activity in cultured neonatal mouse ganglia. Dibutyryl cyclic GMP, however, at a concentration of 1 mM produced increases in T-OH activity comparable with those observed with dbcAMP. The response to dbcAMP was completely abolished by cycloheximide (2 μg/ml).

Our results are in agreement with other recent reports which have shown that addition of dbcAMP leads to increased T-OH activity in cultured neuroblastoma cells (Waymire *et al.*, 1972; Richelson, 1973), and to increased dopamine-β-hydroxylase activity in cultured sympathetic ganglia (Keen and McLean, 1972). *In vivo* results of Guidotti and Costa (1973) have also shown that changes in T-OH activity in rat adrenal medulla may be associated with increases in the cAMP content of this tissue. These results thus favour the view that changes in the intracellular production of cyclic nucleotides may provide the link between membrane depolarization and the control of T-OH synthesis.

6. EFFECTS OF INHIBITION OF RNA POLYMERASE AND PROTEIN SYNTHESIS

The results described so far indicate that depolarizing stimuli and dbcAMP are capable of inducing rises in the T-OH activity of cultured adrenergic neurons, and that these rises are mediated through cycloheximide-sensitive protein synthesis. In further experiments we have attempted to determine whether these stimuli operate directly at a ribosomal level to control the rate of transcription of T-OH molecules or whether the responses are dependent upon a nuclear-directed synthesis of messenger RNA. There is some doubt about the precise site(s) of action of cycloheximide (Cundliffe, 1972), and thus the effects of the specific peptidyl transferase inhibitors anisomycin and sparsomycin were investigated (Grollman, 1967; Cundliffe, 1972). Anisomycin at a concentration of 5 μg/ml completely inhibited the increases in T-OH activity normally evoked by high potassium and by dbcAMP. Sparsomycin at a similar concentration produced a marked diminution of the potassium-evoked rise in T-OH activity (Table 5). This drug, however, penetrates only poorly into mammalian cells, and would thus be expected to be less effective than anisomycin.

Actinomycin D specifically inhibits the nuclear synthesis of messenger RNA from DNA templates. Cultured neonatal ganglia exposed to this drug (5 μg/ml) for 48 h showed an 85% increase in T-OH activity. In the presence of this concentration of actinomycin D, ganglia exposed to high potassium or to dbcAMP failed to show any increases in T-OH activity beyond that evoked by the drug alone. This suggests that the effects of both the high potassium stimulus and dbcAMP require translation of a nuclear message for their expression. The apparently paradoxical effect of actinomycin D in increasing T-OH activity is similar to the effects of this drug on enzyme synthesis in a variety of other mammalian systems and is consistent with a model of post-transcriptional control of enzyme synthesis proposed by Tomkins *et al.* (1972). The hypothesis states that two species of messenger RNA may be involved in the synthesis of enzyme protein. One of these is relatively stable and represents the product of the structural gene for the enzyme protein. The other is more labile and represents the product of a regulatory gene. This substance, either directly or after transcription, normally represses the transcription of the enzyme protein at a ribosomal level. Thus when messenger RNA production is totally blocked by actino-mycin D, the rapid decay of the repressor results in temporarily elevated rates of enzyme

TABLE 5. EFFECTS OF INHIBITORS OF PROTEIN AND RNA
SYNTHESIS ON T-OH ACTIVITY OF CULTURED SYMPATHETIC
GANGLIA

	T-OH %
Culture control	100 ± 9 (12)
X10K	205 ± 10 (18)
dbcAMP (1 mM)	160 ± 5 (12)
Anisomycin (5 µg/ml)	67 ± 9 (12)
Sparsomycin (5 µg/ml)	111 ± 10 (6)
Actinomycin D (5 µg/ml)	180 ± 8 (18)
X10K + Anisomycin	70 ± 5 (12)
X10K + Sparsomycin	161 ± 6 (6)
X10K + Act. D	126 ± 14 (12)
X10K + Act. D + Anisomycin	50 ± 7 (6)
dbcAMP + Anisomycin	65 ± 9 (6)
dbcAMP + Act. D	168 ± 10 (12)
Act. D + Anisomycin	65 ± 7 (6)

Neonatal mouse superior cervical ganglia were
cultured for 48 h in the presence of a tenfold increase in
potassium (K^+) concentration or dibutyryl cyclic-AMP
(dbc AMP) at a concentration of 1 mM. Results represent
total T-OH activity per ganglion and are expressed as
percentages ± SEM relative to the culture control
(absolute T-OH activity 2.1 pmoles DOPA h^{-1} per
ganglion) for numbers of ganglia shown in parentheses.

synthesis. This model predicts that the paradoxical effect of actinomycin D involves on-going protein synthesis, and should thus be prevented by the simultaneous presence of a peptidyl transferase inhibitor such as anisomycin. In agreement with this prediction, anisomycin (5 µg/ml) completely inhibited the actinomycin-D-induced rise in ganglionic T-OH activity.

Neither high potassium nor dbcAMP had any significant effects on total ganglionic protein content. The increases in T-OH activity evoked by these stimuli thus represent increases in the specific activity of this enzyme. This suggests that the nuclear-directed increase in T-OH synthesis is not accompanied by any general increase in ganglion protein synthesis, and this conclusion is supported by the results of experiments in which the rate of incorporation of labelled amino acid into ganglionic protein was measured under these conditions. Under control conditions there was a linear increase in the incorporation of ^{3}H-leucine into TCA-precipitable protein in cultured ganglia over a 48 h period. This incorporation could be completely inhibited by anisomycin (5 µg/ml), and partially inhibited by actinomycin D (5 µg/ml). Exposure of ganglia to high potassium or to dbcAMP, however, did not cause any significant changes in the rate of ^{3}H-leucine incorporation during a 24 h period of culture. Thus the observed rises in T-OH activity appear to represent a specific effect of these stimuli rather than a general increase of ganglionic protein synthesis.

In view of the apparent similarity between the mechanisms involved in the expression of the effects of high potassium and of added dbcAMP, we suggest that increased intracellular production of cyclic AMP (or some similar compound) may enable nuclear recognition of depolarizing events occurring at the membrane of adrenergic neurons.

V. CONCLUSIONS

The results described here do not answer the still important question of the biological role of NGF in regulating the development and maintenance of adrenergic neurons. It is apparent, however, that changes in NGF concentrations in plasma and other tissues can have marked effects on adrenergic neurons even in adult animals. The relationship between the effects of NGF and of depolarizing stimuli on T-OH levels in adrenergic neurons also remains obscure, although the results obtained in isolated cultured ganglia suggest that both of these effects may operate through a similar final common pathway in their expression, although the primary and intermediate molecular events involved may well be different.

The ability to maintain sympathetic ganglia in organ culture for short periods provides a useful *in vitro* model for studies of the mechanisms involved in the long-term regulation of transmitter related enzymes such as T-OH. How far the responses of cultured ganglia to depolarizing stimuli such as high potassium can be taken as a representative model for the *in vivo* trans-synaptic regulation of the synthesis of such enzymes, is not yet clear. The results suggest, however, that membrane depolarization *per se* may be adequate to initiate the train of events leading to changes in the rate of synthesis of T-OH. *In vivo*, such depolarization is probably brought about by the actions of acetylcholine on ganglionic neurons, and it thus seems unnecessary to invoke the occurrence of other unidentified trophic substances to explain the trophic effects of preganglionic sympathetic neurons on post-ganglionic neurons.

REFERENCES

ADDISON, G. M., and HALES, C. N. (1971) Two site assay of human growth hormone. *Horm. Metab. Res.* **3**, 59–60.

ANGELETTI, P., LEVI-MONTALCINI, R., and CALISSANO, P. (1968) The nerve growth factor, chemical properties and metabolic effects. *Adv. Enzymol.* **31**, 51–75.

BLACK, I. B., and GEEN, S. C. (1973) Trans-synaptic regulation of adrenergic neuron development: inhibition by ganglionic blockade. *Brain Res.* **63**, 291–302.

BLACK, I. B., HENDRY, I. A. and IVERSEN, L. L. (1971) Trans-synaptic regulation of growth and development of adrenergic neurones in a mouse sympathetic ganglion. *Brain Res.* **34**, 229–240.

BLACK, I. B., HENDRY, I. A., and IVERSEN, L. L. (1972) Effects of surgical decentralization and nerve growth factor on the maturation of adrenergic neurones in a mouse sympathetic ganglion. *J. Neurochem.* **19**, 1367–1377.

BROWN, G. L., and PASCOE, J. E. (1954) The effect of degenerative section of ganglionic axons on transmission through the ganglion. *J. Physiol. Lond.* **123**, 565–573.

COHEN, S. (1960) Purification of a nerve growth promoting protein from the mouse salivary gland and its neurotoxic antiserum. *Proc. Natn. Acad. Sci. USA* **46**, 302–311.

CUNDLIFFE, E. (1972) Antibiotic inhibitors of ribosomal function. In *The Molecular Basis of Antibiotic Action* (E. F. Gale, E. Cundliffe, P. E. Reynolds, M. H. Richmond, and M. Waring, eds.), Wiley, London.

EDWARDS, D. C., FENTON, E. L., and HENDRY, I. A. (1972) Quantitative aspects of the effects in mice of nerve growth factor and its antiserum. In *Nerve Growth Factor and its Antiserum* (E. Zaimis, ed.), Athlone Press, University of London, pp. 237–252.

FENTON, E. L. (1970) Tissue-culture assay of nerve growth factor and the specific antiserum. *Expl. Cell Res.* **59**, 383–392.

GROLLMAN, A. P. (1967) Structural basis for the inhibition of protein biosynthesis: mode of action of tubulosine. *Science* **157**, 84–85.

GUIDOTTI, A., and COSTA, E. (1973) Involvement of adenosine 3′,5′-monophosphate in the activation of tyrosine hydroxylase elicited by drugs. *Science* **179**, 902–904.

HENDRY, I. A. (1972) Developmental changes in tissue and plasma concentrations of the biologically active species of nerve growth factor in the mouse, by using a two-site radioimmunoassay. *Biochem. J.* **128**, 1265–1272.

HENDRY, I. A. (1973) Trans-synaptic regulation of tyrosine hydroxylase activity in a developing mouse sympathetic ganglion: effects of nerve growth factor (NGF), NGF antiserum and pempidine. *Brain Res.* **56**, 313–320.

HENDRY, I. A., and IVERSEN, L. L. (1971) Effect of nerve growth factor and its antiserum on tyrosine hydroxylase activity in mouse superior cervical ganglion. *Brain Res.* **29**, 159–162.

HENDRY, I. A., and IVERSEN, L. L. (1973) Reduction in nerve growth factor (NGF) concentrations and tyrosine hydroxylase activity in mouse tissues after sialectomy and castration. *Nature* **243**, 500–504.

JARROTT, B., and IVERSEN, L. L. (1971) Modification of an enzyme radiochemical assay procedure for noradrenaline. *Biochem. Pharmac.* **19**, 1841–1843.

JOHNSON, P. G., GORDON, P., and KOPIN, I. J. (1971) A sensitive radioimmunoassay for 7S-nerve growth factor antigen in serum and tissues. *J. Neurochem.* **19**, 2025–2029.

KAKIUCHI, S., RALL, T. W., and McILWAIN, J. (1969) Effect of electrical stimulation upon the accumulation of adenosine 3′,5′-monophosphate in isolated cerebral tissue. *J. Neurochem.* **16**, 485–491.

KEEN, P., and McLEAN, W. G. (1972) Effect of dibutyryl cyclic-AMP on levels of dopamine β-hydroxylase in isolated superior cervical ganglia. *Naunyn-Schmiedeberg's Arch. exp. Path. Pharmak.* **275**, 465–469.

LEVI-MONTALCINI, R., and ANGELETTI, P. (1968) Nerve growth factor. *Physiol. Rev.* **48**, 534–569.

LYON, M. F., HENDRY, I. A., and SHORT, R. V. (1973) The submaxillary glands as test organs for response to androgen in mice with testicular feminization. *J. Endocrinology* **58**, 357–362.

MACAFEE, D. A., SCHORDORET, M., and GREENGARD, P. (1971) Adenosine 3′,5′-monophosphate in nervous tissue: increase associated with synaptic transmission. *Science* **171**, 1156–1158.

MACKAY, A. V. P., and IVERSEN, L. L. (1972a) Trans-synaptic regulation of tyrosine hydroxylase activity in adrenergic neurons: effect of potassium concentration on cultured sympathetic ganglia. *Naunyn-Schmiedeberg's Arch. exp. Path. Pharm.* **272**, 225–229.

MACKAY, A. V. P., and IVERSEN, L. L. (1972b) Increased tyrosine hydroxylase activity of sympathetic ganglia cultured in the presence of dibutyryl cyclic AMP. *Brain Res.* **48**, 424–426.

PATRICK, R. L., and KIRSHNER, N. (1971) Acetylcholine-induced stimulation of catecholamine recovery in denervated rat adrenals after reserpine-induced depletion. *Molec. Pharmac.* **7**, 389–396.

RALL, T. W. (1972) Role of adenosine 3′,5′-monophosphate (cyclic AMP) in actions of catecholamines, *Pharmac. Rev.* **24**, 399–409.

RICHELSON, E. (1973) Stimulation of tyrosine hydroxylase activity in an adrenergic clone of mouse neuroblastoma by dibutyryl cyclic AMP. *Nature New Biol. Lond.* **242**, 175–177.

SHIMIZU, H., and DALY, J. W. (1972) Effect of depolarising agents on accumulation of cyclic adenosine 3′,5′-monophosphate in cerebral cortical slices, *Eur. J. Pharmac.* **17**, 240–252.

SILBERSTEIN, S. D., LEMBERGER, L., KLEIN, D. C., AXELROD, J., and KOPIN, J. (1972a). Induction of adrenal tyrosine hydroxylase in organ culture. *Neuropharmacology* **11**, 721–726.

SILBERSTEIN, S. D., BRIMIJOIN, S., MOLINOFF, P. B., and LEMBERGER, L. (1972b) Induction of dopamine-β-hydroxylase in rat superior cervical ganglia in organ culture. *J. Neurochem.* **19**, 919–921.

THOENEN, H. (1972) Neuronally mediated enzyme induction in adrenergic neurones and adrenal chromaffin cells. In *Neurotransmitters and Metabolic Regulation* (R. M. S. Smellie, ed.), *Biochemical Society Symposia* **36**, 3–15.

THOENEN, H., ANGELETTI, P., LEVI-MONTALCINI, R., and KETTLER, R. (1971) Selective induction by nerve growth factor of tyrosine hydroxylase and dopamine-β-hydroxylase in the rat superior cervical ganglia. *Proc. Natn. Acad. Sci. USA*, **68**, 1598–1602.

THOENEN, H., SANER, A., ANGELETTI, P., and LEVI-MONTALCINI, R. (1972) Increased activity of choline acetyl transferase in sympathetic ganglia after prolonged administration of nerve growth factor. *Nature New Biol. Lond.* **236**, 26–28.

TOMKINS, G. M., LEVINSON, B. B., BAXTER, J. D., and DETHLEFSEN, L. (1972) Further evidence for post-transcriptional control of inducible tyrosine aminotransferase synthesis in cultured hepatoma cells. *Nature New Biol. Lond.* **239**, 9–14.

TROWELL, D. A. (1959) The culture of mature organs in a synthetic medium. *Expl. Cell Res.* **16**, 11–147.

UDENFRIEND, S. (1966) Tyrosine hydroxylase. *Pharmac. Rev.* **18**, 43–51.

VARON, S., NOMURA, J., and SHOOTER, E. (1967) Isolation of mouse nerve growth factor in a high M.W. form. *Biochemistry* **6**, 2202–2209.

VARON, S., NOMURA, J., and SHOOTER, E. (1968) Reversible dissociation of mouse nerve growth factor protein into subunits. *Biochemistry* **7**, 1296–1303.

WAYMIRE, J. C., WEINER, N., and PRASAD, K. N. (1972) Regulation of tyrosine hydroxylase activity in cultured mouse neuroblastoma cells: elevation induced by analogs of adenosine 3′,5′-cyclic monophosphate. *Proc. Natn. Acad. Sci. USA* **69**, 2241–2245.

ZAIMIS, E., and KNIGHT, J. (eds.) (1972) *Nerve Growth Factor and its Antiserum*, Athlone Press, University of London.

THE NERVE GROWTH FACTOR RECEPTOR: DEMONSTRATION OF SPECIFIC BINDING IN SYMPATHETIC GANGLIA

S. H. Snyder, S. P. Banerjee, P. Cuatrecasas, and L. A. Greene*

Departments of Pharmacology and Experimental Therapeutics and Psychiatry and the Behavioral Sciences, The Johns Hopkins University School of Medicine, Baltimore, Maryland 21205

*Laboratory of Biochemical Genetics, National Heart and Lung Institute, National Institutes of Health, Bethesda, Maryland 20014

SUMMARY

Membrane preparations from superior cervical ganglia of the rabbit and calf bind [^{125}I] nerve growth factor (NGF) in a specific fashion indicating that this binding represents an interaction with the physiological NGF receptors. Items of evidence supporting this conclusion include the following:

(1) Of a variety of tissues studied, specific NGF binding has been observed only in the superior cervical ganglia, the presumed target organ for NGF.

(2) [^{125}I] NGF binding is highly specific for the NGF peptide sequence and is not displaced by several other peptide hormones, though it is displaced by low amounts of nonradioactive NGF.

(3) N-bromosuccinimide treatment of NGF preparations produces a decrease in receptor binding which closely parallels the decrease in biological activity.

(4) NGF receptor binding is saturable with an affinity constant of about 2×10^{-10} M, which is similar to reported plasma levels of NGF and to concentrations of NGF which produce biological effects.

INTRODUCTION

Although nerve growth factor (NGF) is well known to have important functions in regulating growth and development of sympathetic neurons, its exact mode of action has not been determined nor is it altogether clear whether its effects are restricted to the sympathetic and sensory nervous system. Several aspects of the action of NGF resemble those of a hormone. In the mouse NGF is stored in the submaxillary salivary glands, whose removal results in a marked decline in plasma levels of NGF (Hendry and Iversen, 1973). Moreover, there is a close parallel between plasma and tissue levels of NGF (Hendry, 1972). As occurs with most hormones, systemically administered NGF tends to localize in its presumed target organ, the sympathetic ganglia (Angeletti *et al.*, 1972). Thus one might

347

conceptualize the behavior of NGF as resembling a hormone in being formed in a discrete organ source, being discharged into the circulation and accumulated in specific target organs. Moreover, removal of a presumed source-organ, the submaxillary gland of the mouse, results in decreased functioning of target tissue, namely tyrosine hydroxylase activity of sympathetic ganglia (Hendry and Iversen, 1973). If NGF were to function like most other peptide hormones, then one might expect that specific receptor sites on the cell surface of target organ tissues would be demonstrable, as is the case with insulin, glucagon, and growth hormone.

Some aspects of the physiological disposition of NGF are unlike those of most hormones. While submaxillary glands of mice store large quantities of NGF, the salivary glands of other species do not have a uniquely high concentration of NGF. Indeed, in most mammalian species there does not appear to be a single organ with high levels of NGF, so that the source of circulating NGF is not clear. Recently, Hendry and Iversen (1973) have obtained evidence that NGF may not reach its target organs via the circulation but might instead be manufactured in sympathetic end organs and then migrate antidromically down sympathetic nerves to the superior cervical ganglia. When they removed submaxillary glands unilaterally from mice, NGF levels declined only in the superior cervical ganglion on the side of the excised salivary gland. This finding is incompatible with a secretion of NGF from the salivary gland into the circulation and thence to the superior cervical ganglia. Hendry and Thoenen (personal communication) have directly demonstrated the movement of radiolabeled NGF from the salivary gland to the superior cervical ganglion.

Whether or not NGF behaves like most peptide hormones, it is reasonable to speculate that there might be specific NGF receptors on the surface of cells in sympathetic ganglia. Similarities between the amino-acid sequences of NGF and of proinsulin (Frazier et al., 1972; Angeletti and Bradshaw, 1971) as well as similarities in some of the biological activities of these two hormones in their respective target cells (Levi-Montalcini and Angeletti, 1968; Frazier et al., 1972) suggested the possibility that tissue receptors for NGF and insulin may possess common features. Accordingly we initiated studies of specific NGF receptor binding to membrane preparations from the sympathetic ganglia (Banerjee et al., 1973a, b). Here we will describe some of the properties of NGF receptor binding in sympathetic ganglia.

Our studies utilized [^{125}I] labeled NGF. NGF was iodinated by procedures similar to those used with insulin (Cuatrecasas, 1971a, b, c) but omitting the addition of sodium metabisulfite. In most experiments, the 2.5 S preparation of NGF, prepared by the procedure of Bocchini and Angeletti (1969) was used and will be henceforth simply referred to as NGF, while other preparations will be specifically designated. In some experiments the β subunit of 7 S NGF was prepared by the method of Varon et al. (1967). It is generally assumed that 2.5 S NGF and the β subunit of NGF are very similar if not identical entities, and in all our studies they behaved in the same way. 2.5 S NGF was employed for binding studies, because it is known to be the active principle of 7 S NGF and because it was unclear what influence other subunits of 7 S NGF might have upon the binding of 2 S NGF.

An important initial question dealt with the most appropriate source of NGF receptors to study. Biological activity of NGF is usually measured on sympathetic or sensory ganglia of chick embryos. However, these are extremely small and would present great difficulties in carrying out extensive binding experiments. Accordingly, we chose to utilize sympathetic ganglia from young rabbits (Pelfreez, Birmingham, Alabama) which could be obtained fresh frozen in large quantities. The crude microsomal fraction was divided into multiple aliquots and stored in liquid nitrogen or at $-30°$. When stored in this way NGF receptor binding did not decline for at least 9 weeks, providing a convenient source of tissue for binding studies. Membrane fractions from these ganglia were obtained by homogenizing the ganglia in 10 volumes of 0.32 N sucrose containing 100 mM NaCl and 0.5 mM $MgSO_4$ with a Brinkmann Polytron. Various subcellular fractions were obtained by differential centrifugation, and the crude microsomal fraction was routinely used for binding studies (Banerjee et al., 1973a, b) because it contained the great majority of all the binding activity of homogenates.

In studies with iodinated peptides it is important to ensure that biological activity is retained in the radioactive hormone. Accordingly the biological activity of all our [^{125}I] NGF preparations was routinely assayed by measuring neurite production in dissociated sympathetic cells of chick embryo (L. Greene, in preparation). In this assay 10 units correspond to 1 unit in conventional assays for NGF (Levi-Montalcini et al., 1954). This assay is more sensitive than the conventional bioassay and permits detection of changes in activity which vary by a factor of less than 2. In the conventional bioassay 1 BU is referred to as the amount of NGF required to give a 4+ response in the tissue culture system. The biological activity of the NGF preparation used in the present study varied from 30 to 40 units per μg protein when the unit is defined as described by Levi-Montalcini et al. (1954).

The assay used to measure specific binding of iodinated NGF to ganglia cell membranes was similar to that previously described to study the binding of [^{125}I] insulin to cell membranes (Cuatrecasas, 1971b, c). The usual assay consisted of incubating ganglia cell membranes at 24° for 40 min with 0.25 ml of Krebs–Tris buffer, pH 7.4, containing 0.1 % (w/v) crystalline bovine serum albumin and [^{125}I] NGF. After incubation 3 ml of ice-cold Krebs–Tris buffer with 0.1 % albumin were added to each tube, which were filtered and washed over EHWP Millipore filters. Corrections were made for nonspecific binding of [^{125}I] NGF to the membrane and to the filters by running incubations in parallel with excess unlabeled NGF (10 μg/ml) added to the membranes prior to [^{125}I] NGF. Specific binding was obtained by subtracting from the total radioactive uptake the amount that was not displaced by native NGF.

CHARACTERISTICS OF NGF BINDING

The binding of [^{125}I] NGF was proportional to the concentration of tissue over a ten-fold range (Fig. 1) and all binding assays were performed in the linear range. NGF binding was saturable. Saturation could be demonstrated both with increasing amounts of iodinated NGF as well as by displacing [^{125}I] NGF with nonradioactive NGF. In experiments in which saturation was studied with [^{125}I] NGF, binding saturated at about 20–30 ng/ml and half-maximal binding occurred at 6 ng/ml (2×10^{-10} M). By contrast, nonspecific binding of [^{125}I] NGF, defined as its binding in the presence of excess nonradioactive NGF, did not saturate but increased linearly with increased amounts of [^{125}I] NGF. The ratio of specific to nonspecific binding was about 10 when assays were performed with NGF concentrations below 5 ng/ml (Fig. 2a).

When the displacement of [^{125}I] NGF was examined with increasing amounts of nonradioactive NGF (Fig. 2b), half-maximal displacement occurred at about 7 ng/ml (2×10^{-10} M), about the same as was obtained with iodinated NGF. These similar values suggest that [^{125}I] NGF is biologically equivalent to native NGF in terms of receptor binding. Moreover it confirms the validity of the specific activity of the preparations of [^{125}I] NGF utilized. In other experiments we examined saturation using [^{125}I] labeled β subunit of 7 S NGF and nonradioactive β subunit and obtained the same values as were obtained with 2.5 S NGF.

By examining the rates of association and dissociation of NGF receptor binding, it was possible to estimate the dissociation constant for binding and compare it with the affinity constant obtained in equilibrium experiments. At 24° specific NGF receptor binding occurred rapidly, attained half-maximal values at about 1 min and plateaued by 12 min (Fig. 3a). The time course of binding was consistent with a bimolecular reaction, which suggests that NGF binds to a single species of receptor. This data permitted calculations of the bimolecular rate constant for NGF receptor association k_1, providing a volume of

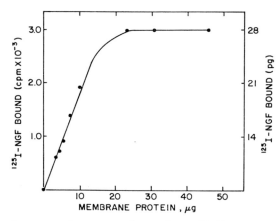

FIG. 1. Effect of membrane protein concentration on the specific binding of [^{125}I] NGF. Varying amounts of microsomal protein obtained from rabbit sympathetic ganglia were incubated for 40 min at 24°C with 6.5 ng/ml of [^{125}I] NGF (30,000 cpm) in a total volume of 0.25 ml. Each point is the mean of duplicate determinations.

4×10^6 mole^{-1} s^{-1}. We were also able to measure the rate of dissociation of the NGF-receptor complex directly both at 24° and at 4° (Fig. 3b). When plotted semilogarithmically, dissociation at 24° was linear with a half-life of about 13 min. The rate constant for dissociation at this temperature was 9×10^{-4} s^{-1}. In contrast dissociation was quite slow at 4° with less than 20% of bound [^{125}I] NGF dissociated in 20 min.

The ratio of dissociation constant to association constant (k_{-1}/k_1) yielded a value of 2.3 $\times$ 10^{-10} M for the dissociation constant of the NGF receptor. This is quite similar to the value of 2×10^{-10} M calculated from the equilibrium data. Interestingly, this value is also quite similar to plasma levels of NGF in mouse serum, which are about 4×10^{-10} M (Hendry and Iversen, 1973).

Some peptide hormones such as glucagon (Desbouqois and Cuatrecasas, 1972) are degraded as a result of interactions with their receptor sites, while others such as insulin (Cuatrecasas, 1971a, b, c) remain intact after binding to the receptor. To examine this phenomenon with NGF we measured the binding capacity of [^{125}I] NGF after it had been bound to ganglia membranes and was eluted with 0.1 N HCl. The eluted NGF bound to ganglia membranes to the same extent as comparable amounts of untreated [^{125}I] NGF. The binding of both preparations was similarly displaced by excess nonradioactive NGF. Thus, like insulin, NGF remains biologically intact after binding to receptors.

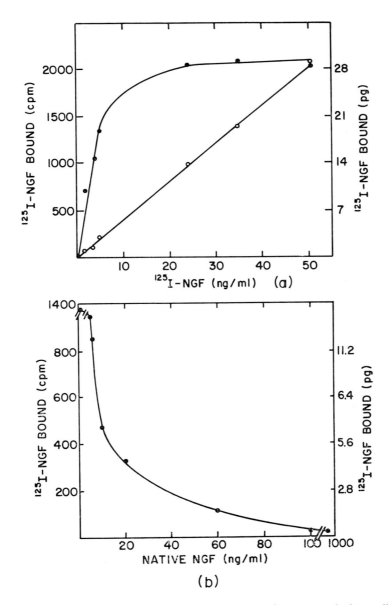

FIG. 2. (a) Saturation of specific NGF binding to membranes from sympathetic ganglia. The binding was measured by incubating varying amounts of [^{125}I] NGF with microsomal preparations of rabbit sympathetic ganglia (8 μg of protein) in a total volume of 0.25 ml of Krebs buffer for 40 min at 24°C. For every concentration of [^{125}I] NGF studied, control incubations were performed in the presence of 10 μg/ml of native NGF to obtain nonspecific binding. This non-specific binding ($\bigcirc$) has been subtracted from the total binding to obtain the specific binding curve ($\bullet$). (b) Competition by native NGF for the specific binding of [^{125}I] NGF to microsomes obtained from rabbit ganglia. Microsomal suspensions (7 μg/ml of protein) were incubated with 6 ng/ml of [^{125}I] NGF (25,000 cpm) and increasing amounts of native NGF at 24°C for 40 min. The nonspecific binding obtained in the presence of 10 μg/ml of native NGF has been subtracted from all experimental points.

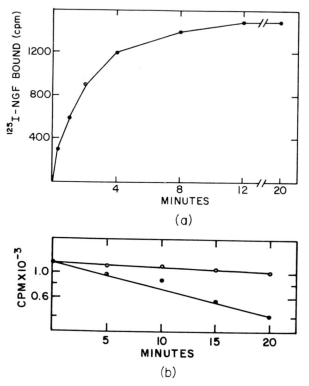

FIG. 3. Rates of association and dissociation of [^{125}I] NGF to microsomes obtained from rabbit sympathetic ganglia. (a) The rate of binding at 24°C of 4 ng/ml of [^{125}I] NGF to microsomes (8 μg/ml of protein). Nonspecific binding has been subtracted from all experimental points. (b) Semilog plot of the dissociation of [^{125}I] NGF bound to microsomes as a function of time at 4°C (○) and 24°C (●). The procedure for determining the rate of dissociation has been described before (Cuatrecasas, 1971a).

SPECIFICITY OF NGF RECEPTOR BINDING

One way of determining whether NGF binding to membranes from sympathetic ganglia represents an interaction with the physiological NGF receptor is to assess whether other peptides which do not possess NGF biological activity are able to compete for binding. We examined a variety of other peptide hormones as potential displacers of [^{125}I] NGF binding to ganglia membranes (Table 1). Even in very high concentrations, glucagon, insulin, proinsulin, desoctapeptide insulin, and growth hormone did not alter binding. At 1 mg/ml, growth hormone did reduce binding by 25% but it did not affect NGF binding when it was employed at 10 or 100 μg/ml.

As another means of examining peptide hormone specificity, we determined whether NGF could interfere with the binding of [^{125}I] epidermal growth factor to sympathetic ganglia or liver membranes (Tables 1 and 2) or of [^{125}I] insulin to fat-cells or liver membranes. We were interested in possible relationships of NGF and epidermal growth factor because both peptides are obtained in greatest abundance from the mouse salivary gland. Very little epidermal growth factor bound to sympathetic ganglia, and the limited amount of binding observed was not displaced by excess amounts of nonradioactive epidermal growth factor or by NGF.

TABLE 1. EFFECT OF PEPTIDE HORMONES ON THE BINDING OF [^{125}I] NGF AND [^{125}I] EPIDERMAL GROWTH FACTOR TO RABBIT GANGLIA MEMBRANE PREPARATIONS

Iodohormone	Tissue	Hormone added	[^{125}I] hormone binding (cpm)
[^{125}I] NGF (4 ng/ml)	Sympathetic ganglia	No addition	3368 ± 33
		NGF (5 μg/ml)	742 ± 7
		Glucagon:	
		(5 μg/ml)	3269 ± 18
		(50 μg/ml)	3156 ± 23
		(500 μg/ml)	3023 ± 21
		Growth hormone:	
		(10 μg/ml)	3241 ± 17
		(100 μg/ml)	3026 ± 26
		(1 mg/ml)	2512 ± 19
		Insulin (500 μg/ml)	3257 ± 28
		Proinsulin (500 μg/ml)	3008 ± 16
		Desoctapeptide insulin (1 mg/ml)	3263 ± 22
[^{125}I] Epidermal growth factor	Sympathetic ganglia	No addition	262 ± 2
		NGF (100 μg/ml)	248 ± 2

Data presented are the mean of four determinations ± SEM.

TABLE 2. EFFECT OF NGF ON THE SPECIFIC BINDING OF [^{125}I] INSULIN AND [^{125}I] EPIDERMAL GROWTH FACTOR TO VARIOUS TISSUES

Tissue	[^{125}I] hormone added	Native hormone		Binding (cpm)
		Hormone	Concentration (μg/ml)	
Fat-cells	Insulin (1.2 × 10⁵ cpm)	None		14,730
		Insulin	0.1	7100
		Insulin	1	4,613
		NGF (7 S)	100	14,680
		NGF (7 S)	1	15,210
		NGF (β subunit)	100	14,280
		NGF (β subunit)	0.1	74,380
Liver membrane	Insulin (9.4 × 10⁴ cpm)	None		5,780
		Insulin	0.1	940
		NGF (7 S)	100	5,860
		NGF (β subunit)	100	5,610
	EGF (6.8 × 10⁴ cpm)	None		28,300
		EGF	0.01	5,220
		NGF (7 S)	100	29,100
		NGF (β subunit)	100	28,530

Fat-cells (1.1 × 10⁵ cells per ml) and liver membranes (210 μg of protein) were incubated at 24° for 30 min in 0.25 ml of Krebs–Ringer bicarbonate buffer, pH 7.4, containing 0.1% albumin and the indicated concentrations of [^{125}I] insulin (140 μCi/μg), [^{125}I] epidermal growth factor (EGF) [96 μCi/μg], and the indicated native hormone. The latter was added to the membranes before addition of the iodohormone. Binding was determined as described earlier (Cuatrecasas, 1971a, b, c); all values are corrected for non-specific binding. Many similar experiments were performed using various concentrations of the iodoproteins with a broad range of concentrations of NGF; in no case did NGF cause significant displacement of binding.

Under a variety of conditions it was not possible to demonstrate significant effects of native NGF on the specific binding of $[^{125}I]$ insulin to intact fat cells or liver membranes (Table 2). In addition, NGF did not alter the specific binding of $[^{125}I]$ epidermal growth factor to liver membranes.

To obtain more precise information correlating NGF receptor binding with biological receptor activity, NGF was treated with N-bromosuccinimide in varying concentrations. This treatment destroys the biological activity of NGF by selectively oxidizing tryptophan residues (Angeletti, 1970). By using different amounts of N-bromosuccinimide, one can obtain NGF derivatives with a wide range of biological activity (Table 3). The reduction in

TABLE 3. NGF SPECIFIC BINDING AND BIOLOGICAL ACTIVITY AFTER N-BROMOSUCCINIMIDE TREATMENT

N-Bromosuccinimide (pmole/μg protein)	Biological activity (units per μg protein)	Tryptophan (% of untreated control)	Percent displacement specific $[^{125}I]$ NGF binding	
			NGF concentration	
			5.5 ng/ml	55.0 ng/ml
None	333	100	52	91
0.30	108	45	—	55
0.43	49	18	17	27
0.57	0	0	8	4

The binding experiment was done as described in the text and native NGF was treated with N-bromosuccinimide by the procedure of Angeletti (1970). The specific binding of $[^{125}I]$ NGF to ganglia microsomal preparation in the absence of N-bromosuccinimide-treated NGF was 3630 cpm.

biological activity of various preparations correlates well with the content of tryptophan. We were able to obtain preparations ranging from complete loss of biological activity to loss of only about 65% of biological activity. One derivative, retaining about 40% of the biological activity of the native hormone, displaced $[^{125}I]$ NGF binding half as well as native NGF, while a sample containing only 14% of control biological activity decreased binding 27% as well as native NGF.

SUBCELLULAR LOCALIZATION

Most peptide hormone receptors are located on the cell membrane. When tissues are subjected to differential centrifugation after homogenization, the cell membranes are usually most enriched in the microsomal fractions. To obtain an estimate of the intracellular localization of NGF receptor binding, we homogenized ganglia and subjected them to differential centrifugation (Table 4). The specific activity of NGF binding was highest in the crude microsomal fraction, almost ten times that of the whole homogenate. Of the total binding activity of the whole homogenate, about 80% was recovered in the microsomal fraction. Essentially all the binding activity of the homogenate could be accounted for by the three subcellular fractions. Thus it is likely that no more than a negligible portion of the total binding activity could be present in the supernatant fraction. However, we did not directly examine the soluble supernatant fraction for NGF receptor binding activity. These results are consistent with NGF receptor binding to the cell membrane. However, it should be borne in mind that the microsomal fraction contains many other membrane fragments, including ribosomes.

TABLE 4. SPECIFIC BINDING OF [^{125}I] NGF TO SUBCELLULAR FRACTIONS OF RABBIT SYMPATHETIC GANGLIA

Fraction	Specific binding (cpm/mg protein)	Total binding per fraction (cpm $\times 10^{-5}$)
Whole homogenate	6880 ± 11	14
Crude nuclear fraction (1000 g × 10 min)	4857 ± 4	2
Crude mitochondrial fraction (7710 g × 10 min)	9043 ± 14	0.9
Crude microsomal fraction (100,000 g × 10 min)	62,931 ± 33	11

The binding of 4 ng/ml of [^{125}I] NGF was assayed in a total volume of 0.25 ml. For each experimental point, nonspecific binding in the presence of 10 µg/ml of native NGF was subtracted. Data for specific binding are the means ± SEM of four samples.

TISSUE DISTRIBUTION

Another way of determining whether NGF binding takes place to the physiological receptor is to evaluate which tissues evince specific NGF binding. Generally, hormone receptors are confined to the target organ of the hormone. In the case of NGF it is conceivable that there might exist target organs other than sympathetic ganglia, so that a study of the tissue distribution of the NGF receptor might reveal new tissues where NGF might exert physiological actions (Table 5). We found a considerable amount of saturable NGF binding to superior cervical ganglia of the rabbit and calf. Although in several other tissues some NGF binding was observed, none of the binding in tissues other than sympathetic ganglia was displaced by excess (10 µg/ml) nonradioactive NGF. Tissues in which we failed to detect specific NGF binding included midbrain, adrenal glands, liver, heart, kidney, and fat-cells.

Since the norepinephrine neurons of the brain behave quite similarly to sympathetic neurons in the periphery, one might conceivably expect NGF to influence cell bodies of

TABLE 5. TISSUE SPECIFICITY OF [^{125}I] NGF BINDING

Tissue	[^{125}] NGF bound (cpm)	
	Without native NGF	10 µg/ml native NGF
Rabbit superior cervical ganglia	4210	326
Calf superior cervical ganglia	3174	628
Midbrain	701	804
Adrenal glands	713	893
Liver	1504	1389
Heart	500	505
Kidney	571	522
Fat-cells	1391	1297

The indicated tissues, obtained from rabbit (except fat-cells and calf ganglia) were homogenized in 10 volumes of 0.32 M sucrose with 100 mM Na$^+$ and 0.5 mM Mg^{++}. The isolated microsomes were suspended in the same volume of Krebs–Tris buffer and 20 µl of this suspension was used in the standard binding assay. The incubation medium contained 6 ng/ml of [^{125}I] NGF in a total volume of 0.25 ml. Fat-cells were obtained from rat and contained about 4 × 10^5 cells per ml. Data are the mean results from three determinations.

norepinephrine neurons in the central nervous system, especially in young animals. Accordingly, in preliminary experiments we measured NGF binding in membrane preparations from the brains of newborn and very young rats. In no case could we demonstrate specific NGF receptor binding. It is still conceivable that NGF receptors might exist in the brain but escape detection because norepinephrine neurons constitute only a small fraction, no more than 2–4%, of the neurons in the brain.

Although NGF receptor binding was not observed in the tissues examined, we did not exhaustively study various organs of the body, and it is conceivable that NGF receptors exist in tissues other than sympathetic ganglia.

NGF AND INSULIN-LIKE ACTIVITY

Because of the similar amino-acid sequences of NGF and proinsulin and because both of these peptides exert trophic effects on their target organs, one might wonder whether NGF might act at insulin-receptive sites and whether insulin might mimic NGF in sympathetic ganglia. It is already well established that insulin lacks the ability of NGF to cause sprouting of neurites from sympathetic and sensory ganglia of chick embryos (L. Greene, unpublished observations). We failed to detect any insulin-like metabolic effects for NGF. Thus whereas insulin (2 ng/ml) increased the conversion of $[^{14}C]$ glucose (0.2 mM) to $[^{14}C]$ CO_2 in a 2 h incubation at 37° (Cuatrecasas, 1969), NGF had no effect in concentrations ranging from 1 ng/ml to 100 μg/ml. Similarly, though insulin (1 ng/ml) inhibited the norepinephrine stimulated release of glycerol from fat-cells, NGF failed to exhibit this effect in concentrations ranging from 10 ng/ml to 20 μg/ml. The 7 S form of NGF also had no effect at concentrations up to 1 μg/ml, though small effects were observed at 2–10 μg/ml (Banerjee et al., 1973b).

CONCLUSIONS

The binding of $[^{125}I]$ NGF to membrane fractions of rabbits superior cervical ganglia we have observed appears to involve an interaction with the physiological receptor for NGF. Of several tissues examined, only superior cervical ganglia preparations displaced significant NGF binding. Binding is saturable over the concentration range of NGF which exists in the circulation and which is biologically effective with in vivo assays. NGF binding is specific for NGF and not modified by high concentrations of several other peptides. Moreover, when NGF is treated with varying amounts of N-bromosuccinimide, the reduction in receptor binding closely parallels the reduction in biological activity.

The ability to measure specific NGF receptor binding by the simple, sensitive, and specific assay that we have employed, provides a valuable tool for measuring NGF receptors in a variety of physiological, pharmacological, and pathological states which could conceivably be associated with a change in the number of NGF receptors. Disease states of interest include hyperthyroidism, hypertension, and malignancy. In this connection we have observed that human lymphocytes stimulated with concanavalin-A develop NGF receptors (manuscript in preparation) at about the same time that they developed new insulin receptors (Krug et al., 1972).

ACKNOWLEDGEMENTS

Supported by USPHS grants MH-18501, AM-14956, NS-07275; the John A. Hartford Foundation; the American Cancer Society; the National Science Foundation (No. GB-34300); and the Kroc Foundation.

S.H.S. and P.C. are recipients of USPHS Research Scientist Development Awards, MH-33128 and AM-31464, respectively. S.P.B. and L.A.G. are post-doctoral fellows of Medical Research Council (Canada) and American Cancer Society, respectively.

REFERENCES

ANGELETTI, R. H. (1970) The role of the tryptophan residues in the activity of the nerve growth factor. *Biochim. biophys. Acta* **214**, 478–482.

ANGELETTI, R. H., and BRADSHAW, R. A. (1971) The amino acid sequence of 2.5 S mouse submaxillary gland nerve growth factor. *Proc. Natn. Acad. Sci. USA* **68**, 2417–2420.

ANGELETTI, R. H., ANGELETTI, P. U., and LEVI-MONTALCINI, R. (1972) Selective accumulation of [^{125}I] labelled nerve growth factor in sympathetic ganglia. *Brain Res.* **46**, 421–425.

BANERJEE, S. P., SNYDER, S. H., CUATRECASAS, P., and GREENE, L. A. (1973a) Identification of specific nerve growth factor binding in superior cervical ganglia. *Fed. Proc.* **32**, 525.

BANERJEE, S. P., SNYDER, S. H., CUATRECASAS, P., and GREENE, L. A. (1973b) Nerve growth factor receptor binding in sympathetic ganglia. Communicated to *Proc. Natn. Acad. Sci. USA*.

BOCCHINI, V., and ANGELETTI, P. U. (1969) The nerve growth factor: purification as a 30,000 molecular weight protein. *Proc. Natn. Acad. Sci. USA* **64**, 787–794.

CUATRECASAS, P. (1969) Interaction of insulin with the cell membrane: The primary action of insulin. *Proc. Natn. Acad. Sci. USA* **63**, 450–457.

CUATRECASAS, P. (1971a) Insulin-receptor interactions in adipose tissue cells: Direct measurement and properties. *Proc. Natn. Acad. Sci. USA* **68**, 1264–1268.

CUATRECASAS, P. (1971b) Perturbation of the insulin receptor of isolated fat cells with proteolytic enzymes: direct measurement of insulin-receptor interactions. *J. Biol. Chem.* **246**, 6522–6531.

CUATRECASAS, P. (1971c) Properties of the insulin receptor of isolated fat cell membranes. *J. Biol. Chem.* **246**, 7265–7274.

DESBOUQOIS, B., and CUATRECASAS, P. (1972) Independence of glucagon receptors and glucagon inactivation in liver cell membranes. *Nature New Biology* **236**, 202–204.

FRAZIER, W. A., ANGELETTI, R. H., and BRADSHAW, R. A. (1972) Nerve growth factor and insulin. *Science* **176**, 482–488.

HENDRY, I. A. (1972) Developmental changes in tissue and plasma, concentrations of the biologically active species of nerve growth factor in the mouse, using a two-site radioimmunoassay. *Biochem. J.* **128**, 1265–1272.

HENDRY, I. A., and IVERSEN, L. L. (1973) Reduction of nerve growth factor (NGF) concentrations and tyrosine hydroxylase activity in mouse tissues after submaxillary gland removal: a hypothesis for the retrograde trophic role of NGF in the sympathetic nervous system. *Nature* (in press).

KRUG, V., KRUG, F., and CUATRECASAS, P. (1972) Emergence of insulin receptors on human lymphocytes during *in vitro* transformation. *Proc. Natn. Acad. Sci. USA* **69**, 2634–2638.

LEVI-MONTALCINI, R., and ANGELETTI, P. U. (1968) Nerve growth factor. *Physiol. Rev.* **48**, 534–569.

LEVI-MONTALCINI, R., MEYER, H., and HAMBURGER, V. (1954) *In vitro* experiments on the effects of mouse sarcoma, 180 and 37 on the spinal and sympathetic ganglia of the chick embryo. *Cancer Res.* **14**, 49–57.

VARON, S., NOMURA, J., and SHOOTER, E. M. (1967) The isolation of the mouse nerve growth factor protein in a high molecular weight form. *Biochemistry* **6**, 2202–2209.

DNA SYNTHESIS AND CELL DIVISION IN DIFFERENTIATING AVIAN ADRENERGIC NEUROBLASTS

ALAN M. COHEN

Department of Anatomy, the Johns Hopkins University School of Medicine, Baltimore, Maryland 21205, *USA*

SUMMARY

Differentiation of avian adrenergic neuroblasts is marked by a stage of rapid formation of cate-cholamine-containing cells. These neuroblasts, identified by formaldehyde-induced fluorescence contribute to development of sympathetic ganglia and adrenal medulla. It is generally believed that the cells arise from an indifferent population of stem cells. Consistent with this is the idea that differentiation begins after cell division ceases. The early appearance of CA fluorescence in neuroblasts and the rapid increase in their number suggest that differentiation, judged by synthesis and storage of CA, might not be incompatible with cell division.

The possibility that differentiating adrenergic neuroblasts could proliferate was tested using autoradiography to follow DNA synthesis and direct observation to identify mitosis. Chick embryos $5\frac{1}{2}$–12 days of development were injected with thymidine-^{3}H, incubated for 1 h, and then prepared for formaldehyde-induced fluorescence to demonstrate CA or electron microscopy to identify dense-core granules. The simultaneous presence of CA fluorescence and silver grains, representative of iso-topically labeled DNA, was examined by combining darkfield-tungsten and reflected ultraviolet illumination.

Incorporation of thymidine-^{3}H by CA fluorescent neuroblasts took place at all stages examined. Labeled neuroblasts were seen in paravertebral, para-aortic, and adrenal medullary positions. Electron microscopic autoradiography revealed isotopically labeled nuclear DNA in cells containing dense-core granules. In addition, mitotic figures were seen in cells identified by the presence of dense-core granules. These observations indicate that initiation of differentiation by adrenergic neuroblasts does not preclude their proliferation. The suggestion that such cells might contribute significantly to multiplicative growth in the sympathetic system is discussed.

INTRODUCTION

Adrenergic neurons and secretory cells are presumed to differentiate from a common stem cell referred to as "the primitive sympathetic cell" (Coupland, 1965; Hervonen, 1971; Hervonen and Kanerva, 1972; Papka, 1972). These small cells are characterized by a baso-philic nucleus, scanty cytoplasm, absence of formaldehyde-induced fluorescence and lack of catecholamine-storage granules. Furthermore, mitosis is routinely observed, implicating primitive sympathetic cells as a precursor population. The primitive sympathetic cells acquire euchromatic nuclei and weakly CA fluorescent cytoplasm containing a few small storage granules. With appearance of these cytoplasmic features, the cells are identified as sympathicoblasts, phaeocromoblasts, or sympathetic neuroblasts, presumably transitional phases in development of adrenergic neurons and storage cells. The blast cells have been observed in mitosis, but with further differentiation and accumulation of dense core granules mitosis ceases (Hervonen, 1971; Kanerva, 1972). Ultimately, proliferation of adrenergic precursors stops, and mitosis cannot be detected in adrenergic neurons or adrenal medullary cells in the adult (Leblond and Walker, 1956).

It would appear that ontogenesis of adrenergic neuroblasts obeys the old embryological dictum "differentiated cells do not divide" or, stated otherwise, "cell division is incompatible with differentiation". This rule fits our understanding of developing neuroblasts in the central nervous system. Accumulation of neurofibrils and outgrowth of axons do not occur until the neuroblasts withdraw from the mitotic cycle and migrate from the ventricular germinal epithelium into the mantle zone (reviewed in Jacobson, 1970). In maturing adrenergic neuroblasts, failure to detect mitosis in granule-containing cells may be due to withdrawal from the mitotic cycle. On the other hand, mitotic activity could continue but might be difficult to detect in routine fine structural investigation. Generally, the period spent in mitosis is short compared to the duration of the cell cycle; therefore, relatively few proliferating cells are accounted for by the presence of metaphase figures (Mitchison, 1971).

The present paper further examines the relationship between proliferation and differentiation by adrenergic cells in avian embryos. Catecholamine-positive cells differentiate relatively early in chicks, rats, mice, rabbits, and humans (Encmar et al., 1965; de Champlain et al., 1970; Hervonen, 1971; Fernholm, 1972; Papka, 1972). The numbers of CA-fluorescent cells rapidly increase and organize to form primary and secondary sympathetic ganglia, paraganglia, and adrenal medulla. The increase in numbers of CA fluorescent cells may reflect (1) differentiation of primitive sympathetic cells, (2) proliferation of cells already synthesizing and storing neurotransmitter, or (3) a combination of these possibilities.

If appearance of CA synthesis and storage mechanisms is incompatible with proliferation, as might be expected from our understanding of neuroblast differentiation in the central nervous system, then CA fluorescent cells would not be expected to synthesize DNA. To test this possibility, autoradiographic methods were combined with fluorescence histochemistry and electron microscopy in order to identify thymidine-^{3}H incorporation in adrenergic neuroblasts. The data demonstrate that the presence of CA and storage granules does not preclude cell division. This raises the possibility that mitotic activity of the CA-positive neuroblasts might account for a significant proportion of proliferation in the adrenergic system.

MATERIALS AND METHODS

White Leghorn chicken embryos, $5\frac{1}{2}$–12 days of incubation (Hamburger–Hamilton stages 28–38) were used for this study. DNA synthesis was examined autoradiographically after injecting 5 μCi (for light microscopy) or 50 μCi (for electron microscopy) thymidine-^{3}H (New England Nuclear Corp., Boston, Mass.) into the vitelline or chorioallantoic veins. Embryos were incubated for 1 h further at 38°C, then tissues were removed and prepared for either CA fluorescence histochemistry or electron microscopy.

The formaldehyde-induced fluorescence technique (Falck and Owman, 1965) was used to identify intracellular CA. Tissues from lower thoracic and lumbar regions were quenched, lyophilized, and gassed as described elsewhere (Cohen, 1972). Spurr low viscosity embedding media (Polysciences, Inc., Warrington, Pennsylvania) was used for infiltration and embedding; infiltration took place at room temperature *in vacuo*, followed by polymerization at 70°C overnight. Sections cut at 3 μ were transferred to gelatin-coated slides, dipped into Ilford K-2 photographic emulsion (Ilford Ltd., Essex, England), and after 1–2 weeks' exposure were developed in Dektol. Silver grains and formaldehyde-induced fluorescence were demonstrated simultaneously by combining darkfield-tungsten and reflected ultraviolet illumination. For this purpose, a Zeiss universal microscope was equipped with a cardioid darkfield condenser, an FL 450 dichroic reflector, an Osram HBO 200 mercury lamp and Schott KG1, BG 12, and 500 μ barrier filters.

Electron microscopic autoradiography was used to follow thymidine-^{3}H incorporation into cells with dense-core vesicles. Tissues were fixed by immersion in Karnovsky's formaldehyde-glutaraldehyde solution (Karnovsky, 1965) for 15 min at room temperature, postosmicated, dehydrated, embedded in Araldite, and sectioned (Hay and Revel, 1969). Silver–gold sections were picked up on grids and coated with Ilford L-4 emulsion by using a chromium wire loop (Caro, 1964). After a period of 2–5 weeks, the autoradiographs were developed in Microdol-X and stained with uranyl acetate and lead citrate.

RESULTS

LIGHT MICROSCOPY

Green to yellow–green formaldehyde-induced fluorescence, characteristic of CA, was observed in sections processed for autoradiography. These sections showed only a slight reduction in intensity of fluorescence as compared with sections not exposed to the aqueous solvents used for autoradiography. Fluorescent cells were identified in paravertebral and para-aortic ganglia, adrenal medulla, and in aggregations of cells forming plexuses of differing morphology (Figs. 1–3). The intensity of fluorescence varied from cell to cell, although cells of para-aortic ganglia and adrenal medulla varied less in intensity than cells of para-vertebral ganglia. Fluorescent cell processes, when present, were generally short and thick and did not exhibit varicosities.

Formaldehyde-induced fluorescence and silver grains were observed simultaneously by combining tungsten and ultraviolet illumination. Autoradiography of tissues fixed 1 h after administration of thymidine-^{3}H showed label over nuclei in fluorescent cells at all stages examined (Figs. 1–3). The number of silver grains over nuclei of sympathetic neuroblasts was estimated to be roughly equivalent to that over other proliferating populations, such as germinal epithelium of the spinal cord. These observations at 5, 9, and 12 days of development were qualitatively similar and will be considered together.

Whereas silver grains show up as black spots in bright-field illumination, in mixed illumination they appear as brilliant orange points of light. In cells without CA or background fluorescence, clusters of these orange spots are seen against an empty black background (Figs. 1 and 2). In CA fluorescent neuroblasts, silver grains are generally restricted to the nonfluorescent area representing the nucleus, but some label is usually seen over adjacent fluorescent regions. These juxtanuclear grains probably represent nuclear DNA synthesis but cannot be resolved as such because either (1) CAs have diffused into the nucleus during histological processing or (2) cytoplasm overlaps the nucleus within the plane of the section. That the label is primarily nuclear in nature is demonstrated by observation of corresponding stained sections after fluorescence analysis.

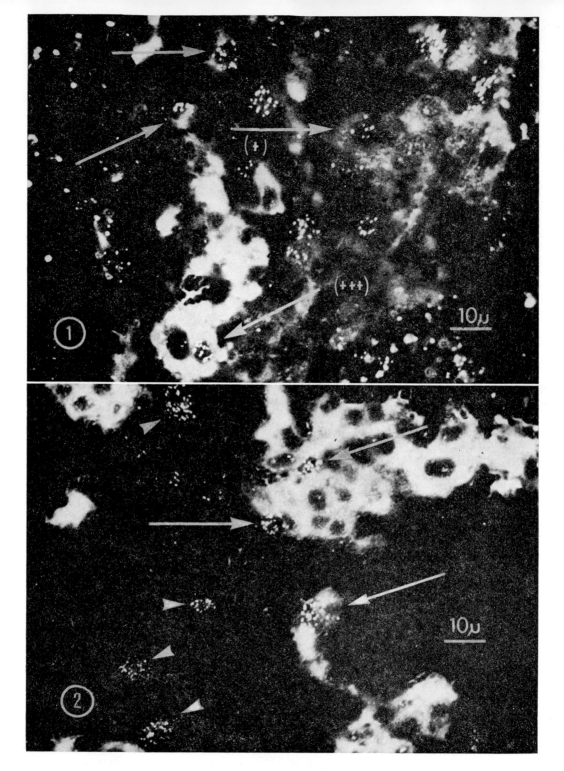

FIG. 1. A light microscopic autoradiograph of a paravertebral ganglion from a 9-day chick embryo exposed to thymidine-^{3}H for 1 h. Darkfield tungsten mixed with reflected ultraviolet illumination demonstrate silver grains and formaldehyde induced fluorescence simultaneously. The presence of silver grains over cells containing CA (arrows) indicates that DNA synthesis is not incompatible with synthesis and storage of neurotransmitter. The label is found primarily over the nonfluorescent nuclear areas. Note labeling in weakly (+) and intensely (+++) fluorescent cells. ($\times$1080).

FIG. 2. This autoradiograph of an adrenal gland from the same embryo shown in Fig. 1 illustrates the incorporation of thymidine-^{3}H into nuclei in medullary cells (arrows). Labeled nuclei are seen both in the center and at the periphery of the cord of CA-containing cells, shown in the upper right-hand corner of the figure. Several labeled cells that do not exhibit formaldehyde-induced fluorescence are identified by arrowheads. ($\times$1080.)

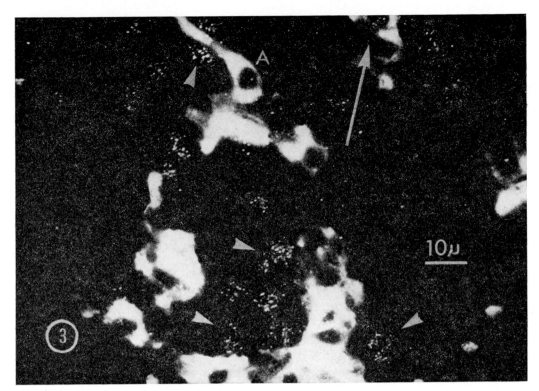

Fig. 3. A group of CA-positive cells from the para-aortic region of a 5½-day embryo incubated with thymidine-³H for 1 h is shown in this autoradiograph. Only 1 adrenergic cell is labeled (arrow). Note labeled nuclei of nonfluorescent cells (arrowheads) adjacent to a group of sympathicoblasts and associated with an adrenergic axon (A). These nonfluorescent cells may represent satellite cells or primitive sympathetic cells. (× 1080.)

The distribution of labeled nuclei in the developing sympathetic nervous system does not suggest an obvious pattern. Both moderately and weakly fluorescent cells synthesize DNA, shown by the distribution of silver grains in the paravertebral ganglia (Fig. 1). The labeled cells are positioned randomly, both in the center and at the periphery of groups of fluorescent cells. The situation is similar in the adrenal gland where labeled nuclei are found at the periphery and in the middle of medullary cords (Fig. 2). The medullary cells exhibit a yellowish fluorescence, indicative of high levels of CA (Norberg *et al.*, 1966). Even so, DNA synthesis is routinely detected in such cells.

Occasionally, groups of labeled nonfluorescent cells are observed adjacent to CA-containing cells in sympathetic ganglia (Fig. 3). These cells may represent primitive sympathetic cells, the suggested sympathetic precursors. On the other hand, satellite cells, fibroblasts, and other connective tissue cells are present and may account for such labeling. Two clusters of silver grains adjacent to a CA-fluorescent axon, by virtue of their position, most likely belong to satellite cells (Fig. 3).

ELECTRON MICROSCOPY

Electron microscopic autoradiography of adrenal tissue from 9-day embryos exposed to thymidine-³H for 1 h prior to fixation, revealed that differentiating medullary cells synthesize DNA (Figs. 4 and 5). The main cytological feature of these cells is their complement of electron opaque granules, measuring 1000–4800 Å in diameter. The density, irregular halo, and secretory membrane of these structures suggests storage of noradrenaline (Coupland and Hopwood, 1966). Label was found over nuclei of medullary cells packed into large clusters (Fig. 4) as well as over granule-containing cells in the connective tissue capsule (Fig. 5). Labeled nuclei in the medullary collections were round or ovoid and regular in shape. The chromatin was usually dispersed and 1 or 2 nucleoli were generally present. In addition to dense-core granules, the cytoplasm contained limited amounts of rough endoplasmic reticulum, Golgi apparatus, and mitochondria, all indicative of secretory activity. These cells would be considered as maturing CA storage cells according to the criteria of Coupland and Weakley (1968) and Hervonen (1971).

Mitoses were occasionally observed in CA-storage cells in the adrenal gland (Fig. 6). The granules usually occupied a peripheral position in the cell, although sometimes they were found centrally, adjacent to chromosomes. A preliminary examination of lumbar paravertebral neuroblasts from a 10-day embryo also revealed mitotic figures in cells with dense-core granules (Fig. 7). Again, the granules were at the margins of the cell, presumably assuming this position due to the central position of the spindle and metaphase chromosomes.

DISCUSSION

The results from this investigation show that synthesis of neurotransmitter by the differentiating sympathetic neuroblasts does not preclude continued proliferation. Thymidine-^{3}H was incorporated into nuclei of CA fluorescent cells as well as into cells with dense-core granules. In addition, mitoses are observed in CA storage cells of the adrenal medulla and in paravertebral neuroblasts with dense-core vesicles. These observations are contrary to the widely held belief that the increase in numbers of CA-containing cells during development is due to proliferation and differentiation of an indifferent population of cells. The labeling index of CA fluorescent cells at 6 days of development may be as high as 25% (Cohen, unpublished data), suggesting that differentiating sympathicoblasts contribute significantly to growth of the sympathetic ganglia and adrenal medulla.

The incorporation of thymidine-^{3}H into nuclei is used in the present study to distinguish cells synthesizing DNA. Such labeling has been shown by others to identify those cells in preparation for division (Mitchison, 1971). An alternative explanation that cannot be ruled out entirely is that the label might represent "differential" replication of certain regions of the chromosome (Ebert and Kaighn, 1966). Silver grains over sympathicoblasts most likely, however, represent DNA synthesized during the S period of the mitotic cycle. This is suggested by the fact that the amount of label over sympathetic nuclei is similar to that over germinal cells of the neuroepithelium and other proliferating cells in the same section.

The old embryological dictum that cell specialization is incompatible with differentiation has been weakened considerably in recent years. Cardiac muscle (Manasek, 1968; Weinstein and Hay, 1970), smooth muscle (Cobb and Bennett, 1970), cartilage (Cahn and Lasher, 1967), white adipose tissue (Pilgrim, 1971), and pancreatic endocrine (von Denffer, 1970) and exocrine (Pictet et al., 1972) cells have been shown to divide after appearance of their respective phenotypic traits. On the other hand, an obligatory relationship exists between the maturation of certain cell characteristics and cessation of DNA synthesis. This is well illustrated in the case with skeletal muscle (Stockdale and Holtzer, 1961), neuroblasts of the central nervous system (Fujita, 1964), and lens fiber cells (Modak et al., 1968).

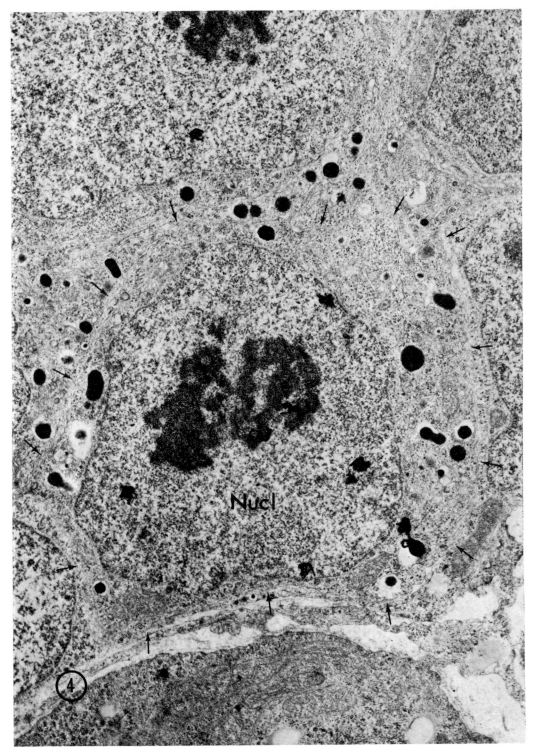

FIG. 4. This electronmicroscopic autoradiograph illustrates silver grains over the nucleus (Nucl) of a sympathicoblast in an adrenal medullary cord. The adrenal gland is from a 12-day embryo that had been exposed to thymidine-^{3}H for 1 h. The silver grains represent isotopically labeled DNA synthesized in a differentiating cell identified by its complement of large CA storage granules. The margins of the cell are indicated by arrows. ($\times$8300.)

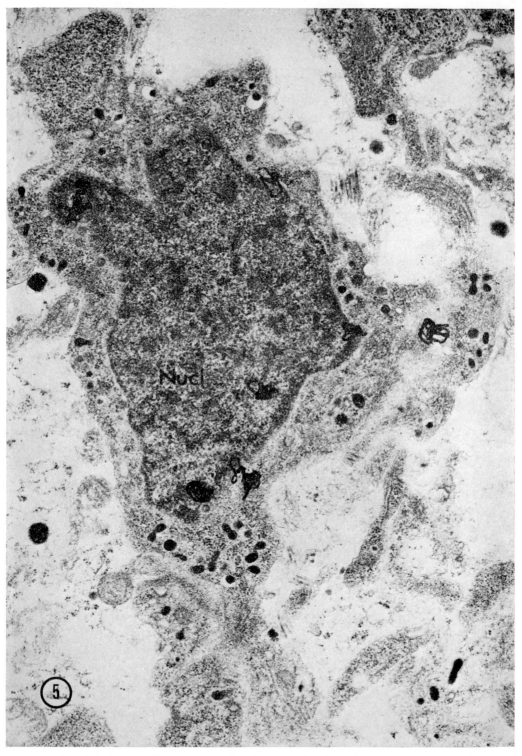

Fig. 5. A CA storage cell in the connective tissue capsule of an adrenal gland from a 12-day embryo after administration of thymidine-³H. Incorporation of the isotopic precursor of DNA is indicated by the moderate number of silver grains over the nucleus (Nucl) in this electron-microscopic autoradiograph. (×11,000.)

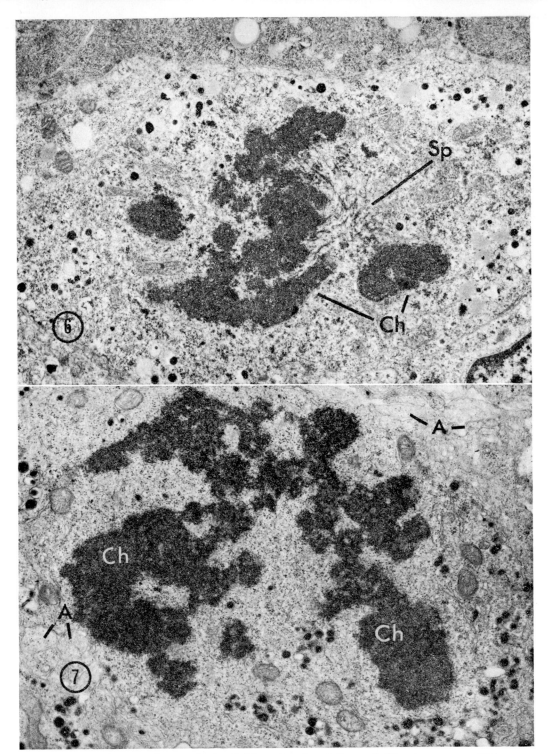

Fig. 6. An electron micrograph of a dividing adrenal medullary cell. The chromosomes (Ch) and mitotic spindle apparatus (Sp) occupy a central position surrounded by dense core granules. The presence of a mitotic figure in this differentiating sympathicoblast indicates that such cells play a role in multiplicative growth of the medullary cords. (×6600.)

Fig. 7. A dividing sympathetic neuroblast is shown in this electron micrograph from a 10-day embryonic paravertebral ganglion. The condensed chromosomes (Ch) are prominent, surrounded by dense core granules in the peripheral cytoplasm. Several axons are present adjacent to the cell. The observation of mitosis in granule-containing cells and the incorporation of thymidine-^{3}H in CA fluorescent cells suggest that sympathetic neurons do not arise entirely from an indifferent population of cells. (×8100.)

Sympathetic neuroblasts eventually stop dividing, indicated by the diminishing mitotic index in sympathetic ganglia during development (Yates, 1961) and the fact that mitoses are not detected in adult sympathetic ganglia and adrenal medulla (Leblond and Walker, 1956). Are there morphological correlates that can be related to withdrawal from the mitotic cycle? The presence of cellular monoamines and storage granules does not appear to prohibit cell division. Contrary to a previous report (Yates, 1961), sympathetic neuroblasts do not cease dividing by 8 days of incubation in the chick. DNA synthesis and cell division in adrenergic elements have been observed in the present study through 12 days of development; older stages have not yet been examined. In addition, mitosis has also been reported in cells containing dense-core granules in rabbits, rats, and humans (Coupland and Weakly, 1968; Mascorro and Yates, 1970; Hervonen, 1971; Hervonen and Kanerva, 1972).

The nature of the sympathetic stem cells is not clear at this time. They originate in the neural crest, migrate ventrally, and localize dorso-lateral to the aorta (Hammond and Yntema, 1947). During this ventral migration, CA fluorescence is not detected but is seen first in the crest cells aggregating to form the primary sympathetic chains (Enemar et al., 1965). Differentiation of the neuroblasts depends, at least in part, on tissue interactions between crest cells and neighboring tissues during the early phases of migration (Cohen, 1972). Somites and ventral half of the spinal cord both play an as yet undefined role in eliciting the appearance of CA. Synthesis of CA in the primary sympathetic neuroblasts is followed by a period of rapid hyperplastic growth in sympathetic ganglia, plexuses, and adrenal medulla. As we have seen, the CA positive sympathicoblasts themselves contribute to this activity, but to what extent is not known.

It may be tempting to infer, as some investigators do, the state of cytodifferentiation from the intensity of formaldehyde-induced fluorescence. In the chick, the first CA fluorescence is weak, but rapidly increases in intensity (Enemar et al., 1965). In mice and rats, young sympathicoblasts exhibit medium to strong fluorescence followed by a decrease later in development (de Champlain et al., 1970; Fernholm, 1972). In humans, the more immature sympathicoblasts are reported to be weakly fluorescent, with differentiation accompanied by increases in intensity (Hervonen, 1971; Hervonen and Kanerva, 1972). These differences could reflect species variation or the fact that monoamines in embryonic cells are more difficult to preserve and demonstrate (Olson, 1967; Björklund et al., 1968). On the other hand, the variations might be due to differences in the state of maturation. For instance, weakly fluorescent cells might represent (1) immature cells with low levels of CA, or (2) differentiating neurons in which axonal transport has displaced monoamines from the cell body. Cells characterized by high levels of CA fluorescence might represent (1) young sympathicoblasts (de Champlain et al., 1970), or (2) differentiating small intensely fluorescent (SIF) cells (Eränkö, 1972). In the present study, DNA synthesis was observed both in strongly and weakly fluorescent cells. Taken together, these observations suggest caution in judging cytodifferentiation on the basis of intensity of CA fluorescence.

In recent years a number of substances have been identified which promote growth of adrenergic nerve elements. Nerve growth factor stimulates mitotic activity in sympathetic ganglia of chick embryos, in addition to accelerating the maturation process of differentiating neuroblasts (Levi-Montalcini and Angeletti, 1968). Guanethidine, a chemical which destroys adrenergic neurons, causes the mean number of SIF cells to increase in the superior cervical ganglion of the newborn rat (Eränkö and Eränkö, 1971). Another growth-promoting substance, hydrocortisone, influences the maintenance and growth of extramedullary chromaffin tissue (Lempinen, 1964) and formation of increased numbers of SIF cells in sympathetic ganglia of the newborn rat, both *in vivo* (Eränkö and Eränkö, 1972) and *in vitro* (Eränkö *et al.*, 1972). The SIF cells, newly formed in response to guanethidine and hydrocortisone (*in vitro*), develop in clusters, which suggested to Eränkö *et al.* that SIF cells divide. The present study supports such a possibility. Examination of cell proliferation and its associated kinetics in sympathetic neuroblasts responding to growth-promoting substances should provide a better understanding of the mechanisms involved in regulation of growth and differentiation in this system.

ACKNOWLEDGEMENTS

This investigation was supported by NIH General Research Support Grant No. RR-5378 from the US Public Health Service.

REFERENCES

BJÖRKLUND, A., ENEMAR, A., and FALCK, B. (1968) Monoamines in the hypothalamo-hypophyseal system of the mouse with special reference to the ontogenetic aspects. *Z. Zellforsch.* **89**, 590–607.

CAHN, R. D. and LASHER, R. (1967) Simultaneous synthesis of DNA and specialized cellular products by differentiating cartilage cells *in vitro*. *Proc. Natn. Acad. Sci. USA* **58**, 1131–1138.

CARO, L. G. (1964) High-resolution autoradiography. In *Methods in Cell Physiology* (D. Prescott, ed.), Academic Press, New York, pp. 327–363.

COBB, J. L. S., and BENNETT, T. (1970) An ultrastructural study of mitotic division in differentiated gastric smooth muscle cells. *Z. Zellforsch.* **108**, 177–189.

COHEN, A. M. (1972) Factors directing the expression of sympathetic nerve traits in cells of neural crest origin. *J. Exp. Zool.* **179**, 167–182.

COUPLAND, R. E. (1965) *The Natural History of the Chromaffin Cell*, Longmans, London.

COUPLAND, R. E., and HOPWOOD, D. (1966) The mechanism of the differential staining reaction for adrenaline- and noradrenaline-storing granules in tissues fixed in glutaraldehyde. *J. Anat.* **100**, 227–243.

COUPLAND, R. E., and WEAKLY, B. S. (1968) Developing chromaffin tissue in the rabbit: an electron microscopic study. *J. Anat.* **102**, 425–455.

DE CHAMPLAIN, J., MALMFORS, T., OLSON, L., and SACHS, CH. (1970) Ontogenesis of peripheral adrenergic neurons in the rat: pre- and postnatal observations. *Acta physiol. scand.* **80**, 276–288.

EBERT, J. D., and KAIGHN, M. E. (1966) The keys to change: factors regulating differentiation. In *Major Problems in Developmental Biology* (M. Locke, ed.), Academic Press, New York, pp. 29–84.

ENEMAR, A., FALCK, B. and HAKANSON, R. (1965) Observations on the appearance of norepinephrine in the sympathetic nervous system of the chick embryo. *Devel. Biol.* **11**, 268–283.

ERÄNKÖ, O. (1972) Light and electron microscopic histochemical evidence of granular and non-granular storage of catecholamines in the sympathetic ganglion of the rat. *Histochem. J.* **4**, 213–224.

ERÄNKÖ, L., and ERÄNKÖ, O. (1971) Effect of guanethidine on nerve cells and small intensely fluorescent cells in sympathetic ganglia of newborn and adult rats. *Acta pharmac. tox.* **30**, 403–416.

ERÄNKÖ, L., and ERÄNKÖ, O. (1972) Effect of hydrocortisone on histochemically demonstrable catecholamines in the sympathetic ganglia and extra-adrenal chromaffin tissue of the rat. *Acta physiol. scand.* **84**, 125–133.

ERÄNKÖ, O., ERÄNKÖ, L., HILL, C. E., and BURNSTOCK, G. (1972) Hydrocortisone-induced increase in the number of small intensely fluorescent cells and their histochemically demonstrable catecholamine content in cultures of sympathetic ganglia of the newborn cat. *Histochem. J.* **4**, 49–58.

FALCK, B., and OWMAN, C. (1965) A detailed methodological description of the fluorescence method for the cellular demonstration of biogenic amines. *Acta Univ. Lund.*, Section II, No. 7, Lund.

FERNHOLM, M. (1972) On the appearance of monoamines in the sympathetic systems and the chromaffin tissue in the mouse embryo. *Z. Anat. Entw. Gesch.* **135**, 350–361.

FUJITA, S. (1964) Analysis of neuron differentiation in the central nervous system by tritiated thymidine autoradiography. *J. Comp. Neurol.* **122**, 311–327.

HAMBURGER, V., and HAMILTON, H. L. (1951) A series of normal stages in the development of the chick embryo. *J. Morph.* **88**, 49–92.

HAMMOND, W. S., and YNTEMA, C. L. (1947) Depletions in the thoraco-lumbar sympathetic system following removal of neural crest in the chick. *J. Comp. Neurol.* **86**, 237–265.

HAY, E. D., and REVEL, J. P. (1969) *Fine Structure of the Developing Avian Cornea*, Vol. 1, *Monographs in Developmental Biology* (A. Wolski and P. S. Chen, eds.), Karger, Basel.

HERVONEN, A. (1971) Development of catecholamine-storing cells in human fetal paraganglia and adrenal medulla. *Acta physiol. scand.*, Suppl. 368.

HERVONEN, A., and KANERVA, L. (1972) Catecholamine storing cells in human fetal superior cervical ganglion. *Acta physiol. scand.* **84**, 538–542.

JACOBSON, M. (1970) *Developmental Neurobiology*, Holt, Rinehart & Winston, New York, pp. 27–33.

KANERVA, L. (1972) Ultrastructure of sympathetic ganglion cells and granule-containing cells in the paracervical (Frankenhäuser) ganglion of the newborn rat. *Z. Zellforsch.* **126**, 25–40.

KARNOVSKY, M. J. (1965) Formaldehyde-glutaraldehyde fixative of high osmolarity for use in electron microscopy. *J. Cell Biol.* **27**, 137A.

LEBLOND, C. P., and WALKER, B. E. (1956) Renewal of cell populations. *Physiol. Rev.* **36**, 255–276.

LEMPINEN, M. (1964) Extra-adrenal chromaffin tissue of the rat and the effect of cortical hormones on it. *Acta physiol. scand.* **62**, Suppl. 231.

LEVI-MONTALCINI, R., and ANGELETTI, P. U. (1968) Nerve growth factor. *Physiol. Rev*, **48**, 534–569.

MANASEK, F. J. (1968) Mitosis in developing cardiac muscle. *J. Cell Biol.* **37**, 191–196.

MASCORRO, J. A., and YATES, R. O. (1970) Microscopic observations on abdominal sympathetic paraganglia. *Texas Rep. Biol. Med.* **28**, 58–68.

MITCHISON, J. M. (1971) *The Biology of the Cell Cycle*, Cambridge University Press, London.

MODAK, S. P., MORRIS, G., and YAMADA, T. (1968) DNA synthesis and mitotic activity during early development of chick lens. *Devel. Biol.* **16**, 545–561.

NORBERG, K.-A., RITZEN, M., and UNGERSTEDT, U. (1966) Histochemical studies on a special catecholamine-containing cell type in sympathetic ganglia. *Acta physiol. scand.* **67**, 260–270.

OLSON, L. (1967) Outgrowth of sympathetic adrenergic neurons in mice treated with a nerve-growth factor (NGF). *Z. Zellforsch.* **81**, 155–173.

PAPKA, R. E. (1972) Ultrastructural and fluorescence histochemical studies of developing sympathetic ganglia in the rabbit. *Am. J. Anat.* **134**, 337–364.

PICTET, R. L., CLARK, W. R., WILLIAMS, R. H., and RUTTER, W. J. (1972) An ultrastructural analysis of the developing embryonic pancreas. *Devel. Biol.* **29**, 436–467.

PILGRIM, C. (1971) DNA synthesis and differentiation in developing white adipose tissue. *Devel. Biol.* **26**, 69–76.

STOCKDALE, F. E., and HOLTZER, H. (1961) DNA synthesis and myogenesis. *Expl. Cell Res.* **24**, 508–520.

VON DENFFER, H. (1970) Autoradiographische und histochemische untersuchungen über das teilungsvermögen von B-Zellen der langerhansschen inseln im pankreas fetaler und neugeborener mäuse. *Histochemie* **21**, 338–352.

WEINSTEIN, R. B., and HAY, E. D. (1970) Deoxyribonucleic acid synthesis and mitosis in differentiated cardiac muscle cells of chick embryos. *J. Cell Biol.* **47**, 310–316.

YATES, R. D. (1961) A study of cell division in chick embryonic ganglia. *J. Exp. Zool.* **147**, 167–182.

GROWTH
SESSION II
Chairman: K. Fuxe

COLLATERAL REINNERVATION IN THE CENTRAL NERVOUS SYSTEM

G. RAISMAN

Department of Human Anatomy, South Parks Road, Oxford, O X1 3Q X, England

SUMMARY

In the adult rat, quantitative electron microscopic studies of synapses in the septal nuclei suggest that selective partial denervation induces a reaction akin to collateral reinnervation in the peripheral nervous system. Deafferented postsynaptic sites are reinnervated by adjacent normal axon terminals which thus acquire additional contacts.

It is a generally accepted view that injury to axons in the central nervous system has quite different effects from injury to axons in the peripheral nervous system. Whereas destruction of a peripheral nerve trunk can be followed by regeneration of the original connections (and hence functional recovery), lesions of central axons in mammals do not lead to regeneration. This has led to the opinion that the neurons of the central nervous system are incapable of regeneration or possibly that the environment of the central nervous system is in some way inimical to growth. In a series of experiments in the septal nuclei of the rat we have obtained some electron microscopical evidence which suggests that after selective partial deafferentation there may occur in this region a form of axonal reaction which results in the formation of new synapses and which results in the reinnervation of deafferented tissue. This is not regeneration of the cut axons but is comparable to the reaction of collateral reinnervation observed in the peripheral nervous system (Liu and Chambers, 1958). The existence of such a reaction suggests that there exists in the central nervous system the potentiality for efficient synaptogenesis even in adult mammals and this observation in turn re-opens the question of why the central nervous system is not therefore capable of true regeneration after injury. The present communication will deal with some of the principal findings in the rat septal nuclei, and for further details the reader is referred to the original publications (Raisman, 1969a; Raisman and Field, 1973).

In the design of the experiments we have been able to take advantage of the fact that there are two known sources of afferent fibres to the septal nuclei—axons of hippocampal origin which travel in the fimbria and axons ascending through the medial forebrain bundle

(Raisman, 1966). By examining the neuropil of the septal nuclei at the electron microscopic level we can identify all the synapses present in a given tissue sample, and these synapses have been classified in various ways. Most useful in respect of the present study have been, firstly, a division of axon terminals into classes according to their site of termination on the postsynaptic surface (i.e. on cell somata, dendritic shafts, or dendritic spines), and, secondly, the use of orthograde terminal degeneration as a method of identifying which terminals belong to axons travelling in either the fimbria or the medial forebrain bundle. Two days after a lesion of the parent axons, the terminals of these fibre systems undergo a form of degeneration which involves increased electron density and collapse of the terminal profile, although at this survival period the majority of terminals are still in apposition with their postsynaptic sites. This is, therefore, a useful technique for identifying the mode of distribution of fibre tracts within the septal neuropil.

By the use of this method (Raisman, 1969b) it was found that the fibres of the fimbria account for a large proportion (about one-third) of all axon terminals in the medial part of the lateral septal nucleus of the same side. These terminals contain principally small clear synaptic vesicles (of around 50 nm diameter) and make contact either with dendritic shafts or with their appendages. The axons of the medial forebrain bundle account for a rather smaller proportion of the synapses in this region, and they also differ from the terminals of the fimbrial fibres in two ways. Firstly, they make contact not only with dendrites but also directly with the cell bodies (axosomatic synapses), and, secondly, they contain in addition to synaptic vesicles a population of larger dense core vesicles (of around 100 nm diameter). Apart from the fimbria and the medial forebrain bundle, none of the remaining population of synapses in the septum have been identified in terms of their tracts of origin although it is clear from Golgi studies that the axons of the septal neurons themselves have profusely branched collaterals within the septal neuropil and these collaterals presumably form intrinsic synapses.

If the fimbria is cut and the survival time extended beyond the 2 days used to elicit the recognizable reaction of orthograde degeneration of terminals (Raisman, 1969a), there is a progressive collapse and dissolution of the degenerating axons which results in a mass of debris which is phagocytosed by astroglial elements. By 2 months after operation almost all traces of the degeneration have been removed as a consequence of this glial reaction. At this time the septal neuropil appears superficially normal although on closer inspection various abnormalities could be seen. Of these the most common was the existence of axon terminals which, in the plane of section, made contact with more than one postsynaptic element. The commonest configuration was a terminal which made contact with two separate postsynaptic profiles, and this has been called a double synapse (a term which is used here in a purely descriptive sense). The extent of this phenomenon was assessed quantitatively by calculating the number of such multiple synaptic contacts per hundred single synaptic contacts, and this figure was called the multiple synapse index. One possible explanation of the appearance of double synapses after a lesion of the fimbria was that the axon terminal involved in the double synapse had originally contacted only one of the two sites and that the other had been contacted by a fimbrial fibre terminal whose parent axon had been destroyed in the lesion. As a consequence of the removal of the degenerating terminal, the remaining adjacent axon terminal had been stimulated to synaptogenesis and had formed an additional synaptic contact which reinnervated the denervated site. This would result in the appearance of a double synapse and a rise in the multiple synapse index of the samples from the neuropil.

The rise in the multiple synapse index itself demonstrates that the remaining axon terminals in the septum have reacted to the original lesion and raises the interesting question of which axon terminals are showing this reaction. In order to investigate this point, we used a double-lesion technique. In animals in which the fimbria had been cut at least 2 months previously (i.e. at a time when all degeneration has been removed and when the double synapses have had time to form), a second lesion was placed in the medial forebrain bundle and after a further survival of 2 days the animals were sacrificed. In these cases it was found that as well as non-degenerating axon terminals participating in double synapse formation, a comparable proportion of the degenerating terminals were engaged in double synapses. This means that the original lesion of the fimbria had caused double synapse formation by axon terminals, some of which belonged to fibres running in the medial forebrain bundle. This, then, was a clear indication that destruction of one fibre tract can cause a direct modification of the fibres of another tract. It does not, however, prove that the second tract is reinnervating sites left vacant by the first lesion.

In order to examine this point, a converse type of double lesion experiment was performed (Raisman, 1969a). It will be recalled that in the normal septal neuropil the fimbrial fibres are never distributed upon cell bodies whereas the fibres of the medial forebrain bundle form direct axosomatic contacts (and account for up to one in four of all axosomatic contacts in some samples). A first lesion was placed in the medial forebrain bundle and a survival period of over 2 months was allowed. At this time the cell bodies had therefore suffered deafferentation and the degenerating products had been removed. In such animals a second lesion was placed in the fimbria, and after a further survival of 2 days the animals were sacrificed. In samples from the septum of these animals the fimbrial fibre terminals can be recognized by the reaction of electron-dense degeneration. Under these circumstances it was found that in addition to the normal distribution of degenerating terminals upon dendritic shafts and spines, the degenerating terminals were now found upon cell bodies. This means that the fimbrial fibres had acquired a new and abnormal distribution upon a site which had suffered deafferentation as a result of the original lesion of the medial forebrain bundle. It was therefore extremely tempting to speculate that the fimbrial fibres had, in thus expanding their distribution, taken over sites which had been denervated by the original lesion.

To test this hypothesis in a different way, we used a slightly different and in some ways simpler experimental design (Raisman and Field, 1973). In this later series of experiments we simply made lesions of the fimbria and examined the total number of synapses in the sampled areas of the septum, but took advantage of the extra dimension afforded by studying a series of animals at gradually increasing survival periods after the fimbrial lesion. After section of the fimbria it was found that the number of terminals showing degeneration rose rapidly in the first few days after operation, reaching a peak which was maintained over about the first week. During this time about one-third of all the synapses in the samples were degenerating. At longer survival times, the amount of degeneration fell until at 1-month postoperatively there were practically no degenerating terminals left. When the multiple synapse index was measured it was found that the double synapses do not appear in any great numbers for the first postoperative week. During the next 3 weeks, however, the multiple synapse index rises to reach a maximum. This is achieved at about 1 month after operation and from this time there is no further increase. This is exactly what would be predicted if the double synapses were formed as a result of the reinnervation of sites left vacant as a result of degeneration. During the first week, while the sites are still occupied by the degenerating terminals, double synapses cannot form; during the next 3 weeks, as the degenerating terminals are removed, the double synapses form in increasing numbers. After 1-month postoperatively, all the degeneration has been removed and there are therefore no further sites to be vacated; it is precisely at this point that the multiple synapse index ceases to rise further. This correspondence of time course, therefore, strongly supports the original hypothesis of collateral reinnervation of denervated sites.

The material used for this study, however, offered an even more convincing and independent piece of evidence favouring the hypothesis of collateral reinnervation. This was gained simply by counting the relative distribution of synapses on dendritic shafts and spines. In the normal septum, approximately two-thirds of all synapses are on dendritic spines and one third on dendritic shafts (ignoring the axosomatic synapses which account for less than 5% of all synapses). By use of the reaction of orthograde degeneration after short-term fimbrial lesions it could be shown that the fimbrial fibres are distributed preferentially upon dendritic spines. Thus, after cutting the fimbria, one-half of the synapses on dendritic spines show degeneration whereas only a small proportion (less than 10%) of those on dendritic shafts degenerate. If we now look at the numbers of normal (i.e. non-degenerating) synapses on dendritic spines at increasing survival times after a lesion of the fimbria, we find a striking reaction. During the first week after operation (when half the spine synapses are degenerating) the number of non-degenerating synapses on dendritic spines falls to half its original value—exactly as would be expected. However, during the next 3 weeks, when the degeneration is being removed (and the multiple synapse index is rising), the number of synapses on dendritic spines begins to rise again. It rises from its low level (of one-half the level found in the intact animals) until by 1 month after operation it has reached normal levels again.

At this point the proportion of synapses on dendritic spines reaches a level which is statistically indistinguishable from the normal animals and it ceases to rise further. As a result, the ultimate distribution of synapses on dendritic shafts and spines in the animals with long-term survivals is exactly the same as that in normal intact animals. Furthermore, the total number of all types of synapse present in the septum of these animals appears to be not less than that of the normal, intact animals. It is difficult to explain these observations in any way other than that the denervated dendritic spine sites persist after the original lesion and that they are reinnervated by the remaining axon terminals in the region.

On the basis of these findings we would suggest that in the septum of the adult rat collateral reinnervation occurs after selective partial deafferentation. When a postsynaptic site is vacated as a result of degeneration it acts in some way as a stimulus for the formation of additional synaptic contacts by adjacent axon terminals. This is not regeneration because the connections formed in this way are abnormal—the reaction can result in axon terminals innervating structures with which they are never normally in contact. However, the reaction is very rapid—following almost immediately after the removal of the degeneration. It is also very efficient in that virtually all the denervated sites are reclaimed by this process. In its time course the process is far from random—it follows a precise pattern which is predictable from one animal to the next.

While accepting that this reaction of collateral reinnervation does not result in true regeneration, and accepting also that these deductions have been drawn from one specific area in the rat brain, it is nonetheless striking that we have here a method of reaction to injury that is far more positive than is usually associated with the central nervous system of mammals. Perhaps most important are the two possibilities—that denervated sites can

persist and that axons can form new synaptic contacts. Given these conclusions it is even more interesting to ask the question, Why then do we not get true regeneration after axonal injuries in the central nervous system?

REFERENCES

LIU, C. N., and CHAMBERS, W. W. (1958) Intraspinal sprouting of dorsal root axons. *Archs. Neurol. Chicago*, **79**, 46–61.

RAISMAN, G. (1966) The connexions of the septum. *Brain* **89**, 317–348.

RAISMAN, G. (1969a) Neuronal plasticity in the septal nuclei of the adult rat. *Brain Res.* **14**, 25–48.

RAISMAN, G. (1969b) A comparison of the mode of termination of the hippocampal and hypothalamic afferents to the septal nuclei as revealed by electron microscopy of degeneration. *Expl. Brain Res.* **7**, 317–343.

RAISMAN, G., and FIELD, P. M. (1973) A quantitative investigation of the development of collateral re-innervation after partial deafferentation of the septal nuclei. *Brain Res.* **50**, 241–264.

GROWTH OF ADRENERGIC NEURONS IN THE ADULT MAMMALIAN NERVOUS SYSTEM

ROBERT Y. MOORE

Department of Pediatrics, Medicine (Neurology) and Anatomy and the Joseph P. Kennedy, Jr., Mental Retardation Research Center, the University of Chicago, Chicago, Illinois 60637, USA

SUMMARY

Central adrenergic neurons are capable of vigorous growth in response to injury. These regenerative reactions may occur either in response to direct insult to the adrenergic neuron, such as in the case of regenerative sprouting following axonal transection, or in response to the loss of other neuronal elements, as collateral sprouting from intact axons. Few examples of collateral sprouting have been shown in the central nervous system. The most clearly established of these is in the partially denervated septal nuclei. The functional significance of collateral sprouting is unknown at present, but it is suggested that it may be a basic biological phenomenon participating not only in responses to injury but also in functional neuronal reorganization in the intact central nervous system.

INTRODUCTION

There are three situations in which growth of neuronal processes may take place in the mammalian central nervous system. The first, and most extensively analyzed, of these is growth during ontogenetic development. The second is growth to provide a modification of neuronal architecture either as this might occur spontaneously or in response to environmental influences during adult life. Little is known of this type of growth, but there are indications that it may take place (Sotelo and Palay, 1971; Moore *et al.*, 1974). The third situation is growth in response to injury or disease. This type of growth, or regeneration, may also occur in the developing central nervous system, but here the process is complicated by interaction with ontogenetic factors (Schneider, 1970; Lund and Lund, 1971), so that its analysis is not so easily undertaken as in the adult. In this review we shall focus upon regenerative growth as this is expressed by monoamine producing neurons in the adult mammal. Regeneration will be defined in this context as any alteration in the morphological organization of the nervous system occurring in response to injury in which there is growth of neuronal processes to form new, functional synaptic contacts. This should not be taken to imply that the regenerative process itself is necessarily restorative of function in a physiologic or behavioral sense but only that the individual regenerating neuronal processes are capable of forming functional contacts and do so. There is an extensive literature on regeneration in the central nervous system, but most of this has centered on regenerative sprouting from severed central axons (cf. Cajal, 1928; Clemente, 1964; Moore et al., 1974, for reviews). Although it is well known in the periphery (Edds, 1953), little attention has been devoted to collateral sprouting from intact central axons (Moore et al., 1974), and the possibility of regenerative dendritic growth is largely unexplored. The events of regenerative axonal growth are not always separate, however, and it now appears that at least some of what has been viewed as regenerative sprouting may be collateral sprouting (Bernstein and Bernstein, 1973). The evidence for collateral sprouting from intact axons in the adult central nervous system largely has been acquired from studies on either the visual (Goodman and Horel, 1967; Bogdassarian and Goodman, 1970; Lund and Lund, 1971; Cunningham, 1972; Ralston and Chow, 1973) or somatic sensory (Liu and Chambers, 1958; Westrum and Black, 1971; Goldberger and Murray, 1972) systems. Even in these systems some components do not exhibit collateral sprouting and not all studies have achieved consistently positive data (Kerr, 1972; Guillery, 1972). A vigorous collateral sprouting has been observed in some connections of the hippocampal-septal system (Raisman, 1969; Moore et al., 1971b; Lynch et al., 1972, 1973; Raisman and Field, 1973), and this will be discussed in part, in greater detail below. Recent studies indicate that central adrenergic neurons are capable of remarkable regenerative responses, both regenerative sprouting and collateral sprouting, and these will be reviewed in subsequent sections.

REGENERATIVE SPROUTING OF CENTRAL ADRENERGIC NEURONS

Regenerative sprouting and collateral sprouting occur as prominent responses to injury from peripheral adrenergic neurons (Olson and Malmfors, 1970). Regenerative sprouting from severed central adrenergic axons was first shown by Katzman et al. (1971). Growing regenerating axons in rostral, basal midbrain formed extensive plexuses of anomalous innervation in and near a lesion and, in some instances, grew anomalously into adjacent blood vessels and roots of cranial nerves. Subsequent studies demonstrated that similar regenerative sprouting occurs from severed axons of serotonin and noradrenaline neurons of the bulbospinal system (Björklund et al., 1971). In addition, in each instance, it was found that growing noradrenaline fibers would innervate transplants of peripheral tissue normally innervated by sympathetic neurons (Björklund et al., 1971; Björklund and Stenevi, 1971). The pattern of innervation produced in the transplanted tissue by the regenerating central axons was, in each instance, typical of the normal innervation of the tissue. Further, dopamine and serotonin axons did not appear extensively to innervate transplanted tissues and some transplants, such as those from diaphragm, which has little normal sympathetic innervation, received little innervation from regenerating central adrenergic neurons when transplanted into the medial forebrain bundle. These observations have established that central adrenergic neurons are capable of vigorous regenerative sprouting, that the growing axons are capable of forming a distinct pattern of innervation, and that this innervation pattern is determined by an interaction between the growing axons and the tissue to be innervated. It has not been established that this newly formed innervation is functional, but the discrete and recognizable patterns of innervation certainly suggest that this is the case. The capacity for regenerative sprouting by central adrenergic neurons demonstrated in these studies (Katzman et al., 1971; Björklund and Stenevi, 1971; Björklund et al., 1971) goes beyond that described for any other group of central neurons. Nevertheless, as pointed out by Cajal (1928) and others (cf. Clemente, 1964), regenerative sprouting of severed central axons appears to have little role to play, at least at the current state of our knowledge, in establishing restoration of function after central nervous system injury. The functional significance of collateral sprouting may be of considerably greater importance than regenerative sprouting since this form of regenerative response would not be impaired by the cicatricial changes that occur so commonly in the vicinity of a destructive lesion and prevent the growth of regenerative sprouts to regions distal to the lesion.

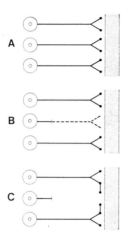

FIG. 1. Diagram representing collateral sprouting. In A, three neurons are shown innervating the structure on the right. In B, the axon of the middle neuron has been transected and degenerates to partially denervate the innervated structure. In C, the adjacent axons have sprouted new collaterals and terminals to reinnervate the denervated area.

COLLATERAL SPROUTING OF CENTRAL ADRENERGIC NEURONS

The basic paradigm for a collateral sprouting experiment is shown schematically in Fig. 1. In this, when part of the innervation to a nucleus is removed by a distant lesion, the severed axons do not grow to reinnervate the nucleus, but the remaining intact axons within the nucleus sprout to innervate the denervated synaptic sites. This phenomenon has been studied very intensively in the rat septal nuclei by Raisman (1969) and Raisman and Field (1973). These studies are reviewed elsewhere in this volume but, in brief, the authors found that removing one source of innervation to the neurons of the septal nuclei, such as that from the hippocampal formation, resulted in a reoccupation of the denervated synaptic sites, presumably from the other major source of afferent input to the medial and lateral septal nuclei, axons of the medial forebrain bundle.

The septal nuclei contain a rather dense adrenergic innervation (Fuxe, 1965) arising from the locus coeruleus and reaching the septal area largely via the medial forebrain bundle, and it appeared worthwhile to determine if this participated in the phenomena described by Raisman (1969). Such a demonstration would have two effects: it would identify the source and system of at least some of the axons participating in those phenomena, and it would provide evidence of the capacity of central adrenergic neurons to participate in collateral sprouting.

An experiment was designed in which rats were subjected to unilateral section of the fornix to partially denervate the medial and lateral septal nuclei ipsilateral to the lesion (Moore *et al.*, 1971b). The contralateral side serves as a control. The distribution of varicose, adrenergic fibers within the septal nuclei and adjacent areas was examined using the Falck–Hillarp histochemical fluorescence method in normal, unoperated animals and at 3, 8, 15, 30, 60, and 100 days after fornix section. No changes in the adrenergic innervation of the septal nuclei were noted at 3 and 8 days after fornix section, but there were some accumulations of amine in swollen, distorted axons located dorsally near the border of the lesion. These were no longer evident beyond 15 days' postoperative survival. By 15 days, however, the distribution of adrenergic innervation appeared greater in the septal nuclei ipsilateral to the fornix lesion and by 30 days, and thereafter, the distinction was clear and consistent. The difference appeared as an increase in the apparent number of fluorescent varicosities without a change in the density of fluorescence (Moore *et al.*, 1971b). No other area in the basal telencephalon or hypothalamus exhibited any such change. For example, the adrenergic innervation of the nucleus of the diagonal band and that of the lateral and medial preoptic areas were indistinguishable in comparing one side of the brain to the other. The changes in septal adrenergic innervation were dependent upon the success of the fornix lesion; when this was misplaced or incomplete the results were variable and did not approach the magnitude of changes obtained with complete denervations (Moore *et al.*, 1971b).

Although these data are in accord with those obtained by Raisman (1969) and Raisman and Field (1973), this does not provide definitive evidence to establish that the apparent change in septal adrenergic innervation following fornix section is a consequence of collateral sprouting. The collateral sprouting concept implies that the increased density of adrenergic varicosities observed following fornix section represents a true increase in the number of terminals and that these are reinnervating the synaptic sites denervated by removal of the hippocampal afferents. This is supported indirectly by the observation that noradrenaline content increases in the denervated septum with a time course equivalent to that obtained in the histochemical studies (Moore *et al.*, 1971b). An alternative explanation would state that the apparent increase in number of fluorescent varicosities and assayable noradrenaline in the denervated septum reflects amine accumulation in septal collaterals of axons passing to the hippocampus rather than collateral sprouting. This recognizes that the septal innervation experiment may not provide a pure situation for collateral sprouting in that the septal and hippocampal adrenergic innervation may each arise as collaterals of the same locus coeruleus neuron axons. It is well known that there is an accumulation of amine proximal to section of an axon, including in collaterals of the axon (Ungerstedt, 1971), but this phenomenon would not appear explanatory of our observations. First, we observed changes only in the lateral and medial septal nuclei, and it would seem unlikely that these are the only nuclei receiving collaterals of locus coeruleus axons passing through the septum to innervate the hippocampus. Second, we observed an increase in the number and distribution of varicosities within the septal nuclei, not an increase in fluorescence intensity of those already present. If this were to be attributed to an increased accumulation in collaterals, those showing the increase would have to be normally not demonstrable in Falck–Hillarp material. There are no data to suggest that such fibers exist. Finally, the time course for amine accumulation usually is brief, whereas the changes noted in our studies appear to be permanent (Moore *et al.*, 1971b, 1973). It is not possible to exclude a type of collateral axonal sprouting occurring in the manner described by Bloom *et al.* (this volume) but, again, in that instance the effect appears self-limited in time.

Nevertheless, we wished to provide some evidence beyond fluorescent histochemistry and amine determinations to support the concept that collateral sprouting was occurring in the partially denervated septum. In one study a unilateral fornix section was performed and 60 days later bilateral, electrolytic lesions produced in the medial forebrain bundle. The animals were sacrificed 5 days later and sections through the septum were prepared using the Fink–Heimer method (cf. Heimer, 1968) for selective demonstration of degenerating axon terminals. Unfortunately all ascending medial forebrain bundle axons were involved, and the silver impregnations proved sufficiently capricious to make this material difficult to interpret. Recently we have undertaken another study in which unilateral fornix section was performed by ablating the anterior hippocampus and waiting for a postoperative survival period of 30 days. The animals were then subjected to bilateral injections of tritiated leucine into the locus coeruleus, the source of noradrenaline neurons innervating the septal nuclei (Ungerstedt, 1971; Moore, unpublished observations). Unoperated control animals were similarly injected for comparison (Table 1). It is now well known that labeled amino acid

TABLE 1. LOCUS COERULEUS INJECTIONS OF LEUCINE-^{3}H-INCORPORATION AND TRANSPORT TO DENERVATED AND INTACT SEPTAL NUCLEI IN THE RAT[a]

Group	Mean dpm/mg tissue		Mean percent difference	Denervated > control side
	Denervated[b] side	Control side		
Control	419.1	398.5	+6.5%	3/6
Hippocampal lesion	907.2	528.8	+61.6%	6/0

[a] Adult female rats were subjected to a unilateral anterior hippocampal ablation as previously described (Moore et al., 1971). Thirty days later bilateral injections of 1 μl ^{3}H-leucine (20 μCi/μl) were made into the locus coeruleus. The animals were sacrificed 24 h later by perfusion with a solution of 10% formaldehyde in 0.9% saline. Septal nuclei from each side were dissected, dissolved in Soluene, and counted.
[b] For injected control animals the right side was arbitrarily designated as "denervated."

injected into a nuclear area will be incorporated into protein within the neurons of the area and transported to the terminals of those neurons (Grafstein, 1969; Cowan et al., 1972). There may be acute changes associated with an immediate neuronal reaction to injury (Grafstein and Murray, 1969), but by 30 days these should have subsided. Therefore one would expect that, if the terminal plexus is increased, this would be reflected in increased rapid transport of labeled protein to that area. This is what is observed (Table 1) following unilateral fornix section. The control animals show no significant difference between sides. The mean disintegrations per minute for the control animals is slightly less than that for the control side of the operated animals, probably reflecting that the two groups were injected with a different batch of labeled amino acid. The denervated septum, that is the one deprived of hippocampal input, shows a markedly increased radioactivity (61.6% greater than the control side) and in no case in this group was the amount of labeled protein transported to the denervated side less than 40% greater than the control side. The placement of the injections within the locus coeruleus was confirmed autoradiographically (Fig. 2). These observations are in accord with those reported above and, taken together with the studies of Raisman (1969) and Raisman and Field (1973), provide substantive evidence that collateral sprouting occurs in the septal area denervated by removal of hippocampal input and that the axons of adrenergic neurons arising in the locus coeruleus participate in this process.

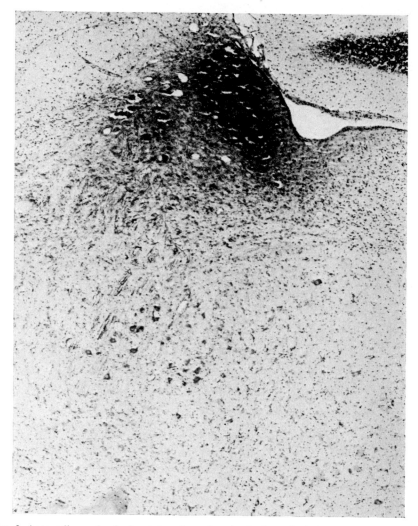

FIG. 2. Autoradiograph of a frontal section of rat brain through the locus coeruleus. One day prior to sacrifice of the animal the locus coeruleus was injected with 20 μCi tritiated leucine in 1 μl normal saline. The cells of the locus coeruleus, lying in the periventricular gray adjacent to the 4th ventricle, are heavily labeled with developed silver grains as are the cells of the adjacent mesencephalic trigeminal nucleus. Some fibers of the mesencephalic root emerging ventrolaterally from the root are also labeled. Cresyl violet stain. ×105.

Thus all the available evidence is in accord with the view that central adrenergic axons will undergo collateral sprouting in response to denervation but it is not known whether this is a phenomenon restricted to noradrenaline neurons or, for that matter, only those innervating the septal area. In order to investigate this problem a series of studies was undertaken. In the original experiment reviewed above (Moore *et al.*, 1971b), other areas than the septum were reviewed and the observations made in these are as follows. After fornix section we did not observe any change in the adrenergic innervation of the nucleus of the diagonal band, lateral preoptic area, or lateral mammillary nucleus. The lateral preoptic area and diagonal band contain a significant number of adrenergic fibers but the hippocampal projection is not heavy (Raisman, 1966). The lateral mammillary nucleus, in contrast, receives a dense hippocampal projection but few adrenergic fibers. The anteroventral thalamic nucleus is heavily innervated by nonadrenergic axons from hippocampus via the fornix and from brainstem adrenergic neurons. Following fornix section there is an apparent increase in the adrenergic innervation of the nucleus, but this observation is preliminary and we cannot rule out the possibility that the observed changes reflect a shrinkage of the nucleus with retrograde degeneration subsequent to incidental interruption of thalamocortical fibers in the lesion. This appears unlikely, however, in view of data obtained from studies on the lateral geniculate. Like the anteroventral nucleus of the dorsal thalamus, the dorsal lateral geniculate nucleus contains quite a rich adrenergic innervation (Fuxe, 1965). Following removal of retinal input to the lateral geniculate, this is unchanged but, after cortical ablation with subsequent retrograde degeneration of geniculate neurons, there is a marked increase in adrenergic innervation (Stenevi et al., 1972). This occurs before significant shrinkage of the nucleus takes place and cannot be attributed to an apparent increase in adrenergic innervation concomitant to a decrease in nuclear volume. When the reactive glial response becomes maximal, however, there is marked shrinkage of the nucleus and the remaining adrenergic innervation is difficult to appreciate in the mass of autofluorescent material which accumulates. This situation would appear, then, to be another in which collateral sprouting of adrenergic axons occurs, in this case only in response to the massive denervation attendant upon degeneration of the dorsal lateral geniculate cell bodies.

A number of other experimental situations have been examined which deserve mention only in passing. Removal of input to the suprachiasmatic hypothalamic nucleus from the retina and from the midbrain raphe does not alter its sparse adrenergic innervation. Similar findings obtain in the superior colliculus upon ablation of the ipsilateral visual cortex, section of the contralateral optic nerve, or both. Again, in this situation the adrenergic fibers to the optic tectum are few and distributed principally to the deep layers, whereas the retinal and corticofugal afferents are distributed principally to superficial layers. Amygdala ablation, with consequent degeneration of the ventral amygdalofugal pathway into the lateral hypothalamus, did not produce any change in the distribution of adrenergic fibers in this area. Olfactory bulb ablation, on the other hand, resulted in a small but significant increase in fluorescence in the olfactory tubercle in Falck–Hillarp material on the denervated side at time intervals from 30 to 180 days after the lesion. This appearance in the fluorescence microscope was confirmed by chemical determinations of dopamine. Dopamine levels in the denervated tubercle are 46 % higher than in controls without any corresponding change in weight (Table 2). Since both the olfactory bulb input (Heimer, 1968) and the ascending dopamine neuron input (Fuxe, 1965) are heavy, and to the same layers of the olfactory tubercle, the observations suggest that the dopamine fibers may exhibit collateral sprouting in response to denervation of olfactory input. This study is open to the same criticisms as the septal study reviewed above, and further data are required before definitive conclusions can be reached.

The focus of these studies has been on adrenergic neurons, and little information is available on the regenerative capacity of indolamine neurons (Björklund et al., 1971; Nygren et al., 1971; Nobin et al., 1973). In order to obtain some information as to whether such neurons may exhibit collateral sprouting, we performed the same experiment with fornix section as had been done before for studying the adrenergic innervation of the septum (Moore et al., 1971b). It did not prove possible to clearly identify serotonin fibers in Falck–

TABLE 2. OLFACTORY TUBERCLE DOPAMINE FOLLOWING OLFACTORY BULB ABLATION IN THE RAT

Sample group	Weight (mg $\pm$ SE)	Olfactory tubercle dopamine (μg $\pm$ SE)	Dopamine content (μg/g $\pm$ SE)
Denervated	130 $\pm$ 11	0.16 $\pm$ 0.03	1.18 $\pm$ 0.20
Control	134 $\pm$ 13	0.11 $\pm$ 0.02	0.81 $\pm$ 0.12
p	NS	<0.05	<0.05

Adult female albino rats were subjected to unilateral ablation, by aspiration, of one olfactory bulb. Thirty days later they were sacrificed and olfactory tubercles dissected from the denervated and control side of the brain. Each group was made up of four samples each containing six pooled olfactory tubercles. Dopamine was analyzed by a method previously described (Moore et al., 1971). The dopamine content of the denervated olfactory tubercle is 46 % greater than that of the control sample. p Values were obtained using a two-tailed t-test for differences. NS refers to $p > 0.05$.

TABLE 3. SEROTONIN CONTENT OF THE RAT SEPTAL NUCLEI FOLLOWING HIPPOCAMPAL ABLATION

Postoperative survival period	Septal serotonin content[a] (μg/g + SE)		Percent difference	p[b]
	Hippocampal group	Sham operated group		
3 days	1.08 $\pm$ 0.15	1.16 $\pm$ 0.07	−7%	NS
15 days	1.09 $\pm$ 0.06	0.93 $\pm$ 0.05	+17%	NS
30 days	1.38 $\pm$ 0.10	1.02 $\pm$ 0.10	+35%	<0.05
60 days	1.34 $\pm$ 0.05	1.03 $\pm$ 0.04	+30%	<0.01

[a] Each sample was made up of the medial and lateral septal nuclei from two rats. Each value in the table represents the mean of 6 samples.
[b] p values were obtained using a two-tailed t-test. NS refers to $p > 0.05$.

Hillarp material in the septum, so that only chemical determinations were performed. The results of this study are shown in Table 3. At 3 days after rostral hippocampal ablation there is only a small difference between denervated and control groups in septal serotonin content. This difference is greater at 15 days, and by 30 days there is a statistically significantly greater serotonin content (35%) in the denervated samples, and this difference appears stable through 60 days after operation. These observations also obviously require confirmation by independent methodology, but they do suggest that the serotonin fibers innervating the septum also participate in a process of collateral sprouting after removal of hippocampal input to the septal nuclei.

The interpretation of studies reviewed above is that the relationship between the extent of denervation and the density of innervation by monoaminergic fibers is critical. For collateral sprouting to take place and be recognized it would appear essential that the denervation of nonmonoaminergic elements must be considerable. This clearly obtains in the septal area studies, the olfactory tubercle study, and the lateral geniculate study. In addition there must be some minimal density of monoaminergic innervation within the denervated area for it to respond to the denervation and to be demonstrable by the methods employed. A corollary of this is that the monoaminergic innervation must be in a sufficient proximity to denervated sites to reinnervate them by collateral sprouting. The stimulus for collateral sprouting is unknown but, as in the periphery (Edds, 1953), the denervated synaptic site would appear the best candidate to promote growth of nearby axons. One cannot exclude the possibility that some continuing "normal" axonal growth contributes to the process, but it appears unlikely to be the whole answer.

There are two further critically important questions which must be put but cannot be answered at this time. First, is collateral sprouting an ubiquitous phenomenon among central axons or is it limited to certain groups or systems? Or does the capacity exist in many central neurons but to a variable extent? Certainly the responses of adrenergic neurons would appear to be greater than those of some components of the visual system (Guillery, 1972) or some cortical neurons (Cajal, 1928; Rutledge et al., 1972), but much more information is required. The process may be extremely important if it occurs as a "normal" phenomenon participating in synaptic reorganization in the adult central nervous system (Sotelo and Palay, 1971; Moore et al., 1971b) as well as in response to injury. Second, one must question the functional significance of collateral sprouting. Again, there are little data to go on. In some situations collateral sprouting may promote neuronal interactions interfering with function (McCouch et al., 1958) whereas in others it may promote function (Goldberger and Murray, 1972). Presumably the effects obtained depend upon the function specified so that in varying situations following neuronal injury collateral sprouting may either lead toward apparent recovery of function, disrupt it, or be functionally insignificant. Obviously, studies of the functional consequences of collateral sprouting are needed.

ACKNOWLEDGEMENTS

This work was supported by grants NS-05002 and HD-04583 from the National Institutes of Health. United States Public Health Service. It was carried out in part in collaboration with Drs. Anders Björklund and Ulf Stenevi, Department of Histology, University of Lund, Lund, Sweden.

REFERENCES

BERNSTEIN, M. E., and BERNSTEIN, J. J. (1973) Regeneration of axons and synaptic complex formation rostral to the site of hemisection in the spinal cord of the monkey, Int. J. Neurosci. 5, 15–26.

BJÖRKLUND, A., and STENEVI, U. (1971) Growth of central catecholamine neurons into smooth muscle grafts in the rat mesencephalon. Brain Res. 31, 7–20.

BJÖRKLUND, A., KATZMAN, R., STENEVI, U., and WEST, K. A. (1971) Development and growth of axonal sprouts from norepinephrine and 5-hydroxytryptamine neurons in the rat spinal cord. Brain Res. 31, 21–33.

BOGDASSARIAN, R. A., and GOODMAN, D. C. (1970) Axonal sprouting of intact retinofugal neurons as a consequence of opposite eye removal: homotypic compared to heterotypic axonal sprouting. Anat. Rec. 166, 280.

CAJAL, S. R. (1928) Degeneration and Regeneration of the Nervous System, Oxford University Press, London.

CLEMENTE, C. D. (1964) Regeneration in the vertebrate central nervous system. Int. Rev. Neurobiol. 6, 257–301.

COWAN, W. M., GOTTLIEB, D. I., HENDRICKSON, A. E., PRICE, J. L., and WOOLSEY, T. A. (1972) The autoradiographic demonstration of axonal connections in the central nervous system. Brain Res. 37, 21–51.

CUNNINGHAM, T. J. (1972) Sprouting of the optic projection after cortical lesions. Anat. Rec. 172, 298.

EDDS, M. V. (1953) Collateral nerve regeneration. Q. Rev. Biol. 28, 260–275.

FUXE, K. (1965) Evidence for the existence of monoamine neurons in the central nervous system: IV, Distribution of monoamine nerve terminals in the central nervous system. Acta physiol. scand., Suppl. 247, 37–85.

GOLDBERGER, M. E., and MURRAY, M. (1972) Recovery of function after partial denervation of the spinal cord: a behavioral and anatomical study. Paper presented at 2nd Society for Neuroscience Meeting, Houston, Texas.

GOODMAN, D. E., and HOREL, J. A. (1967) Sprouting of optic tract projections in the brain stem of the rat J. Comp. Neurol. 127, 71–88.

GRAFSTEIN, B. (1969) Communication between soma and synapse. In *Advances in Biochemical Psychopharmacology* (E. Costa and P. Greengaard, eds.), Raven Press, New York, 1, 11–25.

GRAFSTEIN, B., and MURRAY, M. (1969) Transport of protein in goldfish optic nerve during regeneration. *Expl. Neurol.* 25, 494–508.

GUILLERY, R. W. (1972) Experiments to determine whether retinogeniculate axons can form translaminar collateral sprouts in the dorsal lateral geniculate nucleus of the cat. *J. Comp. Neurol.* 146, 407–420.

HEIMER, L. (1968) Synaptic distribution of centripetal and centrifugal nerve fibers in the olfactory system of the rat: an experimental study. *J. Anat. Lond.* 103, 413–432.

KATZMAN, R., BJÖRKLUND, A., OWMAN, C., STENEVI, U., and WEST, K. A. (1971) Evidence for regenerative sprouting of central catecholamine neurons in the rat mesencephalon following electrolytic lesions. *Brain Res.* 25, 579–596.

KERR, F. L. (1972) The potential of cervical primary afferent to sprout in the spinal nucleus of V following long term trigeminal denervation. *Brain Res.* 43, 547–560.

LIU, C. N., and CHAMBERS, W. W. (1958) Intraspinal sprouting of dorsal root axons. *Archs. Neurol.* 79, 46–61.

LUND, R. D., and LUND, J. S. (1971) Synaptic adjustment after deafferentation of the superior colliculus in the rat. *Science* 171, 804–807.

LYNCH, G. S., MATTHEWS, D. A., MOSKO, S., PARKS, T., and COTMAN, C. (1972) Induced acetylcholinesterase-rich layer in rat dentate gyrus following entorhinal lesions. *Brain Res.* 42, 311–319.

LYNCH, G. S., MOSKO, S., PARKS, T., and COTMAN, C. W. (1973) Relocation and hyperdevelopment of the dentate commissural system after entorhinal lesions in immature rats. *Brain Res.* 49, 57–61.

McCOUCH, G. P., AUSTIN, G. M., LIU, C. N., and LIU, C. Y. (1958) Sprouting as a cause of spasticity. *J. Neurophysiol.* 21, 205–216.

MOORE, R. Y., BHATNAGAR, R. K., and HELLER, A. (1971a) Anatomical and chemical studies of a nigro-neostriatal projection in the cat. *Brain Res.* 30, 119–136.

MOORE, R. Y., BJÖRKLUND, A., and STENEVI, U. (1971b) Plastic changes in the adrenergic innervation of the rat septal area in response to denervation. *Brain Res.* 33, 13–35.

MOORE, R. Y., BJÖRKLUND, A., and STENEVI, U. (1974) Growth and plasticity of adrenergic neurons. In *The Neurosciences—Third Intensive Study Program*, (F. O. Schmitt and F. G. Worden, eds.), MIT Press, Cambridge. pp. 961–977.

NOBIN, A., BAUMGARTEN, H. G., BJÖRKLUND, A., LACHENMEYER, L., and STENEVI, U. (1973) Axonal degeneration and regeneration of the bulbospinal indolamine neurons after 5,6-dihydroxytryptamine treatment. *Brain Res.* 56, 1–24.

NYGREN, L.-G., OLSON, L., and SEIGER, A. (1971) Regeneration of monoamine-containing axons in the developing and adult spinal cord following intraspinal 6-hydroxydopamine injections or transections. *Histochemie* 28, 1–16.

OLSON, L., and MALMFORS, T. (1970) Growth characteristics of adrenergic nerves in the adult rat. *Acta physiol. scand.*, Suppl. 348, 1–112.

RAISMAN, G. (1966) The connections of the septum. *Brain Res.* 89, 317–348.

RAISMAN, G. (1969) Neuronal plasticity in the septal nuclei of the adult rat. *Brain Res.* 14, 25–48.

RAISMAN, G., and FIELD, P. M. (1973) A quantitative investigation of the development of collateral re-innervation after partial deafferentation of the septal nuclei. *Brain Res.* 50, 241–264.

RALSTON, H. J., and CHOW, K. L. (1973) Synaptic reorganization in the degenerating lateral geniculate nucleus of the rabbit. *J. Comp. Neurol.* 147, 321–350.

RUTLEDGE, L. T., DUNCAN, J., and CANT, N. (1972) Long term status of pyramidal cell axon collaterals and apical dendrites in denervated cortex. *Brain Res.* 41, 249–262.

SCHNEIDER, G. E. (1970) Mechanisms of functional recovery following lesions of the visual cortex or superior colliculus in neonate and adult hamsters. *Brain, Behav. Evol.* 3, 295–323.

SOTELO, C., and PALAY, S. L. (1971) Altered axons and axon terminals in the lateral vestibular nucleus of the rat: possible example of axonal remodeling. *Lab. Invest.* 25, 653–672.

STENEVI, U., BJÖRKLUND, A., and MOORE, R. Y. (1972) Growth of intact central adrenergic axons in the denervated lateral geniculate body. *Expl. Neurol.* 35, 290–299.

UNGERSTEDT, U. (1971) Stereotaxic mapping of the monoamine pathways in the rat brain. *Acta physiol. scand.* Suppl. 367, 1–48.

WESTRUM, L. E., and BLACK, R. G. (1971) Fine structural aspects of the synaptic organization of the spinal trigeminal nucleus (pars interpolaris) of the cat. *Brain Res.* 25, 265–288.

HAS NERVE GROWTH FACTOR A ROLE IN THE REGENERATION OF CENTRAL AND PERIPHERAL CATECHOLAMINE NEURONS?

ANDERS BJÖRKLUND, BO BJERRE, AND ULF STENEVI

Departments of Anatomy and Histology, University of Lund, Lund, Sweden

1. INTRODUCTION

Axonal regeneration can be understood as the attempt of a neuron to re-establish axonal connections severed by a lesion. This process implies a series of complex events involving the reaction of the cell body to the injury (referred to as chromatolysis), the formation of new axonal sprouts, the outgrowth of the new sprouts, and, finally, the establishment of new synaptic connections. In the present paper we deal with regeneration in the more restricted meaning of the term, the reformation of a damaged axon part, although it seems likely that also collateral sprouting of intact neurons, in response to a lesion, could be the expression of essentially the same neuronal events (Moore *et al.*, 1973).

Studies of the mechanisms that control axonal regeneration are of particular interest in the central nervous system. Thus, whereas regeneration in the peripheral nervous system usually leads to the reformation of at least part of the severed connections, regeneration in the mammalian brain and spinal cord is usually considered to be very limited, and if regenerative attempts are made, they will be abortive and re-establishment of the original connections will not occur (Cajal, 1928; see Windle, 1955, and Clemente, 1964, for reviews). However, this apparent lack of regeneration in the CNS does not necessarily mean an *inability* of the central neurons to regenerate. In fact the neurons might possess an entirely adequate regenerative capacity, but in the damaged brain tissue the regenerative growth could normally either be actively inhibited, or the mechanisms regulating the process of axonal regeneration could be deficient or inadequately expressed. Very little is known of the conditions necessary to promote the directed growth which could re-establish morphological and functional integrity of lesioned central neurons. From recent studies it seems, however, that the mono-amine-containing neurons provide an excellent model for further studies into the cellular events regulating the process of axonal regeneration in the adult mammalian central nervous system. The catecholamine (CA)-containing and the indolamine (IA)-containing neurons, which are readily and selectively demonstrated with the fluorescence histochemical technique, have thus been found to possess a strong regenerative capacity (Katzman et al., 1971; Björklund et al., 1971, 1973) and in experiments with transplants of denervated peripheral tissue to the brain and the spinal cord, it has been possible to demonstrate that the central CA (noradrenaline (NA) and dopamine (DA)) neurons have an ability to "reinnervate" a denervated tissue that is comparable to that of the peripheral sympathetic noradrenaline neurons (Björklund and Stenevi, 1971; Björklund et al., 1971).

There is much evidence that the nerve growth factor (NGF) proteins play a critical role during ontogenetic growth and differentiation of sympathetic NA neurons (see Levi-Montalcini and Angeletti, 1968; Levi-Montalcini et al., 1972, for reviews). One of the most striking properties of NGF, both in vivo and in vitro, is to support and stimulate axonal outgrowth from the developing sympathetic neurons (Levi-Montalcini and Hamburger, 1953; Levi-Montalcini, 1964; Olson, 1967). In the intact mouse, treatment with NGF during the early neonatal period thus induces an excess axonal outgrowth resulting in adrenergic hyperinnervation of tissues normally innervated by sympathetic fibres (e.g. iris, salivary glands, and blood vessels) and in abnormal sympathetic innervation of such tissues as autonomic ganglia and adrenal cortex that normally more or less lack such innervation (Olson, 1967). There is so far no evidence for a role of NGF during the ontogenetic development of central CA neurons. However, Bjerre and Björklund (1973) found that CA-containing cells differentiated in vitro in explants taken from the cranial neural level of young chick embryos, and that the capacity to form such cells was stimulated by NGF. Although uncertain whether these CA-containing cells are identical with sympathoblasts or represents sympathoblast-like cells or precursor cells to central CA neurons, the findings seem to indicate that not merely the trunk neural crest derived sympathetic and sensory neurons are sensitive to NGF during ontogenesis.

In view of the important role of NGF during ontogenesis, it would be of considerable interest to know whether NGF continues to play a role also in the adult animal and whether NGF has any role in regenerative growth of adult neurons. The series of investigations reviewed in the present paper has attempted to study the possible effects of NGF and its antiserum on axonal regeneration of peripheral and central adult CA neurons. The results support the idea that NGF or NGF-like proteins might participate in the process of axonal regeneration of these neurons and perhaps play a role in the mechanisms regulating the regenerative cellular events.

2. REGENERATIVE CAPACITY OF PERIPHERAL AND CENTRAL CA NEURONS

Similar to other peripheral axons, the sympathetic NA axons regenerate well after damage (see Guth, 1956; Olson and Malmfors, 1970; and Kirpekar et al., 1970, for reviews). The rate at which these axons regenerate is comparable to that of peripheral motor and sensory nerves (Olson, 1969; Kirpekar et al., 1970), and if the lesion is made at a distance from the cell bodies, the sympathetic reinnervation of the denervated tissue appears to be complete or almost complete. In the rat sciatic nerve, Olson (1969) found that after axonal damage the distal portion of the NA-containing axons degenerate rapidly, and NA-containing growth cones and sprouts from the lesioned axons are demonstrable within 2–3 days. These new sprouts were estimated to grow along the nerve at a rate of about 1.4 mm/day during the first week after lesion and about 2.9 mm/day during the second week. In the cat spleen, Kirpekar et al. (1970) demonstrated a partial return of the adrenergic innervation within 4–8 weeks after a crush lesion of the sympathetic nerves, and the reinnervation of the spleen was almost complete after 6 months.

The high capacity for regeneration of peripheral adrenergic nerves is also demonstrated in animals subjected to chemical sympathectomy by 6-hydroxydopamine (6-OH-DA) (Haeusler *et al.*, 1969; Tranzer and Richards, 1971; de Champlain, 1971; Jonsson and Sachs, 1972). In the adult animal, systemic treatment with low to moderate doses of 6-OH-DA causes degeneration primarily of the terminal and paraterminal adrenergic axonal networks, and after such lesions the regrowth of normal or almost normal terminal adrenergic networks is complete within 2–3 months (see below).

Also within the adult central nervous system, it has been demonstrated that CA neurons— both NA-containing and DA-containing ones—as well as IA neurons, have a high capacity for regenerative sprouting (Katzman *et al.*, 1971; Björklund and Stenevi, 1971; Björklund *et al.*, 1971, 1973). Thus after mechanical or electrolytic lesions of preterminal monoamine axon bundles in the brain or the spinal cord, new axonal sprouts are seen to develop within a few days (2–3 days in the spinal cord), and after 2–3 weeks they form abundant fibre systems in the necrosis of the lesion and in the seemingly intact brain tissue surrounding the lesioned axons (Katzman *et al.*, 1971; Björklund *et al.*, 1971). After a substantial lesion, the growing sprouts apparently do not reach across the necrosis into their original pathways; instead, they grow abundantly into abnormal sites, where they also persist for at least several months. The most conspicuous example of such abnormal growth is the invasion of abundant sprouting CA fibres into intracerebral blood vessels and myelinated fibre bundles (Katzman *et al.*, 1971; Björklund and Stenevi, 1971).

The capacity of the adult central CA neurons to "reinnervate" a denervated tissue has been demonstrated in experiments with transplants of peripheral tissue to the brain and the spinal cord (Björklund and Stenevi, 1971; Björklund *et al.*, 1971). Thus after the placement of an iris—which is normally richly innervated by peripheral adrenergic nerves—within the pathways of the major ascending DA and NA neuron systems, the iris transplant will be invaded by regenerating sprouts from the lesioned NA and DA axons. Within 3–4 weeks after transplantation, the entire iris will be covered by the regenerated fibres, and within some areas this new central innervation will have the characteristic pattern of its original peripheral sympathetic innervation (Björklund and Stenevi, 1971; Bjerre *et al.*, 1973a).

From these studies two conclusions can be drawn. First, when the regenerating central CA axons are given the same growth conditions as those of regenerating peripheral CA neurons (i.e. a peripheral tissue denervated of its normal adrenergic innervation) they will readily innervate the denervated tissue. The time course by which this is accomplished, moreover, is similar to, or only slightly less than, that by which peripheral adrenergic neurons reinnervate an iris transplanted to the anterior chamber of the eye (Olson and Malmfors, 1970). Second, the pattern formed by the "reinnervating" central NA fibres is often remarkably similar to that exhibited by the normal, sympathetic innervation.

3. EFFECTS OF NGF AND ITS ANTISERUM ON THE REGENERATION OF PERIPHERAL CA NEURONS

The effects of exogenous NGF and of anti-NGF serum were tested on the process of regeneration after axonal degeneration induced by 6-OH-DA (Bjerre *et al.*, 1973b, 1974a). In the adult animal, 6-OH-DA in low to moderate doses is known to induce a selective degeneration of the terminal and paraterminal axon parts of the sympathetic neurons (Tranzer and Thoenen, 1967, 1968; Malmfors and Sachs, 1968; for reviews see Tranzer and Richards, 1971; Malmfors, 1971); therefore this drug offers a very useful tool for reproducible and widespread lesioning of peripheral adrenergic axons. The 6-OH-DA-lesioned axons regenerate efficiently and almost completely within 2–3 months (Haeusler et al., 1969; de Champlain 1971; Jonsson and Sachs, 1972) and because of its high reproducibility this regeneration process was found to be most favourable for studying the effects of NGF and its antiserum on axonal regeneration.

EFFECTS OF NGF

The study by Bjerre et al. (1973b) was carried out on 4–5-week-old male and female mice, i.e. at an age when the adrenergic innervation of the peripheral organs is fully established (cf. de Champlain et al., 1970; Owman et al., 1971; Mirkin, 1972). The animals were treated with one injection of 60 or 220 mg/kg of 6-OH-DA given intravenously. This treatment was followed either by six daily injections of 1000 or 3000 BU/g of NGF (subcutaneously), the animals being killed 9 days after the 6-OH-DA injection, or by 15 daily injections of 1000 BU/g of NGF (s.c.), the animals being killed 21 days after the 6-OH-DA injection. The extent of regeneration was evaluated in several organs by fluorescence histochemistry and by measurements of the NA content.

At 1 day after the 6-OH-DA treatment, there was a complete disappearance of the adrenergic terminal axonal ramifications in all tissues investigated, i.e. iris, heart, salivary glands, intestine, spleen, and pancreas. In addition, the higher dose of 6-OH-DA (220 mg/kg) caused a complete or almost complete disappearance of the adrenergic terminals also in the vas deferens and the accessory male genital glands. (Bjerre and Rosengren, unpublished). This was accompanied by a reduction of the endogenous NA content to 10% or less of normal. In all peripheral tissues investigated, bundles of preterminal NA-containing axons persisted, and they generally exhibited a higher than normal fluorescence intensity. Thus the 6-OH-DA-induced degeneration seemed to be confined mainly to the terminal and paraterminal ramifications of the axons within the terminal regions, whereas the preterminal axon parts were probably largely intact up to a point near to, or within, the target organs.

In most of the studied organs (iris, salivary glands, heart atria, intestine, and pancreas) the NGF treatment caused a marked stimulation of the axonal regeneration, as observed at both 9 and 21 days after the 6-OH-DA-induced axonal damage (Figs. 1–3). Although there was some variation in the magnitude of the NGF-induced effects (both between different organs within the same animal, and between different animals with respect to the same organ), the effect was usually seen both in the number and in the extent of the ramifications of the regenerating axons (Figs. 1a, b and 3), as well as in the thickness, number, and length of bundles of regenerating axons extending into the organs (Figs. 2 and 3). In addition, the fluorescence intensity—being reduced compared with normal in the regenerating axons of the 6-OH-DA-treated control animals—was generally clearly elevated in the NGF-treated animals (Figs. 1a, b and 2). The histochemical findings were paralleled by an increase in the rate of recovery of endogenous NA in the NGF-treated mice, as illustrated for the salivary glands in Fig. 4.

In interpreting these findings (Bjerre et al., 1973b) it seems that NGF stimulates the regrowth process of peripheral adrenergic neurons in several, and perhaps different, ways (cf. Fig. 3). First, NGF appeared to have a stimulatory effect on the process of sprouting

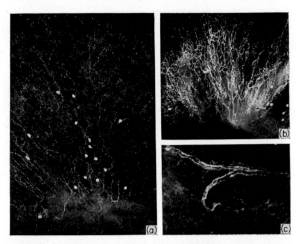

FIG. 1. (a), (b), and (c) Stretch preparations of irises from 4-week-old female mice treated with 60 mg/kg of 6-OH-DA and examined 21 days later. In (a) almost the whole width of the iris is shown; in (b) the sphincter and the inner part of the dilatator (corresponding to the lower half of (a)). The adrenergic innervation of the sphincter is seen at the bottom of the pictures. (a) Control treated with saline. Sparse elementary ground plexus of adrenergic fibres over the dilatator muscle. A few fibres extend a short distance radially into the sphincter ($\times 70$). (b) and (c) NGF specimens treated with 15 daily injections of 1000 BU/g of NGF from the day after the 6-OH-DA treatment and onwards. Note in (b) the dense but irregular ground plexus, the increased fluorescence intensity compared with the control (a), the frequent strands of two or more fibres in the plexus, and the frequent fibres extending into the sphincter ($\times 70$). In (c) a thin bundle of preterminal adrenergic axons is shown on the external edge of the iris at the level of insertion with the ciliary body (usually such bundles were not observed in the control specimens). Note the beginning formation of an adrenergic fibre plexus in the walls of an artery running below the bundle ($\times 110$). (From Bjerre et al., 1973b).

from the lesioned axons. This was observed as an increase in thickness and number of the regenerating fibre bundles, suggesting that NGF increased the number of sprouts growing out from the lesioned axons. Second, NGF was in some organs observed to increase the rate of growth of the sprouting fibres, resulting in a more advanced regeneration in the NGF-stimulated animals. Thus, in some organs, such as the salivary glands and the pancreas, the degree of reinnervation after NGF treatment at 9 days was as advanced as, or even more advanced than, that seen in the 21-day control animals given the same dose of 6-OH-DA. Third, the NGF-treatment was observed to restore the intra-axonal NA concentration in the regenerating axons. It seems possible that this could be due to the ability of NGF to increase the NA synthetic enzymes tyrosine hydroxylase and dopamine-β-hydroxylase, as demonstrated in the superior cervical ganglion of newborn rats and mice by Thoenen et al. (1971), Thoenen (1972), and Hendry and Iversen (1971). This interpretation is supported by the finding of Brimijoin and Molinoff (1971) that the dopamine-β-hydroxylase activity (but not the tyrosine hydroxylase activity) is markedly reduced in sympathetic ganglia of 6-OH-DA-treated adult rats (measured between 1 and 7 days after 6-OH-DA treatment).

In most peripheral organs studied, the effect of NGF was clearly established both by fluorescence histochemistry and by measurements of the endogenous NA content. Interestingly, a slight effect was observed fluorescence microscopically also on the so-called short adrenergic neurons innervating the vas deferens and the accessory genital glands (Bjerre and Rosengren, unpublished). In contrast to the pronounced effects obtained in the

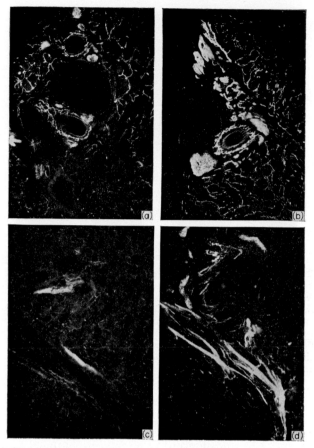

FIG. 2. (a) and (b) (×70) Hilum region of submaxillary-sublingual gland complex from 4-week-old female mice treated with 60 mg/kg of 6-OH-DA and examined 21 days later. (a) Control specimen. (b) NGF specimen treated with 15 daily injections of 1000 BU/g of NGF from the day after the 6-OH-DA injection and onwards. Note the increased number and size of bundles and their increased fluorescence intensity compared with the control picture in (a) showing an otherwise very similar part of the hilum region. (c) and (d) (×70) Bundles of preterminal adrenergic axons demonstrated within the submaxillary glands of 4-week-old female mice treated with 60 mg/kg of 6-OH-DA and killed 9 days later. The bundles run together with arteries and close to excretory ducts in the interlobular septa. (c) Control specimen. (d) NGF specimen treated with daily injections of NGF (1000 BU/g) for 6 consecutive days from the day after the 6-OH-DA treatment and onwards. Note the increased number and size of bundles and the increased fluorescence intensity in the NGF specimen. (From Bjerre et al., 1973b.)

atria of the heart, no clear-cut stimulatory effect of NGF was observed either histochemically or chemically in the heart ventricles, a finding that seems to parallel the observation made by Olson (1967) on intact newborn mice. It is conceivable that the lack of an observable effect on the adrenergic innervation of the ventricles could be due to a lower sensitivity to NGF of the neurons supplying them. The effect, though slight, observed histochemically on the regeneration of the so-called short adrenergic neurons supplying the vas deferens is notable as, in the newborn mouse, these neurons do not show any clear response to NGF (Olson, 1967; Levi-Montalcini and Angeletti, 1968).

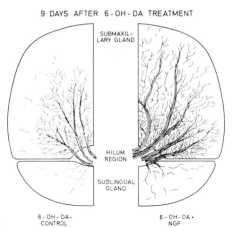

EFFECTS OF NGF AND ANTI-NGF SERUM ON THE
REGENERATIVE GROWTH OF ADRENERGIC FIBRES
INTO THE SALIVARY GLANDS

9 DAYS AFTER 6-OH-DA TREATMENT

SUBMAXIL-
LARY GLAND

HILUM
REGION

SUBLINGUAL
GLAND

6-OH-DA-
CONTROL

6-OH-DA+
NGF

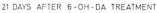

21 DAYS AFTER 6-OH-DA TREATMENT

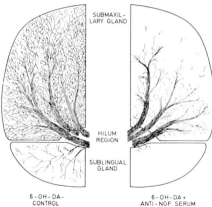

SUBMAXIL-
LARY GLAND

HILUM
REGION

SUBLINGUAL
GLAND

6-OH-DA-
CONTROL

6-OH-DA+
ANTI-NGF SERUM

FIG. 3. Schematic representation of the principal regenerative events in the adrenergic innervation of the salivary (submaxillary and sublingual) glands after 6-OH-DA treatment, as
interpreted from the fluorescence histochemical findings. The drawings represent longitudinal
sections through the glands, including the hilum region of the submaxillary-sublingual gland
complex. Main bundles of preterminal NA-containing axons entering at the hilum, together
with the vessels, branch together with arteries in the interlobular septa in the sub-maxillary gland
and give rise to para-terminal and terminal ramifications of the axons within the terminal regions.
The diagrams do not claim to be accurate with respect to all details (e.g. exact number and positions of bundles and their branches). *Above:* the morphological picture of the adrenergic innervation as observed 9 days after treatment with 6-OH-DA (220 mg/kg) of 5-week-old male mice.
The NGF specimen was given daily injections of NGF (1000 BU/g) for 6 consecutive days from
the first day after the 6-OH-DA treatment and onwards. The control was given saline similarly.
(From Bjerre *et al.*, 1973b.) *Below:* the adrenergic innervation within the salivary glands, as
demonstrated histochemically, 21 days after treatment with 6-OH-DA (60 mg/kg) of 5-week-
old male mice. Horse anti-NGF serum and normal horse serum were given in a single dose of
0.1 ml/g the day after 6-OH-DA treatment. The pattern of the adrenergic innervation within
the terminal areas is more or less restored to normal in the submaxillary, but not the sublingual, gland of the control specimen. In contrast, very few adrenergic terminal fibres are seen
in the anti-NGF serum treated specimen. (From Bjerre *et al.*, 1974a.)

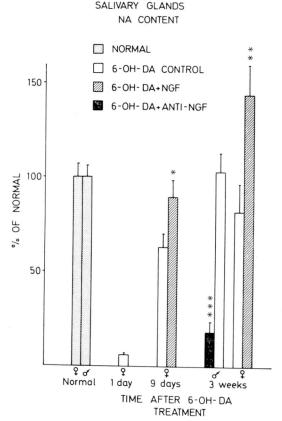

FIG. 4. Effects of NGF and anti-NGF serum on the noradrenaline (NA) content in the salivary glands of mice treated with 6-OH-DA (60 mg/kg, i.v.). Female mice (4 weeks old) were treated with 6-OH-DA and then treated with 1000 BU/g (s.c.) daily for 6 or 15 days. The animals were killed 9 or 21 days after the 6-OH-DA injection. Controls were given 6-OH-DA plus saline similarly. Male mice (5 weeks old) were given 6-OH-DA, followed by one injection (s.c.) of 0.1 ml/g horse anti-NGF serum or normal horse serum the day after 6-OH-DA treatment; they were killed 21 days after the 6-OH-DA injection. NA values are given as per cent of the NA content of untreated animals (1.46 μg NA/g tissue—females; 1.83 μg NA/g tissue—males); means + SEM of 6–12 determinations. Differences between control and experimental values *** $p < 0.001$; ** $0.01 > p > 0.001$; * $0.05 > p > 0.01$. Student's t-test.

EFFECTS OF ANTI-NGF SERUM

A study of the effects of anti-NGF serum on the axonal regeneration in peripheral adrenergic neurons after 6-OH-DA is now in progress (Bjerre *et al.*, 1974a) and only some preliminary observations will be reported here.

One injection of 0.1 ml/g of anti-NGF serum (s.c.) given the day after the 6-OH-DA treatment (60 mg/kg; 5-week-old male mice) caused a strongly inhibited regrowth of adrenergic fibres into all peripheral organs investigated, including the vas deferens and the accessory male genital glands (Bjerre and Rosengren, unpublished). This was observed both fluorescence histochemically as a strong reduction in the reappearance of adrenergic terminals (Figs. 3 and 5), and fluorometrically as a much reduced return of NA in the assayed organs (Fig. 4). The number, size, and length of the preterminal axon bundles seemed to be un-affected by the anti-NGF serum treatment, however, suggesting that this treatment did not

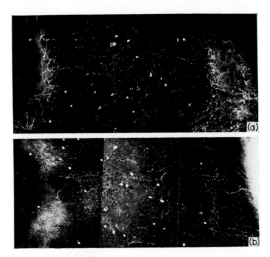

FIG. 5. (a) and (b) (×65) Stretch preparations of irises from 5-week-old male mice treated with 60 mg/kg of 6-OH-DA and examined 21 days later. The whole width of the iris is shown in (a) and almost the whole width in (b). The sphincter is seen to the left in both pictures. (a) Control given 0.1 ml/g of normal horse serum one day after the 6-OH-DA treatment. A sparse, but fairly regular, elementary ground plexus of adrenergic fibres is developed over the whole width of this area of the dilatator muscle. Note the fairly frequent fibres running both radially and circularly in the sphincter. (b) Specimen given 0.1 ml/g of horse anti-NGF serum one day after the 6-OH-DA treatment. A few fibres are branching over the dilatator muscle without developing an obvious elementary ground plexus. A few fibres reach the sphincter without extending into it.

further increase the extent of the axonal damage as observed in the fluorescence microscope, but rather impaired the regrowth of the sprouting fibres.

4. EFFECTS OF NGF AND ITS ANTISERUM ON THE REGENERATION OF CENTRAL CA AND IA NEURONS

The effects of NGF and anti-NGF serum were studied on the process of regeneration of lesioned central NA, DA, and IA neurons into an autologous iris transplant placed in the caudal diencephalon according to the technique of Björklund and Stenevi (1971) (Björklund and Stenevi, 1972; Bjerre et al., 1973a, 1974b; Stenevi et al., 1974). This growth process is sufficiently constant and reproducible to allow reliable quantitative evaluations in the fluorescence microscope of the rate and extent of axonal regeneration. The position of the transplant, as shown in Fig. 6, in close contact with the transected axons in the so-called dorsal catecholamine bundle (DCB) and the medial forebrain bundle (MFB), makes it possible to observe growth from three monoamine neuron types: the ascending CA (predominantly NA-containing) neurons in the DCB, and the ascending DA and IA (and to a minor extent also NA) neurons in the MFB (for anatomical details, see Ungerstedt, 1971). In untreated control animals, the iris, within 3–4 weeks, will be covered by regenerating NA and DA sprouts originating from the lesioned axons of the DCB and the MFB, whereas the sprouting IA fibres will normally enter the transplant only to a very limited extent. At 7 days after transplantation, the first few sprouting NA and DA fibres have entered the transplant, as illustrated schematically in Fig. 7. This survival time was therefore found suitable for observations on possible growth stimulating effects of NGF.

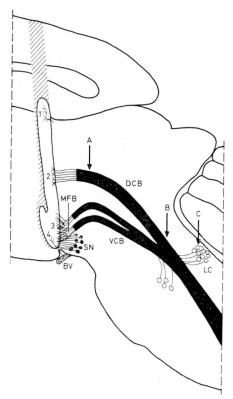

FIG. 6. Position of the iris transplant in the caudal diencephalon. The lesion produced by the transplantation (cross-hatched area) transects the two major ascending monoamine fibre systems, the dorsal catecholamine bundle (DCB) containing predominantly NA axons, and the medial forebrain bundle (MFB) containing IA axons (not represented in the diagram), DA axons (originating, *inter alia*, in the substantia nigra, SN), and also some NA axons (originating in the ventral catecholamine bundle, VCB). In the specimens used for the present study, the transplant is in direct contact with the growing monoamine fibres in these two bundles. The magnitude of ingrowth into the transplant illustrated in the diagram is that observed in control specimens 7 days after the transplantation. Filled circles: DA-containing cell bodies; open circles: NA-containing cell bodies. Arrows indicate sites of injections; close to the NA cell bodies in the locus coeruleus (C); close to the NA axons in the DCB (B), about 3 mm caudal to the site of the lesion; and close to the DCB (A), about 1 mm caudal to the lesion. When the transplant is placed in this position, fibres will grow into it from different locations: 1, the habenula region; 2, the DCB; 3, the MFB; 4, blood vessels at the base of the brain. Note: this is a schematic drawing of a transplant in a non-sympathectomized animal. (From Stenevi *et al.*, 1974.)

Proteins such as NGF and its antibodies will probably pass the blood–brain barrier only to a very limited extent (Angeletti *et al.*, 1972), and their systemic administration can therefore be expected to have exceedingly small possibilities for producing effects in the CNS. To circumvent this problem, NGF and anti-NGF serum were administered stereotaxically either into the cerebrospinal fluid via the lateral ventricle (Björklund and Stenevi, 1972; Bjerre *et al.*, 1973a, 1974b), or directly into the brain parenchyma (Fig. 6; Stenevi, *et al.*, 1974; Bjerre *et al.*, 1974b). In addition, experiments were made with incubations of the iris in NGF or anti-NGF serum before its transplantation into the diencephalon (Stenevi *et al.*, 1974; Bjerre *et al.*, 1974b).

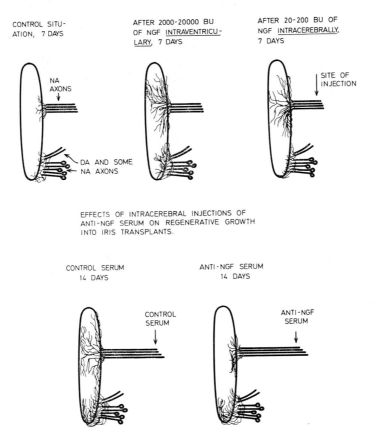

EFFECTS OF IV OR IC INJECTIONS OF NGF
ON REGENERATIVE GROWTH INTO IRIS
TRANSPLANTS.

CONTROL SITU-
ATION, 7 DAYS

AFTER 2000-20000 BU
OF NGF INTRAVENTRICU-
LARY, 7 DAYS

AFTER 20-200 BU OF
NGF INTRACEREBRALLY,
7 DAYS

NA
AXONS

SITE OF
INJECTION

DA AND SOME
NA AXONS

EFFECTS OF INTRACEREBRAL INJECTIONS OF
ANTI-NGF SERUM ON REGENERATIVE GROWTH
INTO IRIS TRANSPLANTS.

CONTROL SERUM
14 DAYS

ANTI-NGF SERUM
14 DAYS

CONTROL
SERUM

ANTI-NGF
SERUM

FIG. 7. Schematic representation of the effect of NGF given intraventricularly and intra-cerebrally as studied on the "reinnervation" of iris transplants to the caudal diencephalon (cf. Fig. 6). Note that 2000–20,000 BU of NGF given intraventricularly roughly correspond to 20–200 BU given intracerebrally, and that intracerebral injections of NGF close to the locus coeruleus neuron system only affects the regenerating fibres in the DCB. Also compared is the effect of intracerebral injections of anti-NGF serum and control serum as observed 14 days after transplantation. Note that anti-NGF serum has reduced the number of fibres and the area covered by these fibres within the transplant, so that the situation within the transplant here appears similar to that in a control specimen at 7 days. The figures also show the similar appearance within the transplant of an NGF-treated specimen at 7 days and a control specimen at 14 days.

EFFECTS OF INTRAVENTRICULARLY OR INTRACEREBRALLY ADMINISTERED NGF

When given at the time of transplantation, one injection of 2000–20,000 BU intraventricularly (i.v.) or one injection of 20–200 BU close to the axons or cell bodies of the locus coeruleus neuron system running in the DCB (Fig. 6) resulted in a markedly increased ingrowth of regenerating CA sprouts into the transplant, as observed 7 days after transplantation (Figs. 7–10; Bjerre *et al.*, 1973a; Stenevi *et al.*, 1974). After intracerebral (i.c.)

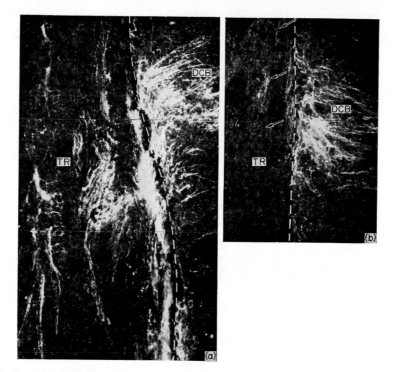

FIG. 8. Growth of CA fibres from the transected DCB into the transplant (TR) 7 days after transplantation (cf. Fig. 6). (a) In a specimen treated with 2000 BU of 7 S NGF intraventricularly at the time of transplantation. (b) in a control specimen given saline. In the NGF-treated specimen, extensive bundles and irregular networks of CA fibres have grown into the transplant, whereas only few such fibres (arrows) are present in the control specimen at this stage. The dashed lines indicate the caudal border of the transplants (×70). Abbreviations as in Fig. 6. (Bjerre *et al.*, 1973a.)

injections, the effect was restricted to the CA (mainly NA-containing) axons in the DCB lying close to the site of injection, whereas after intraventricular injections, strong effects were obtained on both the NA axons in the DCB and the DA axons in the MFB, and in some animals also on the IA axons in the MFB (see Figs. 9a and 10a).

As illustrated in Fig. 7, the NGF-induced effect was observed as an increase in the number of fibres that had grown into the transplant as well as in the distance and area covered by the ingrowing fibres. Generally, the magnitude of the NGF-induced growth response was greater from the NA axons in the DCB than from the DA and IA axons in the MFB. From the DCB (in the i.c.- or the i.v.-treated animals), bundles of smooth or varicose fibres invaded the transplant (Fig. 9c), and within the transplant the fibres branched to form loose networks (Fig. 9a) similar to those observed in control specimens at 2–3 weeks after transplantation. These networks partly resembled the autonomic ground plexus characteristic for the normal sympathetic innervation of the intact iris. From the MFB (in the i.v.-treated animals), the ingrowing DA and IA fibres were more delicate and formed dense patterns or bundles that sometimes penetrated deeply into the transplant (Figs. 9 a and 10a). With both routes of administration, the effect was clearly dose-dependent. After intraventricular injections, the ingrowth from the DCB and the MFB was gradually less after 200

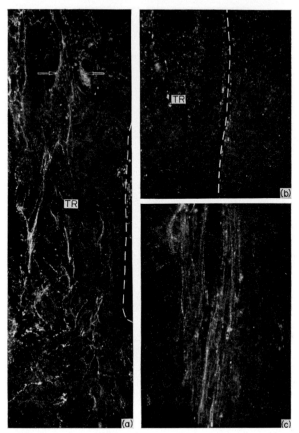

FIG. 9. (a), (b), and (c) (×65) Details of fibre patterns formed within transplants at 7 days survival. (a): Photomontage of a transplant in an animal given 2000 BU of 7 S NGF intraventricularly at the time of transplantation. All three types of fibres, the NA, DA, and IA fibres (IA fibre bundles indicated by arrows), from both the DCB and the MFB, had invaded the transplant (TR) (cf. Fig. 8b showing the situation in a control specimen). NA fibres originating from the DCB partly form a loose, irregular network within the transplant. The caudal border of the transplant is indicated by the dashed line. (b): control specimen that at the day of transplantation was given 2 μl saline intracerebrally close to the NA cell bodies in the locus coeruleus as shown by arrow C in Fig. 6. The picture shows a part of the transplant (TR) immediately ventral to the DCB. No fluorescent fibres are demonstrated within the transplant. The caudal border of the transplant is indicated by the dashed line. (c): specimen given 200 BU of 7 S NGF intracerebrally in a volume of 2 μl at the day of transplantation close to the NA cell bodies in the locus coeruleus. Thick bundles of CA fibres growing in the surface zone of the transplant from the DCB in a ventral direction. Abbreviations as in Fig. 6.

and 20 BU of NGF; similarly, 2 BU of NGF given intracerebrally close to the DCB had much less effect than 20 or 200 BU.

The effect of NGF varied between specimens, although treated similarly, when the protein was administered intraventricularly (Bjerre *et al.*, 1973a). The variations were of two kinds. First, occasional NGF-treated specimens did not clearly differ from the untreated controls; second, the NGF-induced effect on the growth from the two bundles, MFB and DCB, was not always the same. As the effects were more reproducible in the series of investigations with intracerebral administration (Stenevi *et al.*, 1974), it seems highly probable that the

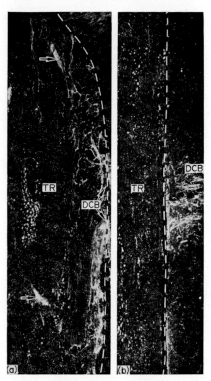

Fig. 10. (a) and (b) Photomontages of iris transplants to the caudal diencephalon (a): Transplant in an animal given 2000 BU of 7 S NGF intraventricularly at the time of transplantation, 7 days survival. The transplant (TR) had been invaded by all three types of monoamine fibres, the NA, DA, and IA fibres (IA fibre bundles indicated by arrows), from both the DCB and the MFB (cf. Fig. 8b showing the situation in a control specimen). The caudal border of the transplant is indicated by the dashed line ($\times 50$). (From Bjerre *et al.*, 1973a.) (b): Transplant in an animal given 2 μl of anti-NGF serum at the time of transplantation locally close to the NA axons in the DCB as shown by arrow B in Fig. 6. The animal was killed 14 days after transplantation. Note the markedly inhibited growth into the transplant (TR) of fibres from the DCB. Only a few CA fibres, indicated by arrows, are demonstrated within the transplant. The caudal border of the transplant is indicated by the dashed line ($\times 55$). (From Bjerre *et al.*, 1974b). Abbreviations as in Fig. 6.

variations seen with the i.v. route of administration were partly due to technical problems related to the distribution of the injected material. Perhaps the accessibility of the i.v.-administered NGF depends very much on the state of the ventricular walls. As the damage of the wall of the third ventricle caused by the transplantation varies considerably, this could greatly influence the effectiveness of the NGF injection and lessen the reproducibility of the effects.

An interesting property of the NGF-induced growth response was that a maximum stimulatory effect was registered when the NGF injection was given at the time of transplantation. Thus one injection of 2000 BU i.v. or 20 BU i.c. had much less effect when given 2 days before, or 2 or 4 days after, the transplantation. It is also notable that the effect of NGF given at the time of transplantation did not become prominent until 7 days later.

The local i.c. route of administration will result in an exposure to the substance that will be much stronger close to the site of injection than at some distance from it. For this reason it should be possible to expose different sites of the regenerating neurons to NGF by injecting it at different sites. The effect of such local injections of NGF has been tested with respect to the NA neurons having their cell bodies in the local coeruleus and many of their axons ascending within the DCB (Stenevi *et al.*, 1974; Fig. 6). Twenty biological units of NGF were injected in a volume of 2 μl at three different sites (see Fig. 6): C, close to the NA cell bodies in the locus coeruleus; B, close to the NA axons in the DCB, about 3 mm caudal to the site of lesion; A, close to the DCB about 1 mm caudal to the site of lesion. Controls received saline similarly. All injections were given at the time of transplantation, and the regeneration into the transplant was evaluated 7 days later.

The effects of the three types of injections were similar and in all cases confined to the NA fibres growing from the DCB. The magnitude of the growth stimulation on the locus coeruleus NA neurons after 20 BU of NGF injected into these sites was similar to that induced by 2000 BU of NGF injected into the cerebrospinal fluid.

EFFECTS OF PREINCUBATION OF THE TRANSPLANT IN NGF

In order to further test whether the stimulation of the growth of new axonal sprouts could be induced by NGF at the level of the lesioned axon stumps and the sprouting fibres, NGF was administered through preincubation of the iris transplant (Stenevi *et al.*, 1974). The incubation was carried out for 15 min at room temperature in a solution of NGF (100,000 BU/ml) in phosphate buffer (pH 7.4), and the iris was then directly transplanted into the brain. This procedure was supposed to make the NGF that was attached to or accumulated in the transplant accessible to the regenerating axons and the sprouting fibres in the MFB and the DCB.

The results suggested that such preincubation in NGF, indeed, results in a stimulation of the ingrowth of sprouting CA (probably NA-containing) fibres into the transplant from the DCB, evaluated 7 days after transplantation. The amount of fibres and the area of the transplant covered by the ingrowing fibres from the DCB varied somewhat, but they were generally less than after i.v. (2000 BU) or i.c. (20–200 BU) injections of NGF, and no certain effect was observed on the growth of fibres (mainly of the DA- and IA-containing types) in the MFB.

EFFECTS OF ANTI-NGF SERUM

The possible inhibitory effect of anti-NGF serum on the regeneration processes was evaluated at 2 and 4 weeks after transplantation (Bjerre *et al.*, 1974b). As illustrated schematically in Fig. 7, there is at two weeks after transplantation a substantial ingrowth of NA fibres from the DCB and (predominantly) DA fibres from the MFB into large areas of the transplant.

Intraventricular injections of the anti-NGF serum did not have any observable effect on the growth into the transplant, as observed 14 days later. In contrast, one injection of 2 μl anti-NGF serum, given locally close to the lesioned axons in the DCB at the time of transplantation, resulted in a marked reduction in the growth from the DCB (Fig. 10b), but not from the MFB. Thus at 14 days after transplantation, there was much less sprouting around the lesioned NA fibres in the DCB, and within the transplant, the growing fibres were limited to the area bordering the DCB. To check the possible role of non-specific inhibitory effects of the rabbit anti-NGF serum, two types of control sera were tested in parallel: normal rabbit serum and another hyperimmune rabbit, anti-mouse lymphocyte serum.

These control injections did not produce any observable inhibitory effects on the axonal sprouting, and thus the inhibition appeared to be specific for the anti-NGF serum.

Also a short preincubation (15 min at room temperature) of the transplant in anti-NGF serum, but not in control sera, caused a significant reduction in the growth of NA fibres from the DCB. However, the effect on the DA and IA fibres in the MFB was uncertain.

5. INTERPRETATION OF THE NGF AND THE ANTI-NGF SERUM EXPERIMENTS

From the studies summarized in the previous sections it seems possible to offer some general statements concerning the effects of NGF and its antiserum on the process of axonal regeneration:

(1) Both peripheral NA-containing neurons and central NA-, DA-, and IA-containing neurons are sensitive to exogenous NGF during regeneration, and among the central monoamine neurons the NA-containing neurons showed the strongest NGF-induced responses.

(2) Both in the periphery and in the brain, the effect of exogenous NGF was observed as an increase in the amount of regenerating sprouts, as well as an acceleration of their growth. In the regenerating peripheral adrenergic axons, the NGF treatment also resulted in a restoration of the axonal NA levels towards normal.

(3) Anti-serum towards NGF strongly reduced the outgrowth of new axonal sprouts from lesioned peripheral, as well as central, NA neurons. No certain effect on the sprouting from central DA and IA neurons could be established.

These observations point to a possible role of NGF or NGF-like proteins in the process of axonal regeneration of fully developed or adult peripheral and central NA neurons. NGF occurs with a wide-spread distribution also in adult animals, as determined either with bioassay (Bueker et al., 1960; Levi-Montalcini and Angeletti, 1961) or immunoassay techniques (Angeletti and Vigneti, 1971; Johnson et al., 1971). As NGF probably cannot enter the brain from the blood stream (Angeletti et al., 1972), it is of particular interest that—although in very low concentrations—7S NGF-antigens are detectable by radioimmunoassay also in the brain (Johnson et al., 1971). The prerequisites for a role of NGF in the adult animal thus seem to exist both in the peripheral and the central nervous system.

It seems reasonable to interpret the experiments with localized i.c. injections of NGF and with transplants of irises preincubated in NGF to signify that the NGF-induced growth response can be elicited at several levels of the regenerating central NA neurons, i.e. at the level of the cell bodies, at the level of the non-terminal axons, as well as at the level of the sprouting fibres. This is interesting in view of the recent findings of Thoenen et al. (1974) that intraocularly injected I^{125} NGF is partly taken up by the adrenergic axons and transported in a retrograde direction to the cell bodies in the superior cervical ganglion. As destruction of the adrenergic terminals with 6-OH-DA did not impair this transport process (in contrast to a complete transection of the postganglionic axons) it seems probable that also the surviving non-terminal parts of the lesioned axons are able to take up NGF. Hendry and Iversen (1974) have suggested that NGF might act on the cell body as a trophic factor carried via the retrograde transport system of the axon. Such a possible mode of function of NGF would seem possible also in the present experiments on regenerating neurons, although uptake and transport of NGF has so far not been demonstrated in central NA neurons. In the experiments with local application of anti-NGF serum close to the lesioned locus coeruleus axons, or with preincubation of the iris transplant in the antiserum, it seems possible that the inhibitory effects were exerted primarily through a blocking of NGF or NGF-like substances locally in the brain tissue, or in the target tissue (i.e. the tissue that was "reinnervated" by the sprouting fibres). If so, the growth impairment could have resulted from the removal of a normally acting growth stimulating principle. This could point to a possible role of NGF or NGF-like substances in the interactions between the axons of CA neurons and their surrounding tissue elements, phenomena that are of central importance in the process of axonal regeneration.

The mechanism or mechanisms by which NGF stimulates the sprouting process of CA axons is not entirely clear. NGF is essential for the survival of sympathetic ganglion neurons in tissue culture (Levi-Montalcini and Angeletti, 1968) and Jacobson (1970) and Larrabee (1972) have suggested that a physiological role of NGF during the ontogenetic development could be to promote the survival and growth of neurons that would otherwise have degenerated. The action of NGF antiserum can then be viewed as removing a factor that permitted the survival of certain neuronal elements. *In vitro*, NGF has extensive metabolic effects on developing ganglia (Angeletti *et al.*, 1964 a and b, 1965; Partlow and Larrabee, 1971). These effects have been described by Partlow and Larrabee (1971) and Larrabee (1972) as a maintenance role of exogenous NGF on the cultured ganglion cells, NGF thus sustaining the initial rates of metabolism in the *in vitro* situation. A possible supportive or permissive role also of *endogenous* NGF on sympathetic neurons *in vivo* is strongly suggested by the dramatic effects observed after administration of the antiserum against NGF to newborn animals, resulting in a rapid degeneration of the neurons (Levi-Montalcini and Booker, 1960; Levi-Montalcini and Angeletti, 1966).

With respect to the process of axonal regeneration of the fully developed central and peripheral NA neurons, it does not seem possible to interpret the observed effects of exogenous NGF and NGF antiserum in terms of the degree of survival of the lesioned neurons, i.e. the number of nerve cells that survive after lesion. As described above, the effects of NGF and anti-NGF serum appears rather as an acceleration or potentiation, and a retardation or impairment, respectively, of the sprouting process. In view of the potent anabolic effects of exogenous NGF observed on developing ganglia *in vitro*, mentioned above, the simplest way to regard its actions on the regenerating neuron would be in terms of effects on the ability of the lesioned neuron to respond to axonal damage, i.e. to form or sustain axonal sprouts. This is supported by the observations of Angeletti *et al.* (1971) and by unpublished observations in our own laboratory that, in the intact adult mouse, the degenerative effects of anti-NGF serum seems to be confined primarily to the axons. Thus in contrast to the permanent destruction of most sympathetic neurons in the newborn animal, Angeletti *et al.* (1971) reported that the most striking effect of the antiserum in the adult mouse was a reduction in NA content and NA uptake in peripheral tissues. The effects were transient, and a few weeks after treatment a progressive recovery of the sympathetic neurons occurred. These data lend support to the idea that NGF is essential for the maintenance of the axons or axon terminals of CA neurons in the adult animal.

One aspect of the effects induced by NGF in developing ganglia that is of particular interest with respect to its stimulation of axonal outgrowth and regenerative sprouting is the very significant alterations in neurotubules and neurofilaments that are induced by both NGF and anti-NGF serum treatments. Thus, *in vitro*, NGF has been reported both to induce *de novo* synthesis of neurotubule protein (Hier *et al.*, 1972) and to enhance the assembly of neurotubules from pre-existing subunits (Roisen and Murphy, 1973) in embryonic chick sensory ganglia. Electron microscopically, NGF induces a massive accumulation of neurotubules and neurofilaments in the cell bodies in developing sensory ganglia *in vitro* (Levi-Montalcini *et al.*, 1968) and in developing and adult sympathetic ganglia *in vivo* (Angeletti *et al.*, 1971a). Conversely, one of the most striking ultrastructural alterations induced by anti-NGF serum treatment in the sympathetic nerve cells in the adult mouse has been reported to be the loss of neurotubules and neurofilaments in the cell bodies (Angeletti *et al.*, 1971b). There is much evidence—particularly from morphological studies on the effects of colchicine, which is known to disrupt the neurotubules—that the neurotubules play an important role in axonal outgrowth. Colchicine treatment of embryonic sensory ganglia *in vitro* results in a retraction of the outgrowing neurites (Daniels, 1968; Yamada *et al.*, 1970), a phenomenon that has been reported to occur also after removal of NGF from the culture medium (Kumar and Steward, 1970). In fact, disruption of the neurotubules by the colchicine-like drug vincristine has been reported to inhibit the effects of NGF on neurite outgrowth *in vitro* (Hier *et al.*, 1972).

From these various observations it would seem possible to explain the effects of exogenous NGF and anti-NGF serum on axonal regeneration on the basis of a role of NGF in the metabolic response of the NA neurons to axonal damage. Axotomy is well known to trigger a retrograde anabolic reaction in the neuron cell bodies, characterized by increases in RNA and protein synthesis, followed by increases in RNA and protein contents (Brattgård *et al.*, 1957; Watson, 1970). This is often accompanied by a chromatolytic reaction, which in the adult sympathetic ganglion cell is chiefly characterized by dispersion of the endoplasmic reticulum, increase in dense bodies, and displacement of the nucleus with a folding of the nuclear membrane (Matthews and Raisman, 1972). The retrograde anabolic response is probably an expression of neuronal repair, chiefly related to the regeneration of the lesioned axon and, as a mere speculation, one might perhaps regard the effects of NGF and anti-NGF serum on the regenerating neuron as an augmentation or diminution, respectively, of this retrograde response. Thus, on excised developing ganglia *in vitro* NGF stimulates RNA and protein synthesis, resulting in increased RNA and protein contents (Angeletti *et al.*, 1965; Burdman, 1967; Partlow and Larrabee, 1971), and anti-NGF serum has, *in vivo*, the opposite effects (Halstead and Larrabee, 1972). At the ultrastructural level, as mentioned above, the most conspicuous effects of NGF and its antiserum on the mature sympathetic ganglion cell seem to be in the accumulation and disappearance, respectively, of the neurofilaments and neurotubules in the cell bodies (Angeletti *et al.*, 1971a, b). Though inconspicuous in the cell bodies of chromatolytic sympathetic neurons (Matthews and Raisman, 1972) neurofilament proliferation is a prominent feature in their regenerating axons (Kapeller and Mayor, 1969), and here they are by all probability an expression of the regenerative efforts, intimately related to the sprouting process (cf. Yamada *et al.*, 1971; Hier *et al.*, 1972). Also in this respect the NGF effect might thus be possible to regard as an exaggeration of the retrograde regenerative response in the axotomized neuron.

It is interesting that in the experiments on the regenerating locus coeruleus neurons the effects of the NGF and the NGF antiserum injections were most pronounced when given at the time of axonal damage, and considerably less when given 4 days after operation, i.e. at a time when the axonal sprouting had already started (see above). When viewed in relation to the retrograde neuronal response, this could point to a role of NGF during regeneration of lesioned NA neurons that is of particular significance during the very early stages, or the triggering, of the sprouting process.

Burnham, Raiborn and Varon (1972) have provided evidence that, *in vitro* at least, non-neuronal cells (e.g. satellite cells, Schwann cells, glial cells) are of importance for the survival and growth of adrenergic neurons, and they have hypothesized that the neuronal support provided by the non-neuronal cell elements might be mediated by NGF-like substances produced by these cells. Such a possible role of NGF or NGF-like substances in the inter-action between neuronal and non-neuronal elements in the tissue is highly interesting in relation to many of the complex cellular events underlying a successful re-establishment of axonal connections. In view of the present findings in transplants preincubated in NGF or anti-NGF serum it should be of great interest to test whether NGF might play a normal physiological role also in the regulatory processes controlling and guiding axonal regrowth during regeneration of central and peripheral CA neurons.

ACKNOWLEDGEMENTS

The studies were supported by grants from the Swedish Medical Research Council (Nos. 04X-3874, 04X-712, and 04X-56); and from the National Institutes of Health, USPHS (No. 06701-07).

REFERENCES

ANGELETTI, P. U., and VIGNETI, (1971) Assay of nerve growth factor (NGF) in subcellular fractionations of peripheral tissue by micro complement fixation. *Brain Res.* **33**, 601–604.

ANGELETTI, P. U., LEVI-MONTALCINI, R., and CARAMIA, F. (1971a) Ultrastructural changes in sympathetic neurons of newborn and adult mice treated with nerve growth factor. *J. Ultrastruct. Res.* **36**, 24–36.

ANGELETTI, P. U., LIUZZI, A., and LEVI-MONTALCINI, R. (1964a) Stimulation of lipid biosynthesis in sympathetic and sensory ganglia by a specific nerve growth factor. *Biochim. biophys. Acta* **84**, 778–781.

ANGELETTI, P. U., LIUZZI, A., LEVI-MONTALCINI, R., and GAUDINI-ATTARDI, D. G. (1964b) Effects of nerve growth factor on glucose metabolism by sympathetic and sensory nerve cells. *Biochim. biophys. Acta* **90**, 445–450.

ANGELETTI, P. U., GAUDINI-ATTARDI, D., TOSCHI, G., SALVI, M. L., and LEVI-MONTALCINI, R. (1965) Metabolic aspects of the effect of nerve growth factor on sympathetic and sensory ganglia in protein and ribonucleic acid synthesis. *Biochim. biophys. Acta* **95**, 111–120.

ANGELETTI, P. U., LEVI-MONTALCINI, R., and CARAMIA, F. (1971b) Analysis of the effects of the antiserum to the nerve growth factor in adult mice. *Brain Res.* **27**, 343–355.

ANGELETTI, R. H., ANGELETTI, P. U., and LEVI-MONTALCINI, R. (1972) Selective accumulation of ^{125}I labelled nerve growth factor in sympathetic ganglia. *Brain Res.* **46**, 421–425.

BJERRE, B., and BJÖRKLUND, A. (1973) The production of catecholamine-containing cells *in vitro* by young chick embryos: Effects of 'nerve growth factor' (NGF) and its antiserum. *Neurobiology* **3**, 140–161.

BJERRE, B., BJÖRKLUND, A., and STENEVI, U. (1973a) Stimulation of growth of new axonal sprouts from lesioned monoamine neurons in adult rat brain by nerve growth factor. *Brain Res.* **50**, 161–176.

BJERRE, B., BJÖRKLUND, A., and MOBLEY, W. (1973b) A stimulatory effect by nerve growth factor on the regrowth of adrenergic nerve fibres in the mouse peripheral tissues after chemical sympathectomy with 6-hydroxydopamine. *Z. Zellforsch.* **146**, 15–43.

BJERRE, B., BJÖRKLUND, A., and EDWARDS, D. C. (1974a) Axonal regeneration of peripheral adrenergic neurons: Effects of antiserum to nerve growth factor in mouse. *Z. Zellforsch.* (in press).

BJERRE, B., BJÖRKLUND, A., and STENEVI, U. (1974b) Inhibition of regenerative growth of central noradrenergic neurones by intracerebrally administered anti-NGF serum. *Brain Res.* (in press).

BJÖRKLUND, A., and STENEVI, U. (1971) Growth of central catecholamine neurones into smooth muscle grafts in the rat mesencephalon. *Brain Res.* **31**, 1–20.

BJÖRKLUND, A., and STENEVI, U. (1972) Nerve Growth Factor: Stimulation of regenerative growth of central noradrenergic neurons. *Science* **175**, 1251–1253.

BJÖRKLUND, A., KATZMAN, R., STENEVI, U., and WEST, K. A. (1971) Development and growth of axonal sprouts from noradrenaline and 5-hydroxytryptamine neurones in the rat spinal cord. *Brain Res.* **31**, 21–33.

BJÖRKLUND, A., NOBIN, A., and STENEVI, U. (1973) Regeneration of central serotonin neurons after axonal degeneration induced by 5,6-dihydroxytryptamine. *Brain Res.* **50**, 214–220.

BRATTGÅRD, S.-O., EDSTRÖM, J.-E., and HYDÉN, H. (1957) The chemical changes in regenerating neurons. *J. Neurochem.* **1**, 316–325.

BRIMIJOIN, S., and MOLINOFF, P. B. (1971) Effects of 6-hydroxydopamine on the activity of tyrosine hydroxylase and dopamine-β-hydroxylase in sympathetic ganglia of the rat. *J. Pharmac. Exp. Ther.* **178**, 417–424.

BUEKER, E. D., SCHENKEIN, I., and BONE, J. L. (1960) The problem of distribution of a nerve growth factor specific for spinal and sympathetic ganglia. *Cancer Res.* **20**, 1220–1228.

BURDMAN, J. A. (1967) Early effects of a nerve growth factor on RNA content and base ratios of isolated chick embryo sensory ganglia neuroblasts in tissue culture. *J. Neurochem.* **14**, 367–371.

BURNHAM, P., RAIBORN, C., and VARON, S. (1972) Replacement of nerve growth factor by ganglionic non-neuronal cells for the survival *in vitro* of dissociated ganglionic neurons. *Proc. Natn. Acad. Sci. USA* **69**, 3556–3660.

CAJAL, S. R. Y. (1928) *Degeneration and Regeneration of the Nervous System*, vol. 2 (translated and edited by R M. May), Oxford University Press, London.

CLEMENTE, C. D. (1964) Regeneration in the vertebrate central nervous system. *Int. Rev. Neurobiol.* **6**, 257–301.

DANIELS, M. P. J. (1968) *J. Cell Biol.* **39**, 31, Abstr.

DE CHAMPLAIN, J. (1971) Degeneration and regrowth of adrenergic nerve fibres in the rat peripheral tissues after 6-hydroxydopamine. *Can. J. Physiol. Pharmac.* **49**, 345–355.

DE CHAMPLAIN, J., MALMFORS, T., OLSON, L., and SACHS, CH. (1970) Ontogenesis of peripheral adrenergic neurons in the rat: pre- and postnatal observations. *Acta physiol. scand.* **80**, 276–288.

GUTH, L. (1956) Regeneration in the mammalian peripheral nervous system. *Physiol. Rev.* **36**, 441–478.

HAEUSLER, G., HAEFELY, W., and THOENEN, H. (1969) Chemical sympathectomy of the cat with 6-hydroxydopamine. *J. Pharmac. Exp. Ther.* **170**, 50–61.

HALSTEAD, D. C., and LARRABEE, M. G. (1972) Early effects of antiserum to the nerve growth factor on metabolism and transmission in superior cervical ganglia of mice. In: *Immunosympathectomy* (G. Steiner and E. Schönbaum, eds.), Amsterdam–London–New York: Elsevier Publ. Comp. pp. 221–236.

HENDRY, I. A., and IVERSEN, L. L. (1971) Effect of nerve growth factor and its antiserum on tyrosine hydroxylase activity in mouse superior cervical sympathetic ganglion. *Brain Res.* **29**, 159–162.

HENDRY, I. A., and IVERSEN, L. L. (1973) Changes in tissue and plasma concentrations of nerve growth factor following removal of the submaxillary glands in adult mice and their effects on the sympathetic nervous system. *Nature* (in press).

HIER, D. B., ARNASON, B. G. W., and YOUNG, M. (1972) Studies on the mechanism of action of nerve growth factor. *Proc. Natn. Acad. Sci., USA* **69**, 2268–2272.

JACOBSON, M. (1970) *Developmental Neurobiology*, Holt, Rinehart & Winston, New York, p. 213.

JOHNSON, D. G., GORDEN, P., and KOPIN, I. J. (1971) A sensitive radioimmunoassay for 7 S nerve growth factor antigens in serum and tissues. *J. Neurochem.* **18**, 2355–2362.

JONSSON, G., and SACHS, CH. (1972) Neurochemical properties of adrenergic nerves regenerated after 6-hydroxydopamine. *J. Neurochem.* **19**, 2577–2585.

KAPELLER, K. and MAYOR, D. (1969) An electron microscopic study of the early changes proximal to a constriction in sympathetic nerves. *Proc. Roy. Soc.* (*London*), ser. B, **172**, 39–51.

KATZMAN, R., BJÖRKLUND, A., OWMAN, CH., STENEVI, U., and WEST, K. A. (1971) Evidence for regenerative axon sprouting of central catecholamine neurons in the rat mesencephalon following electrolytic lesions. *Brain Res.* **25**, 579–596.

KIRPEKAR, S. M., WAKADE, A. R., and PRAT, J. C. (1970) Regeneration of sympathetic nerves to the vas deferens and spleen of the cat. *J. Pharmac. Exp. Ther.* **175**, 197–205.

KUMAR, S., and STEWARD, J. K. (1970) A possible site of action of the nerve growth factor. *Expl. Cell Res.* **63**, 200–201.

LARRABEE, M. G. (1972) Metabolism During Development in Sympathetic Ganglia of Chickens: Effects of Age, Nerve Growth Factor, and Metabolic Inhibitors: *Nerve Growth Factor* and its Antiserum, (E. Zaimis and J. Knight, eds.), Athlone Press, London, pp. 71–88.

LEVI-MONTALCINI, R. (1964) The nerve growth factor. *Ann. NY Acad. Sci.* **118**, 149–168.

LEVI-MONTALCINI, R., and ANGELETTI, P. U. (1961) Biological properties of a nerve-growth promoting protein and its antiserum. In: *Regional Neurochemistry, Proc. 4th Intern. Neurochemical Symp.* (S. S. Kety, and J. Elkes, eds.), Pergamon Press, New York, pp. 362–376.

LEVI-MONTALCINI, R., and ANGELETTI, P. U. (1966) Immunosympathectomy. *Pharmac. Rev.* **18**, 619–628.

LEVI-MONTALCINI, R., and ANGELETTI, P. U. (1968) Nerve growth factor. *Physiol. Rev.* **48**, 534–569.

LEVI-MONTALCINI, R., and BOOKER, B. (1960) Destruction of the sympathetic ganglia in mammals by an antiserum to the nerve-growth promoting factor. *Proc. Natn. Acad. Sci. USA* **42**, 384–391.

LEVI-MONTALCINI, R., and HAMBURGER, V. (1953) A diffusable agent of mouse sarcoma producing hyperplasia of sympathetic ganglia and hyperneurotization of the chick embryo. *J. Exp. Zool.* **123**, 233–288.

LEVI-MONTALCINI, R., CARAMIA, F., LUSE, S. A., and ANGELETTI, P. U. (1968) *In vitro* effects of the nerve growth factor on the fine structure of the sensory nerve cells. *Brain Res.* **8**, 347–362.

LEVI-MONTALCINI, R., ANGELETTI, R. H., and ANGELETTI, P. U. (1972) The Nerve Growth Factor. In: *The Structure and Function of Nervous Tissue*, vol. V, (G. H. Bourne ed.), Academic Press, New York and London, pp. 1–38.

MALMFORS, T. (1971) The effects of 6-hydroxydopamine on the adrenergic nerves as revealed by the fluorescence histochemical method. In: 6-*Hydroxydopamine and Catecholamine Neurons* (T. Malmfors and H. Thoenen, eds.), North-Holland, Amsterdam and London, pp. 47–58.

MALMFORS, T., and SACHS, CH. (1968) Degeneration of adrenergic nerves produced by 6-hydroxydopamine. *Eur. J. Pharmac.* **3**, 89–92.

MATTHEWS, M. R., and RAISMAN, G. (1972) A light and electron microscopic study of the cellular response to axonal injury in the superior cervical ganglion of the rat. *Proc. Roy. Soc. (London)*, ser. B, **181**, 43–79.

MIRKIN, B. L. (1972) Ontogenesis of the adrenergic neuron. In: *Immunosympathectomy* (G. Steiner and E. Schönbaum, eds.), North-Holland, Amsterdam and London, pp. 79–89.

MOORE, R. Y., BJÖRKLUND, A., and STENEVI, U. (1973) Growth of adrenergic neurons. *The Neurosciences, 3rd Study Program* (F. O. Schmitt, ed.), New York: Rockefeller University Press.

OLSON, L. (1967) Outgrowth of sympathetic adrenergic neurons in mice treated with a nerve growth factor (NGF). *Z. Zellforsch.* **81**, 155–173.

OLSON, L. (1969) Intact and regenerating sympathetic noradrenaline axons in the rat sciatic nerve. *Histochemie* **17**, 349–367.

OLSON, L., and MALMFORS, T. (1970) Growth characteristics of adrenergic nerves in the adult rat. *Acta physiol. scand.*, Suppl. 348, 1–112.

OWMAN, CH., SJÖBERG, N.-O., and SWEDIN, G. (1971) Histochemical and chemical studies on pre- and postnatal development of the different systems of "short" and "long" adrenergic neurons in peripheral organs of the rat. *Z. Zellforsch.* **116**, 319–341.

PARTLOW, L. M., and LARRABEE, M. G. (1971) Effects of a nerve-growth factor, embryo, age and metabolic inhibitors on growth of fibres and on synthesis of ribonucleic acid and protein in embryonic sympathetic ganglia. *J. Neurochem.* **18**, 2101–2118.

ROISEN, F. J., and MURPHY, R. A. (1973) Neurite development *in vitro*: II. The role of microfilaments and microtubules in dibutyryl adenosine 3′,5′-cyclic monophosphate and nerve growth factor stimulated maturation. *J. Neurobiol.* **4**, 397–412.

STENEVI, U., BJERRE, B., BJÖRKLUND, A., and MOBLEY, W. (1974) Effects of localized intracerebral injections of nerve growth factor on the regenerative growth of central noradrenergic neurons. *Brain Res.* **69**, 217–234.

THOENEN, H. (1972) Comparison between the effect of neuronal activity and nerve growth factor on the enzymes involved in the synthesis of norepinephrine. *Pharmac. Rev.* **24**, 255–267.

THOENEN, H., and TRANZER, J. P. (1968) Chemical sympathectomy by selective destruction of adrenergic nerve endings with 6-hydroxydopamine. *Naunyn-Schmiedeberg's Arch. exp. Path. Pharmak.* **261**, 271–288.

THOENEN, H., ANGELETTI, P. U., LEVI-MONTALCINI, R., and KETTLER, R. (1971) Selective induction by nerve growth factor of tyrosine hydroxylase and dopamine-β-hydroxylase in the rat superior cervical ganglia. *Proc. Natn. Acad. Sci. USA* **68**, 1598–1602.

THOENEN, H., HENDRY, I. A., STÖCKEL, K., PARAVICINI, V., and OESCH, F. (1974) Regulation of enzyme synthesis by neuronal activity and by nerve growth factor. In: *Dynamics of Degeneration and Growth in Neurons* (K. Fuxe, Olsson and Y. Zotterman, eds.), pp. 315–328.

TRANZER, J. P., and RICHARDS, J. G. (1971) Fine structural aspects of the effect of 6-hydroxydopamine on peripheral adrenergic neurons. In: 6-*Hydroxydopamine and Catecholamine Neurons* (T. Malmfors and H. Thoenen, eds.), North-Holland, Amsterdam and London, pp. 15–31.

TRANZER, J. P., and THOENEN, H. (1967) Ultramorphologische Veränderung der sympatischen Nervenendigungen der Katze nach Vorbehandlung mit 5- und 6-Hydroxy-Dopamin. *Naunyn-Schmiedebergs Arch. exp. Path. Pharmak.* **257**, 343–344.

UNGERSTEDT, U. (1971) Stereotoxic mapping of the monoamine pathways in the rat brain. *Acta physiol. scand.*, Suppl. 367, 1–48.

WATSON, W. E. (1970) Some metabolic responses of axotomized neurones to contact between their axons and denervated muscle. *J. Physiol.* **210**, 321–343.

WINDLE, W. F. (1955) *Regeneration in the Central Nervous System*. Charles C. Thomas, Springfield, Ill., USA.

YAMADA, K. M., SPOONER, B. S., and WESSELS, N. K. (1970) Axon growth: roles of microfilaments and microtubules. *Proc. Natn. Acad. Sci. USA* **66**, 1206.

GROWTH

SESSION III

Chairman: K. FUXE

THE NORADRENERGIC INNERVATION OF CEREBELLAR PURKINJE CELLS: LOCALIZATION, FUNCTION, SYNAPTOGENESIS, AND AXONAL SPROUTING OF LOCUS COERULEUS

F. E. Bloom, H. Krebs, J. Nicholson, and V. Pickel

Laboratory of Neuropharmacology, Division of Special Mental Health Research, National Institute of Mental Health, St. Elizabeth's Hospital, Washington DC 20032, USA

SUMMARY

The norepinephrine-containing afferents to the cerebellum arise from subpopulations within the locus coeruleus cell group A6 and from cell group A4. The axons project to the cerebellum by means of separated fascicles within the superior cerebellar peduncle. After partial lesions of the superior peduncle, intact NE cerebellar afferent fibers are triggered into axon collateral proliferation which results in cytological and physiological evidence of a hyperinnervation of cerebellar Purkinje cells by locus coeruleus NE fibers within 25–35 days. In contrast to other regions of the brain employed to study NE axon collateral proliferation and reinnervation, the changes observed in cerebellum regress towards normal within 60–90 days and are not induced by extensive destruction of non-adrenergic inputs. In ontogenetic studies locus coeruleus neurons begin to differentiate on gestational days 10 and 11, but synapses to these neurons are extremely sparse until after birth. The detailed foundation of knowledge regarding the histology, pharmacology, and physiology of this pathway makes it a valuable test system for the analysis of the dynamics of central axon growth regulation.

INTRODUCTION

In order to explore the exciting biology of the growth and regeneration of central neurons we have based our experiments on a particular defined pathway. Through combinations of light and electron microscopy, iontophoretic pharmacology, and a broad spectrum of electrophysiological tests, our previous data have indicated that cerebellar Purkinje cells in the rat receive a unique inhibitory input from the norepinephrine-containing pontine nucleus, the locus coeruleus (LC), which results in a hyperpolarization of Purkinje cells accompanied by generally increased input impedance of the membrane. The action of the locus coeruleus pathway on Purkinje cells is mimicked by iontophoresis of cyclic 3'5'-adenosine monophosphate (cyclic AMP), potentiated by iontophoresis of phosphodiesterase inhibitors, blocked by iontophoresis of prostaglandins of the E series and by inhibition of

413

tyrosine hydroxylase, as well as by 6-hydroxydopamine-induced destruction of the NE-containing fibers which project to the cerebellum. Cyclic AMP applied iontophoretically to Purkinje cells produces a similar hyperpolarizing action to iontophoretically applied NE and to activation of the LC. All these data have been recently reviewed (Bloom *et al.*, 1973) and extended (Hoffer *et al.*, 1973). In addition, immunocytochemical localization of cyclic AMP in cerebellar neurons (Bloom *et al.*, 1972) indicates that only electrical stimulation of the LC and topical application of NE will increase the cyclic AMP of cerebellar Purkinje cells (Siggins *et al.*, 1973).

Based upon this interdisciplinary foundation of mutually supportive observations, we feel that it is reasonable to speak of a defined noradrenergic central synaptic pathway from LC neurons to cerebellar Purkinje cells, the function of which is to produce an inhibition which can be mediated by cyclic AMP and modulated by prostaglandins. Although the extent of the cerebellar NE innervation may be considered "sparse" when viewed by the neurochemical index of the NE content of the hypothalamus, it is clear that the functional potency of the projection becomes greatly enhanced by the dual amplifications achieved by the NE activation of adenylate cyclase (see Rall, 1972) and by the cyclic AMP activation of cyclic AMP-dependent protein kinases (Greengard *et al.*, 1973). Furthermore, the cytological estimations of the extent of the innervation have probably been extremely conservative due to the deficiencies in the detection of the extremely fine fiber systems (see below). This system, then, would seem particularly well suited for an extended study of axonal dynamics, in view of the detailed information of the noradrenergic innervation and in view of the very convenient gross morphology of the cerebellum which permits direct neurosurgical manipulation of the cerebellar peduncles for selective destruction of all afferent and efferent connections without damage to the cortex.

Using the LC to cerebellar Purkinje cell pathway, we have explored four aspects relevant to the goals of this conference: (1) a detailed mapping of the LC neurons and their projections into the cerebellum (Krebs *et al.*, in preparation); (2) the induction of enhanced axonal arborizations from LC to cerebellar Purkinje cells (Pickel *et al.*, 1973; Krebs and Bloom, in preparation); (3) the changes in the physiology and pharmacology of the pathway under these conditions (Krebs and Bloom, in preparation); and (4) the ontogenesis and synaptogenesis of LC neurons (Nicholson and Bloom, 1973).

LOCUS COERULEUS PROJECTIONS TO CEREBELLAR CORTEX

Since the original descriptions of the cerebellar NE innervation indicated an extremely sparse network of fine fibers (Fuxe, 1965) which were thought to originate from the somewhat diffusely arranged NE cell bodies of the lateral reticular formation, extended reinvestigations of the pathway were required. Utilizing novel methods for circuit analysis including incubation of slices in more fluorescent congeners of NE (Hokfelt and Fuxe, 1969), autoradiography after labeling with H^3NE (Bloom *et al.*, 1971), destruction after exposure to 6-hydroxydopamine (Bloom *et al.*, 1971), formaldehyde perfusion on sections sliced by the vibratome (Hokfelt and Ljungdahl, 1972; Fig. 1), and fine adjustments in the application of the freeze-dry technique as well as using surgical lesions of the dorsal ascending bundle of LC fibers (Ungerstedt, 1971) to enhance the fluorescence of the projection to cerebellum (Olson and Fuxe, 1971), it was possible to trace the preterminal axons from LC into the brachium conjunctivum (superior cerebellar peduncle (SP)), through the cerebellar juxtafastigial white matter, into every folia of the cortex, where these axons then branch

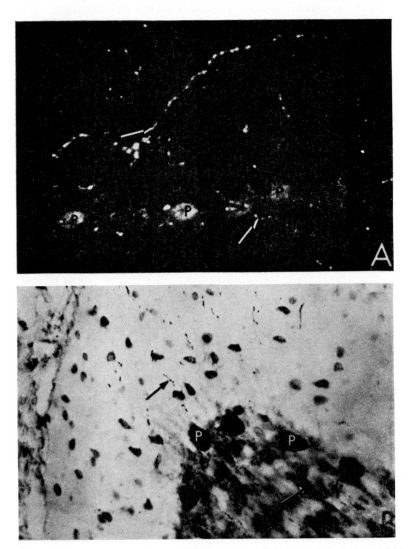

Fig. 1. Comparison of methods for localizing norepinephrine-containing axons within the molecular layer of the cerebellar cortex of the rat. A, Fluorescence histochemistry in a vibratome section from formaldehyde perfused material (see Hokfelt and Ljungdahl, 1972). Note long varicose fibers running parallel to the apical dendrite of the Purkinje cells (P); smaller varicose fibers are also present within the granular layer. B, Autoradiograph of cerebellar cortex from tissue perfused with formaldehyde 24 h after microinjection of H^3proline into the LC. The distribution of labeled transported material is highly similar to the distribution of fluorescent axons within the molecular layer and the granule cell layer (arrows). The autoradiographic localization method confirms the origin of the projection as locus coeruleus. (From Segal et al., 1973.)

and course through the granule cell layer, around Purkinje cells to "climb" along the apical dendrites toward the pial surface, exhibiting multiple terminal arborizations of the axon which generally come to lie parallel to the surface in the sagittal plane (Bloom et al., 1971). A similar cytological pattern of NE fibers within the cerebellar cortex has been observed in the cat, rabbit, monkey, and mouse cerebellum (Hoffer et al., 1972; Jacobowitz and Kostrzewa, 1972; Nelson et al., 1973).

Two questions seemed worthy of additional pursuit: do all LC neurons project equally to the cerebellum and are the cerebellar NE fibers wholly within the SP? Earlier studies from our group (see Hoffer et al., 1973) employed the methodology of Olson and Fuxe (1971) in which neonatal cerebella were examined after partial cerebellar ablations; these experiments indicated that the most marked retrograde cell body changes appeared in the neurons of the ventrolateral pole of the anterior LC subnucleus. This question has been re-investigated in detail in adult animals in experiments using fluorescence histochemistry and autoradiography to trace the pathway from the cell bodies in the pons. After micro-injections of H^3-proline or 6-hydroxydopamine into the LC, and after discrete minor transections of the peduncles (see below), as well as repeated observations on the results of ascending bundle transections or 6-hydroxydopamine micro-injections (Ungerstedt, 1971) into the fascicles of NE fibers, our results indicate that rat LC is less homogeneous than previously conceived. It is our interpretation that the posterior cells of the LC (which would include the nucleus termed A4 and the posterior lateral groups of A6 in the terminology of Dahlström and Fuxe (1964) and Ungerstedt (1971), project chiefly to the cerebellum through a fascicle of fibers which runs through the posterior-lateral portion of the SP (Krebs and Bloom, in preparation). In addition, axon collaterals also project to cerebellum from neurons in the anterior half of the LC, and their axon collaterals aggregate into a more medial fascicle within the SP (Krebs and Bloom, in preparation). A similar conception of the projections has been achieved by micro-injections of H^3proline into the LC and following the distribution of autoradiographically detected axons and terminals (see Cowan et al., 1972) into the cerebellum and forebrain (Segal et al., 1973). The distribution of the projection seems similar—if not identical—by both methods (see Figs. 1 and 2).

This subnuclear organization of the LC and its efferent projections is borne out by cytological studies in the cat (Chu and Bloom, 1974) and by electrophysiological studies in the rat (see Hoffer et al., 1973, and below) in which placement of the LC stimulating electrode in the position of maximal effectiveness for the cerebellar inhibition is generally ineffective in inhibiting hippocampal neurons (Segal and Bloom, 1973) while placements in the anterior pole or ascending bundle region do inhibit the hippocampal pyramidal neurons.

ENHANCEMENT OF THE CEREBELLAR NE PROJECTION BY EXPERIMENTAL NEUROSURGERY

Based almost exclusively on the fluorescence histochemical methodology, it has been demonstrated that central NE axons possess a striking capacity to give off collateral sprouts and produce enlarged terminal arborizations under certain experimental conditions. Björklund and Stenevi (1971) and Katzman et al. (1971) showed that collateral sprouting of NE axons would follow electrolytic destruction of the ascending projections sufficient to partially denervate diencephalic areas, and that the sprouted NE axons would also re-innervate the properly receptive smooth muscle grafted into the mesencephalon. Moore

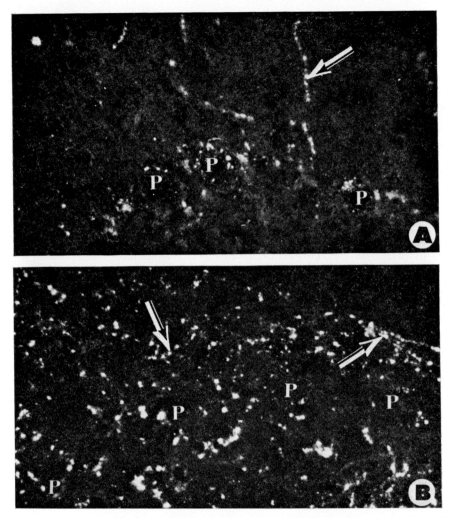

FIG. 2. Fluorescence photomicrograph illustrating the catecholamine fluorescent terminals (arrows) in cerebellar slices incubated with α-m-NE from: A, unlesioned rat, sagittal section with terminals in the molecular layer above the Purkinje cells (P); B, bilateral SP lesioned rat, tangential section with terminals in molecular layer above numerous Purkinje cells (P). The labeled Purkinje cells indicate the superior border of the Purkinje cell layer which constitutes more than one layer of cells in this tangential section.

et al. (1971) and Stenevi *et al.* (1972) have reported that central NE fibers will proliferate into the septum and lateral geniculate nucleus after removal of nonadrenergic inputs to these areas, according to the experimental paradigm devised by Raisman (1969) to analyze for central plasticity. We have performed experiments to determine if enhanced axonal arborizations of the NE cerebellar afferent system could be induced, since this system seemed a suitable test system for an examination of the functional properties of the synapses which might be expected to derive from the sprouted axons.

Lesions of the superior (SP), middle (MP), and inferior (IP) cerebellar peduncles were placed in rats weighing approximately 150–180 g. These lesions included various combinations of unilateral and bilateral transections of the SP, IP, and MP (indicated as SPX, IPX, and MPX, respectively). Animals with the cerebellum lifted but not lesioned served as controls. Direct "stab" lesions of the LC were also made unilaterally. Details of the neurosurgical procedures employed are described elsewhere (Pickel et al., 1973).

During the first week after the surgery, rats with unilateral IPX and MPX exhibited ataxia and rolling movements toward the transected side. Animals with bilateral SPX, presumably due to the balanced effects on each side, showed fewer motor symptoms. Within 2 weeks a large proportion of the animals with IPX and MPX regained coordinated movements and demonstrated only minor unilateral muscle deficiencies. Rats with SPX moved like controls. Only the animals showing maximal recovery from the surgical procedure were used in the subsequent histological studies of catecholamine fluorescence and fiber degeneration.

The Falck–Hillarp histochemical technique was used for the demonstration of catecholamines in both control and lesioned animals at time intervals ranging from 5 to 60 days following surgery, and the Fink–Heimer (1967) staining method was used in order to ascertain the extent of the terminal degeneration 2–7 days following peduncle lesions. In order to differentiate between true growth of NE fibers after surgical denervation and enhanced ease of detection of NE fibers due to metabolic factors arising secondary to the surgical lesions, precisely timed analysis was required. At the shortest time interval (5 days) after sectioning of the NE fibers in the SP, there is indeed an accumulation of fluorescent products in the preterminal axons proximal to the lesion and in intact collaterals of the severed axons as previously described for other adrenergic pathways (Andén et al., 1966; Ungerstedt, 1971). This "pile-up" of fluorescent material is almost completely removed by 15 days after the lesion.

When evaluated at intervals of 25 or more days after peduncle transection, lesions of the major afferent fibers entering the cerebellum through either the inferior or the middle peduncles produced no increase in the density of NE terminal fluorescence in the cerebellar cortex above the sham-operated controls (Table 1). However, when lesions of either the IP

TABLE 1.[a] HISTOFLUORESCENCE IN CEREBELLAR CORTEX

Terminal density of NE fibers after transection of superior (SPX), middle (MPX), or inferior (IPX) cerebellar peduncles bilaterally (bilat.) or unilaterally (unilat.)

Experimental conditions	NE terminal density	Number of animals observed	Number of animals with enhanced density
Control	$+$[b]	6	—
Uni/IPX	$+$	17	—
Uni/MPX	$+$	2	—
Uni/SPX	$++$	27	11
Uni /SPX IPX	$++$	13	7
Uni/SPX MPX IPX	$++$	5	2
Uni/Part. SPX	$+++$	25	18
Unilat. LC	$+++$	5	5
Bilat./Part. SPX	$++++$	15	13
Bilateral/SPX-MPX-IPX	0[c]	0	

[a] Modified from Pickel et al. (1973).
[b] $+$, $++$, $+++$, $++++$ = increasing density of NE terminals.
[c] 0 = Absence of fluorescent terminals.

or MP and IP are combined with lesions of the SP, the NE terminal density was increased in about half of the animals observed. Approximately the same amount of terminal fluorescence is also produced when only the SP is transected unilaterally (Table 1). These results indicated that the increased number of NE axon collaterals observed in the combination peduncle lesions could be due to manipulation of superior peduncle.

The involvement of the SPX in the proliferation of NE terminals in the cerebellar cortex was further substantiated by the results of partial lesions of the SP. Partial, unilateral SPX is followed by an increased terminal fluorescence in almost 70% of the animals observed. The fluorescent NE terminal density is greatest in the cerebellar cortex on the same side as the partial SPX, but is also above control on the contralateral side. A similar degree of NE fiber axon collateral formation occurs in the cerebellar cortex following unilateral lesions produced by knife-stabs into the LC. The maximum terminal fluorescence is induced by partial bilateral SPX (Table 1). This proliferation of fluorescence appeared to be brightest and most dense 25–40 days after the lesion. Complete bilateral lesions of the three cerebellar peduncles abolishes the NE fluorescence in the cerebellum. The green NE fluorescent terminals also disappear when the sections are treated with sodium borohydride.

In animals with partial SPX, the entire pathway of LC to cerebellar cortex could be visualized far more easily than in other described preparations (see Pickel et al., 1973).

Since the standard Falck–Hillarp procedure does not necessarily reveal all NE fibers present at the time of freezing (see Hokfelt and Ljungdahl, 1972), we felt compelled to demonstrate that the peduncle lesions had induced increased numbers of NE fibers rather than merely increasing the likelihood of visualizing them. The maximum fluorescence and density of NE fibers in the cerebellum occurred about 35 days after the lesion, and this time interval was chosen for further studies in vitro. Sagittal slices of the cerebellum and brainstem from lesioned and control rats were incubated either in Krebs–Bicarbonate Ringers alone or in combination with a monoamine congener known to enhance fluorescence of the catecholamine fibers. The congeners included alpha-methyl-norepinephrine (a-m-NE) and 6-hydroxytryptamine (6-HT) in concentrations of 1×10^{-6} M. During the 15 minute incubation period, the slices were continuously agitated in a water bath at 37°C, and the atmosphere above the section was saturated with 95% O_2 and 5% CO_2 (Hokfelt and Fuxe, 1969).

The incubation studies with a-m-NE and 6-HT confirm that partial SPX induces a true proliferation of NE terminals in the cerebellum. In comparison, the NE terminal density around the Purkinje cells and into the molecular layer is far greater than control in rats with partial unilateral SPX and greatest in animals with bilateral SPX (Fig. 2). The intensity and density of the terminal fluorescence appears to be greater with a-m-NE than with 6-HT, but the distribution of terminals was similar with both compounds.

With Fink–Heimer silver staining, degenerating axon terminals were seen in both the granular and molecular layers of the cerebellum from IPX and SPX rats. In animals with unilateral IPX, the silver deposits are widespread, diffusely arranged in the granular and molecular layer of the homolateral cerebellar hemisphere. In contrast, animals with unilateral SPX often showed degenerating axon terminals in the molecular layer arranged in parallel series. This degeneration (see at 5 days postsurgery) is most extensive on the lesioned side. The distribution of these silver deposits is similar to the distribution of the NE terminals observed in the molecular layer of the cerebellum 35 days after partial SPX (see Pickel et al., 1973). The similarity of this distribution suggests that the newly formed NE terminals may in part be filling the sites vacated by the degenerated NE axons. The pattern of the silver staining following SPX resembles the histofluorescence pattern of NE terminals in the normal rat cerebellum; however, the degenerating axon terminals appear to have a much greater density than the terminals revealed by histofluorescence.

These observations on the cytology of the lesions which will induce axonal proliferation within the cerebellar cortex have been the subject of continuing analysis which will be presented in detail elsewhere (Krebs and Bloom, in preparation). All of the results obtained thus far suggest that LC neurons which project to the cerebellum do exhibit the capacity to produce extensive axonal sprouting within the cerebellum, that the primary condition which must be satisfied to evoke this response is direct injury to either of the existing NE afferent fascicles within the SP or the LC itself, and that selective and extensive denervation of non-adrenergic cerebellar afferents is insufficient to induce sprouting of the NE fiber system.

PHYSIOLOGY AND PHARMACOLOGY OF LC—PURKINJE CELL CONNECTIONS AFTER INDUCTION OF AXON COLLATERAL FORMATION

We next turned our attention to the physiological actions of the pathway under conditions which produce sprouting, namely partial SPX (Krebs and Bloom, in preparation). When cerebellar Purkinje cells from animals prepared in the manner described above are analyzed for discharge patterns with microelectrodes at 25–35 days after surgery (the time of maximal terminal density increase and of visualization of axonal collaterals), the spontaneous discharge pattern is distinctly abnormal with respect to the normal animal or that examined 1 week after surgery. The effects seen are directly interpretable in light of the previously described actions of LC stimulation, and NE iontophoresis on Purkinje cell discharge patterns (see review, Bloom et al., 1973).

In normal animals, NE slows the mean discharge rate of Purkinje cells (Siggins et al., 1969) by prolonging the spontaneous pauses which occur between bursts of single action potentials. Analysis by the method of interspike interval measurements thus shows reduced rates, but retention of the modal interspike interval. Similarly, when the NE fibers have been eradicated by chronic exposure to 6-hydroxydopamine (Hoffer et al., 1971) the mean discharge rate of Purkinje cells is increased at the expense of the almost total elimination of the long interburst pauses. Animals examined approximately 1 week after complete unilateral SPX exhibit discharge rates and patterns like 6-hydroxydopamine-treated rats (Krebs and Bloom, in preparation). On the other hand, animals recorded at 25–35 days after partial SPX show discharge rates which are slower, and interspike intervals which demonstrate longer pauses between single spike bursts.

These results indicated that the period of enhanced axonal proliferation in the cerebellar cortex correlated with changes in discharge rate and pattern identical to the actions of NE, suggesting that the increased axonal sprouts could form functional synapses. To verify this suggestion, Purkinje cell recordings were made and the effects of LC stimulation were examined after partial bilateral SPX (Krebs and Bloom, in preparation). Preliminary results of these latter experiments confirm that the presence of increased numbers of NE afferents from LC to cerebellar Purkinje cells correlates extremely well with increased ease of inhibiting Purkinje cell discharge upon LC stimulation. The effects are not only more potent and more prolonged in duration, but are elicitable with lower stimulating currents. In addition, the actions produced by LC stimulations are no longer restricted to the ipsi-lateral cerebellar cortex, but extend well across the midline, as does the cytological evidence of axonal proliferation. In further correlation with the effects of partial bilateral SPX on NE cerebellar afferent fibers, both the NE fiber density and the effects of LC stimulation are reduced to normal levels by 60–90 days after the surgery.

In retrospect, it appears that the procedures which successfully induce cytological and functional enhancement of NE afferents to the cerebellum have certain characteristics not described in the heterotypic reinnervation of the septal area and mesencephalon (see Moore and Björklund, this Volume). Destruction of septal afferents by ablation of portions of the hippocampus (presumed to be exclusively nonadrenergic fibers) induced sprouting of the NE fibers in the medial forebrain bundle (Moore *et al.*, 1971). On the other hand, the major nonadrenergic cerebellar afferent fibers from the spinal cord, inferior olive, medullary and pontine reticular nuclei pass through the IP and MP (see Fox and Snider, 1967), but removal of these nonadrenergic fibers by IPX and MPX did not enhance the NE terminals in the cerebellar cortex. Moreover, the SP contains only a few nonadrenergic afferent fibers, arising from the spinal cord, tectum, and red nucleus, and yet partial transections of SP induced proliferation of the intact NE fibers. Since the massive removal of the nonadrenergic afferents by the IPX and MPX did not produce any change in the NE terminal density, it seems unlikely that the removal of the nonadrenergic fibers by SPX could account for the fiber proliferation unless these nonadrenergic afferents in the SP were to have certain unique spatial and topologic relations to the NE terminals on Purkinje cells. However, these nonadrenergic SP afferent axons are generally thought to end in cerebellar cortex as mossy fibers, and a common target cell with the NE fibers would thus seem only a remote possibility.

The passage of the NE fibers from the LC through the SP to the cerebellar cortex was clearly mapped in animals with partial SPX, excluding the MP and IP as access routes for the adrenergic afferent fibers. Moreover, complete transection of SP abolishes all cerebellar NE fibers and all effects of LC stimulation (Krebs and Bloom, in preparation). Damage to the NE fibers in rats with SPX could directly induce axonal growth and branching by retrograde changes in the neuron. In this case, the neuronal cell bodies or intact collaterals of severed axons might produce additional NE fibers in excess of the number necessary to replace the vacated adrenergic sites. The cytologically demonstrated overshoot or hyper-innervation was indicated by the greater intensity and density of the terminal fluorescence 25–40 days after SPX and correlates with increased potency of the LC projection onto Purkinje cells. Furthermore, direct mechanical damage to the LC did result in enhancement of cerebellar NE fiber arborization almost as extensive as that produced by SPX.

These results indicate that the induction of axon collaterals in NE afferents to the cerebellum can produce functionally increased potency of the pathway, and additional experiments are now in progress to determine the biological and chemical events which trigger and modulate this provocative physiological change.

ONTOGENY AND SYNAPTOGENESIS OF THE LC

To gain a better understanding of the time course of the development of the LC, we have examined the neonatal development of the nucleus and of the synapses which contact these cells (Nicholson and Bloom, 1973). Using the techniques of thymidine incorporation and autoradiography, it appears that the LC begins its differentiation on the 10–11th days of gestation and shortly thereafter begins to synthesize norepinephrine (Olson and Seiger, 1972; Coyle and Axelrod, 1973). Thus these neurons must be one of the earliest populations of transmitter-forming cells in the developing brain; clearly they are 2–4 days earlier in differentiation time than the dopamine-forming cells of the substantia nigra, and the serotonin-forming cells of the median raphe nucleus (Nicholson and Bloom, 1973). Even though they differentiate early and appear able to synthesize histochemically demonstrable catecholamines early in gestation, formation of synapses onto the LC neurons, as revealed by the technique of ethanolic phosphotungstic acid staining (Bloom and Aghajanian, 1966, 1968), does not begin to accelerate toward adult levels until after birth (Nicholson and Bloom, 1973). Thus if the system is functioning early in neurogenesis as a trophic system to activate or regulate the development of other groups of target cells, one would have to assume that the neurons are able to generate activity spontaneously long before they receive the normal inputs of the adult brain, or, alternatively, that their bioelectrical activity (see Chu and Bloom, 1974) postdates their secretory function.

REFERENCES

ANDÉN, N.-E., DAHLSTRÖM, A., FUXE, K., LARSSON, L., OLSON, L., and UNGERSTEDT, U. (1966) Ascending monoamine neurons to the telencephalon and diencephalon. *Acta physiol. scand.* **67**, 313–326.

BJÖRKLUND, A., and STENEVI, U. (1971) Growth of central catecholamine neurons into smooth muscle grafts in the rat mesencephalon. *Brain Res.* **31**, 1–20.

BLOOM, F. E., and AGHAJANIAN, G. K. (1966) Cytochemistry of synapses: selective staining for electron microscopy. *Science* **154**, 1575–1577.

BLOOM, F. E., and AGHAJANIAN, G. K. (1968) Fine structural and cytochemical analysis of the staining of synaptic junctions with phosphotungstic acid. *J. Ultrastruct. Res.* **22**, 361–376.

BLOOM, F. E., HOFFER, B. J., and SIGGINS, G. R. (1971) Studies on norepinephrine-containing afferents to Purkinje cells of rat cerebellum: I, Localization of the fibers and their synapses. *Brain Res.* **25**, 501–521.

BLOOM, F. E., HOFFER, B. J., BATTENBERG, E. F., SIGGINS, G. R., STEINER, A. L., PARKER, C. W., and WEDNER, H. J. (1972) Adenosine 3′,5′-monophosphate is localized in cerebellar neurons: immunofluorescence evidence. *Science* **177**, 436–438.

BLOOM, F. E., CHU, N-S., HOFFER, B. J., NELSON, C. N., and SIGGINS, G. R. (1973) Studies on the function of central noradrenergic neurons. *Neurosci. Res.* (In press.)

CHU, N-S., and BLOOM, F. E. (1974) The catecholamine-containing neurons in the cat dorso-lateral pontine tegmentum: distribution of the cell bodies and some axonal projections. *Brain Res.* (In press.)

COWAN, W. M., GOTTLIEB, D. I., HENDRICKSON, A. E., PRICE, J. L., and WOOLSEY, T. A. (1972) The autoradiographic demonstration of axonal connections in the central nervous system. *Brain Res.* **37**, 21–35.

COYLE, J. T., and AXELROD, J. (1973) Studies on the ontogeny of central monoamine neurons. This volume.

DAHLSTRÖM, A., and FUXE, K. (1964) Evidence for the existence of monoamine-containing neurons in the central nervous system: I, Demonstration of monoamines in the cell bodies of brain stem neurons. *Acta physiol. scand.* **62**, 1–55.

FINK, R., and HEIMER, L. (1967) Two methods for selective silver impregnation of degenerating axons and their synaptic endings in the central nervous system. *Brain Res.* **4**, 369–374.

FOX, C. A., and SNIDER, S. (eds.) (1967) *The Cerebellum, Prog. Brain Res.*, vol. 25, Elsevier.

FUXE, K. (1965) Evidence for the existence of monoamine-containing neurons in the central nervous system: IV, Distribution of monoamine-containing nerve terminals in the central nervous system. *Acta physiol. scand.* **64**, 39–85.

GREENGARD, P., KEBABIAN, J. W., and McAFFEE, D. A. (1973) Studies on the role of cyclic AMP in neuronal function. In *Proc. Vth Int. Congr. Pharmacol.* (G. Acheson, ed.), S. Karger, Basel (in press).

HOFFER, B. J., SIGGINS, G. R., WOODWARD, D. J., and BLOOM, F. E. (1971) Spontaneous discharge of Purkinje neurons after destruction of catecholamine-containing afferents by 6-hydroxydopamine. *Brain Res.* **30**, 425–430.

HOFFER, B. J., SIGGINS, G. R., OLIVER, A. P., and BLOOM, F. E. (1972) Cyclic adenosine monophosphate mediated adrenergic synapses to cerebellar Purkinje cells. *Adv. Cyclic Nucleotide Res.* **1**, 411–423, Raven Press.

HOFFER, B. J., SIGGINS, G. R., OLIVER, A. P., and BLOM, F. E. (1973) Activation of the pathway from locus coeruleus to rat cerebellar Purkinje neurons: Pharmacological evidence of noradrenergic central inhibition. *J. Pharmac.* **184**, 553–569.

HOKFELT, T., and FUXE, K. (1969) Cerebellar monoamine nerve terminals, a new type of afferent fiber to the cortex cerebelli. *Expl. Brain Res.* **9**, 63–72.

HOKFELT, T., and LJUNGDAHL, A. (1972) Modification of the Falck–Hillarp formaldehyde fluorescence method using the vibratome: simple, rapid and sensitive localization of catecholamines in sections of unfixed or formalin fixed brain tissue. *Histochemie* **29**, 324–339.

JACOBOWITZ, D., and KOSTRZEWA, R. (1972) Selective action of 6-hydroxydopa on noradrenergic terminals: mapping of preterminal axons of the brain. *Life Sci.* **23**, 1329–1342.

KATZMAN, R., BJÖRKLUND, A., OWMAN, C. H., STENEVI, U., and WEST, K. (1971) Evidence for regenerative axon sprouting of central catecholamine neurons in the rat mesencephalon following electrolytic lesions. *Brain Res.* **25**, 589–596.

MOORE, R. Y., BJÖRKLUND, A., and STENEVI, U. (1971) Plastic changes in the adrenergic innervation of the rat septal area in response to denervation. *Brain Res.* **33**, 13–35.

NELSON, C. N., HOFFER, B. J., CHU, N.-S., and BLOOM, F. E. (1973) Cytochemical and pharmacological studies on polysensory neurons in the primate frontal cortex. *Brain Res.* (In press.)

NICHOLSON, J., and BLOOM, F. E. (1973) Cell differentiation and synaptogenesis in the locus coeruleus, raphe nuclei, and substantia nigra of the rat. *Anat. Rec.* **175**, 398.

OLSON, L., and FUXE, K. (1971) On the projection from the locus coeruleus noradrenaline neurons: the cerebellar innervation. *Brain Res.* **28**, 165–171.

OLSON, L., and SEIGER, A. (1972) Early prenatal ontogeny of central monoamine neurons in the rat: fluorescence histochemical observations. *Z. Anat. EntwGesch.* **137**, 301–316.

PICKEL, V. M., KREBS, W. H., and BLOOM, F. E. (1973) Proliferation of norepinephrine-containing axons in rat cerebellar cortex after peduncle lesions. *Brain Res.* **59**, 169–179.

RAISMAN, G. (1969) Neuronal plasticity in the septal nuclei of the adult rat. *Brain Res.* **14**, 25–48.

RALL, T. (1972) Role of adenosine 3′-5′ monophosphate (cyclic AMP) in actions of catecholamines. *Pharmac. Rev.* **24**, 399–410.

SEGAL, M., and BLOOM, F. E. (1973) A projection of the nucleus locus coeruleus to the hippocampus of the rat. *Abstr. IIIrd Ann. Meet. Soc. Neurosci.* p. 371.

SEGAL, M., PICKEL, V. M., and BLOOM, F. E. (1973) The projections of the nucleus locus coeruleus: an autoradiographic study. *Life Sci.* **13**, 817–821.

SIGGINS, G. R., HOFFER, B. J., and BLOOM, F. E. (1969) Cyclic 3′5′ adenosine monophosphate: possible mediator for the response of cerebellar Purkinje cells to microelectrophoresis of norepinephrine. *Science* **165**, 1018–1020.

SIGGINS, G. R., BATTENBERG, E. F., HOFFER, B. J., BLOOM, F. E., and STEINER, A. L. (1973) Noradrenergic stimulation of cyclic adenosine monophosphate in rat Purkinje neurons: an immuno-cytochemical study. *Science* **179**, 585–588.

STENEVI, U., BJÖRKLUND, A., and MOORE, R. Y. (1972) Growth of intact central adrenergic axons in the denervated lateral geniculate body. *Expl. Neurol.* **35**, 290–304.

UNGERSTEDT, U. (1971) Stereotaxic mapping of the monoamine pathways in the rat brain. *Acta physiol. scand.* Suppl. 367, 1–48.

BIOCHEMICAL ASPECTS OF THE CATECHOLAMINERGIC NEURONS IN THE BRAIN OF THE FETAL AND NEONATAL RAT

Joseph T. Coyle

Laboratory of Clinical Science, National Institute of Mental Health, Bethesda, Maryland 20014

SUMMARY

Histologic, autoradiographic, and biochemical studies are in agreement that the catecholaminergic neurons appear in the fetal rat brain by 15 days of gestation. Regional and subcellular distribution of the enzymes in the synthesis pathway for catecholamines indicates that axonal processes have grown from these neurons as early as 8 days before birth. By birth, all major regions of the brain contain catecholaminergic terminals as demonstrated by the presence of the biosynthetic enzymes as well as endogenous catecholamines. Pharmacologic manipulation of the central catecholaminergic neurons of the fetal rat at 18 days of gestation indicates that the neurotransmitters are under controls similar to those known to occur in the adult. Since catecholaminergic receptors are functional at birth, it is suggested that significant interactions may transpire between the catecholaminergic neurons and other neurons of the brain well before birth of the rat.

INTRODUCTION

The catecholamines, dopamine, and norepinephrine, are present in neurons of a number of invertebrates including Echinodermata, Mollusca, and Crustacea (Cottrell, 1967). Recently, Bartels (1971) has examined the development of the central aminergic neurons of the frog. Catecholamine fluorescence is apparent within specific neurons of the central nervous system early in the tadpole stage. These studies underline two important facts: (1) that catecholaminergic neurons appear phylogenetically quite early, and (2) that even in lower phyla, these neurons appear ontogenetically rather early. According to Haeckel's dictum that ontogeny recapitulates phylogeny, one would anticipate that the catecholaminergic neurons would be formed quite early in the development of the mammalian brain.

A considerable amount of evidence derived from both histologic and biochemical studies indicates that the catecholaminergic neurons in the rat brain exhibit their major phase of differentiation postnatally (Breese and Traylor, 1972; Loizou, 1972; Porcher and Heller,

1972). These investigations, however, do suggest that a significant and functionally import-ant aminergic neuronal system is already present in the rat brain at birth. The antenatal period of development has received little attention until recently, perhaps because of the methodologic difficulties involved. This fetal stage is of particular interest because herein lie clues to the mechanisms involved in the formation and initial differentiation of the catecholaminergic neurons as well as to the primordial neuronal relationships that may occur in the developing brain (Jacobson, 1970).

HISTOLOGY OF CATECHOLAMINERGIC NEURONS IN FETAL AND NEONATAL BRAIN

Olson and Seiger (1972) have examined the prenatal development of the central catechol-aminergic neurons of the rat with the histofluorescent technique. Presumptive dopaminergic neurons appear at about 13 days of gestation and noradrenergic neurons at 14 days of gestation. As early as 15 days of gestation axonal projections can be observed emanating for a considerable distance from the nascent neurones. By birth, most of the regions of the brain including the telencephalon have some catecholaminergic terminals although they may be quite scarce (Loizou, 1972). Another approach for documenting the time of form-ation of the catecholaminergic neurons is by means of ^{3}H-thymidine autoradiography. By injecting a single dose of ^{3}H-thymidine into a pregnant rat at a specific stage of pregnancy and examining the catecholaminergic neurons of the locus coeruleus and substantia nigra 30 days after birth by autoradiography, Nicholson and Bloom (1973) have determined when these aminergic neurons undergo cell division. As has been established for other major nuclei in the brainstem of the rat, the dopaminergic and noradrenergic neurons in these two nuclei exhibit a period of cell division that peaks between 12–14 days of gestation and is terminated at 16 days of gestation. Thus the appearance of catecholamine fluorescence in these neurons coincides closely with the period when these neurons are undergoing their terminal phase of cell division.

ENZYMES INVOLVED IN THE SYNTHESIS AND DEGRADATION OF CATECHOLAMINES

The noradrenergic and dopaminergic neurons possess in common two enzymes in the biosynthetic pathway for their neurotransmitters, tyrosine hydroxylase, and dopa decarb-oxylase (Molinoff and Axelrod, 1971). The noradrenergic neurons have, in addition, dopamine-β-hydroxylase, which catalyzes the conversion of dopamine to norepinephrine. Since tyrosine hydroxylase is localized in both types of catecholaminergic neurons (Uretsky and Iversen, 1970) and dopamine-β-hydroxylase is limited to the noradrenergic neurons in the brain (Hartman *et al.*, 1972), these two enzymes can be used as specific biochemical markers for the catecholaminergic neurons and their axonal processes.

All three enzymes in the biosynthetic pathway for catecholamines are present in the fetal rat brain at 15 days of gestation (Coyle and Axelrod, 1972a, b; Lamprecht and Coyle, 1972). The whole brain, at this stage, contains about 0.2% of the enzyme activity of the adult brain (Fig. 1). During the last 8 days of gestation, the activity of tyrosine hydroxylase, dopa decarboxylase and dopamine-β-hydroxylase in the whole brain increases approximately twenty-five fold in a rather linear fashion. Regression of the linear increase in enzyme activity back to zero suggests that the enzymes would appear in the fetal brain at 14 days of

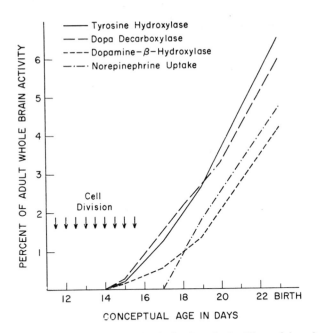

FIG. 1. Development of biosynthetic enzymes in fetal rat brain. The activity of the norepine-phrine uptake mechanism (Coyle and Axelrod, 1971), tyrosine hydroxylase (Coyle and Axelrod, 1972b), dopa decarboxylase (Lamprecht and Coyle, 1972) and dopamine-β-hydroxylase (Coyle and Axelrod, 1972a) is expressed in terms of percent of whole brain activity of the adult. Dates at which cell division of the noradrenergic and dopaminergic neurons takes place are indicated by arrows (Nicholson and Bloom, 1973).

gestation. This date agrees closely with that established by the histofluorescent and auto-radiographic studies as to when the central catecholaminergic neurons appear in the fetal rat brain. Furthermore, since the total number of catecholaminergic neurons is established in the brain by 16 days of gestation, expressing enzymatic values in terms of whole brain activity most accurately reflects the developmental increase in the enzymes that takes place in this fixed population of neurons.

Regional and subcellular studies of the enzymes in the biosynthetic pathway for catechol-amines indicate that there is a translocation of these enzymes during maturation that correlates with the outgrowth of the neuronal processes as documented by the histo-fluorescent technique (Coyle, 1973). As early as 15 days of gestation, one-seventh of the activity of tyrosine hydroxylase and dopamine-β-hydroxylase sediments with the synapto-somal fraction, whereas in the adult brain, two-thirds of the enzyme activity sediments with this fraction (Coyle and Axelrod, 1972a, b). In addition, the demonstration of the activity of these two enzymes in regions of the brain that do not contain catecholaminergic cell bodies as early as 8 days before birth is in agreement with Olson and Seiger's (1972) observ-ation that significant axonal growth has occurred by this early stage of development.

By birth, activity of tyrosine hydroxylase, dopa decarboxylase, and dopamine-β-hydroxylase can be demonstrated in all major regions of the rat brain (Table 1). Notably, the regions of the brain that contain the cell bodies (Dahlström and Fuxe, 1964) or are in close proximity to their source of innervation exhibit relatively small increases in the specific activities of their biosynthetic enzymes between birth and adulthood. In contrast,

TABLE 1. ENZYME ACTIVITY IN VARIOUS REGIONS OF THE RAT BRAIN AT BIRTH

Region	Percent of specific activity in adulthood		
	Tyrosine hydroxylase	Dopa decarboxylase	Dopamine-β-hydroxylase
Medulla-pons	61 ± 3	53 ± 3	32 ± 2
Cerebellum	46 ± 7	19 ± 2	33 ± 2
Midbrain-hypothalamus	67 ± 2	53 ± 2	17 ± 1
Striatum	9 ± 1	13 ± 2	—
Cerebral cortex	17 ± 2	16 ± 2	6 ± 2

Values are expressed in terms of the percentages of the specific activity of the enzymes in each region of the adult brain and are a mean ± SEM from at least eight determinations as reported by Coyle and Axelrod (1972a, b) and Lamprecht and Coyle (1972).

the rostral regions such as the cerebral cortex and corpus striatum, show large increases in their specific activity. The disparity between the activity of tyrosine hydroxylase and dopamine-β-hydroxylase in the midbrain-hypothalamus reflects the large amount of tyrosine hydroxylase that is localized in dopaminergic neurons of the nigral-striatal pathway (Coyle, 1972). This early biochemical maturation of the caudal regions of the brain correlates well with the regional distribution of catecholaminergic terminals as demonstrated by the histo-fluorescent technique (Loizou, 1972).

Monoamine oxidase is the enzyme that is primarily responsible for the intraneuronal catabolism of catecholamines and, therefore, plays a major role in modulating the levels of the neurotransmitters (Molinoff and Axelrod, 1971). Monoamine oxidase is present in the rat brain at 15 days of gestation (Table 2). The specific activity of the enzyme increases threefold during the last 8 days of gestation, whereas between birth and adulthood, the specific activity increases only an additional threefold. Histochemical and biochemical studies indicate that the caudal regions of the brain develop higher activities of monoamine oxidase prior to the rostral regions (Shimizu and Morikawa, 1959; Porcher and Heller, 1972). Although the levels of activity of the enzyme are apparently low in the immature brain, they may be relatively high in the regions of the brain where catecholaminergic neurons are localized.

TABLE 2. MONOAMINE OXIDASE ACTIVITY IN DEVELOPING RAT BRAIN

Age	nmole/mg wet weight/h
15 days gestation	0.12 ± 0.01
18 days gestation	0.21 ± 0.01
20 days gestation	0.30 ± 0.01
Birth	0.33 ± 0.01
Adult	1.16 ± 0.01

Monoamine oxidase was assayed by the method of Wurtman and Axelrod (1963). Values are a mean ± SEM derived from six brains.

LEVELS OF ENDOGENOUS CATECHOLAMINES AND COTRANSMITTERS

The histofluorescent studies indicate that catecholamines are localized in specific neuronal systems in the fetal rat brain by at least 15 days of gestation; and biochemical studies indicate that the brain, at this stage, contains all the enzymes in the biosynthetic pathway for catecholamines. A number of factors including the vesicular storage capacity, activity of processes involved in the catabolism of the neurotransmitters, and the activity of the various regenerative systems for the cofactors utilized by the biosynthetic enzymes could significantly influence the steady state levels of the catecholamines in the neurons of the fetal brain. Quantitative measurements of the amine levels at this stage of development could provide information about the functional characteristics of the differentiating neurons.

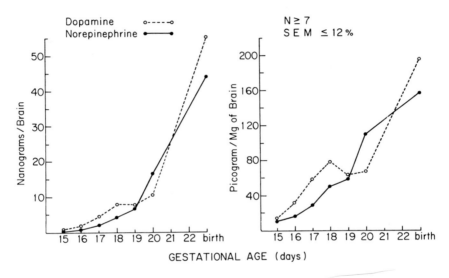

FIG. 2. Levels of endogenous norepinephrine and dopamine in fetal rat brain. Values are expressed in terms of concentration and total content of the brain. (Coyle and Henry, 1973.)

By means of a sensitive, enzymatic-radiometric method, it has been possible to accurately measure the low levels of catecholamines in the milligram amounts of tissue of the fetal rat brain (Coyle and Henry, 1973). Both norepinephrine and dopamine are present at 15 days of gestation, although their levels are considerably below what would be anticipated on the basis of the activity of their biosynthetic enzymes (Fig. 2). The concentration of norepinephrine increases fifteenfold during the last 8 days of gestation, nearly doubling every 24 h. In contrast, the concentration of dopamine exhibits a rapid rise between 15 and 17 days of gestation, remains stable for the next 72 h, and finally increases threefold more by birth. The different developmental profiles for norepinephrine and dopamine are reminiscent of the developmental increases in the specific activity of dopamine-β-hydroxylase and tyrosine hydroxylase. Dopamine-β-hydroxylase, like norepinephrine, exhibits a relatively linear increase in specific activity throughout the last 8 days of gestation, whereas tyrosine hydroxylase, as dopamine, shows an initial rapid increase in specific activity and then a much slower rate of rise during the last 5 days of gestation. After birth, the levels of

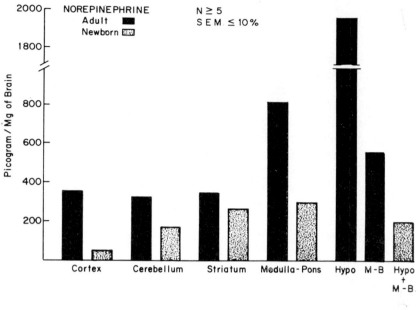

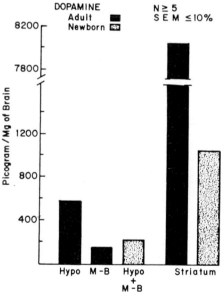

FIG. 3a and b. Levels of endogenous norepinephrine and dopamine in various regions of rat brain at birth and in adulthood. (Coyle and Henry, 1973.)

the neurotransmitters and the activity of the biosynthetic enzymes increase in a coordinate fashion in the whole brain (Breese and Traylor, 1972; Coyle and Axelrod, 1972a, b).

By means of sensitive radiometric-enzymatic assays, the levels of endogenous β-phenyl-ethanolamine and octopamine (Saavedra and Axelrod, 1973) have been determined in the fetal rat brain (Saavedra et al., in preparation). At 15 and 16 days of gestation, the concentration of both putative cotransmitters is relatively high, being over fourfold greater than observed in the adult rat brain. At this early stage of development, the levels of β-phenyl-ethanolamine and octopamine are even higher than the levels of endogenous norepinephrine. During the last week of gestation, the content of norepinephrine rises as the levels of the other biogenic amines decrease by birth to concentrations comparable to that of the adult brain. Studies in the adult rat suggest that β-phenylethanolamine and octopamine are localized in adrenergic neurons (Molinoff and Axelrod, 1971; Saavedra and Axelrod, 1973). However, octopamine is a neurotransmitter in its own right in invertebrates (Nathanson and Greengard, 1973). The extremely high levels of these amines in the fetal brain is perhaps a situation in which ontogeny recapitulates phylogeny in the development of the nervous system of the rodent.

By birth, catecholamines are present in all regions of the rat brain (Fig. 3). The cerebral cortex, midbrain, and hypothalamus exhibit severalfold increases in the concentration of norepinephrine between birth and adulthood, whereas the medulla-pons shows a more modest elevation. As suggested from the activity of the biosynthetic enzymes, the concentration of norepinephrine increases only twofold in the cerebellum between birth and adulthood. The modest 30% increase in the concentration of norepinephrine in the striatum suggests that noradrenergic neurons achieve a full development of innervation in this region early. Although the concentration of dopamine is already quite high in the striatum at birth, it increases eightfold during subsequent maturation. In general, the regional distribution of the neurotransmitters in the brain at birth correlates well with the distribution of their biosynthetic enzymes.

CONTROL OF CATECHOLAMINE LEVELS IN FETAL BRAIN

Pharmacologic perturbations of the amine levels *in vivo* can provide information about the dynamic characteristics of the catecholaminergic neurons. Therefore we have examined the effects of various agents on the levels of dopamine and norepinephrine in the rat brain at 18 days of gestation. Although the wet weight of the brain is only 90 mg at this stage, the catecholaminergic neurons possess not only the biosynthetic enzymes and monoamine oxidase but also the high affinity uptake mechanism and the vesicular storage process (Coyle and Axelrod, 1971).

Reserpine, a drug that blocks vesicular storage (Iversen, 1967), causes a profound depletion of endogenous dopamine and norepinephrine (Table 3). Thus vesicular storage plays an important role in maintaining the levels of the amines in the fetal brain. Amphetamine, which acts by displacing catecholamines from their storage sites as well as by inhibiting the re-uptake process (Axelrod, 1970), causes a 70% decrement in the amine levels. It is noteworthy that this depletion by amphetamine is considerably greater than that reported for the brain of the adult rat (Lewander, 1971).

Inhibition of monoamine oxidase results in a 35% increase in the levels of dopamine and norepinephrine within 3 h. Histofluorescent studies in the fetal brain concur in this observation that monoamine oxidase plays a significant role in modulating amine levels in the fetal brain (Olson and Seiger, 1972; Loizou, 1971).

Administration of the precursor, L-DOPA, circumvents the rate-limiting step in the biosynthetic pathway for catecholamine, tyrosine hydroxylase. In the adult rat, large doses of L-DOPA have relatively modest effects on the concentration of norepinephrine and dopamine (Romero *et al.*, 1972). This appears to be related to the regulation of catecholamine synthesis by feedback inhibition but is also influenced by the storage capacity of the

TABLE 3

Treatment	Duration (h)	Percent of control	
		Norepinephrine	Dopamine
Control		100 ± 4	100 ± 3
Reserpine (4 mg/kg)	5	8 ± 1	5 ± 1
D-Amphetamine (20 mg/kg)	3	27 ± 3	31 ± 6
α-Methyl-p-tyrosine (400 mg/kg)	3	55 ± 3	60 ± 3
Diethyldithiocarbamate (500 mg/kg)	3	60 ± 2	141 ± 6
Pheniprazine (20 mg/kg)	4	134 ± 6	134 ± 6
L-DOPA (300 mg/kg) + MK-486 (150 mg/kg)	4	160 ± 11	7460 ± 230

Drugs were administered to pregnant rats at 18 days of gestation. Results are expressed in terms of the mean percentage of the untreated control ± SEM. Levels in controls are 51 pg/mg for norepinephrine and 97 pg/mg for dopamine. Each value is derived from at least seven fetuses from two or more litters. Degree of significance for all treated fetuses as compared to controls: $p < 0.001$. (Reported in part in Coyle and Henry, 1973.)

neurons and the activity of monoamine oxidase. Administration of L-DOPA in conjunction with a peripheral decarboxylase inhibitor to pregnant mothers causes a 60% increase in the levels of norepinephrine and an eightyfold increase in the levels of dopamine in the fetal brain. Using the fluorometric assay, Kellogg and Lundborg (1972) have observed comparable effects of L-DOPA on the neonatal rat brain. Their study indicates that this dramatic effect on amine levels becomes attenuated with postnatal maturation. The effects of amphetamine, of inhibition of monoamine oxidase and of L-DOPA at 18 days of gestation suggest that the catecholamine levels are less stringently controlled in the fetal brain than in the adult brain.

Inhibition of tyrosine hydroxylase, the initial enzyme in the synthesis pathway for catecholamines, with α-methyl-p-tyrosine results in a 40% decrement in the levels of dopamine and norepinephrine in 3 h in the fetal brain. Inhibition of dopamine-β-hydroxylase with diethyldithiocarbamate causes a 40% decrease in the levels of norepinephrine but a 40% increase in the levels of dopamine in 3 h. The fact that inhibition of the first and last enzymes in the synthesis pathway for norepinephrine causes the same decrement in the levels of the amine indicates that there are negligible amounts of the intermediates, DOPA, and dopamine in the fetal noradrenergic neurons. Thus even in the fetal brain there is biochemical as well as anatomical evidence that dopamine and norepinephrine are localized in distinctly different neuronal populations.

In the brain of the adult rat, the fall in the levels of catecholamines after inhibition of their biosynthetic enzymes is related to the neuronal activity of the catecholaminergic neurons (Andén et al., 1967). The half-lives for dopamine and norepinephrine in the rat brain at 18 days of gestation are slightly in excess of 3 h, a value that is similar to that reported for the brain of the adult rat (Goldstein and Nakajima, 1967). In contrast, inhibition of norepinephrine synthesis for 4 h at 16 days of gestation results in only a slight (20 ± 7%) decrement in the levels of the amine. Thus the rapid, adult-type turnover develops in the ensuing 48 h (unpublished observation, Coyle). Axosomatic synapses are present on the central catecholaminergic neurons at least by 20 days of gestation (Nicholson and Bloom, 1973); and the earliest electrical recordings from the noradrenergic neurons in the locus coeruleus demonstrate that they already exhibit spontaneous electrical activity by birth (Hoffer *et al.*, 1972). Thus the central catecholaminergic neurons are most probably physiological by functional by 18 days of gestation.

POSSIBLE FUNCTIONAL INTERACTION OF CENTRAL CATECHOLAMINERGIC NEURONS IN FETAL BRAIN

Since the central catecholaminergic neurons already possess well extended axonal processes and appear to be releasing neurotransmitter at 18 days of gestation, it is relevant to consider what functional significance this has in the fetal brain. Birth is the earliest point in the development of the rat that has been examined with regards to the presence of catecholamine receptors. β-Adrenergic receptors are present on the Purkinje cells of the cerebellum by birth, which is well before synaptogenesis has occurred (Woodward *et al.*, 1971). Schmidt *et al.* (1970) have shown that in slices prepared from whole rat brain cyclic AMP levels increase in response to norepinephrine within a few days after birth. A number of behavioral studies, which depend upon a substratum of complex neuronal circuitry, indicate that noradrenergic and dopaminergic receptors are functional in the neonatal rat (Fibiger *et al.*, 1970; McGeer *et al.*, 1971; Kellogg and Lundborg, 1972).

During the development of innervation of the rat diaphragm, muscle fibers become less sensitive to acetylcholine with synaptogenesis; thus, prior to innervation, the muscle exhibits supersensitivity to neurotransmitter analogous to that observed in the denervated muscle of the adult (Diamond and Miledi, 1962). Deguchi and Axelrod (1973) have recently shown that the β-adrenergic receptor of the denervated pineal becomes supersensitive to norepinephrine, responding to hundredfold lower concentrations of the amine. Ungerstedt (1971) has obtained indirect evidence that the dopaminergic receptors in the striatum may also exhibit denervation supersensitivity. If receptor neurons in the fetal brain are likewise supersensitive to neurotransmitter prior to innervation as is the muscle fiber, central catecholaminergic neurons may be interacting with neurons in proximity to their axonal processes even before synaptogenesis has occurred.

ACKNOWLEDGEMENT

The author gratefully acknowledges the advice, support, and encouragement of Dr. Julius Axelrod, who made these studies possible.

REFERENCES

ANDÉN, N.-E., CORRODI, H., FUXE, K., and HOKFELT, T. (1967) Increased impulse flow in bulbospinal noradrenaline neurons produced by catecholamine receptor blocking agents. *Eur. J. Pharmac.* **2**, 59–64.

AXELROD, J. (1970) Amphetamine: metabolism, physiological disposition and its effects on catecholamine storage. In *Amphetamines and Related Compounds*. Raven Press, New York, pp. 207–216.

BARTELS, W. (1971) Die ontogenese der aminhaltigen neurone-systeme im gehirn von Rana temporaria. *Z. Zellforsch.* **116**, 94–118.

BREESE, G. R., and TRAYLOR, T. D. (1972) Developmental characteristics of brain catecholamines and tyrosine hydroxylase in the rat: effects of 6-hydroxydopamine. *Br. J. Pharmac.* **44**, 210–222.

COTTRELL, G. A. (1967) Occurrence of dopamine and noradrenaline in the nervous tissues of some invertebrate species. *Br. J. Pharmac.* **29**, 63–69.

COYLE, J. T. (1972) Tyrosine hydroxylase in rat brain—cofactor requirements, regional and subcellular distribution. *Biochem. Pharmac.* **21**, 1935–1944.

COYLE, J. T. (1973) Development of the central catecholaminergic neurons. In *The Neurosciences, Third Study Program* (in press).

COYLE, J. T., and AXELROD, J. (1971) Development of the uptake and storage of L-^{3}H-norepinephrine in the rat brain. *J. Neurochem.* **18**, 2061–2075.

434 J. T. COYLE

COYLE, J. T., and AXELROD, J. (1972a) Dopamine-β-hydroxylase in the rat brain: developmental characteristics. *J. Neurochem.* **19**, 449–459.

COYLE, J. T., and AXELROD, J. (1972b) Tyrosine hydroxylase in rat brain: developmental characteristics. *J. Neurochem.* **19**, 1117–1123.

COYLE, J. T. and HENRY, D. (1973) Catecholamines in fetal and newborn rat brain. *J. Neurochem.* (in press).

DAHLSTRÖM, A., and FUXE, K. (1964) Evidence for the existence of monoamine-containing neurons in the central nervous system. *Acta physiol. scand.* **62**, Suppl. 232.

DEGUCHI, T., and AXELROD, J. (1973) Superinduction of serotonin *N*-acetyltransferase and supersensitivity of adenyl cyclase to catecholamines in denervated pineal gland. *Molec. Pharmac.* (in press).

DIAMOND, J., and MILEDI, R. (1962) A study of fetal and newborn rat muscle fibers. *J. Physiol. Lond.* **206**, 437–455.

FIBIGER, H. C., LYTLE, L. D., and CAMPBELL, B. A. (1970) Cholinergic modulation of adrenergic arousal in the developing rat. *J. Comp. Physiol. Psychol.* **72**, 384–389.

GOLDSTEIN, M., and NAKAJIMA, K. (1967) Effects of disulfiram on catecholamine levels in the brain. *J. Pharmac. Exp. Ther.* **157**, 96–102.

HARTMAN, B. K., ZIDE, D., and UDENFRIEND, S. (1972) The use of dopamine-β-hydroxylase as a marker for central noradrenergic nervous system in rat brain. *Proc. Natn. Acad. Sci. USA* **69**, 2722–2726.

HOFFER, B. J., CHU, N-S., and OLIVER, A.-P. (1972) Cytochemical and electrophysiological studies on central catecholamine-containing neurons. *Abst. Vol. Papers, 5th Int. Cong. Pharmac., San Francisco*, p. 103 (618 Abst.)

IVERSEN, L. L. (1967) *The Uptake and Storage of Noradrenaline*, University Press, Cambridge.

JACOBSON, M. (1970) *Developmental Neurobiology*, Holt, Rinehart & Winston, New York.

KELLOGG, C., and LUNDBORG, P. (1972) Ontogenic variations in responses to L-DOPA and monoamine receptor-stimulating agents. *Psychopharmacologia* **23**, 187–200.

LAMPRECHT, F., and COYLE, J. T. (1972) DOPA decarboxylase in the developing rat brain. *Brain Res.* **41**, 503–506.

LEWANDER, T. (1971) On the presence of *p*-hydroxynorepinephrine in rat brain and heart in relation to changes in catecholamine levels after administration of amphetamine. *Acta pharmac. tox.* **29**, 33–48.

LOIZOU, L. A. (1971) The effect of inhibition of catecholamine synthesis on central catecholamine-containing neurones in the developing albino rat. *Br. J. Pharmac.* **41**, 41–48.

LOIZOU, L. A. (1972) The postnatal ontogeny of monoamine-containing neurones in the central nervous system of the albino rat. *Brain Res.* **40**, 395–418.

MCGEER, E. G., FIBIGER, H. C., and WICKSON, V. (1971) Differential development of caudate enzymes in neonatal rat. *Brain Res.* **32**, 433–440.

MOLINOFF, P. B., and AXELROD, J. (1971) Biochemistry of catecholamines. *A. Rev. Biochem.* **40**, 465–500.

MOLINOFF, P. B., and AXELROD, J. (1972) Distribution and turnover of octopamine in tissues. *J. Neurochem.* **19**, 157–163.

NATHANSON, J. A., and GREENGARD, P. (1973) Octopamine-sensitive adenylate cyclase: evidence for a biological role of octopamine in nervous tissue. *Science* **180**, 308–310.

NICHOLSON, J. L., and BLOOM, F. E. (1973) Cell differentiation and synaptogenesis in the locus coeruleus, raphe nuclei, and substantia nigra of the rat. *Anat. Rec.* **175**, 398–399.

OLSON, L., and SEIGER, A. (1972) Early prenatal ontogeny of central monoamine neurons in the rat: fluorescence histochemical observations. *Z. Anat. Ent-Gesch.* **137**, 301–316.

PORCHER, W., and HELLER, A. (1972) Regional development of catecholamine biosynthesis in rat brain. *J. Neurochem.* **19**, 1917–1930.

ROMERO, J. A., CHALMERS, J. P., COTTMAN, K., LYTLE, L. D., and WURTMAN, R. J. (1972) Regional effects of L-dihydroxyphenylalanine (L-DOPA) on norepinephrine metabolism in rat brain. *J. Pharmac. exp. Ther.* **180**, 277–285.

SAAVEDRA, J., and AXELROD, J. (1973) Demonstration and distribution of phenyl-ethanolamine in brain and other tissues. *Proc. Natn. Acad. Sci. USA* **70**, 769–772.

SCHMIDT, M. J., PALMER, E. C., DETTBORN, W. D. and ROBISON, G. A. (1970) Cyclic AMP and adenyl cyclase in developing rat brain. *Devel. Psychobiol.* **3**, 53–67.

SHIMIZU, N., and MORIKAWA, N. (1959) Histochemical study of monoamine oxidase in developing rat brain. *Nature* **184**, 650–651.

UNGERSTEDT, U. (1971) Postsynaptic supersensitivity after 6-hydroxydopamine induced degeneration of the nigra-striatal dopamine system. *Acta physiol. scand.* Suppl. 367, 69–93.

URETSKY, N. J., and IVERSEN, L. L. (1970) Effects of 6-hydroxydopamine on catecholamine containing neurones in rat brain. *J. Neurochem.* **17**, 269–278.

WOODWARD, D. J., HOFFER, B. J., SIGGINS, G. R., and BLOOM, F. E. (1971) The ontogenetic development of synaptic junctions, synaptic activation and responsiveness to neurotransmitter substances in rat cerebellar Purkinje cells. *Brain Res.* **34**, 73–97.

WURTMAN, R. J., and AXELROD, J. (1963) A sensitive and specific assay for the estimation of monoamine oxidase. *Biochem. Pharmacol.* **12**, 1439–1441.

ONTOGENESIS OF CENTRAL AND PERIPHERAL ADRENERGIC NEURONS IN THE RAT FOLLOWING NEONATAL TREATMENT WITH 6-HYDROXYDOPAMINE

JACQUES DE CHAMPLAIN† AND BEATA SINGH

Centre de Recherche en Sciences Neurologiques, Département de Physiologie, Faculté de Médecine, Université de Montréal, Canada

SUMMARY

The ontogenesis of peripheral and central noradrenergic neurons was studied in the rat following subcutaneous injections of 6-hydroxydopamine (6-OH-DA, 100 mg/kg) 1, 3, and 5 days after birth. This treatment caused severe and long-lasting depletions of the NA content in various peripheral organs. One year after treatment, the endogenous norepinephrine content in the submaxillary gland and spleen was 85% lower, 70% lower in the duodenum, 60% lower in the heart, and 25% lower in the large intestine, compared to age-matched normal animals. In contrast, the catecholamine content in the adrenal gland was totally unaffected by this treatment. The adrenergic cell population of the sympathetic ganglia was greatly diminished by the neonatal 6-OH-DA treatment, but some of these cells survived and were responsible for the partial growth of fibers in the various organs examined.

Neonatal treatment with 6-OH-DA also caused marked alterations in the ontogenesis of central noradrenergic neurons. The results suggest that 6-OH-DA, administered during the first week after birth, crosses the blood–brain barrier, thereby causing an important impairment of terminal fiber growth in the anterior portion of the brain, whereas, the cell bodies localized in the brain stem seem unaffected by the treatment.

One year after treatment, the endogenous norepinephrine levels in the telediencephalic portion of the brain, were 35% lower, whereas in the brain stem the norepinephrine levels were about 80% higher than in control animals. The gradual increase in the norepinephrine concentration in the brain stem during ontogenesis appears to be due to a backward accumulation of this amine subsequent to terminal fiber destruction in the telediencephalon.

INTRODUCTION

The peripheral administration of 6-hydroxydopamine (6-OH-DA) to various adult animal species has been found to produce a selective degeneration of peripheral terminal adrenergic fibers leaving intact sympathetic ganglion cell bodies and adrenal medullary cells (Thoenen and Tranzer, 1968; Tranzer and Thoenen, 1968; Mueller *et al.*, 1969; de

† Member of the Medical Research Council Group (Canada) in Neurological Sciences at the Université de Montréal.

Champlain and Nadeau, 1971). Electron microscopic as well as histochemical fluorescence studies revealed that the effect of 6-OH-DA was not permanent. Adrenergic fibers were seen to regenerate within a few days and a normal adrenergic innervation was restored in various peripheral organs 2–4 months after initial treatment (Malmfors and Sachs, 1968; Thoenen and Tranzer, 1968; de Champlain, 1971).

It was later suggested that the administration of 6-OH-DA to newborn mice could result in a selective and permanent sympathectomy following the observation that this compound caused the degeneration of sympathetic ganglion cell bodies when administered during the perinatal period (Angeletti and Levi-Montalcini, 1970; Angeletti, 1971). However, no systematic studies have thus far been undertaken to study the pattern of growth of peripheral noradrenergic fibers following neonatal treatment with 6-OH-DA. Moreover, since the blood–brain barrier in rats is not completely mature at birth (Dobbing, 1968), and since the development of central adrenergic fibers takes place mainly after birth (Glowinski et al., 1964; Karki et al., 1962; Agrawal et al., 1966; Loizou and Salt, 1970), the study of the ontogenesis of this system after 6-OH-DA treatment was justified. In the present study, using biochemical and histochemical techniques, the ontogenesis of central and peripheral adrenergic fibers was investigated for as long as 1 year following treatment with 6-OH-DA during the first week after birth.

METHODS

Sprague–Dawley rats were treated with three subcutaneous injections of 6-OH-DA-HCl (Kistner Labtjänst, Göteborg) 100 mg/kg, on days 1, 3, and 5 after birth. Control animals received injections of physiological saline according to the same treatment schedule. The animals were killed at 2-week intervals during a period of 4 months except at the beginning of the experiment when groups of animals were killed on the day of birth and 1 week later. Two additional groups of animals were also killed 13 months after the beginning of the experiment. The animals were rapidly killed by decapitation and the tissues were either prepared for biochemical analysis or for histofluorescence examination.

Norepinephrine (NE) was extracted from peripheral tissues and brain, on alumina columns, according to the technique of Anton and Sayre (1962) and assayed fluorometrically by a modification of the technique of von Euler and Lishajko (1961) as previously described (de Champlain et al., 1967).

Tissues were prepared for histofluorescence examination by treatment with paraformaldehyde according to the technique of Falck et al. (1962).

To study the permeability of the blood–brain barrier (BBB) to amines, groups of animals were given subcutaneous injections of 0.25 μCi/g body weight of tritiated norepinephrine (DL-3H NE, New England Nuclear, Boston, s.a. 10 Ci/mmole) on days 1, 8, and 1 month after birth. Animals were killed 1 h after the injection. The brains were homogenized in 0.4 N perchloric acid and 3H NE was isolated by passage on an alumina column as previously described (de Champlain et al., 1967).

RESULTS

BODY AND ORGAN GROWTH

Following 6-OH-DA treatment in the first week after birth, the rats showed a body growth curve comparable to that of age-matched control animals. Moreover, the growth

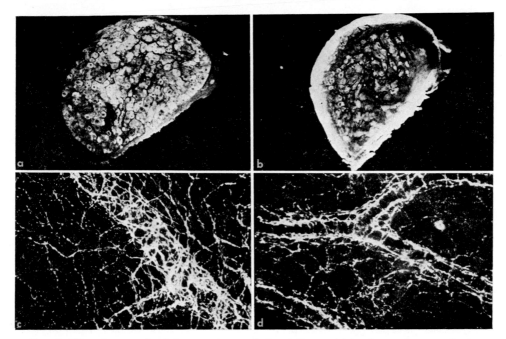

FIG. 1. Microphotograph of the superior cervical ganglion and iris of normal rats and rats treated with 6-OH-DA 100 mg/kg s.c. on days 1, 3 and 5 after birth. (a) Superior cervical ganglion of a normal 3½ month-old rat. Densely packed ganglion cells are easily identifiable by their strong fluorescence intensities. (×60.) (b) Superior cervical ganglion of an age-matched treated animal. The ganglion is atrophied, but a few cell bodies of normal appearance are visible. (×60.) (c) Normal innervation of the dilator muscle and a blood vessel of the iris in an 8-month-old rat. (×150.) (d) Innervation of the dilator muscle and a blood vessel 8 months after treatment. (×150.)

curve of brain, salivary gland, and heart did not differ consistently between the treated and control groups of rats at the various times studied. However, the spleen was significantly bigger and the adrenal glands were significantly smaller in the older groups of treated animals.

ONTOGENESIS OF PERIPHERAL SYMPATHETIC SYSTEM

Sympathetic ganglia. Neonatal treatment with 6-OH-DA caused the destruction of sympathetic ganglion cell bodies in the superior and inferior sympathetic ganglia which were more specifically examined with the fluorescence technique (Fig. 1). In these ganglia, the cell population was considerably reduced and the ganglia were atrophied. However, in all animals studied, the presence of apparently normal cell bodies could, nevertheless, be observed.

Iris. In the iris of treated rats, the growth of a limited number of adrenergic fibers could be observed. These fibers increased with age, distributing partly to the parenchyma and partly to the wall of small arteries (Fig. 1). In the older groups of rats, the number of fibers was less than 25% of the fibers normally present in the iris of control animals.

Salivary gland (submaxillary), heart, spleen. The increase of the NE content in the salivary gland, spleen, and heart of control animals during development was comparable to that reported previously (Iversen *et al.*, 1967; de Champlain *et al.*, 1970). In the treated animals, however, the rate of increase was considerably reduced (Table 1). Nevertheless, a gradual increase of NE, at a diminished rate, was observed in these tissues. More than one year after treatment, the endogenous levels amounted to only 15% of the control values in the spleen and submaxillary gland. In the heart, however, the growth rate was less affected and 1 year after treatment, endogenous levels amounted to about 40% of the control values. The histofluorescence examination of these tissues revealed the presence and growth of adrenergic fibers in proportion to the endogenous levels (Singh and de Champlain, 1974).

TABLE 1. NOREPINEPHRINE LEVELS IN VARIOUS PERIPHERAL TISSUES OF NORMAL AND 6-OH-DA-TREATED RATS DURING DEVELOPMENT

Time after 6-OH-DA injection (weeks)	Group	Salivary gland NE (ng/tissue)	Heart NE (ng/tissue)	Spleen NE (ng/tissue)	Duodenum NE (ng/g)	Intestine NE (ng/g)
Birth	Control	4 ± 0.4	3 ± 1	2 ± 0.3	160 ± 17	497 ± 90
1	Control	20 ± 0	12 ± 1	9 ± 1	416 ± 41	466 ± 59
	6-OH-DA	$7 \pm 1^*$	$6 \pm 1^*$	6 ± 1	$148 \pm 17^*$	453 ± 56
$2\frac{1}{2}$	Control	74 ± 4	100 ± 7	52 ± 6	774 ± 53	449 ± 40
	6-OH-DA	$13 \pm 2^*$	$30 \pm 3^*$	$12 \pm 3^*$	$227 \pm 51^*$	381 ± 28
4	Control	101 ± 3	215 ± 6	171 ± 27	368 ± 41	201 ± 20
	6-OH-DA	$2 \pm 1^*$	$45 \pm 3^*$	$8 \pm 1^*$	$59 \pm 17^*$	$142 \pm 12^{**}$
6	Control	131 ± 4	431 ± 19	319 ± 14	445 ± 44	184 ± 17
	6-OH-DA	$16 \pm 2^*$	$114 \pm 10^*$	$31 \pm 2^*$	$171 \pm 13^*$	150 ± 12
8	Control	157 ± 20	237 ± 25	120 ± 9	285 ± 19	225 ± 24
	6-OH-DA	$26 \pm 6^*$	$88 \pm 8^*$	$24 \pm 4^*$	$155 \pm 9^*$	232 ± 17
10	Control	203 ± 33	513 ± 31	365 ± 48	753 ± 51	345 ± 36
	6-OH-DA	$15 \pm 4^*$	$149 \pm 31^*$	$23 \pm 3^*$	$261 \pm 30^*$	$239 \pm 34^{**}$
12	Control	301 ± 14	528 ± 17	427 ± 23	732 ± 67	290 ± 15
	6-OH-DA	$34 \pm 7^*$	$112 \pm 11^*$	$65 \pm 18^*$	216 ± 21	253 ± 12
14	Control	148 ± 15	557 ± 40	496 ± 32	556 ± 66	448 ± 59
	6-OH-DA	$38 \pm 3^*$	$155 \pm 10^*$	$40 \pm 3^*$	$187 \pm 14^*$	$324 \pm 30^{**}$
16	Control	248 ± 19	427 ± 19	496 ± 26	947 ± 52	378 ± 72
	6-OH-DA	$15 \pm 3^*$	$137 \pm 6^*$	$83 \pm 4^*$	$288 \pm 44^*$	$260 \pm 17^*$
56	Control	440 ± 33	636 ± 41	694 ± 76	1239 ± 123	636 ± 98
	6-OH-DA	$75 \pm 21^*$	$263 \pm 40^*$	$91 \pm 8^*$	$408 \pm 51^*$	$476 \pm 56^*$

Each value represents the mean $\pm$ SEM of tissues taken from 5 to 10 animals except at birth and at 1 week when 30 animals were used to allow for pooling of three tissues per determination.
* $p < 0.01$. ** $p < 0.05$—compared to age-matched control values.

Small and large intestine. The small intestine corresponded to a piece of duodenum sampled from the stomach to the pancreatic angle and the large intestine consisted of a piece of the descending segment. The growth of adrenergic fibers differed markedly between these two segments in the treated animals (Table 1). The growth rate was considerably delayed in the small intestine so that more than 1 year after the treatment the NE had increased to only 30% of the control levels. In contrast, in the large intestine, the perinatal 6-OH-DA treatment affected the growth of sympathetic fibers only minimally. In that tissue, the NE concentration in the treated animals was only slightly but not significantly lower than the concentration in control animals. It is interesting to note that in the large intestine, the NE concentration was already at adult levels in the newborn animals, thus suggesting a normal density of adrenergic fibers at birth. However, during the growth of the intestine, the nonnervous elements developed at a faster rate so that the NE concentration fell during a few weeks. Thereafter the density of fibers increased gradually to adult levels. The histochemical examination of these tissues corroborated the biochemical findings (Singh and de Champlain J., 1974).

Adrenal medulla. The development of the adrenal medulla did not seem to be impaired by neonatal treatment with 6-OH-DA. The pattern of increase in both NE and epinephrine as well as the ratio of E/NE were almost identical in the groups of control and treated animals (Table 2).

TABLE 2. EPINEPHRINE (E) AND NOREPINEPHRINE (NE) IN THE ADRENAL GLANDS OF NORMAL AND 6-OH-DA TREATED RATS DURING DEVELOPMENT

Time after 6-OH-DA injection (weeks)	Group	E (μg/pair)	NE (μg/pair)	Ratio E/NE
Birth	Control	0.4 $\pm$ 0.1	0.4 $\pm$ 0.1	1.0
1	Control	2.3 $\pm$ 0.2	1.2 $\pm$ 0.3	1.9
	6-OH-DA	2.6 $\pm$ 0.1	1.7 $\pm$ 0.1	1.6
2½	Control	2.1 $\pm$ 0.2	1.6 $\pm$ 0.2	1.3
	6-OH-DA	2.8 $\pm$ 0.3*	1.0 $\pm$ 0.2	2.8
4	Control	20.1 $\pm$ 1.4	3.9 $\pm$ 0.8	5.2
	6-OH-DA	17.0 $\pm$ 1.2	4.6 $\pm$ 0.8	3.7
6	Control	8.1 $\pm$ 0.2	2.8 $\pm$ 0.4	2.9
	6-OH-DA	7.2 $\pm$ 0.3*	2.6 $\pm$ 0.5	2.8
8	Control	13.3 $\pm$ 0.9	6.7 $\pm$ 1.4	2.0
	6-OH-DA	16.2 $\pm$ 1.7	6.3 $\pm$ 1.9	2.6
10	Control	29.1 $\pm$ 1.8	5.9 $\pm$ 1.0	4.9
	6-OH-DA	28.5 $\pm$ 2.8	5.1 $\pm$ 1.8	5.6
12	Control	16.2 $\pm$ 1.8	4.1 $\pm$ 0.7	4.0
	6-OH-DA	12.7 $\pm$ 1.2	3.0 $\pm$ 1.0	4.2
14	Control	15.5 $\pm$ 3.3	12.0 $\pm$ 5.0	1.3
	6-OH-DA	15.6 $\pm$ 1.6	3.7 $\pm$ 0.9	4.2
16	Control	27.7 $\pm$ 1.2	9.0 $\pm$ 1.1	3.1
	6-OH-DA	21.1 $\pm$ 1.0	9.5 $\pm$ 0.7	2.2
56	Control	41.6 $\pm$ 3.1	9.9 $\pm$ 1.8	4.2
	6-OH-DA	37.3 $\pm$ 2.9	10.3 $\pm$ 4.4	3.6

Each value represents the mean $\pm$ SEM of tissues taken from 5 to 10 animals except at birth and at 1 week when 30 animals were used to allow for pooling of three tissues per determination.
* $p < 0.05$—compared to age-matched control values.

ONTOGENESIS OF CENTRAL ADRENERGIC FIBERS

The brain was separated into two portions, namely the telediencephalon and brain stem, by an oblique section at the level of the inferior colliculi to include most of the mesencephalon in the brain stem portion. With this arbitrary separation, it was assumed that the telediencephalic portion of the brain contained almost exclusively adrenergic fibers, whereas the brain stem portion contained almost all noradrenergic cell bodies.

Telediencephalon. The pattern of increase of the endogenous NE content or concentration confirmed that the development of the central adrenergic fibers occurred mainly after birth in the rat (Fig. 2). It appeared that neonatal peripheral treatment with 6-OH-DA significantly impaired the growth of adrenergic fibers in the brain. Shortly after treatment (i.e. 1 week

TELEDIENCEPHALON

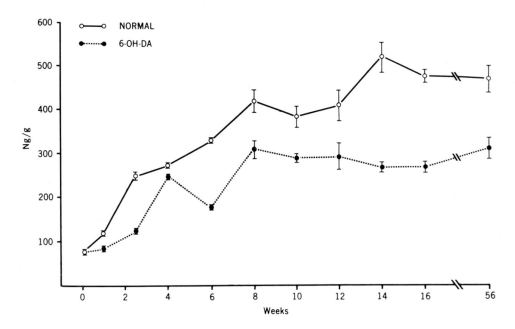

FIG. 2. Norepinephrine concentration in the telediencephalon of normal rats and 6-OH-DA-treated rats. Treatment given, same as described in Fig. 1. Observations were made at various times during development. Each point represents the mean ± SEM of tissues taken from ten animals with the exception of the points on day 1 and 1 week when thirty animals were used to allow for the pooling of three tissues per determination.

after birth), the difference between the NE concentration of control and treated animals was already significant, and this difference appeared to increase in the following months. More than 1 year after treatment, the endogenous concentration or content was about 35% lower in the telediencephalon of treated animals. In contrast, the concentration of dopamine in the same brain portion was not affected by neonatal treatment with 6-OH-DA (Singh and de Champlain, 1972).

Brain stem. The NE content and concentration of the brain stem reached a plateau earlier than in the telediencephalon, thus suggesting a faster maturation of the noradrenergic system at this level (Fig. 3). In contrast to the findings in the telediencephalon, the accumulation of NE occurred faster and reached much higher levels in the brain stem of treated animals. In 1- and 2.5-week-old animals, the NE concentration did not differ significantly, but as the animals grew older the NE increased at a higher rate in the treated animals. One year after treatment, the endogenous NE content was more than 100% greater (Singh and de Champlain, 1972), and the concentration about 80% higher (Fig. 3) in the brain stem of the 6-OH-DA treated animals.

Permeability of blood–brain barrier to amines during development. It appeared that the BBB was more permeable to amines during the first week after birth. One hour after subcutaneous injection of tritiated NE, the concentration of NE in the telediencephalon and

BRAIN STEM

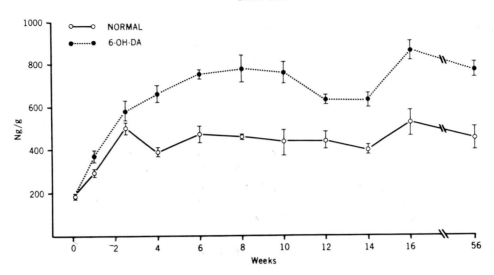

FIG. 3. Norepinephrine concentration in the brain stem of normal rats and 6-OH-DA-treated rats. Treatment given, same as described in Fig. 1. Number of animals per point same as described in Fig. 2.

brain stem was greater in newborn animals than in 8-day and 1-month-old rats, indicating a greater uptake of amines at this stage of development (Table 3). At 8 days, the amount of NE remaining in the brain was minimal and corresponded to the levels found in 1-month-old rats.

TABLE 3. RETENTION OF TRITIATED NOREPINEPHRINE 1 HOUR AFTER SUBCUTANEOUS INJECTION OF A DOSE OF 0.25 μCi/g

TELEDIENCEPHALON

Group	Weight (mg)	3H NE (CPM/g)	Endogenous NE (ng/g)
1 day	209 ± 5*	396 ± 54*	77 ± 1*
8 days	717 ± 7*	198 ± 21	98 ± 4*
1 month	1343 ± 14	180 ± 29	286 ± 7

BRAIN STEM

Group	Weight (mg)	3H NE (CPM/g)	Endogenous NE (n g/g)
1 day	78 ± 2*	789 ± 161*	113 ± 5*
8 days	191 ± 4**	181 ± 50	203 ± 5*
1 month	203 ± 4	145 ± 33	394 ± 17

Each value represents the mean ± SE of tissues taken from 5 to 10 animals.
* $p < 0.01$.   ** $p < 0.05$—compared to values at 1 month.

DISCUSSION

The development of adrenergic fibers in various peripheral organs and in the brain was studied in normal rats and in animals which were treated subcutaneously with 6-OH-DA during the first week after birth. This treatment affected the ontogenesis of adrenergic fibers in the various peripheral organs to different extents, causing severe impairments in the iris, spleen, and salivary gland, moderate impairment in the heart and small intestine, and only minimal impairment in the large intestine. However, whatever the degree of impairment, perinatal 6-OH-DA treatment did not prevent the partial growth of adrenergic fibers in all organs studied as estimated by the measurement of endogenous NE levels and direct observation of the adrenergic fibers with the histofluorescence technique.

Although the variable depleting effect of neonatal 6-OH-DA treatment has also been observed in various peripheral tissues by others (Jaim-Etcheverry and Zieher, 1971; Clark et al., 1972), no systematic studies have been made on the ontogenesis of adrenergic fibers after such treatment. Jaim-Etcheverry and Zieher (1971) reported a 10% increase in the NE content of the heart between the second and tenth week after 6-OH-DA treatment, suggestive of a partial outgrowth of fibers in that organ. However, these investigators could not detect any increase in the NE content of the salivary gland or spleen during the same period.

At the dose used in the present study, an important number of ganglion cell bodies disappeared, suggesting that in newborn animals 6-OH-DA has the ability to destroy adrenergic cell bodies. However, the fluorescence microscopic examination of certain ganglia revealed the presence of morphologically normal adrenergic cell bodies which were most likely responsible for the partial growth of adrenergic fibers. The present findings are in contradiction with the initial study of Angeletti and Levi-Montalcini (1970) who reported that a comparable dose of 6-OH-DA administered during the first week after birth caused irreversible damage to sympathetic neuroblasts, resulting in a total and permanent sympathectomy. However, in a more recent study, Angeletti (1971) found structurally intact cell bodies within the sympathetic ganglia of rats examined 6 months after neonatal 6-OH-DA treatment. Moreover, several recent studies have also reported the presence of structurally intact cell bodies in the sympathetic ganglia of animals treated neonatally with 6-OH-DA (Jaim-Etcheverry and Zieher, 1971; Clark et al., 1972; Barka et al., 1972; Eränkö and Eränkö, 1972).

The difference in the growth pattern of sympathetic fibers in the various organs suggests that 6-OH-DA has a variable effect on sympathetic ganglia. These variations in the effect of 6-OH-DA could probably be explained by a difference in the degree of maturation of sympathetic neuroblasts at the time of the treatment. It is possible that immature sympathetic ganglion cells might be more sensitive to the toxic effect of 6-OH-DA. This hypothesis is supported by the observation that the growth of fibers is less affected in the large intestine where the sympathetic innervation is more developed at birth. This could also explain the lack of effect of 6-OH-DA on sympathetic ganglion cells of adult animals as well as the more complete regrowth of fibers in adult animals compared to that seen in newborn animals (Malmfors and Sachs, 1968; Tranzer and Thoenen, 1968; Jonsson and Sachs, 1970; de Champlain, 1971; Gauthier et al., 1972).

The lack of effect of 6-OH-DA on the adrenal medullary cells, observed in the present study, has also been reported by others in young and adult rats (Mueller et al., 1969; Thoenen, 1971; de Champlain and Nadeau, 1971; Clark et al., 1972; Eränkö and Eränkö,

1972). The apparent insensitivity of these cells to the toxic effects of 6-OH-DA could be due to a higher degree of maturity, to a weaker amine uptake mechanism in the chromaffin cells, or to a smaller fractional blood flow. The adrenal medulla could play an important compensatory role on the maintenance of cardiovascular function after neonatal 6-OH-DA treatment as was observed in adult dogs and rats (Gauthier et al., 1972; de Champlain and van Ameringen, 1972). In these studies it was found that following chemical sympathectomy, the cardiovascular functions were mostly maintained by the adrenal catecholamines. On the other hand, in intact animals, the adrenal medulla did not seem to contribute significantly to the maintenance of these functions. The observations by Mueller et al. (1969) that the catecholamine synthesis rate increased markedly in the adrenal medulla of animals treated with 6-OH-DA, also support the capacity of the adrenal medulla to compensate in the absence of sympathetic fibers.

In addition to the peripheral findings, in the present series of studies it was also found that neonatal peripheral treatment with 6-OH-DA markedly altered the ontogenesis of central adrenergic neurons (Singh and de Champlain, 1972; Jacks et al., 1972). Part of the impairment in the ontogenesis of central fibers could be explained by a direct toxic effect of 6-OH-DA on adrenergic fibers. Previous studies have demonstrated that the BBB is not fully developed at birth in rats and that the barrier matures in the first few weeks following birth (Donahue and Pappas, 1961; Dobbing, 1968). Moreover, it was shown that catecholamines which do not cross the BBB in adult rats, can penetrate into the brain tissue after peripheral injections given in the first few days after birth (Glowinski et al., 1964; Loizou, 1970). The present study using tritium labeled norepinephrine also suggested a greater permeability of the BBB to circulating catecholamines during the first week after birth. Since 6-OH-DA has the same stereochemical characteristics as NE, it is likely that, injected at this stage of development, this compound would cross the BBB as well.

The dissimilar effect of 6-OH-DA on the brain stem and telediencephalon cannot be explained solely on the basis of regional differences in BBB permeability since the barrier appears to be as permeable to catecholamines in both regions in newborn rats. In the telediencephalon, the decrease in NE content and concentration is most likely due to a direct toxic effect of 6-OH-DA on central noradrenergic fibers. The NE levels in this region decreased immediately following treatment suggesting direct fiber destruction. The slower rate of increase in NE levels during the development of 6-OH-DA-treated rats indicated a partial adrenergic innervation in this part of the brain. In the brain stem, where most of the adrenergic cell bodies are localized, the NE content or concentration remained normal for as long as 1.5 weeks following 6-OH-DA treatment, indicating that the subsequent greater increase in the NE content of this region is probably not due to a direct effect of the drug on the noradrenergic structures but is rather secondary. Previous studies have shown that the interruption of axonal flow by ligature or by lesions leads to an accumulation of catecholamines proximal to the site of interruption. (Dahlström and Häggendal, 1966). It is, therefore, possible that the increased accumulation of NE in the brain stem portion could be the consequence of terminal fiber destruction in the anterior portion of the brain followed by a retrograde accumulation in the cell bodies. However, the possibility of new fibers sprouting in the vicinity of the cell bodies has yet to be excluded by direct examination with the histofluorescence technique. Similar differences in the distribution of NE between the telediencephalon and the brain stem have also been observed in the adult brain of animals treated with 6-OH-DA during the perinatal period, by various groups of investigators (Jacks et al., 1972; Pappas and Sobrian, 1972; Taylor et al., 1972).

In conclusion, the administration of 6-OH-DA during the first week after birth caused variable impairment in the pattern of adrenergic fibers growth in various peripheral organs. Although the effects of 6-OH-DA produced by such treatment are longer lasting than those observed after a similar treatment in adult animals, the chemical sympathectomy produced by neonatal treatment was far from being complete or permanent as originally proposed. Moreover, although the functional significance of the changes in the regional distribution of NE in the brain have not yet been established, these alterations should be taken into consideration when interpreting findings using this preparation.

ACKNOWLEDGEMENTS

This study was supported by grants of the Medical Research Council of Canada given to the Research Group in the Neurological Sciences at the Université de Montréal. The authors are grateful to Miss Solange Imbeault and to Miss Lise Farley for their skilful assistance in these studies.

REFERENCES

AGRAWAL, H. C., GLISSON, S. N., and HIMWICH, W. A. (1966) Changes in monoamines of rat brain during postnatal ontogeny. *Biochim. biophys. Acta* **130**, 511–513.

ANGELETTI, P. U. (1971) Chemical sympathectomy in newborn animals. *Neuropharmacology* **10**, 55–59.

ANGELETTI, P. U., and LEVI-MONTALCINI, R. (1970) Sympathetic nerve cell destruction in newborn mammals by 6-hydroxydopamine. *Proc. Natn. Acad. Sci. USA* **65**, 114–121.

ANTON, A. W., and SAYRE, D. F. (1962) Study of the factors affecting the aluminium oxide-trihydroxyindole procedure for the analysis of catecholamines. *J. Pharmac. Exp. Ther.* **138**, 360–375.

BARKA, T., CHANG, W. W. L., and VAN DER NOEN, H. (1972) The effect of 6-hydroxydopamine on rat salivary glands and on their response to isoproterenol. *Lab. Res.* **27**, 594–599.

CLARK, D. W. J., LAVERTY, R., and PHELAN, E. L. (1972) Long-lasting peripheral and central effects of 6-hydroxydopamine in rats. *Br. J. Pharmac.* **44**, 233–243.

DAHLSTRÖM, A., and HÄGGENDAL, J. (1966) Studies on the transport and life-span of amine storage granules in a peripheral adrenergic neuron system. *Acta physiol. scand.* **67**, 278–288.

DE CHAMPLAIN, J. (1971) Degeneration and regrowth of adrenergic nerve fibers in the rat peripheral tissues after 6-hydroxydopamine. *Can. J. Physiol. Pharmac.* **49**, 343–355.

DE CHAMPLAIN, J., and NADEAU, R. (1971) 6-hydroxydopamine, 6-hydroxydopa and degeneration of adrenergic nerves. *Fedn. Proc.* **30**, 877–885.

DE CHAMPLAIN, J., and VAN AMERINGEN, M. R. (1972) Regulation of blood pressure by sympathetic nerve fibers and adrenal medulla in normotensive and hypertensive rats. *Circulat. Res.* **31**, 617–628.

DE CHAMPLAIN, J., KRAKOFF, L. R., and AXELROD, J. (1967) Catecholamine metabolism in experimental hypertension in the rat. *Circulat. Res.* **20**, 136–145.

DE CHAMPLAIN, J., MALMFORS, T., OLSON, L., and SACHS, CH. (1970) Ontogenesis of peripheral adrenergic neurons in the rat: pre- and postnatal observations. *Acta physiol. scand.* **80**, 276–288.

DOBBING, J. (1968) The development of the blood brain barrier. In A. Lajtha, *Brain Barrier Systems* (A. Lajtha and D. H. Ford, eds.), *Progr. Brain Res.* **29**, 417.

DONAHUE, A., and PAPPAS, G. D. (1961) The fine structure of capillaries in the cerebral cortex of the rat at various stages of development. *Am. J. Anat.* **108**, 331–344.

ERÄNKÖ, L., and ERÄNKÖ, O. (1972) Effect of 6-hydroxydopamine on the ganglion cells and the small intensely fluorescent cells of the superior cervical ganglion of the rat. *Acta physiol. scand.* **84**, 115–124.

FALCK, B., HILLARP, N. A., THIEME, G., and TORP, A. (1962) Fluorescence of catecholamines and related compounds condensed with formaldehyde. *J. Histochem. Cytochem.* **10**, 348–354.

GAUTHIER, P., NADEAU, R., and DE CHAMPLAIN, J. (1972) Acute and chronic cardiovascular effects of 6-hydroxydopamine in dogs. *Circulat. Res.* **31**, 207–217.

GLOWINSKI, J., AXELROD, J., KOPIN, I., and WURTMAN, R. (1964) Physiological disposition of H^3-norepinephrine in the developing rat. *J. Pharmac. Exp. Ther.* **146**, 48–53.

IVERSEN, L., DE CHAMPLAIN, J., GLOWINSKI, J., and AXELROD, J. (1967) Uptake, storage and metabolism of norepinephrine in tissues of the developing rat. *J. Pharmac. Exp. Ther.* **157**, 509–516.

JACKS, B. R., DE CHAMPLAIN, J., and CORDEAU, J. P. (1972) Effects of 6-hydroxydopamine on putative transmitter substances in the central nervous system. *Eur. J. Pharmac.* **18**, 353–360.

JAIM-ETCHEVERRY, G., and ZIEHER, L. M. (1971) Permanent depletion of peripheral norepinephrine in rats treated at birth with 6-hydroxydopamine. *Eur. J. Pharmac.* **13**, 272–276.

JONSSON, G., and SACHS, CH. (1970) Effects of 6-hydroxydopamine on the uptake and storage of noradrenaline in sympathetic adrenergic neurons. *Eur. J. Pharmac.* **9**, 141–155.

KARKI, N., KONTZMAN, R., and BRODIE, B. B. (1962) Storage, synthesis and metabolism of monoamines in the developing rat. *J. Neurochem.* **9**, 53–58.

LOIZOU, L. A. (1970) Uptake of monoamines into central neurons and the blood brain barrier in the infant rat. *Br. J. Pharmac.* **40**, 800–813.

LOIZOU, L. A., and SALT, P. (1970) Regional changes in monoamine of the rat brain during postnatal development. *Brain Res.* **20**, 467–470.

MALMFORS, T., and SACHS, CH. (1968) Degeneration of adrenergic nerves produced by 6-hydroxydopamine. *Eur. J. Pharmac.* **3**, 89–92.

MUELLER, T., THOENEN, H., and AXELROD, J. (1969) Adrenal tyrosine hydroxylase: compensatory increase in activity after chemical sympathectomy. *Science* **163**, 468–469.

PAPPAS, B. A., and SOBRIAN, S. K. (1972) Neonatal sympathectomy by 6-hydroxydopamine in the rat: no effects on behaviour but changes in endogenous brain norepinephrine. *Life Sci.* **11**, 653–659.

SINGH, B., and DE CHAMPLAIN, J. (1972) Altered ontogenesis of central noradrenergic neurons following neonatal treatment with 6-hydroxydopamine. *Brain Res.* **48**, 432–437.

SINGH, B., and DE CHAMPLAIN, J. (1974) Ontogenesis of sympathetic fibers after noenatal 6-hydroxydopamine treatment in the rat. *Can. J. Physiol. Pharmac.* (In press).

TAYLOR, K. M., CLARK, D. W. J., LAVERTY, R., and PHELAN, E. L. (1972) Specific noradrenergic neurons destroyed by 6-hydroxydopamine injection into newborn rats. *Nature New Biol.* **239**, 247–248.

THOENEN, H. (1971) Biochemical alterations induced by 6-hydroxydopamine in peripheral adrenergic neurons. In *6-Hydroxydopamine and Catecholamine Neurons* (T. Malmfors and H. Thoenen, eds.), North-Holland, Amsterdam and London, pp. 75.

THOENEN, H., and TRANZER, J. P. (1968) Chemical sympathectomy by selective destruction of adrenergic nerve endings with 6-hydroxydopamine. *Arch. Pharm. Exp. Pathol.* **261**, 271–288.

TRANZER, J. P., and THOENEN, H. (1968) An electron microscopic study of selective acute degeneration of sympathetic nerve terminals after administration of 6-hydroxydopamine. *Experientia* **24**, 155–156.

VON EULER, U. S., and LISHAJKO, F. (1961) Improved technique for the fluorometric estimation of catecholamines. *Acta physiol. scand.* **51**, 348–356.

GROWTH

SESSION IV

Chairman: G. Burnstock

AGGLUTININS OF FORMALINIZED ERYTHROCYTES: CHANGES IN ACTIVITY WITH DEVELOPMENT OF *DICTYOSTELIUM DISCOIDEUM* AND EMBRYONIC CHICK BRAIN

S. H. Barondes, S. D. Rosen, D. L. Simpson, and J. A. Kafka

Department of Psychiatry, University of California, San Diego, La Jolla, California 92037

INTRODUCTION

It is generally believed that cell surface molecules determine specific cellular associations. A number of studies indicate that some of these are soluble factors which are relatively easily dissociable from cell surfaces (Humphreys, 1963; Moscona, 1963, 1968) rather than tightly bound to membranes. For example, a soluble factor is obtained from sponge cells by dispersing tissue in sea water from which calcium and magnesium have been removed (Humphreys, 1963; Moscona, 1963). Addition of this factor to the dissociated sponge cells in complete sea water promotes their aggregation. This factor shows a striking specificity since it promotes aggregation of sponge cells of the species from which it is derived but not that of another species (Humphreys, 1963; Moscona, 1963). It is believed to act as a "ligand" which holds two cells of the same species together (Moscona, 1968), but the mechanism of this reaction is obscure. Soluble factors have also been obtained from embryonic vertebrate brain which may play a role in the association of cells from specific brain regions (Garber and Moscona, 1972a,b).

An additional body of evidence implicates carbohydrate containing macromolecules on the cell surface in specific cellular interactions. For example, the sponge factor mentioned above is a glycoprotein (Moscona, 1968; Humphreys, 1970). More direct evidence of participation of glycoproteins in specific cellular interactions comes from demonstration of their role in association of male and female gametes in the mating of yeast (Crandall and Brock, 1968) and *Chlamydomonas* (Wiese and Hayward, 1972). Additional evidence which implicates carbohydrate containing molecules in specific cell interactions has been reviewed (Kalckar, 1965; Ginsburg and Neufeld, 1969; Barondes, 1970; Winzler, 1970).

A major problem in studies of the participation of cell surface molecules in intercellular interactions is the difficulty of assaying this interaction. This is generally accomplished by adding putative adhesion factors to dissociated cells which have been stripped of their endogenous ones, and observing aggregation. An alternative strategy makes use of antibodies prepared to putative adhesion factors, and studies the effect of monovalent fragments derived from these antibodies on specific intercellular association. If monovalent antibody fragments bind to specific surface molecules which participate in cell adhesion, the cells are prevented from associating. With this approach a specific cell surface component which participates in intercellular association in the cellular slime mold has been identified (Beug et al., 1970, 1973). Sugar residues appear to play a role in its activity (Beug et al., 1970).

The present report describes preliminary results with an alternative strategy which may prove useful in identifying molecules which participate in cell adhesion. It is based on the finding that soluble extracts of a variety of tissues agglutinate formalinized erythrocytes (Rosen, 1972). Although this agglutination might have been due to nonspecific nonphysiological interactions, it seemed possible that molecules whose natural function was cell adhesion might be particularly active as agglutinins. The work which will be reported indicates that this speculation merits further exploration.

STUDIES WITH THE CELLULAR SLIME MOLD
DICTYOSTELIUM DISCOIDEUM

The cellular slime mold is a favorite for studies of differentiation because of its unusual life cycle. The organism exists in two distinct phases: a nonsocial vegetative state in which separate amoeba feed on bacteria and divide every few hours, and a social phase, initiated by a period of starvation, in which the amoeba aggregate to form a multicellular structure (Bonner, 1967; Gerisch, 1968). Under standard culture conditions the entire life cycle takes 24 h during which time the nonassociating vegetative cells develop the capacity to relay and respond to chemotactic signals and the capacity to form stable intercellular contacts (Gerisch, 1968; Robertson and Cohen, 1972). These contacts appear to be species specific since amoebae of different species do not coaggregate (Raper and Thom, 1941). For these reasons this system is ideally suited for studies of the development of the factors which mediate specific cell association.

In the course of an investigation of the potency of extracts of various tissues to agglutinate formalinized sheep erythrocytes, extracts of vegetative and differentiated slime mold cells were tested. It was found that vegetative slime mold cells contain trace levels of agglutination factor whereas differentiated slime mold cells had 400 times as much (Rosen, 1972). Further study indicated the cohesiveness of the slime mold cells and the presence of this factor correlated very well (Fig. 1) (Rosen et al., 1973). This suggested that the agglutination factor and cellular cohesiveness might be related.

Further investigations were influenced by the great contemporary interest in lectins. These are a class of specific carbohydrate-binding proteins of unknown function, isolated from a wide variety of plant and animal sources, which are readily identified by their ability to agglutinate erythrocytes and other cell types (Sharon and Lis, 1972). It seemed possible that the agglutination produced by the factor from *D. discoideum* like that produced by lectins, was due to binding of the factor to sugars on adjacent erythrocyte surfaces. For this reason, the effect of simple sugars on the agglutination reaction was tested. These experiments showed that N-acetyl-D-galactosamine, D-galactose, and L-fucose (6,deoxy-L-galactose) markedly inhibited the reaction, whereas other monosaccharides had little or no activity (Table 1) (Rosen et al., 1973). The selective inhibition by monosaccharides with a

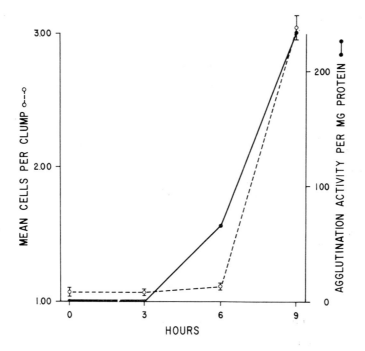

FIG. 1. Specific activity of agglutination factor and cell cohesiveness in differentiating *D. discoideum*. Development was initiated by washing growth phase NC-4 cells free of bacteria and distributing them on Millipore filters and supports. At intervals after plating, cells were assayed for cohesiveness (dashed line) by rolling cells for 30 min and determining the mean cells per clump using a Coulter Electronic Particle Counter, as described by Rosen *et al.* (1973). Extracts of the cells were also assayed for agglutination activity (solid line) with formalinized sheep erythrocytes, as described by Rosen *et al.* (1973). The vertical bars denote two standard errors of the mean.

galactose configuration supported the hypothesis that the agglutination is based on association of the slime mold factor with specific carbohydrate residues on the surface of sheep erythrocytes. The specific carbohydrate-binding property of the agglutination factor was also shown by the finding that it bound quantitatively to a column of Sepharose which is a linear polymer of D-galactose and 3,6,anhydro-L-galactose. The factor was quantitatively eluted from the column with D-galactose and a single pure protein was thereby obtained (Simpson *et al.*, 1974).

Since cohesiveness of slime mold cells could be mediated by the carbohydrate-binding protein which we have identified, attempts were made to determine if the agglutination factor was detectable on the surface of cohesive slime mold cells. It was found that addition of intact cohesive slime mold cells to formalinized sheep erythrocytes produced agglutination of the latter, whereas addition of sixteen times as many vegetative cells were required to produce agglutination (Rosen *et al.*, 1973). The agglutination produced by the cohesive cells was specifically blocked by *N*-acetyl-D-galactosamine but not by *N*-acetyl-D-glucosamine. These experiments indicate that a substance with the same sugar specificity as the soluble agglutination factor is detectable on the surface of cohesive slime mold cells. Localization on the cell surface is, of course, a prerequisite for an intercellular adhesion factor.

TABLE 1. THE EFFECTS OF MONOSACCHARIDES AND DISACCHARIDES ON THE AGGLUTINATION OF FORMALINIZED SHEEP RED BLOOD CELLS BY *D. discoideum* FACTOR

Sugar	Agglutination activity (units/ml) in 0.15 M sugar	Concentration for 50% inhibition of agglutination ($\times 10^{-3}$ M)
No sugar	256	—
N-Acetyl-D-galactosamine	0	2
6,Deoxy-L-galactose (L-fucose)	16	9
D-Galactose	32	19
D-Galactosamine	32	19
Lactose	32	19
Sucrose	128	150
D-Mannose	128	150
D-Glucose	256	>150
N-Acetyl-D-glucosamine	256	>150
N-Acetyl-D-mannosamine	256	>150

For methods of extraction and assay, see Rosen *et al.* (1973).

AGGLUTINATION FACTOR FROM DEVELOPING CHICK BRAIN

In view of the usefulness of the agglutination reaction in identifying a developmentally regulated, carbohydrate-binding protein from slime mold, agglutination activity in extracts of embryonic chick brain of different ages was studied. When formalinized sheep red blood cells were treated with extracts of embryonic chick brain, agglutination was observed. When formalinized chicken erythrocytes were used, agglutination occurred at a lower concentration of factor. Therefore this cell was used for studies of the relative potency of this factor in embryos of various ages and for further work. It should be noted that agglutination of formalinized chicken cells by embryonic chick brain factor distinguishes it from the slime mold factor which does not agglutinate this cell type.

Studies of the concentration of factor in brain at various times after onset of incubation indicated that the factor was highest early in brain development and declined at later stages (Fig. 2). Agglutination activity was not unique to brain since extracts of heart from 11- or 14-day-old chick embryos had agglutination activity, although this was about one-eighth as potent per milligram as the factor from brain. Extracts of liver prepared from these same embryos had no agglutination activity.

Because of our findings with slime mold factor, the effects of monosaccharides on the agglutination reaction were studied. None of the monosaccharides tested had any effect on the agglutination activity. However, glycopeptides derived by Pronase digestion or trypsin digestion of embryonic chick brain inhibited agglutination. The efficacy of the glycopeptides in inhibiting the reaction was reduced by mild treatment with periodate, which oxidizes vicinal hydroxyl groups of monosaccharides. This finding is preliminary evidence that the embryonic chick brain factor may bind to oligosaccharides.

CONCLUSION

The results of these studies indicate that soluble factors which are agglutinins of form-alinized erythrocytes can be extracted from both developing slime mold cells and embryonic

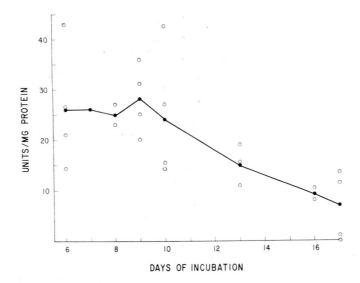

FIG. 2. Specific activity of agglutination factor from embryonic chick brain. The whole brain was removed from embryos after the indicated period of incubation, homogenized in cold water and the homogenate was centrifuged at 150,000 g for 30 min. The supernatant was assayed for agglutination activity with formalinized chicken erythrocytes by the method of Rosen *et al.* (1973).

chick brain. The factor from slime mold agglutinates formalinized sheep erythrocytes but not chicken erythrocytes; is present in very low concentrations in vegetative cells and in high concentrations as the cells become cohesive; and has been shown to be a carbohydrate-binding protein with an affinity for carbohydrates with a galactose configuration. It has been isolated as a pure protein by adsorption on a Sepharose column and elution with D-galactose. The factor appears to be present on the surface of cohesive but not vegetative cells.

The factor from embryonic chick brain is less well defined. It agglutinates both chicken and sheep erythrocytes although the former are agglutinated at lower protein concentrations; it is present in higher concentration early in embryogenesis than at later times; interaction with simple monosaccharides has not been detected; glycopeptides derived from embryonic chick brain appear to interact with it.

Neither of these studies shows that the function of these factors is the mediation of intercellular association. Nevertheless, they are sufficiently encouraging to merit further study.

ACKNOWLEDGEMENTS

This work was supported by grants from the USPHS (MH 18282) and the Alfred P. Sloan Foundation

REFERENCES

BARONDES, S. H. (1970) Brain glycomacromolecules and interneuronal recognition in *Neurosciences: A. Second Study Program* (F. O. Schmitt, ed.) Rockefeller University Press, New York, pp. 747–760.

BEUG, H., GERISCH, G., KEMPFF, S., RIEDEL, V., and CREMER, E. (1970) Specific inhibition of cell contact formation in *Dictyostelium* by univalent antibodies. *Expl. Cell Res.* **63**, 147–158.

BEUG, H., KATZ, F., and GERISCH, G. (1973) Dynamics of antigenic membrane sites relating to cell aggregation in *Dictyostelium discoideum*. *J. Cell Biol.* **56**, 647–658.

BONNER, J. T. (1967) *The Cellular Slime Molds*, 2nd edn., Princeton University Press, Princeton, New Jersey.

CRANDALL, M. A., and BROCK, T. D. (1968) Molecular aspects of specific cell contact. *Science* **161**, 473–475.

GARBER, B., and MOSCONA, A. (1972a). Reconstruction of brain tissue from cell suspensions: I. Aggregation patterns of cells dissociated from different regions of developing brain. *Devel. Biol.* **27**, 217–234.

GARBER, B., and MOSCONA, A. (1972b) Reconstruction of brain tissue from cell suspensions. II. Specific enhancement of aggregation of embryonic cerebral cells by supernatant from homologous cell cultures. *Devel. Biol.* **27**, 235–243.

GERISCH, G. (1968) Cell aggregation and differentiation in *Dictyostelium*. In *Current Topics in Developmental Biology* (A. Monroy and A. A. Moscona, eds.), Academic Press, New York, vol. 3, pp. 157–197.

GINSBURG, V., and NEUFELD, E. F. (1969) Complex heterosaccharides of animals. *A. Rev. Biochem.* **38**, 371–388.

HUMPHREYS, T. (1963) Chemical dissolution and *in vitro* reconstruction of sponge cell adhesions. I. Isolation and functional demonstration of the components involved. *Devel. Biol.* **8**, 27–47.

HUMPHREYS, T. (1970) Biochemical analysis of sponge cell aggregation. *Symp. Zool. Soc. Lond.* **25**, 325–334.

KALCKAR, H. M. (1965) Galactose metabolism and cell "sociology". *Science* **150**, 305–313.

MOSCONA, A. (1963) Studies on cell aggregation: demonstration of materials with selective cell-binding activity. *Proc. Natn. Acad. Sci. USA* **49**, 742–747.

MOSCONA, A. (1968) Cell aggregation: properties of specific cell-ligands and their role in the formation of multicellular systems. *Devel. Biol.* **18**, 250–277.

RAPER, K. B., and THOM, C. (1941) Interspecific mixtures in the *Dictyosteliaceae*. *Am. J. Bot.* **28**, 69–78.

ROBERTSON, A., and COHEN, M. H. (1972) Control of developing fields. *A. Rev. Biophys. Bioeng.* **1**, 409–464.

ROSEN, S. D. (1972) A possible assay for intercellular adhesion molecules. Ph.D. thesis, Cornell University.

ROSEN, S. D., KAFKA, J. A., SIMPSON, D. L., and BARONDES, S. H. (1973) Developmentally regulated carbohydrate-binding protein in *Dictyostelium discoideum*. *Proc. Natn. Acad. Sci. USA* **70**, 2554–2557.

SHARON, N., and LIS, H. (1972) Lectins: cell-agglutinating and sugar specific proteins. *Science* **177**, 949–959.

SIMPSON, D. L., ROSEN, S. D., and BARONDES, S. H. (1974) Properties of a purified carbohydrate-binding protein synthesized during the development of *Dictyostelium discoideum* (submitted for publication).

WIESE, L., and HAYWARD, P. C. (1972) On sexual agglutination and mating-type substances in isogamous dioecious chlamydomonads. III. The sensitivity of cell contact to various enzymes. *Am. J. Bot.* **59**, 530–536.

WINZLER, R. (1970) Carbohydrates in cell surfaces. *Int. Rev. Cytol.* **29**, 77–125.

GROWTH AND DEVELOPMENT OF CHOLINERGIC AND ADRENERGIC NEURONS IN A SYMPATHETIC GANGLION: RECIPROCAL REGULATION AT THE SYNAPSE

IRA B. BLACK

Department of Neurology and Laboratory of Neurobiology, Cornell University Medical College, New York, NY, USA

SUMMARY

The superior cervical ganglion (SCG) in the neonatal mouse is employed as a model system to discuss the regulation of development of presynaptic cholinergic nerves and postsynaptic adrenergic neurons. During the course of maturation, presynaptic choline acetyltransferase (ChAc) activity increases thirty- to forty-fold, whereas postsynaptic tyrosine hydroxylase (T-OH) activity rises six- to eight-fold. Transection of the presynaptic cholinergic nerves which innervate the ganglion prevents the normal development of postsynaptic T-OH activity, suggesting that trans-synaptic influences are necessary for normal postsynaptic maturation. Furthermore, pharmacologic ganglionic blockade reproduces the effects of decentralization, implying that depolarization is necessary for normal postsynaptic development and, further, that presynaptic acetylcholine itself may constitute the trans-synaptic message.

Conversely, the postsynaptic neuron appears to contribute to the normal development of presynaptic cholinergic fibers in SCG. Selective destruction of adrenergic neurons in neonatal mice with either 6-hydroxydopamine or antiserum to nerve growth factor prevents the normal maturation of ChAc activity in presynaptic terminals of SCG. Thus presynaptic and postsynaptic neurons appear to exert reciprocal regulatory influences during ontogeny.

INTRODUCTION

Study of neuronal growth and development is essential for understanding mechanisms controlling orderly maturation and specialization within the nervous system. Such knowledge may, in addition, lead to a more precise definition of synaptic plasticity and elucidation of the biochemistry of communication between nerve cells. Although it has been established that development of innervation is necessary for normal maturation of organs such as skeletal muscles (Guth, 1968), little is known about mechanisms by which developing neurons interact to regulate the maturation of each other.

Developmental milestones in the mammalian central nervous system have been documented using anatomical (Eayrs and Goodhead, 1959; Peters and Flexner, 1950), ultrastructural (Aghajanian and Bloom, 1967; Bunge and Bunge, 1965), electrophysiological (Deza and Eidelberg, 1967), and biochemical (Lognado and Hardy, 1967; Hebb, 1956) approaches. However, due to the complexity of the central nervous system, such studies have been largely descriptive. Even the simplest brain nuclei contain heterogeneous groupings of cells which differ morphologically, biochemically, and probably functionally.

THE SYMPATHETIC GANGLION: A MODEL SYSTEM

Studies in the periphery (Giacobini et al., 1970; Giacobini, 1970) provide simpler models of neural ontogeny. Sympathetic ganglia in mouse, rat, and cat contain primarily two neural elements in synaptic contact: presynaptic cholinergic nerve terminals and postsynaptic adrenergic neurons (Giacobini, 1970). Specifically the well defined, relatively noncomplex superior cervical ganglion (SCG) is ideal for the study of neuronal growth and development because the SCG is composed of biochemically distinct, well defined neural elements consisting primarily of the cholinergic–adrenergic neural unit defined above. In addition, recent studies have indicated the presence of low numbers of small neurons (Williams and Palay, 1969), adrenergic fibers (Hamberger et al., 1963), and scattered cholinergic cells (Sjoqvist, 1962) in sympathetic ganglia. The SCG is anatomically discrete and easily accessible, and its bilaterally symmetric nature allows rigorously controlled experiments within a single animal (Black et al., 1971a). Ontogenetically and anatomically there is no fundamental difference between the autonomic and somatic systems, neurons of the latter arising uninterruptedly from the neural crest (Monnier, 1968). Hence, while the SCG is less complex than central models, data derived from its study may define mechanisms governing growth and development throughout the nervous system.

In the present communication the maturation of mouse SCG in vivo will be described utilizing a combination of biochemical and morphological parameters. Choline acetyltransferase (ChAc), the enzyme catalyzing the conversion of acetyl CoA and choline to the neurotransmitter acetylcholine, is used as a marker for the development of presynaptic cholinergic fibers. The enzyme is highly localized to these presynaptic terminals (Hebb and Waites, 1956). Maturation of postsynaptic neurons is followed by measuring the activity of tyrosine hydroxylase (T-OH), the rate-limiting enzyme in the biosynthesis of noradrenaline (Levitt et al., 1965), the postganglionic neurotransmitter. Visualization of ganglion synapses with the electron microscope is used to estimate the development of synaptic connections.

ENZYME DEVELOPMENT IN THE SUPERIOR CERVICAL GANGLION

ChAc activity increases thirty- to forty-fold during the course of development (Black et al., 1971b). From low levels on day 1, enzyme activity rises rapidly during the first 2 weeks of life reaching a hyperbolic plateau by approximately 3 weeks (Black et al., 1971b) (Fig. 1). This increase in enzyme activity may reflect either ongoing invasion of the ganglion by presynaptic nerve endings and/or transport of the enzyme to nerve endings already present in the ganglion.

The developmental curve for T-OH activity differs significantly from that of ChAc. T-OH activity increases six- to eight-fold from birth to adulthood (Black et al., 1971b). The major increase occurs during the second week of development when enzyme activity

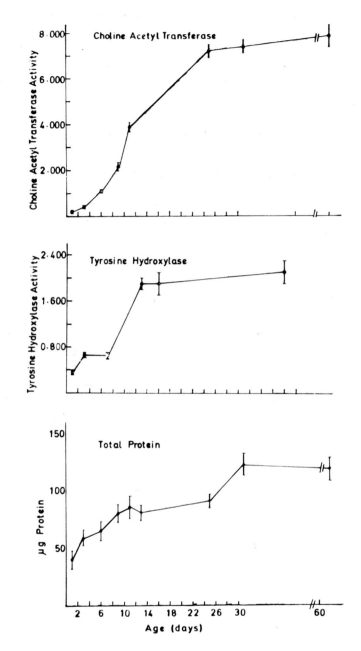

FIG. 1. Developmental increases of transmitter enzyme activities and total protein in mouse superior cervical ganglia. Groups of six mice were taken from litters of varying ages and ganglion pairs from each animal were assayed for enzyme activities and total protein. Choline acetyltransferase activity is expressed as mean (nmoles product per ganglion pair) per hour $\pm$ SEM (vertical bars). Tyrosine hydroxylase activity is expressed as (10^{-11} moles product per ganglion pair) per hour. Total protein is expressed as mean micrograms per ganglion pair $\pm$ SEM (Black et al., 1971b.)

undergoes nearly a three-fold rise with little subsequent elevation to the thirty-eighth day of life (Black *et al.*, 1971b) (Fig. 1).

During development total ganglion protein increases only three-fold, rendering the rises in enzyme specific activities highly significant (Black *et al.*, 1971b) (Fig. 1). This relatively modest increase in total protein has been observed previously during the development of ganglia (Cohen, 1960).

MECHANISM OF THE DEVELOPMENTAL INCREASE OF ENZYME ACTIVITY

These increases in enzyme activity could be due either to the activation of pre-existent enzyme molecules or to the synthesis of new enzyme protein. To distinguish between these alternatives neonatal mice were treated with the protein synthesis inhibitor cycloheximide (Trakatellis *et al.*, 1965). Such treatment prevents the normal developmental increase in T-OH activity (Black *et al.*, 1972b), suggesting that the developmental T-OH rise is dependent on the ongoing synthesis of new enzyme molecules.

DEVELOPMENTAL FORMATION OF SYNAPTIC JUNCTIONS

To appreciate the functional significance of these biochemical correlates of maturation, their temporal relation to the development of interneural connections was defined (Black *et al.*, 1971b). Synaptic junctions were identified and counted, as described by Bloom and Aghajanian (1968), in ganglia of mice aged 1–60 days. During this period total synapses per ganglion increase from approximately 8000 on day 1 to 3,000,000 by day 60 (Fig. 2) (Black *et al.*, 1971b). The number of synapses remains relatively constant during the first 2 days after birth, but rises dramatically between days 5 and 11 to an asymptotic plateau (Fig. 2).

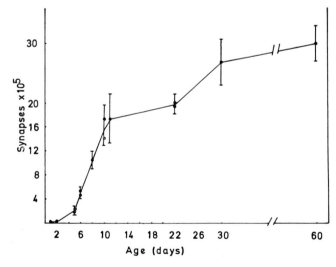

FIG. 2. Development of ganglion synapses. Total synapses per ganglion were estimated in mice of different ages by electron microscopy. Each point represents the estimated total synapses in a superior cervical ganglion from a single mouse. Vertical bars represent SE of determinations of synapse numbers in the ten grid squares sampled for each ganglion. (Black *et al.*, 1971b.)

From day 11 to day 60 the further increase in the number of synapses just reached statistical significance.

Comparison of synapse development with the developmental pattern of ChAc activity reveals some similarities (Black *et al.*, 1971b). Both functions display roughly hyperbolic curves with relatively modest increases during the first 3–4 days of life, and rapid rises early in the second week of development.

The development of T-OH activity contrasts interestingly with synapse formation. The early rise in T-OH activity precedes the increase in synapses. Enzyme activity remains at plateau levels during the initial phase of synaptic rise, days 5–7. Immediately following the steep increase in synapse formation, however, T-OH activity increases markedly to adult levels. These observations suggest that the development of T-OH activity in postsynaptic neurons might be dependent on contact with presynaptic nerve endings.

EFFECT OF DECENTRALIZATION OF THE SUPERIOR CERVICAL GANGLION

To determine whether the presynaptic cholinergic nerve terminals regulate the development of T-OH activity in the postsynaptic neuron, ganglia were decentralized in neonatal mice. The preganglionic trunk was transected unilaterally in mice aged 5–6 days. The contralateral normal ganglion served as control. Mice were killed at varying times postoperatively, ipsilateral ptosis and reduced ganglion ChAc activity indicating success of the procedure. As expected, ChAc activity was reduced to less than 10% of control values. T-OH activity failed to increase above normal 7-day levels, remaining at approximately 30% of the activity of contralateral unoperated ganglia (Black *et al.*, 1971b, 1972b) (Fig. 3). These findings suggest that the increase in T-OH activity occurring during the second week of development (Fig. 1) is dependent on innervation of the postsynaptic neuron.

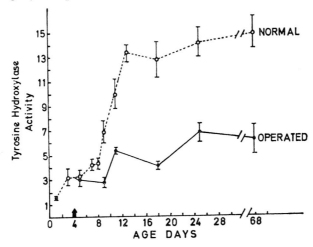

FIG. 3. Effect of surgical decentralization on development of tyrosine hydroxylase activity in mouse superior cervical ganglion. Groups of six mice were killed at various times postoperatively and tyrosine hydroxylase activity (pmoles per ganglion per hour) was measured in control and contralateral decentralized ganglia. The value obtained 1 day after surgery does not differ significantly from control, all other values are significantly lower than respective controls at $p < 0.01$. (Black *et al.*, 1972b.)

In additional studies, sham operations were performed in which ganglia were exposed unilaterally without transection of the preganglionic trunk. This procedure did not alter the normal pattern of development of ChAc of T-OH activities.

THE TRANS-SYNAPTIC MESSAGE

Treatment of neonatal mice and rats with nerve growth factor (NGF) results in profound hyperplasia and hypertrophy of adrenergic neurons throughout the animal (Levi-Montalcini and Angeletti, 1968). Consequently, this substance was considered a prime candidate

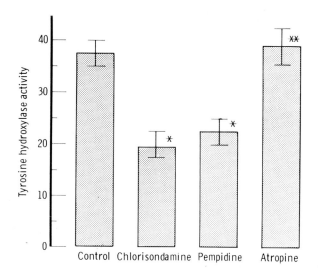

Fig. 4. Effect of ganglion blockade on the development of tyrosine hydroxylase activity in mouse superior cervical ganglion. Groups of six to eight mice were treated with chlorisondamine 5 μg/g, pempidine 50 μg/g, or atropine 5 μg/g every 12 h from day 2 of life and were killed at age 2 weeks. Tyrosine hydroxylase activity is expressed as in Fig. 1. *Chlorisondamine and pempidine groups differ from control and atropine groups at $p < 0.001$. Atropine group does not differ significantly from control.

for the trans-synaptic message. However, treatment with NGF does not fully reverse the effects of decentralization on ganglion T-OH development (Black et al., 1972a), and therefore, NGF cannot completely replace presynaptic terminals during maturation. On this basis NGF cannot be considered alone as the presynaptic message.

Another approach to the problem of identifying the trans-synaptic factor(s) regulating adrenergic neuron development has involved the use of long-acting ganglionic blocking agents (Hendry and Iversen, 1972; Black, 1973). These compounds prevent depolarization of postsynaptic neurons in sympathetic ganglia by competing with acetylcholine for receptor sites. Indeed, the structurally dissimilar, long-acting ganglionic blocking agents, chlorisondamine and pempidine (Corne and Edge, 1958; Grimson et al., 1955), prevent the normal development of T-OH activity in postsynaptic neurons of the superior cervical ganglion (Fig. 4) (Hendry and Iversen, 1972; Black, 1973; Black and Geen, 1973). Atropine, a muscarinic blocking agent, had no effect on enzyme development (Fig. 4). These observations suggest that acetylcholine itself may constitute the trans-synaptic message.

REGULATION OF PRESYNAPTIC DEVELOPMENT BY POSTSYNAPTIC NEURONS

The studies described above suggest that presynaptic cholinergic nerve terminals regulate the growth of postsynaptic neurons in SCG. To determine whether, conversely, postsynaptic neurons regulate the development of presynaptic nerves, adrenergic cells were selectively destroyed in neonatal mice. Animals were treated with 6-OH-DA according to the regimen described by Angeletti and Levi-Montalcini (1970), to destroy peripheral adrenergic neurons of the sympathetic nervous system. The resulting 94% decrease in ganglionic T-OH activity indicated virtually complete destruction of the adrenergic cells in

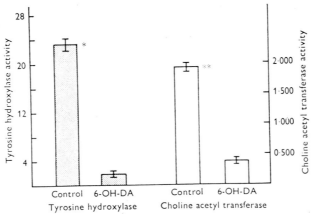

FIG. 5. Effect of 6-hydroxydopamine on the developing ganglion. Six mice were injected with 6-hydroxydopamine in 0.2% ascorbic acid, 150 mg/kg subcutaneously, on days 2, 4, 6, and 8 of life and were killed on day 13. Six littermate controls were treated with vehicle at appropriate times. Ganglia pairs were removed and assayed as indicated in the text. Results are expressed as mean nmole product per ganglion pair per hour $\pm$ SE (vertical bars) for choline acetyltransferase and as pmoles product per pair per hour for tyrosine hydroxylase. *, ** Control differs from appropriate treated groups at $p < 0.001$. (Black et al., 1972a.)

the ganglion (Black et al., 1972a) (Fig. 5). This was confirmed by histological studies demonstrating a 92% decrease in ganglion neuron numbers after 6-OH-DA treatment. ChAc activity failed to develop normally after destruction of adrenergic neurons and remained at levels observed in the normal 1- to 3-day-old mouse (Black et al., 1972a). These findings suggested that destruction of postsynaptic neurons prevented normal development of presynaptic terminals.

These results suggested that the absence of intact sympathetic neurons in the ganglia prevented normal presynaptic development. Alternatively, toxic substances released from degenerating adrenergic neurons might have been responsible for inhibiting the development of the presynaptic terminals. To distinguish between these possibilities, ChAc activity was examined in the ganglia of mice treated with a single dose of 6-OH-DA on day 2 of life and killed 1 week later. The major increase in ChAc activity and the bulk of synapse formation occur between days 5 and 11 in the normal SCG; thus the adrenergic neurons in these animals were destroyed by 6-OH-DA well before this stage. One week after a single injection of 6-OH-DA, ChAc activity failed to develop normally and was not significantly different from the values observed in mice treated with a series of injections of 6-OH-DA on days 2, 4, and 6 (Black et al., 1972a).

Destruction of adrenergic neurons in the superior cervical ganglion was also accomplished by immunological means. Four-day-old mice were treated with a single injection of NGF antiserum and were killed at 28 days of age. A marked diminution of T-OH activity indicated the efficacy of this procedure. ChAc activity again failed to develop normally after destruction of postsynaptic neurons in this manner (Black et al., 1972a).

To determine the duration of the effects of postsynaptic neuron destruction, other experiments were performed in which mice were killed 2 months after injection of NGF-antiserum at 2 days of age. ChAc activity remained depressed even 2 months after treatment, with control values of 8.4 ± 0.32 and treated values of 5.6 ± 0.43 nmoles acetylcholine/ganglion pair/h (Black et al., 1972a). Since NGF-antiserum does not destroy adrenergic neurons in mature animals (Levi-Montalcini and Angeletti, 1968) its effects in the neonate were compared with those in the adult. NGF-antiserum failed to alter T-OH activity in adult animals and ChAc activity was also unaffected, suggesting the absence of any direct effect of NGF-antiserum on presynaptic cholinergic terminals (Black et al., 1972a).

DISCUSSION

DEVELOPMENT OF THE PREGANGLIONIC NEURON

The SCG receives presynaptic innervation from axons arising in the intermediolateral column of the lateral horn of thoracic spinal segments 1–3 (Monnier, 1968). ChAc is, presumably, synthesized within these spinal neuron cell bodies and transported peripherally as in other cholinergic neuron systems (Frizell et al., 1970). Since no natural activator or inhibitor [except possibly acetylcholine itself (Kaita and Goldberg, 1969)] of ChAc has been identified (Fonnum, 1970), it is likely that the increased ganglionic enzyme activity observed during maturation represents an actual increase in numbers of enzyme molecules. Thus the increase in ChAc activity in the ganglion during development may represent a summation of the rates of enzyme synthesis and degradation in the spinal cell body, the rate of transport of ChAc along the axon, and the rates of ingrowth of cholinergic nerve terminals, and degradation of enzyme in the nerve endings.

The marked increase in ChAc activity, and most probably in ChAc molecules, closely approximates adult levels by the second to third week of life. At this time the capacity for neurotransmitter synthesis is thus present. These results also suggest that acetylcholine synthesis does not suddenly appear, in an all or none fashion, but increases progressively over the first few postnatal weeks.

The similarities in the patterns of ChAc activity and synapse development suggest that the increased activity of this enzyme reflects functional cholinergic neuron maturation. Such a formulation is consistent with that of Burt (1968), who has noted association of ChAc activity with the development of motor activity in embryonic chick spinal cord. In addition, since ChAc activity appears shortly after acetylcholine storage vesicles are present (Burt, 1968), and since enzyme is associated with cholinergic nerve terminals in the ganglion (Hebb, 1956), ChAc activity may reflect functional synaptic development as well as neurotransmitter synthesis.

DEVELOPMENT OF THE POSTGANGLIONIC NEURON

The developmental pattern of ganglionic T-OH activity occurs in a context different from that of ChAc. T-OH is largely restricted to postsynaptic cell bodies (Black et al., 1971a), and thus the activity measured directly reflects development of the noradrenergic neuron, and is dependent on enzyme turnover within that neuron. The initial rise occurs prior to the period of synapse formation and before ChAc activity has increased to any significant degree. Hence it is unlikely that this initial phase is regulated by the presynaptic neuron. This elevation of T-OH may occur in perikarya which later respond to synaptic influences. However, it is possible that the early elevation of T-OH activity reflects a separate enzyme pool whose turnover is regulated by other factors.

TRANS-SYNAPTIC REGULATION OF POSTGANGLIONIC DEVELOPMENT

The virtually synchronous increase of ganglionic synapses and T-OH activity suggested that maturation of the noradrenergic neurons depends on synapse formation. Abolition of the major increase in T-OH activity by transection of the preganglionic nerve trunk supports this view. Thus the presynaptic cholinergic nerve terminals influence the development of the postsynaptic cells.

These studies further suggest that, in some sense, the synapses demonstrated by electron microscopy are functional. That is, surgical destruction of the synaptic junctions prevents normal T-OH development. However, the observations presented do not indicate whether the demonstration of synapses morphologically can be correlated with the onset of cholinergic synaptic transmission.

Synapse numbers remain at basal level for at least the first 5 days of life. Preliminary investigations also indicate that a similar number of synapses exist in the superior cervical ganglion in the foetus near full term. After day 5, however, there is an abrupt and marked increase in synapses. Thus, once again, there is a striking degree of synchrony in a developmental parameter, suggesting an almost simultaneous staging of many cell functions within the ganglion. The development of synapses in the mouse sympathetic ganglion exhibits interesting similarities to that previously described in various regions of brain (Aghajanian and Bloom, 1967). In both cases an early plateau phase in synapse density is replaced by a sudden steep increase in synapse numbers to near adult values within a few days. Such a pattern may thus be typical of synapse formation during development in the peripheral as well as the central nervous system.

THE TRANS-SYNAPTIC MESSAGE

The studies described above employing ganglionic blocking agents suggest that blockade of acetylcholine-induced depolarization of adrenergic neurons prevents the normal development of tyrosine hydroxylase activity in these cells. Thus ganglionic blockade reproduces the effects of ganglionic decentralization in preventing normal adrenergic development. The administration of these agents is not associated with the appearance of inhibitors or disappearance of activators, and chlorisondamine itself does not alter enzyme activity *in vitro* (Black, 1973; Black and Geen, 1973). Consequently, the failure of maturation is most probably secondary to decreased T-OH enzyme protein in the SCG and not a result of enzyme inhibition. It would appear that trans-synaptic regulation of the development of T-OH in the adrenergic neurons of SCG requires depolarization of these cells. On this basis, acetylcholine itself may constitute the trans-synaptic message. Consequently, it may not be necessary to postulate the existence of some as yet unidentifiable trans-synaptic "trophic" factor(s), since the normal presynaptic neurotransmitter may also regulate maturation of the postsynaptic neuron. It should be stressed that while presynaptic acetyl-choline may be *necessary* for the normal development of ganglionic neurons, it may not be *sufficient*, and other unidentified mechanisms may also participate. In the rat (Thoenen, 1972; Thoenen *et al.*, 1972a, b), for example, and most probably to a lesser extent in the mouse, NGF also appears to contribute to the regulation of adrenergic neuron development. In some sense, then, the synapses demonstrated by electron microscopy are functional, since surgical destruction of the synaptic junctions prevents normal T-OH development. Moreover, prevention of development by ganglionic blockade suggests that synapses demonstrated morphologically may be correlated with the onset of cholinergic synaptic transmission.

POSTSYNAPTIC REGULATION OF PRESYNAPTIC DEVELOPMENT

On the basis of the studies performed with 6-OH-DA and NGF antiserum it can be concluded that destruction of postsynaptic adrenergic neurons in the SCG prevents the normal biochemical maturation of presynaptic cholinergic nerves.

After the administration of either 6-OH-DA or NGF antiserum to neonatal mice, the expected decrease in postsynaptic T-OH activity is associated with inhibition of the normal developmental increase in ChAc activity. A single injection of 6-OH-DA on day 2 is as effective as a series of doses in preventing the normal development of ChAc activity between birth and 9 days of age. Hence it appears that it is the *absence* of normally function-ing adrenergic neurons *per se*, and not the presence of degenerating neurons which inhibits the maturation of presynaptic terminals.

The precise nature of the developmental defect induced in the presynaptic neuron has not been identified. As described above, ChAc activity in presynaptic fibers in the developing ganglion may reflect enzyme synthesis and degradation in the preganglionic neuron peri-karya, axoplasmic transport of the enzyme to the ganglion terminals, degradation of the enzyme within the nerve endings, and invasion of the ganglion by cholinergic terminals. The decrease in ChAc activity observed in the present studies may reflect alteration of any or all of these processes. Reference to analogous investigations in other neural systems may help to distinguish among these alternatives.

The early work of Hamberger (1934) demonstrated that limb amputation results in increased degeneration of motor cells in the developing chick central nervous system. Prestige (1965, 1967a), has investigated the regulation of cell numbers in *Xenopus* dorsal root ganglion during development. During maturation extensive cell degeneration normally occurs. Amputation of a leg, the field of innervation for these neurons, can lead to an irreversible fall in the number of ganglion cells. Similarly, amputation results in increased degeneration of anterior horn cells which innervate the limb (Prestige, 1967b). These results suggest that in the somatic and sensory system, end organ cells regulate neuron develop-ment. The present studies are consistent with these findings, and suggest that the post-synaptic neurons in the autonomic ganglion may serve a function analogous to the end organ in the somatic system. Thus destruction of the postsynaptic adrenergic neurons in sympathetic ganglion may result in degeneration of preganglionic neurons. Preliminary electron microscopic studies of the preganglionic nerve trunks 1–2 mm away from normal and 6-OH-DA-treated superior cervical ganglia in 14-day-old mice, however, did not show any obvious damage or loss of axons as a result of 6-OH-DA treatment.

The studies involving NGF antiserum indicate that the destruction of adrenergic ganglion cells exerts a long term effect on cholinergic nerves. When NGF antiserum was given on day 4, ChAc activity remained depressed for at least 2 months, suggesting an irreversible alteration of the presynaptic nerves which may reflect an arrest of development of cholinergic fibers in the ganglion.

The regulation of maturation of presynaptic neurons by postsynaptic cells may be mediated either by a direct feedback of information between the post- and presynaptic cells and/or through central reflex neural connections involving end organs and their afferent connections. The latter alternative appears unlikely since the organs innervated by the SCG have not yet received a functional mature nerve supply during the first week of life, when these studies were performed (Iversen et al., 1967). It would appear, then, that in the SCG a retrograde flow of information from postsynaptic to presynaptic cell constitutes the regulatory route.

CONCLUSIONS AND IMPLICATIONS

The above studies suggest that there is a reciprocal regulatory relationship between cholinergic and adrenergic neurons at the synapse during development. Such a flow of regulatory information may also occur in the central nervous system and may constitute a major mechanism governing neuronal development. Considerable evidence indicates that an intact innervation is necessary for the normal maturation of neurons in a number of brain areas. The visual system provides an excellent example of this phenomenon. After eye removal in fetal guinea-pigs, the contralateral superior colliculus does not develop normally (Hess, 1958), suggesting a critical role for trans-synaptic influences. Furthermore, Weisel and Hubel (1963), in elegant studies employing kittens, have observed that unilateral visual deprivation results in arrested development of lateral geniculate neurons receiving fibers from the deprived eye. Thus physiologic presynaptic activity appears necessary for normal growth and differentiation of postsynaptic geniculate neurons. This mode of regulation is strikingly similar to that in the SCG where denervation or ganglionic blockade prevents normal postsynaptic development. Such trans-synaptic regulation of maturation is not restricted to the visual pathways in brain. Torvik (1956), for example, has demonstrated that diencephalic and mesencephalic lesions in kittens results in cell loss and chromatolytic changes in the inferior olive. It is apparent that trans-synaptic regulation of development occurs in the central nervous system as well as in the periphery, although in the former this may be more difficult to analyze due to the multiplicity of afferent inputs for any given neuron.

While trans-synaptic influences participate in neuronal development, it is clear that other factors also play critical roles. Nerve growth factor (Thoenen, 1972; Thoenen et al., 1972a, b), for example, exerts a profound effect on neuronal growth in sympathetic and sensory ganglia. It is thus probable that trans-synaptic influences constitute one of several mechanisms regulating the expression of information already encoded in the developing neuron.

REFERENCES

AGHAJANIAN, G., and BLOOM, F. E. (1967) The formation of synaptic junctions in developing rat brain: a quantitative electron microscopic study. *Brain Res.* **6,** 716–727.

ANGELETTI, P., and LEVI-MONTALCINI, R. (1970) Sympathetic nerve cell destruction in new-born mammals by 6-hydroxydopamine. *Proc. Natn. Acad. Sci. USA* **56,** 114–121.

BLACK, I. B. (1973) Development of adrenergic neurons *in vivo*: inhibition by ganglionic blockade. *J. Neurochem.* **20,** 1265–1267.

BLACK, I. B., and GEEN, S. C. (1973) Trans-synaptic regulation of adrenergic neuron development: inhibition by ganglionic blockade. *Brain Res.* **63**, 291–302.

BLACK, I. B., HENDRY, I. A., and IVERSEN, L. L. (1971a) Differences in the regulation of tyrosine hydroxylase and DOPA-decarboxylase in sympathetic ganglia and adrenal. *Nature* **231**, 27–29.

BLACK, I. B., HENDRY, I. A., and IVERSEN, L. L. (1971b) Trans-synaptic regulation of growth and development of adrenergic neurons in a mouse sympathetic ganglion. *Brain Res.* **34**, 229–240.

BLACK, I. B., HENDRY, I. A., and IVERSEN, L. L. (1972a) The role of post-synaptic neurons in the biochemical maturation of pre-synaptic cholinergic nerve terminals in a mouse sympathetic ganglion. *J. Physiol.* **221**, 149–159.

BLACK, I. B., HENDRY, I. A., and IVERSEN, L. L. (1972b) Effects of surgical decentralization and nerve growth factor on the maturation of adrenergic neurons in a mouse sympathetic ganglion. *J. Neurochem.* **19**, 1367–1377.

BLOOM, F. E., and AGHAJANIAN, G. K. (1968) Fine structural and cytochemical analysis of the staining of synaptic junctions with phosphotungstic acid. *J. Ultrastruct. Res.* **22**, 361–375.

BUNGE, R. P., and BUNGE, M. B. (1965) Ultrastructural characteristics of synapses forming in cultured spinal cord. *Anat. Rec.* **151**, 329.

BURT, A. M. (1968) Acetylcholinesterase and choline acetyltransferase activity in the developing chick spinal cord. *J. Exp. Zool.* **169**, 107–112.

COHEN, S. (1960) Purification of a nerve-growth promoting protein from the mouse salivary gland and its neuro-cytotoxic antiserum. *Proc. Natn. Acad. Sci. USA* **46**, 302–311.

CORNE, S. J., and EDGE, N. D. (1958) Pharmacological properties of pempidine (1:2:2:6:6-pentamethyl piperidine), a new ganglion-blocking compound. *Br. J. Pharmac.* **13**, 339.

DEZA, L., and EIDELBERG, E. (1967) Development of cortical electrical activity in the rat. *Expl. Neurol.* **17**, 425–438.

EAYRS, J. T., and GOODHEAD, B. (1959) Postnatal development of the cerebral cortex in the rat. *J. Anat. Lond.* **93**, 385–402.

FONNUM, F. (1970) *Studies of Choline Acetyltransferase with Particular Reference to its Subcellular localization*, Norwegian Defence Research Establishment Report No. 58.

FRIZELL, M., HASSELGRAN, P. O., and SJÖSTRAND, J. (1970) Axoplasmic transport of acetylcholinesterase and choline acetyltransferase in the vagus and hypoglossal nerve of the rabbit. *Expl. Brain Res.* **10**, 524–531.

GIACOBINI, E. (1970) Biochemistry of synaptic plasticity studies in single neurons in *Biochemistry of Simple Neuronal Models, Advances in Biochemical Psychopharmacology*, vol. 2, Raven Press, New York.

GIACOBINI, G., MARCHISIO, P. C., GIACOBINI, E., and KOSLOW, S. H. (1970) Developmental changes of cholinesterases and monoamine oxidase in chick embryo spinal and sympathetic ganglia. *J. Neurochem.* **17**, 1177.

GRIMSON, K. S., TARAZI, A. K., and FRAZER, J. W. (1955) A new orally active quaternary ammonium ganglion blocking drug capable of reducing blood pressure, SU-3088. *Circulation* **11**, 733–741.

GUTH, L. (1968) "Trophic" influences on nerve on muscle. *Physiol. Rev.* **48**, 645–687.

HAMBERGER, V. (1934) The effects of wing bud extirpation on the development of the central nervous system in chick embryos. *J. Exp. Zool.* **68**, 49–494.

HAMBERGER, B., NORBERG, K. A., and SJOQVIST, F. (1963) Evidence for adrenergic nerve terminals and synapses in sympathetic ganglia. *Int. J. Neuropharmac.* **2**, 279–282.

HEBB, C. O. (1956) Choline acetylase in the developing nervous system of the rabbit and guinea pig. *J. Physiol. Lond.* **133**, 566–570.

HEBB, C. O., and WAITES, G. M. H. (1956) Choline acetylase in antero- and retrograde degeneration of a cholinergic nerve. *J. Physiol. Lond.* **132**, 667–671.

HENDRY, I. A., and IVERSEN, L. L. (1972) Effect of nerve growth factor and ganglion blockade on the normal development of the superior cervical ganglion in the mouse. *Proc. Fifth Int. Cong. Pharmacol. San Francisco*, p. 100.

HESS, A. (1958) Optic centers and pathways after eye removal in fetal guinea pigs. *J. Comp. Neurol.* **109**, 91–115.

IVERSEN, L. L., DE CHAMPLAIN, J., GLOWINSKI, J., and AXELROD, J. (1967) Uptake, storage and metabolism of norepinephrine in tissues of the developing rat. *J. Pharmac. Exp. Ther.* **157**, 509–516.

KAITA, A. A., and GOLDBERG, A. M. (1969) Control of acetylcholine synthesis: the inhibition of choline acetyltransferase by acetylcholine. *J. Neurochem.* **16**, 1185–1191.

LEVI-MONTALCINI, R., and ANGELETTI, P. U. (1968) Nerve growth factor. *Physiol. Rev.* **48**, 534–569.

LEVITT, M., SPECTOR, S., SJOERDSMA, A., and UDENFRIEND, S. (1965) Elucidation of the rate-limiting step in norepinephrine biosynthesis in the perfused guinea pig heart. *J. Pharmac. Exp. Ther.* **148**, 1–8.

LOGNADO, J. R., and HARDY, M. (1967) Brain esterases during development. *Nature* **214**, 1207–1210.

MONNIER, M. (1968) Functions of the nervous system, *General Physiology, Autonomic Functions*, vol. 1, Elsevier, Amsterdam, pp. 91–129.

PETERS, V. B., and FLEXNER, L. B. (1950) Biochemical and physiological differentiation during morphogenesis: VIII, Quantitative morphologic studies on the developing cerebral cortex of the fetal guinea pig. *Am. J. Anat.* **86,** 133–157.

PRESTIGE, M. C. (1965) Cell turnover in the spinal ganglia of *Xenopus laevis* tadpoles. *J. Embryol. Exp. Morph.* **13,** 63–72.

PRESTIGE, M. C. (1967a) The control of cell number in the lumbar spinal ganglia during the development of *Xenopus laevis* tadpoles. *J. Embryol. Exp. Morph.* **17,** 453–471.

PRESTIGE, M. C. (1967b) The control of cell numbers in the lumbar ventral horns during development of *Xenopus laevis* tadpoles. *J. Embryol. Exp. Morph.* **18,** 359–387.

SJOQVIST, F. (1962) *Cholinergic Sympathetic Ganglion Cells.* Kungl. Boktryekeriet P.A. Norstedt and Soner, Stockholm.

THOENEN, H. (1972) Comparison between the effect of neuronal activity and nerve growth factor on the enzymes involved in the synthesis of norepinephrine. *Pharmac. Rev.* **24,** 255–267.

THOENEN, H., SANER, A., ANGELETTI, P. U., and LEVI-MONTALCINI, R. (1972a) Increased activity of choline acetyltransferase in sympathetic ganglia after prolonged administration of nerve growth factor. *Nature New Biol.* **236,** 26–27.

THOENEN, H., SANER, A., KETTLED, R., and ANGELETTI, P. U. (1972b) Nerve growth factor and preganglionic cholinergic nerves; their relative importance to the development of the terminal adrenergic neurone. *Brain Res.* **44,** 593–602.

TORVIK, A. (1956) Transneuronal changes in the inferior olive and pontine nuclei in kittens. *J. Neuropathol. Expl. Neurol.* **15,** 119–145.

TRAKATELLIS, A. C., MONTJAR, M., and AXELROD, A. E. (1965) Effect of cycloheximide on polysomes and protein synthesis in the mouse liver. *Biochemistry* **4,** 2065.

WEISEL, T. M., and HUBEL, D. H. (1963) Effects of visual deprivation on morphology and physiology of cells in the cat's lateral geniculate body. *J. Neurophysiol.* **26,** 978–993.

WILLIAMS, T. H., and PALAY, S. L. (1969) Ultrastructure of the small neurons in the superior cervical ganglion. *Brain Res.* **15,** 17–34.

HETEROGENOUS REINNERVATION OF SYMPATHETIC LUMBAR GANGLIA WITH SYMPATHETIC POSTGANGLIONIC NERVES

Amin Suria and Stephen H. Koslow

Laboratory of Preclinical Pharmacology, National Institute of Mental Health, Saint Elizabeth's Hospital, Washington DC 20032, USA

SUMMARY

Replacement of the normal input (cholinergic) to the lumbar (L_4) sympathetic chain ganglia with the splenic nerve (adrenergic) results in a successful reinnervation in approximately 70% of the preparations. On the basis of the neurotransmitter released during stimulation, these functioning reinnervated ganglia can be classified into two groups. Those termed adrenergic released nor-epinephrine and dopamine-β-hydroxylase and dopamine, while those defined as cholinergic did not release any of these three compounds; in this way the cholinergic ganglia were similar to normal control ganglia which also failed to release any of these compounds.

These classifications were further substantiated by testing these ganglia with pharmacological agents known to alter the synaptic response. Acetylcholine and curare both had the predicted effects on the cholinergic ganglia. Acetylcholine had a dual action, initially a facilitation of the synaptic response followed by inhibition, while curare blocked the evoked synaptic potential. These compounds were unable to alter the response in the adrenergic ganglia. Similarly, Dibenamine was without effect on the synaptic response of the adrenergic ganglia.

These data support the contention of the *de novo* formation of a noradrenergic synapse in place of the normal cholinergic synapse and also suggest that the postganglionic receptor site has been altered by the novel neuronal input.

INTRODUCTION

Heterogenous reinnervation studies on the peripheral nervous system by Langley (1898) were carried out long before the concept of the chemical mediation of nerve impulses. Langley and Anderson (1904a, b) classified the peripheral nerves into different groups depending upon their ability to replace each other. It later became apparent that these classifications coincided with the cholinergic or adrenergic groupings of Dale (1935).

This problem of heterogenous reinnervation was again extensively studied by Hillarp (1946). In studies on anastomosis between postganglionic and preganglionic nerves he concluded that no synapses developed. He did find, using light microscopy, that many postganglionic nerve fibers regenerated, but there was no direct connection with the ganglionic cells.

We have approached this problem of heterogenous reinnervation using two different models. The first and most successful is reinnervation of the normally adrenergically innervated nictitating membrane with cholinergic hypoglossal nerves (Koslow *et al.*, 1972b). In these studies, monoamine-containing fluorescent fibers are no longer seen to innervate the musculature of the membrane, and there is a significant decrease in the monoamine oxidase activity. These changes indicate the loss of the normally present sympathetic adrenergic innervation. The reinnervated nictitating membranes instead contain cholineacetylase. In addition, some nerve fibers stain positive for cholinesterase, and the contraction in response to electrical stimulation is blocked by atropine. These results supported the view that a functional cholinergic innervation of the membrane is established in the absence of any detectable adrenergic innervation as a consequence of the heterogenous anastomosis of the nictitating membrane with a cholinergic nerve.

The second model is the reinnervation of the normally cholinergically innervated lumbar ganglia with adrenergic splenic nerve (the postganglionic fibers of the coeliac ganglion) (Koslow *et al.*, 1971). In approximately 15% of these preparations there was a unique depolarizing wave in response to electrical stimulation. In these reinnervated ganglia there was a dependence on 3,4-1-dihydroxyphenylalanine (L-DOPA) and pyridoxal phosphate for continued synaptic transmission when the preparation was subjected to prolonged stimulation. Using fluorescence microscopy it was demonstrated that numerous norepinephrine containing axons bridged the site of anastomosis. These findings suggested that in these preparations the synaptic transmission was adrenergic.

The present study is a continuation of the splenic reinnervated lumbar ganglia. If this reinnervation is adrenergic then it should be possible by using the GC-MS assay for catecholamines (Koslow *et al.*, 1972a) to detect the release of a monoamine neurotransmitter. Furthermore, using specific pharmacological agents known to affect cholinergic synaptic transmission, i.e. acetylcholine, curare, dibenamine, we could probe the characteristics of the postsynaptic receptor involved.

MATERIALS AND METHODS

Cats of either sex weighing 2–3 kg were used for all experiments. The splenic-lumbar anastomosis was accomplished using sterile surgical conditions. The sympathetic chain was cut between the lumbar-3 (L_3) and lumbar-4 (L_4) ganglion and, following splenectomy, the splenic nerve was sutured to the proximal L_4 stump (Koslow *et al.*, 1971).

Approximately 2 years after the surgery, cats were anesthetized with 20% urethane (w/v; 500 mg/kg) and the L_4 ganglion with its splenic nerve homograft and distal segment of the sympathetic chain was isolated. The isolated preparation was mounted in a plexiglas chamber and superfused with Krebs-bicarbonate buffer (Umbriet *et al.*, 1951). The buffer was continuously aerated with 95% O_2 and 5% CO_2 mixture. Temperature was maintained at 37°C.

ELECTROPHYSIOLOGY

Bioelectric potentials were recorded by placing the indifferent electrode on the distal end of the preparation (postganglionic) and the recording electrode (Ag-AgCl) on the body of the L_4 ganglion. Platinum stimulating electrodes were placed on the splenic nerve proximal to site of anastomosis, in the case of reinnervated ganglion, or on the preganglionic end of the nerve in normal preparations.

The potentials were displayed on a cathode ray oscilloscope and recorded with a Grass C4 camera. After the ganglion was mounted in a chamber it was superfused with buffer for at least 1 h before any tests were conducted. At the end of an hour the preparation was subjected to a single supramaximal shock to obtain the initial control potential. Thereafter the ganglion was superfused with the buffer medium containing 1 mg/ml ascorbic acid for 30 min. The potentials generated in the presence of ascorbic acid were unchanged. The perfusion chamber was then totally emptied of any fluid, superfusion stopped, and 500 μl of the oxygenated bicarbonate buffer containing ascorbic acid were pipetted directly into the chamber. The preparation was allowed to stay in this environment for 15 mins. After 15 mins, 200 μl of the fluid were collected for catecholamines estimation, and 200 μl were collected for dopamine-β-hydroxylase (DBH) determination. To determine the amount of catecholamines and DBH released after stimulation, 500 μl of the buffer were added directly to the chamber again and the preparation was stimulated continuously for 15 min (30 Hz; 8–10 V; 0.3 ms duration pulses). This stimulation and collection procedure was repeated four times, the total time of stimulation being 1 h. Ascorbic acid was added to prevent the oxidation of catecholamines. Bioelectric potentials were always recorded before and after the stimulation periods. After these studies, the ganglion was allowed to rest (continuous superfusion without ascorbate) for 1 h. All drug studies were then carried out. Drugs were added directly from the stock solutions into the superfusion medium to give the desired concentrations and the ganglion was allowed to bathe in this medium for the times indicated in the results section of this report.

Norepinephrine (NE) and dopamine (DA) were determined by gas chromatography–mass spectrometry (LKB 9000, GC-MS) (Koslow et al., 1972a). DBH was estimated by the method described by Weinshilboum and Axelrod (1971) with some modifications.

Identical studies were performed on the L_4 ganglion isolated from normal unoperated cats.

RESULTS AND DISCUSSION

Of the eight preparations in which the splenic nerve was anastomosed to the L_4 ganglion, six exhibited evoked potentials having characteristics of synaptic transmission. In five normal control L_4 ganglion tested, no NE, DA, or DBH was detected in the fluid collected. Four of the six successfully reinnervated preparations failed to show any release of NE, DA, or DBH in response to stimulation. These ganglion will hereafter be referred to as cholinergic reinnervated ganglion. Of the remaining two splenic reinnervated ganglia, one was found to release NE and DBH, and the second NE, DBH, and DA. The ganglion releasing only NE and DBH will be termed adrenergic-I and the one releasing all three compounds, adrenergic-II.

In the adrenergic-I preparation there was a release of both NE and DBH during the stimulation (Fig. 1). During 1 h of stimulation 482 pmoles NE was released. This 1 h stimulation period was divided in four 15 min periods; the amount of NE collected during each stimulation period was consistent as was the evoked potential recorded between each successive 15 min stimulation period. It would thus appear that in this adrenergic preparation, the catecholamine terminals are functioning in terms of their ability to maintain and release their NE content.

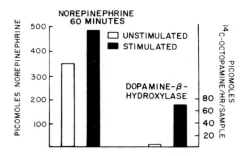

FIG. 1. Stimulation-induced release of norepinephrine and dopamine-β-hydroxylase from the adrenergic-I splenic reinnervated preparation.

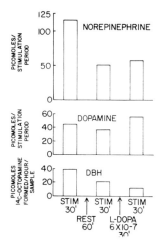

FIG. 2. Stimulation induced release of norepinephrine, dopamine and dopamine-β-hydroxylase from the adrenergic-II splenic reinnervated preparation.

Similarly, in the adrenergic-II preparation, NE and DBH were released; however, there was, in addition, the "release" of DA (Fig. 2). In contrast to the adrenergic-I preparation in this preparation, there was a significant change in the concentrations of these compounds released during two successive stimulation periods; 66% decrease NE, 16% decrease DA, and 46% decrease DBH. Between these two stimulation periods there was a 60 min period of no stimulation. The evoked potential although diminished after the first 30 min period was restored at the end of 60 min of rest. At the end of the second stimulation period, the adrenergic component was severely depressed and only restored after the ganglion was superfused with L-DOPA. In the last 30 min stimulation period (Fig. 2), which followed the L-DOPA superfusion, there was a 12% increase in NE released, a 34% increase in DA released, and a 43% decrease in DBH. The increase in the catecholamines release may be due to the previous addition of the biosynthetic precursor L-DOPA to the bath resulting in an increased synthesis of DA and NE. The continuous decrease in the DBH content and the threefold greater increase in the DA released over that of the NE indicates a malfunctioning adrenergic terminal, probably low in DBH and synaptic vesicles capable of synthesizing and storing NE.

ELECTROPHYSIOLOGY

The response of the cholinergic reinnervated ganglion showed marked similarity to the evoked potential recorded from the normal L_4 ganglion (Fig. 3(A)); indicative of some through fibers and a large synaptic depolarization (Fig. 3(B)). In the adrenergic-I preparation the waveform was similar to that previously reported (Type II; Koslow *et al.*, 1971): (1) the voltage of the response is lower than that of normal controls and the cholinergic reinnervated ganglion, (2) the time course of the rise of the evoked potential was slower than that of controls, and (3) the response was unstable and made up of a number of peaks, the pattern of which is irregular (Fig. 3(D)). In the adrenergic-II reinnervated ganglion, the

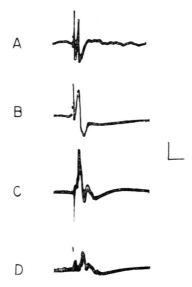

FIG. 3. Control responses (orthodromic stimulation). Normal L_4 ganglia (A); cholinergic reinnervated (B); adrenergic-II (C); adrenergic-I (D). Time scale 50 ms; reinnervated amplitude calibration A and B 0.1 mV and C and D 0.05 mV.

evoked potential showed an initial synaptic potential reminiscent of the normal and cholinergic ganglia, and a second slower component of labile amplitude and exhibited marked fatigue to repetitive stimulation (Fig. 3(C)).

NEUROPHARMACOLOGY

A major test for adrenergic synaptic transmission in the splenic reinnervated ganglion was prolonged stimulation (20–30 Hz, 60 min). Following such a stimulation period in an adrenergic preparation the synaptic potential was elicited again if L-DOPA, the biosynthetic precursor for NE and DA was added to the solution superfusing the ganglion (Koslow *et al.*, 1971). In the reinnervated cholinergic preparations, the use of this experimental protocol did not alter the synaptic potential. This potential was, however, modified by pharmacological agents known to alter the normal cholinergic synapse. Acetylcholine (ACh) in high concentrations (5×10^{-4} M) has been shown to produce an initial facilitation of the synaptic stimulation followed by inhibition (Nishi and Koketsu, 1968). The facilit-

ation may be due to sustained depolarizing action of ACh on the ganglion cells that spontaneously subsides leaving the postsynaptic cholinoceptive sites desensitized. In the cholinergic
reinnervated preparation this dual effect of ACh was recorded (Fig. 4). Furthermore, with
D-tubocurarine (1.4×10^{-7}) the action potential of the reinnervated cholinergic ganglion
was diminished. It is believed that this is due to the blockade of cholinergic nicotinic sites
by curare (Eccles and Libet, 1961). Eccles and Libet (1961) showed that after a conditioning
train the excitatory postsynaptic potential (EPSP) is facilitated and at the same time a late
hyperpolarization is elicited (inhibitory postsynaptic potential, IPSP), this IPSP is blocked
by dibenamine. In the splenic cholinergic ganglia, curare (1.4×10^{-7} M) suppressed the
action potential, and a single test shock following a conditioning train resulted in the

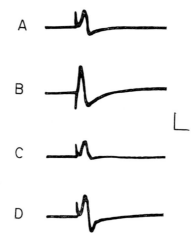

FIG. 4. Acetylcholine facilitation and inhibition of cholinergic reinnervated L_4 ganglia. Control
response (A); 30 min infusion of acetylcholine (B), 60 min infusion of acetylcholine (C); acetylcholine wash out, 30 min (D); acetylcholine was superfused at a concentration of 5×10^{-4} M.
Calibration 0.05 mV, 50 ms.

initial depolarization response followed by a hyperpolarization. The hyperpolarization was
blocked by dibenamine (1.4×10^{-7} M). It thus appears from this data that these four
splenic reinnervated preparations termed cholinergic release ACh that acts at a cholinoceptive postsynaptic site. The inability to alter the potentials by prolonged stimulation and
L-DOPA shows that the depolarization response does not contain any adrenergic depolarizing component.

The splenic-L_4 ganglion termed adrenergic-I, although exhibiting the three electrophysiological characteristics representative of adrenergic function did not, however, show
fatigue to prolonged stimulation (2 h; 30 Hz; 3 ms) and the addition of L-DOPA failed to
facilitate the evoked synaptic potential. The superfusion of the preparation for 45 min
with ACh (1×10^{-3} M) did not result in any change in the evoked potential (Fig. 5(A),
5(C)). The inability of ACh to enhance or decrease the synaptic potentials would indicate
that the depolarizing wave recorded may be due to a noncholinergic pre- and postsynaptic
system (Nishi and Koketsu, 1968). This contention of a noncholinergic synapse is further
supported by the failure of curare (1.4×10^{-7} M, 60 min) to block the electrical response
(Fig. 5(D)). In the presence of curare the application of a single test shock following a

conditioning train resulted in depolarizing wave which was followed by a hyperpolariz-ation (Fig. 5(E)). Furthermore, the addition of dibenamine failed to alter the response to either a single test stimulus (Fig. 5(F)) or a single test shock following a conditioning train (Fig. 5(G)). The inability of dibenamine to block either of these evoked potentials would indicate that if the transmission process is monoaminergic there may be an alteration in postsynaptic receptor. On the basis of these neuropharmacological data it appears that the synaptic elements are not cholinergic and that the neurotransmitter may be a monoamine. In addition, the finding that the potential was not abolished by prolonged stimulation nor facilitated by L-DOPA may indicate the completeness of the new synapses with appropriate functioning storage and reuptake mechanisms.

Abolishment of one of the synaptic waves with prolonged stimulation was possible in adrenergic-II preparation. That this potential is due to a monoamine was substantiated by

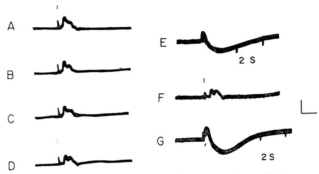

FIG. 5. Effects of acetylcholine, curare, and dibenamine on adrenergic-I preparation. Control response (A); acetylcholine (1×10^{-3} M) superfusion 30 min (B); acetylcholine superfusion 45 min (C); curare (1.4×10^{-7} M) superfusion 60 min (D); in the presence of curare response to a single test shock given at 200 ms following a conditioning train (30 Hz, 10 s) (E); in the presence of curare and dibenamine (1.4×10^{-7} M) 30 min single shock (F); (G) same as F. Response to a single test shock delivered at 100 ms following a conditioning train. Calibration 0.05 mV, 50 ms unless otherwise shown.

the restoration of the signal by superfusing L-DOPA (6.6×10^{-7} M). In an attempt to replete the monoaminergic response by the neurotransmitter directly, solutions of epinephrine (E) (6×10^{-7} M) and DA (6.6×10^{-7} M) were used to superfuse the ganglion after prolonged stimulation periods. Both of these compounds failed to restore the second wave and, in fact, resulted in suppression of both potentials. The addition of DOPA however, once again restored the adrenergic component and in the absence of E and DA, the first depolarizing wave was normal. Failure of E or DA to restore the adrenergic component may be explained by their poor penetration into the ganglion. The diminution produced by these compounds may be explained by the direct hyperpolarizing action of these compounds on the ganglion (de Groat, 1967; Christ and Nishi, 1971).

CONCLUSIONS

In suturing the splenic nerve to the cut preganglionic nerve trunk entering the L_4 ganglion, one would expect that if new synapses were formed, they would clearly be of an adrenergic nature. This assumption is based on the fact that the splenic nerve is made up almost entirely of adrenergic postganglion fibers (Rexed and von Euler, 1951). There is also, however, a low concentration of ACh in the splenic nerve (von Euler, 1947). Since a number of the reinnervated ganglion are cholinergic, one could speculate that it is these ACh-containing fibers which reinnervate the ganglion, resulting in the cholinergic synapse. The possibility also exists that the fibers may be of a preganglionic origin, that is those that originally innervate the Coeliac ganglion, and have now grown past the Coeliac and into the L_4 ganglion resulting in the new cholinergic synapse. Although the origin of the cholinergic fibers is at this time unknown, it is clear that the synapse is cholinergic since in all tests the responses are identical to those obtained from normal control ganglion. (1) No release of catecholamines or DBH during stimulation, (2) ACh both facilitates and desensitizes the response to presynaptic stimulation, (3) after curare only an initial depolarization is recorded and following a conditioning train the response to a single shock shows in addition a hyperpolarizing wave, and (4) the hyperpolarizing wave is blocked by dibenamine.

In normal ganglionic transmission it is believed that the hyperpolarizing wave blocked by dibenamine is due to release of a catecholamine, possibly from the small intensely fluorescent cells (Eccles and Libet, 1961). The hyperpolarizing wave seen in curarized normal ganglia is believed to have a modulating effect on ganglionic transmission (Costa et al., 1961; Eccles and Libet, 1961). The fact that we did not measure any catecholamines released does not dispute this theory. The amount of catecholamines released under these circumstances would be small and thus to be measured would have to be protected from enzymatic destruction. The only postulated receptor for catecholamines is one which results in hyperpolarization and not depolarization. It therefore seems plausible to state that in the adrenergic-I and adrenergic-II splenic reinnervated L_4 ganglia there is an alteration in the postsynaptic receptor site.

That those reinnervated ganglia termed adrenergic truly have an adrenergic synapse is suggested by the release of NE and DBH. The additional release of DA in the adrenergic-II ganglion is probably indicative of a malfunctioning membrane and explains the ability of some of these adrenergic preparations (Koslow et al., 1971) to be depleted by prolonged stimulation. This in itself supports the adrenergic synapse since the signal could be restored if the ganglion was provided with the biosynthetic precursor, DOPA. The inability of ACh, curare, or dibenamine to alter the adrenergic response further support the contention of an adrenergic synapse and also suggests that the postganglionic receptor site has been altered.

The evidence presented is in favor of the *de novo* formation of noradrenergic synapses in place of the normal cholinergic synapse. This only occurs in a small percentage of the anastomosed preparations and it is impossible at this time to say whether or not there is an endogenous factor which is necessary for the transformation or if the success rate is dependent on the surgical procedure. It is conclusive, however, that the peripheral nervous system has sufficient plasticity to alter itself when challenged with a new neurotransmitter.

REFERENCES

CHRIST, D. D., and NISHI, S. (1971) Site of adrenaline blockade in the superior cervical ganglion of the rabbit. *J. Physiol. Lond.* **213**, 107–117.

COSTA, E., REVZIN, A. M., KUNTZMAN, R., SPECTOR, S., and BRODIE, B. B. (1961) Role for ganglionic norepinephrine in sympathetic synaptic transmission. *Science* **133**, 1822–1823.

DALE, H. (1935) Walter Ernest Dixon memorial lecture; pharmacology and nerve endings, *Proc. R. Soc. Med.* **28**, 319–332.

DE GROAT, W. C. (1967) Actions of the catecholamines in sympathetic ganglia. *Circ. Res.* **20**, Suppl. 111, 111–135.

ECCLES, R. M., and LIBET, B. (1961) Origin and blockade of synaptic responses of cararized sympathetic ganglia. *J. Physiol. Lond.* **157**, 484–503.

HILLARP, N.-Å. (1946) Structure of the synapse and the peripheral innervation apparatus of the autonomic nervous system. *Acta Anat.*, Suppl. IV.

KOSLOW, S. H., STEPITA-KLAUCO, M., OLSON, L., and GIACOBINI, E. (1971) Functional reinnervation of cat sympathetic ganglia with splenic nerve homografts. *Experientia* **27**, 799–801.

KOSLOW, S. H., CATTABENI, F., and COSTA, E. (1972a) Norepinephrine and dopamine: assay by mass fragmentography in the picomole range. *Science* **176**, 177–180.

KOSLOW, S. H., GIACOBINI, E., KERPEL-FRONIUS, S., and OLSON, L. (1972b) Cholinergic transmission in the hypoglossal reinnervated nictitating membrane of the cat: an enzymatic histochemical and physiological study. *J. Pharmac. Exp. Ther.* **180**, 664–671.

LANGLEY, J. N. (1898) On the union of cranial autonomic (visceral) fibers with the nerve cells of the superior cervical ganglion. *J. Physiol. Lond.* **23**, 240–270.

LANGLEY, J. N., and ANDERSON, H. K. (1904a) On the union of the fifth cervical nerve with the superior cervical ganglion. *J. Physiology* **30**, 439–442.

LANGLEY, J. N., and ANDERSON, H. K. (1904b) The union of different kinds of nerve fibers. *J. Physiology* **31**, 365–391.

NISHI, S., and KOKETSU, K. (1968) Early and late afterdischarges of amphibian sympathetic ganglion cells. *J. Neurophysiol.* **31**, 109–121.

REXED, B., and VON EULER, U. S. (1951) The presence of histamine and noradrenaline in nerves as related to their content of myelinated and unmyelinated fibers. *Acta psychiat. neurol. scand.* **26**, 61–65.

UNBREIT, W. W., BURNS, R. H., and STAUFFER, J. F. (1951) *Manometric Techniques and Tissue Metabolism*, Burgess, Minneapolis, p. 119.

VON EULER, U. S. (1947) Sympathin, histamine and acetylcholine in mammalian fibers. *J. Physiol. Lond.* **107**, 10P.

WEINSHILBOUM, R., and AXELROD, J. (1971) Serum dopamine-β-hydroxylase activity. *Circ. Res.* **28**, 307–315.

ONTOGENESIS OF CENTRAL NORADRENALINE NEURONS AFTER 6-HYDROXYDOPAMINE TREATMENT AT BIRTH

Charlotte Sachs, Chris Pycock[†], and Gösta Jonsson

Department of Histology, Karolinska Institutet, S-104 01 Stockholm 60, Sweden

Systemic administration of 6-hydroxydopamine (6-OH-DA) to neonate rats causes a selective and permanent decrease of the noradrenaline (NA) levels in several forebrain regions, especially in the cerebral cortex, which is associated with a degeneration of the NA nerve terminals (Sachs and Jonsson, 1972; Clark *et al.*, 1972). However, the same treatment leads in addition to a considerable increase of the NA concentration in the pons-medulla region (Clark *et al.*, 1972; Pappas and Sobrian, 1972; Taylor *et al.*, 1972; Singh and de Champlain, 1972; Jonsson *et al.*, 1974). Although the reason for this NA increase is not quite clear, recent studies indicate that it may be related to both a "collateral accumulation" of NA and an increased outgrowth of NA nerve terminals (Jonsson *et al.*, 1974; see also Fig. 5). The aim of the present study has been to follow the postnatal development of the changes in the NA neurons after 6-OH-DA, given at birth, by fluorescence histochemistry (according to Falck and Hillarp), chemical-analytical NA determinations and ^{3}H-NA uptake studies *in vitro*.

The rats (Sprague–Dawley) were injected with 6-OH-DA (3×100 mg/kg s.c.) on the day of birth and on the two following days and were sacrificed after 7, 21, 42, or 70 days. Littermate controls were injected with saline. Cerebral cortex and pons-medulla were dissected out, homogenized in 10 volumes 0.25 M sucrose and centrifuged 1000 g for 10 min. Aliquots (100 μl) of the supernatant containing NA nerve terminals (varicosities) were taken for *in vitro* incubation in ^{3}H-NA (0.05 μM, 5 min) using a Krebs–Ringer bicarbonate buffer as incubation medium (see Jonsson *et al.*, 1974). The rest of the supernatant was taken for determination of endogenous NA according to Bertler *et al.* (1958). Aliquots of the supernatant were also taken for protein determination (Lowry *et al.*, 1951), and ^{3}H-NA uptake was expressed as dpm/mg protein and endogenous NA as μg/mg protein. Brains were also taken for fluorescence histochemical studies of the monoamine neurons (Falck

† Wellcome Trust Fellow.

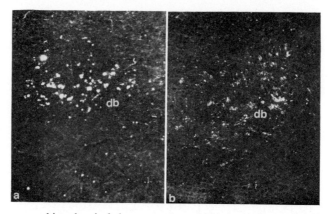

FIG. 1. Fluorescence histochemical demonstration of NA in sections of rat brain. ($\times 100$.) (a): 6-OH-DA (3×100 mg/kg s.c., 24 h intervals) was injected at birth and the animals were sacrificed at an age of 21 days. Strongly fluorescent accumulations of transmitter are seen in axons of the dorsal NA bundle (db) in the mesencephalon. (b): Control, 21-day-old rat. The NA axons of the dorsal bundle are faintly fluorescent. The animals were treated with the mono-amine oxidase inhibitor nialamide (100 mg/kg i.p.) 2 h before death in order to facilitate the histochemical demonstration of NA.

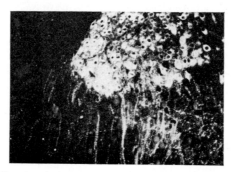

FIG. 2. Fluorescence histochemical demonstration of NA in a section of rat brain. The rats were treated as in Fig. 1a and sacrificed on the seventh day after birth. The NA cell bodies of the locus coeruleus are strongly fluorescent and show a similar appearance as in the controls. ($\times 160$).

et al., 1962; Corrodi and Jonsson, 1967; and Fuxe *et al.*, 1970). In order to optimize the histochemical demonstration of NA, the rats were treated with nialamide (100 mg/kg i.p.) 2 h before death.

Fluorescence histochemical studies of the 7- and 21-day-old 6-OH-DA-treated rats showed strongly fluorescent accumulations of transmitter in ascending axons of the dorsal NA bundle, originating from cell bodies in the locus coeruleus (Fig. 1). The dorsal NA bundle supplies NA nerve terminals to *inter alia* the cerebral cortex (Ungerstedt, 1971). Practically no such accumulations of transmitter were found in the 42- and 70-day-old rats. Accumulations of transmitter after 6-OH-DA are signs of neuronal damage and degeneration, which may be related to a pile up of NA in the lesioned axon and/or possibly to a more diffuse destruction of the axoplasma transport mechanism (see Jonsson and Sachs, 1972a; Sachs *et al.*, 1973). The NA cell bodies of the locus coeruleus were well developed at 7 days and had, after 6-OH-DA treatment at birth, the same appearance as in the litter mate control (Fig. 2; see Seiger and Olson, 1973). The fluorescence morphology of NA cell bodies did not apparently differ from control at any of the times studied. An increased number of NA nerve terminals, often with an increased fluorescence intensity compared to control, in areas normally innervated by NA nerve terminals in the pons-medulla could be observed in 21-, 42-, and 70-day-old rats treated with 6-OH-DA at birth (cf. Jonsson *et al.*, 1974). In these animals also a marked decrease in the number of NA nerve terminals in the cerebral cortex could be seen. No notable changes in the fluorescence morphology of the dopamine and 5-hydroxytryptamine neurons were observed after the 6-OH-DA treatment.

In agreement with previous studies (Jonsson *et al.*, 1974), the 6-OH-DA treatment leads to a marked decrease in endogenous NA and ^{3}H-NA uptake in the cerebral cortex, whereas

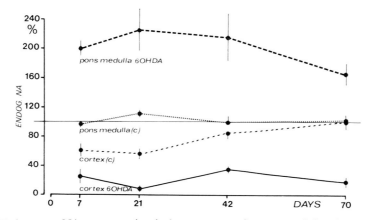

FIG. 3. Endogenous NA concentration in homogenates of cortex cerebri and pons-medulla from 6-OH-DA treated and control (c) rats. The rats were injected with 6-OH-DA (3 × 100 mg/kg s.c., 24 h intervals) at birth and sacrificed after various periods of time. Each point represents the mean ± SEM of four determinations and is expressed as per cent of adult control.

these parameters are considerably increased in the pons-medulla (Figs. 3 and 4). These changes are observed already in 7-day-old rats. In a recent publication Singh and de Champlain (1972) have also reported an early decrease in forebrain NA and increase in pons-medulla NA during the development after 6-OH-DA treatment at birth. The changes in ^{3}H-NA uptake observed are in all probability associated with changes in the number of NA nerve terminals, since previous studies have clearly shown that there is a good correlation between ^{3}H-NA uptake and nerve density (Jonsson and Sachs, 1972a, b). Thus the increases in ^{3}H-NA uptake and endogenous NA in the pons-medulla would point to an increased outgrowth of NA nerve terminals in this region after 6-OH-DA treatment at birth, while the reductions in the cerebral cortex are related to a degeneration of NA nerve terminals. However, the increase in ^{3}H-NA uptake was less pronounced than that of the endogenous NA in the pons-medulla, whereas in the cerebral cortex the situation was the reverse. The latter observation may be related to the existence of other structures than NA nerve terminals in the cerebral cortex being able to take up ^{3}H-NA and insensitive to 6-OH-DA, e.g. DA nerve terminals (see Lidbrink, this symposium; and Thierry *et al.*, 1973). The more pronounced increase in endogenous NA than in ^{3}H-NA uptake in the pons-medulla indicate that here the NA nerve terminals contain higher concentrations of NA than normally. This is consistent with the fluorescence histochemical results and also with

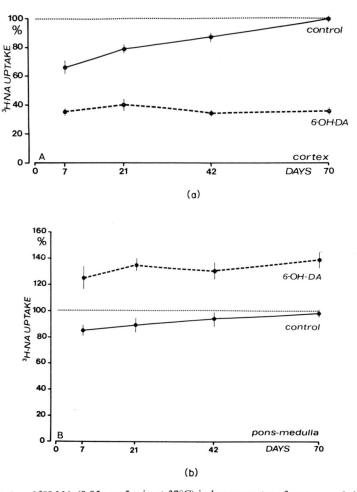

FIG. 4. Uptake of ³H-NA (0.05 μM, 5 min at 37°C) in homogenates of cortex cerebri (a), and pons-medulla (b). The rats were treated with 6-OH-DA as in Fig. 3 and sacrificed after various periods of time. Each point is the mean ±SEM of 10–16 determinations and is expressed as per cent of adult control. The ³H-NA uptake at 0°C has been subtracted from the uptake values obtained at +37°C.

previously reported subcellular distribution results (Jonsson *et al.*, 1974). This increase is best explained by assuming that the synthesis and transport of NA storage granules is unaltered after the 6-OH-DA treatment in the locus coeruleus perikarya. Since the total nerve terminal volume of these neurons is reduced after 6-OH-DA (degeneration of NA nerve terminals in the forebrain), this would lead to a redistribution of granules and an increase in NA concentration in the remaining NA nerve terminals, e.g. in the pons-medulla. Such a "collateral accumulation" of NA might partly explain the increases in endogenous NA in the pons-medulla after 6-OH-DA at birth.

    The present study thus shows that 6-OH-DA administration to neonate rats leads to a permanent and marked reduction in endogenous NA and ³H-NA uptake in the cerebral cortex, certainly related to degeneration of NA nerve terminals. Concomitantly there is a rapidly developing increase in these parameters in the pons-medulla, probably as a result of a "collateral accumulation" and an increased outgrowth of NA terminals in the region (see Fig. 5). These changes in forebrain and pons-medulla are seen very early during the development, already 7 days after birth. Although the definite proof for an increased growth is lacking, the ^{3}H-NA uptake data strongly support this view. Then the question arises whether this increased growth is related to the damage of the terminal areas in the forebrain, to a partial damage initially of the terminals in the pons-medulla followed by massive regeneration or to both these phenomena. The answer to these questions has to await further investigations.

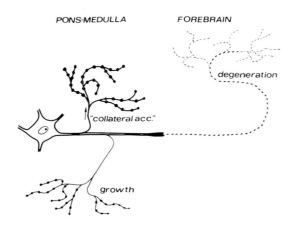

FIG. 5. Schematic representation of a locus coeruleus neuron with hypothetical indications of what may occur after administration of 6-OH-DA at birth. A considerable number of NA nerve terminals in the forebrain has degenerated, while in the pons-medulla region there is an increased number of NA nerve terminals (due to increased outgrowth) with increased NA concentration (due to "collateral accumulation" of NA).

ACKNOWLEDGEMENTS

This work was supported by grants from the Swedish Medical Research Council (04X-3881 and 04X-2295), C.-B. Nathorst, and Svenska Livförsäkringsbolaget.

REFERENCES

BERTLER, Å., CARLSSON, A., and ROSENGREN, E. (1958) A method for the fluorimetric determination of adrenaline and noradrenaline in tissues. *Acta physiol. scand.* **44,** 273–292.

CLARK, D. W., LAVERTY, R., and PHELAN, E. L. (1972) Longlasting peripheral and central effects of 6-hydroxydopamine in rats. *Br. J. Pharmac.* **44,** 233–243.

CORRODI, H., and JONSSON, G. (1967) The formaldehyde fluorescence method for the histochemical demonstration of biogenic monoamines: a review of the methodology. *J. Histochem. Cytochem.* **15,** 65–78.

FALCK, B., HILLARP, N.-Å., THIEME, G., and TORP, A. (1962) Fluorescence of catecholamines and related compounds condensed with formaldehyde. *J. Histochem. Cytochem.* **10,** 348–354.

FUXE, K., HÖKFELT, T., JONSSON, G., and UNGERSTEDT, U. (1970) Fluorescence microscopy in neuroanatomy. In *Contemporary Research in Neuroanatomy* (W. J. H. Nauta and S. O. E. Ebbesson, eds.), Springer-Verlag, Berlin, Heidelberg, and New York, pp. 275–314.

JONSSON, G., and SACHS, CH. (1972a) Neurochemical properties of adrenergic nerves regenerated after 6-hydroxydopamine. *J. Neurochem.* **18,** 2577–2585.

JONSSON, G., and SACHS, CH. (1972b) Degenerative and nondegenerative effects of 6-hydroxydopamine on adrenergic nerves. *J. Pharmac. Exp. Ther.* **180,** 625–635.

JONSSON, G., PYCOCK, CH., FUXE, K., and SACHS, CH. (1974) Changes in the development of central noradrenaline neurons following neonatal administration of 6-hydroxydopamine. *J. Neurochem.* (in press).

LOWRY, O. H., ROSEBROUGH, N. J., FARR, A. L., and RANDALL, R. J. (1951) Protein measurement with the folin phenol reagent. *J. Biol. Chem.* **193**, 265–275.

PAPPAS, B. A., and SOBRIAN, S. K. (1972) Neonatal sympathectomy by 6-hydroxydopamine in the rat: no effects on behaviour but changes in endogenous brain noradrenaline. *Life Sci.* **11**, 653–659.

SACHS, CH., and JONSSON, G. (1972) Degeneration of central noradrenaline neurons after 6-hydroxydopamine in newborn animals. *Res. Communs. Chem. Path. Pharmac.* **4**, 203–220.

SACHS, CH., JONSSON, G., and FUXE, K. (1973) Mapping of central noradrenaline pathways with 6-hydroxy-DOPA. *Brain Res.* **63**, 249–261.

SEIGER, Å., and OLSON, L. (1973) Late prenatal ontogeny of central monoamine neurons in the rat: fluorescence histochemical observations. *Z. Anat. Entw. Gesch.* **140**, 281–318.

SINGH, B., and DE CHAMPLAIN, J. (1972) Altered ontogenesis of central noradrenergic neurons following neonatal treatment with 6-hydroxydopamine. *Brain Res.* **48**, 432–437.

TAYLOR, K. M., CLARK, D. W., LAVERTY, R., and PELAN, E. L. (1972) Specific noradrenergic neurones destroyed by 6-hydroxydopamine injection into newborn rats. *Nature New Biol.* **239**, 247–248.

THIERRY, A. M., STINUS, L., BLANC, G., and GLOWINSKI, J. (1973) Some evidence for the existence of dopaminergic neurons in the rat cortex. *Brain Res.* **50**, 230–234.

UNGERSTEDT, U. (1971) Stereotoxic mapping of the monoamine pathways in the rat brain. *Acta physiol. scand.*, Suppl. 367, 1–48.

EFFECTS OF VINBLASTINE ON PERIPHERAL AUTONOMIC NERVES: DEGENERATION AND FORMATION OF NEW NERVE FIBERS

Ingeborg Hanbauer, Irwin J. Kopin, and David M. Jacobowitz

Laboratory of Clinical Science, National Institute of Mental Health, Bethesda, Maryland 20014, USA

SUMMARY

The present investigation attempts to correlate histochemical changes observed in autonomic nerves of the superior cervical ganglion (SCG) with biochemical parameters which reflect the survival and function of the sympathetic neurons within the ganglion after vinblastine application. In addition, the question of the influence of vinblastine on peripheral nerves is explored after vinblastine application to the SCG. The present results reveal that interpretation of biochemical data obtained from the effect of neurotoxic drugs on sympathetic ganglia must consider the changes observed, not only in the cell body but also in the postganglionic axonal processes, the intraganglionic system of adrenergic varicosities, and the preganglionic cholinergic terminals.

INTRODUCTION

The vinca alkaloids, vinblastine and vincristine, were introduced in cancer therapy in 1958 (Noble *et al.*, 1958). Both alkaloids cause arrest of mitosis in metaphase by interfering with spindle formation (Marmont and Damasio, 1967), and they both inhibit the polymerization of microtubular protein (Malawista *et al.*, 1968; Bensch *et al.*, 1969; Marantz *et al.*, 1969). Schmitt (1968) suggested that microtubules play a role in the regulation of axonal flow of various molecular aggregates including noradrenaline (NA) storage vesicles. In line with this hypothesis, Dahlström (1970) has shown that vinblastine, applied locally to adrenergic neurons, inhibits transport of NA-containing storage vesicles. Keen and Livingstone (1970) observed that vinblastine injected intravenously decreases NA concentration in peripheral tissues without affecting the axonal transport. Cheney *et al.* (1973) have shown that intravenously administered vinblastine fails to decrease the acetylcholine concentration in salivary glands and heart although the NA content of these tissues is decreased. In the present report an attempt is made to correlate histochemical changes with biochemical parameters of sympathetic neuronal function after local application of vinblastine.

LOCAL APPLICATION OF VINBLASTINE

A. CATECHOLAMINE HISTOCHEMISTRY

The superior cervical ganglion (SCG) was studied histochemically (Falck, 1962; Falck *et al.*, 1962) from 6 h to 47 days after local application of vinblastine. In the ganglion, attention was focused on three structures: adrenergic cell bodies, smooth axonal processes, and intraganglionic system of adrenergic varicosities. The end-organ effect of vinblastine applied locally to the SCG was examined in the iris and submaxillary gland. The results of this experiment are summarized in a quantitative manner in Table 1.

TABLE 1. SUMMARY OF THE EFFECT OF LOCAL APPLICATION OF VINBLASTINE ON THE SUPERIOR CERVICAL GANGLION

Histochemical observation of the catecholamine fluorescence intensity in the cell body, axonal processes, and the number of intraganglionic varicosities is indicated by an increase (↑), decrease (↓), or no change (N). The origin of the varicosities in the ganglion is unknown (?). Semiquantitation of the number of adrenergic varicosities is indicated by 0 to +4 ratings: 0 = no nerves; +1 = few fibers; +2 = a low to moderate number; +3 = moderate to many; +4 = normal. The number of observations is indicated in the Table.

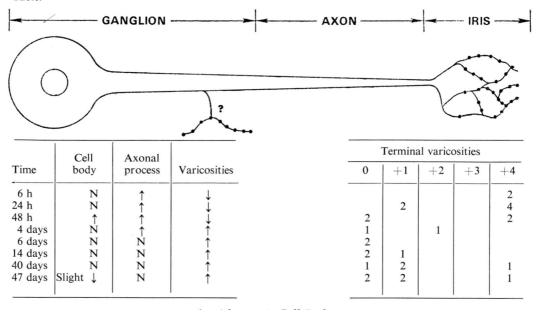

Time	Cell body	Axonal process	Varicosities	Terminal varicosities				
				0	+1	+2	+3	+4
6 h	N	↑	↓					2
24 h	N	↑	↓		2			4
48 h	↑	↑	↓	2		1		2
4 days	N	↑	↑	1		1		
6 days	N	N	↑	2				
14 days	N	N	↑	2	1			
40 days	N	N	↑	1	2			1
47 days	Slight ↓	N	↑	2	2			1

1. *Adrenergic Cell Bodies*

Normal ganglion cell bodies vary in intensity of fluorescence, but most of the perikarya exhibit a moderate intensity. Up to 24 h after vinblastine application, no clear change in the intensity of fluorescence could be observed. Only at 48 h after vinblastine, however, was there a moderate to marked increase in the fluorescence intensity within the cell bodies (Figs. 3c and 3d).

2. *Smooth Axonal Processes*

Six hours to 4 days after vinblastine application, there was a marked increase in the intensity of fluorescence of the smooth axonal processes. The axons were observed singly or as fascicles among the cell bodies and eventually joined to form the postganglionic trunks, which emanate from the ganglion (Figs. 1–3a, b). After 6 days the smooth axonal processes were normal in fluorescence intensity (Fig. 6).

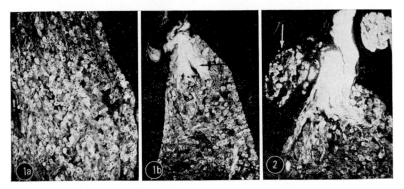

FIG. 1. SCG, 6 h after treatment with vinblastine. (×100.) (a) Control. Normal variations in fluorescence intensity of adrenergic cell bodies. (b) Vinblastine-treated. Note increase in fluorescence intensity of the postganglionic axonal trunks (arrow, above) and fascicles among the cell bodies (arrow, below). A decrease in the number of intraganglionic varicosities is also observed.

FIG. 2. SCG, 24 h after vinblastine treatment. (×85.) A marked increase in the intensity of fluorescence of the postganglionic trunk is noted. The position of the normal intense green fluorescent chromaffin cells of the carotid body is indicated (arrow).

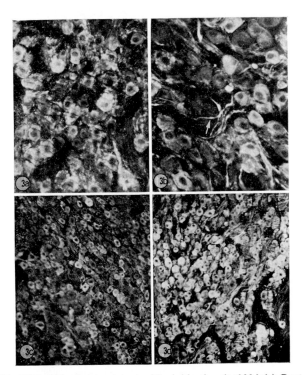

FIG. 3. (a) and (b): SCG, 24 h after treatment with vinblastine. (×330.) (a) Control. Normal cell bodies and intraganglionic varicosities. (b) Vinblastine-treated. The cell body fluorescence appears normal. Note the increased fluorescence intensity of the smooth axonal fascicles between the perikarya (arrow) and the decrease in the number of varicosities. (c) and (d): SCG, 48 h after treatment with vinblastine. (×155.) (c) Control. Normal variations in cell body fluorescence intensity. (d) Vinblastine-treated. Note the marked increase in the intensity of fluorescence of the cell bodies and the reduced number of varicosities.

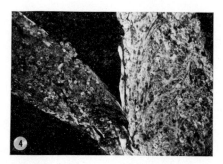

FIG. 4. SCG, 4 days after treatment with vinblastine. (×85.) Control ganglion (right) and vinblastine-treated (left). A marked increase in the number of varicose terminals is noted in the drug-treated ganglion.

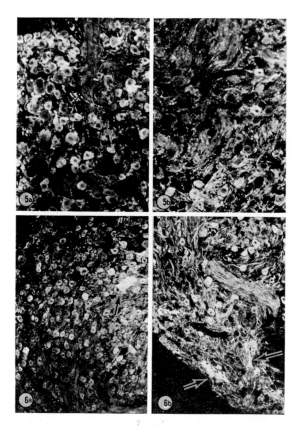

FIG. 5. SCG, 6 days after treatment with vinblastine. (×250.) (a) Control (left). Normal cell bodies and varicosities. (b) Vinblastine-treated. A marked increase in the number of varicosities is noted in proximity to the cell bodies and within the large smooth nerve fascicles.

FIG. 6. SCG, 14 days after treatment with vinblastine. (×155.) (a) Control (left). Normal ganglion with small cluster of intense fluorescent chromaffin cells (arrow). (b) Vinblastine-treated. Note the marked increase in the number of varicose processes in proximity to ganglion cell bodies and within large nerve trunks. Two clusters of chromaffin cells are also noted (arrows).

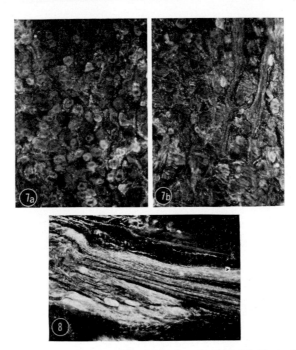

FIG. 7. SCG, 47 days after treatment with vinblastine. (×210.) (a) Control (b) Vinblastine-treated. Note increase in the number of varicose terminals and slight decrease in the fluorescence intensity of cell bodies.

FIG. 8. Cervical sympathetic preganglionic nerve trunk, 47 days after vinblastine treatment. (×210.) A marked increase in the number of varicose processes is noted just caudal to the ganglion.

3. Intraganglionic Varicosities

At 6 and 24 h after vinblastine application, there was a moderate decrease in the number of intraganglionic varicosities. A marked increase in the number of varicose terminal processes was noted at 4 days, and the number of varicose terminal processes continued to remain increased for up to 47 days (Figs. 4 and 7). The varicosities were observed in close proximity to the cell bodies and within the intracellular fascicles along the smooth axonal processes (Figs. 5–7). The cervical sympathetic preganglionic nerve trunk, located just caudal to the ganglion, was examined only at 47 days after drug application, at which time a marked increase in the number of fine varicose fibers was observed (Fig. 8). Vinblastine treatment did not appear to influence the number of small intensely fluorescent chromaffin-like cells (Fig. 6) or the processes which emanate from clusters of these cells. Vinblastine application did not affect the fluorescence intensity of the chromaffin-like cells in the carotid body located just outside the capsule which encloses the SCG (Fig. 2).

4. Peripheral Adrenergic Plexus

The degree of depletion of fluorescent nerve fibers in the iris is shown in Table 1. Between 4 and 14 days after local application of vinblastine, no irises were found to contain more than a fraction of the fibers. After about 6 weeks, while most irises were almost devoid of nerve fibers (Fig. 9), two were found to be almost normal. Forty-seven days after drug

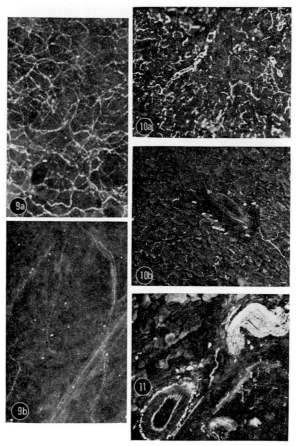

Fig. 9. Iris, 47 days after treatment with vinblastine. (×250.) (a) Normal, control. (b) Iris on the side of vinblastine-treated ganglion. Mostly no nerve terminals, with only rare fiber processes.

Fig. 10. Submaxillary gland, 47 days after treatment with vinblastine. (×155.) (a) Normal, control. Abundant number of adrenergic nerves around the acini. (b) Gland on the side of the vinblastine-treated ganglion. A marked decrease in the number of nerves is noted.

Fig. 11. Submaxillary gland, 47 days after application of vinblastine to the SCG. (×155.) No nerve terminals were found in the acini regions. A large nerve trunk with varicose processes is observed in addition to a large artery with surrounding adrenergic nerves.

treatment, the submaxillary gland of one rat had a moderate decrease in the number of adrenergic nerves (Fig. 10) although the iris had a very sparse number of nerves. In another rat, the submaxillary gland had many nerve fibers surrounding blood vessels and several intensely fluorescent preterminal trunks around the acini (Fig. 11). In a third rat, the submaxillary gland had a slight decrease in the number of nerves which were present around blood vessels and acini. Preterminal nerve trunks containing varicose fibers were also present. Very few nerves were seen in the iris of the third rat (Fig. 9b).

B. ACETYLCHOLINESTERASE

Histochemical observations were made of the acetylcholinesterase-containing fibers and cell bodies of the SCG 1 day to 9 weeks after unilateral application of vinblastine. A

moderate decrease in the number of acetylcholinesterase-staining fibers (mostly preganglionic) was observed 1 day after vinblastine application. A marked decrease in the acetylcholinesterase-staining fibers was seen at 9, 21, and 26 days (Fig. 12). The irises of the above
vinblastine-treated rats were studied for their content of fluorescent adrenergic nerves. Very
few or no adrenergic nerves were present in the irises 1 or 9 days after vinblastine application to the SCG. There was only a slight decrease in the density of acetylcholinesterase-
staining nerves 8 and 9 weeks after vinblastine. The irises of these rats appeared to contain
a normal complement of fluorescent nerves.

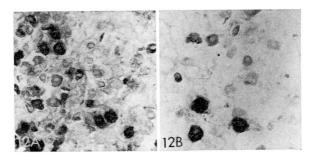

FIG. 12. SCG. Acetylcholinesterase stain (Koelle, 1955) 9 days after treatment (1 h incubation).
(×250.) (a) Control. Normal staining of mostly preganglionic cholinergic terminals in proximity to the ganglion cell bodies. (b) Vinblastine-treated. A marked reduction in the number of
preganglionic cholinergic fibers is noted.

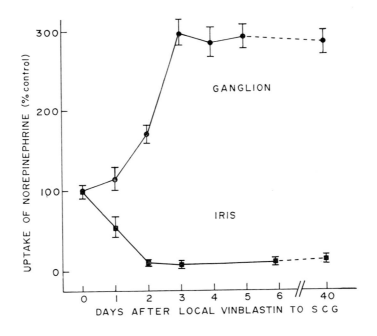

FIG. 13.

C. BIOCHEMICAL STUDIES

1. *Uptake of* ^3H-NA

(a) *SCG*. Uptake of ^{3}H-NA was used as an index of the specific amine transport mechanism of sympathetic nerve terminal membranes. Two days after local application of 20 μg vinblastine to the ganglion, there was a 70% increase of ^{3}H-NA uptake. On the third day a further increase to 300% of control uptake was apparent (Fig. 13). At this time there was no change in the inulin space (untreated 26 $\pm$ 3%; vinblastine-treated 25 $\pm$ 3%).

(b) *Nerve terminals*. The uptake of ^{3}H-NA by irises decreased rather rapidly after local application of the alkaloid to the ganglion (Fig. 13). One day after drug application the uptake of NA was reduced to 54% and 2 days later to 10% of the uptake of NA by contra-lateral untreated iris. After 40 days there was no evidence of recovery of NA uptake. Pargyline treatment enhanced the uptake of ^{3}H-NA by irises from reserpine-treated rats but had no effect on the diminished uptake of the catecholamine uptake by irises from vinblastine-treated animals (Table 2).

TABLE 2. EFFECT OF PARGYLINE ON NORADRENALINE UPTAKE BY IRISES OF
VINBLASTINE- OR RESERPINE-TREATED RATS

Pargyline	Control	Reserpine[a]	Vinblastine[b]
Without	2.8 $\pm$ 0.50 (4)	0.17 $\pm$ 0.02 (8)	0.41 $\pm$ 0.25 (4)
With	2.5 $\pm$ 0.13 (4)	0.68 $\pm$ 0.08*(8)	0.24 $\pm$ 0.14 (4)

L-^{3}H-Noradrenaline uptake was measured as described by Silberstein *et al.* (1971). Number of observations per experiment is indicated in parentheses.

[a] Reserpine (5 mg/kg, i.v.) was injected 5 h before injection of pargyline (30 mg/kg i.p.).

[b] Vinblastine (20 μg) was applied on SCG 48 h before injection of pargyline (30 mg/kg i.p.). The animals were killed 1 h after injection of pargyline.

* $p < 0.01$.

2. *Concentration of Catecholamines in SCG*

Three days after application of vinblastine the dopamine concentration in SCG was increased nearly twofold whereas the increase in NA content did not attain significance. At 8 days the NA concentration was increased about twofold whereas the dopamine content had returned to normal (Table 3).

TABLE 3. CATECHOLAMINE CONCENTRATIONS[a] IN SUPERIOR CERVICAL GANGLION AT VARIOUS TIMES AFTER
VINBLASTINE

Catecholamine	Control	Days after vinblastine		
		3	8	47
Dopamine (pmoles/ganglion)	30 $\pm$ 4 (5)	52 $\pm$ 8 (5)*	39 $\pm$ 3 (6)	—
Noradrenaline (pmoles/ganglion)	129 $\pm$ 13 (5)	172 $\pm$ 16 (5)	251 $\pm$ 19 (6)**	245 $\pm$ 1 (6)**

[a] Dopamine and noradrenaline concentrations were assayed by a sensitive isotopic assay developed in our laboratory by Dr. D. Henry (in preparation).

* $0.05 > p > 0.025$.

** $0.001 > p$.

3. *Activities of Tyrosine Hydroxylase and Dopamine-β-hydroxylase*

It has previously been reported that, initially, the activities of both tyrosine hydroxylase and dopamine-β-hydroxylase increase. Dopamine-β-hydroxylase activity peaks between 12 and 24 h, and tyrosine hydroxylase activity peaks at about 36 h (Lamprecht *et al.*, 1972). At 48 h, the activities of both enzymes had returned to normal and successively declined to about 50% of normal (Table 4). The decreased enzyme activities were maintained for at least 47 days after local application of vinblastine.

TABLE 4. TIME COURSE OF THE EFFECT OF VINBLASTINE APPLICATION ON SUPERIOR CERVICAL GANGLION (SCG) ON TYROSINE HYDROXYLASE, AND DOPAMINE-β-HYDROXYLASE ACTIVITY

Enzyme	Control	Vinblastine (2 days)	Vinblastine (12 days)	Vinblastine (49 days)
Tyrosine hydroxylase (nmole Dopa/SCG/h)	39.4 ± 1.8 (6)	33.3 ± 1.5 (6)	—	17.2 ± 2 (6)*
Dopamine-β-hydroxylase (nmole product/SCG/h)	52.1 ± 3.3 (6)	50.9 ± 3.3 (6)	20.4 ± 0.4 (6)*	26.9 ± 1.5 (6)*

* $0.001 > p$.

Tyrosine hydroxylase activity was measured in 150 μl of SCG homogenates (0.005 M Tris buffer pH 7.5, Triton X-100, 0.02%) by a modification of the Shiman *et al.* method (1971). Dopamine β-hydroxylase activity was measured in 100 μl of the same homogenate according to the method of Molinoff *et al.* (1971).

4. *Choline Acetyltransferase*

One day after local application of vinblastine, the activity of choline acetyltransferase in the SCG was unchanged; after 3 or 12 days, however, a 56% or 80% reduction occurred (Table 5).

TABLE 5. TIME COURSE OF THE EFFECT OF VINBLASTINE APPLICATION ON SUPERIOR CERVICAL GANGLION ON THE CHOLINE ACETYLTRANSFERASE ACTIVITY[a] OF THE SUPERIOR CERVICAL GANGLION

Enzyme	Control	Vinblastine			
		1 day	3 days	12 days	72 days
Choline acetyl-transferase (nmoles/SCG/h)	34.1 ± 5.2 (6)	36.0 ± 3 (6)	15.2 ± 3.6(7)*	7.0 ± 0.8 (6)**	25.2 ± 2.5 (5)

[a] Choline acetyltransferase activity was measured in 50 μl SCG homogenate (0.01 M Tris buffer pH 7.0 Triton X-100, 0.02%) by a radiochemical assay described by Schrier and Schuster (1967).
* $0.02 > p > 0.01$.
** $0.001 > p$.

DISCUSSION

Histochemical observations of the SCG after local vinblastine treatment show that by 6 h there is a large accumulation of catecholamine within the postganglionic axonal processes which lasts for 4 days. This buildup of catecholamine within adrenergic neurons after axonal section or constriction has been extensively studied (Dahlström and Fuxe, 1964; Dahlström, 1965). The accumulation of the amine above a ligature is a reflection of blockade of axoplasmic flow towards the periphery. This blockade has also been documented with the use of vinblastine on lumbar sympathetic ganglia (Dahlström, 1968; Hökfelt and Dahlström, 1971).

The present study demonstrates that there is also an accumulation of catecholamine within cell bodies 2 days after local vinblastine application. This accumulation was no longer observed on the fourth day. A similar accumulation was previously observed in the cat SCG 3 days after ligation of the postganglionic trunk (Jacobowitz and Woodward, 1968; Jacobowitz, 1970). In addition to the changes observed in the cell bodies and axonal processes, a reduction in the number of adrenergic varicosities occurred between 6 and 48 h after local vinblastine treatment. It would appear that the reduction in the intraganglionic varicosities may be a reflection of an initial depletion of amine followed by a possible degeneration of the terminals. The long term disappearance of terminal varicosities in the iris would tend to support the above hypothesis. A blockade of axoplasmic flow of essential substances could cause destruction of axonal or dendritic collaterals within the ganglion and in the terminals of the iris.

The dramatic increase in the number of intraganglionic varicosities 4 days after vinblastine application persisted for 47 days. This increase was correlated with a 200 % increase in uptake of ^{3}H-NA *in vitro* between 3 and 47 days. In addition, there was an increase in the NA content of the ganglion between 3 and 47 days after vinblastine placement. These histochemical and biochemical data strongly suggest sprouting of new varicosities. It would seem that the initial destruction of varicose terminals, both in the ganglion and peripheral organs, triggers an extremely efficient mechanism for the sprouting of new fibers with catecholamine-containing varicosities. The persistent enhanced uptake of ^{3}H-NA (Fig. 13) and the twofold increase of NA content further suggests that there is a permanent increase in new stores of NA. Electron microscopic studies of the SCG of rats 3–7 days following postganglionic nerve trunk ligation revealed many tiny processes, some of which appeared to arise from the neuron. These processes were thought to be the result of a type of sprouting reaction of the cell surface (Matthews and Raisman, 1972).

The long term reduction of the number of acetylcholinesterase-staining nerves, correlated with a marked decrease in choline acetyltransferase, suggests that local vinblastine treatment results in the degeneration of the preganglionic terminals. Regeneration of the terminals, although not complete, had occurred after 2 months. Choline acetyltransferase was still reduced by about 25 % after 10 weeks.

In the brain, electron microscopic studies of the septal area after lesions of hippocampal nonadrenergic pathways to the septal nuclei (Raisman, 1969a, b), Raisman has inferred that axons which emanate from the medial forebrain bundle occupy the vacant synaptic sites in the denervated septal area. Fluroescent microscopic studies have demonstrated that new terminals are derived from collateral sprouting of NA-containing axons derived from the median forebrain bundle (Moore *et al.*, 1971). These observations support the view that degeneration of the cholinergic terminals may further trigger the mechanism for sprouting of catecholamine-containing fibers. Terminal sprouting of adrenergic (Olson and Malmfors, 1970) and cholinergic (Tsukahara *et al.*, 1972) nerves was observed in iris transplants placed in the anterior chamber of the eye. The present observation of an abundant number of catecholamine varicose fibers in the cervical sympathetic preganglionic trunk 47 days after vinblastine application to the ganglion further supports the contention that sprouting of catecholamine-containing fibers results following drug treatment. In a previous study, ligation of the preganglionic trunk of the cat also resulted in the sprouting of catecholamine-containing varicose fibers in a caudal direction toward the ligature (Jacobowitz and Woodward, 1968). It would therefore appear that sprouting of a particular fiber system may occur with or without injury to that neuronal system. It is tempting to suggest that the initiation of nerve sprouting results from neuronal breakdown products. Whether these factors include the nerve growth factor of Levi-Montalcini and Angeletti (1968) remains to be elucidated.

It is of interest that the dopamine content of the ganglion increased twofold 3 days after vinblastine application. This increase may be a reflection of the NA precursor synthesized during the early period of formation of catecholaminergic sprouts. On the other hand, the possibility that the increase in dopamine content is a reflection of an increase in the number of chromaffin cell processes cannot be excluded. Several lines of evidence indicate that the small intensely fluorescent chromaffin cells within the SCG of the rat are dopaminergic (Björklund et al., 1970; Fuxe et al., 1970; Kebabian and Greengard, 1971). Recent observations of chromaffin cells from cultures of dissociated chick embryo sympathetic ganglia (Jacobowitz and Greene, 1974) reveal that extensive fluorescent varicose processes sprout from these chromaffin cells. It was suggested that at least part of the intraganglionic system of adrenergic varicose terminals arises from the chromaffin cells. These chromaffin cells have been shown to contain NA and adrenaline but not dopamine. In view of the above observations, the ganglion chromaffin cells must be considered as a possible source of at least part of the intraganglionic system of varicosities. Ganglionic varicosities may therefore represent axonal collaterals, dendritic collaterals, and/or chromaffin cell processes.

Eight days after vinblastine treatment the dopamine content of the SCG was normal at a time when the NA content was twice the control level. Since this observation would tend to negate an involvement of dopamine-containing cells in the sprouting of varicosities, its significance is not clear.

Following local application of vinblastine, there is an initial increase in the activities of tyrosine hydroxylase and dopamine-β-hydroxylase (Lamprecht et al., 1972). This increase is consistent with a blockade of axonal transport while enzyme synthesis is not altered. Repair and sprouting catecholamine-containing terminals within the SCG are associated with enhanced uptake of ^{3}H-NA and decreased levels of tyrosine hydroxylase and dopamine-β-hydroxylase. After 2 days, when the NA uptake was increasing (by 30%), no change was observed in either enzyme activity. Later, both enzyme activities decline successively, and a 50% reduction was still observed at 47 days. It would seem that the marked increase in the NA content (200%) may cause a feedback inhibition of the formation of the synthetic enzymes (Axelrod, 1972) or synthesis of structural protein may preferentially occur in place of synthesis of functional enzymes (Kopin and Silberstein, 1972).

Histofluorescent observations of the sympathetic terminal plexus of the iris was made in an attempt to reveal whether the adrenergic fibers were destroyed or merely depleted of the aminergic neurotransmitter. Marked depletion of varicose terminals was first observed between 24 and 48 h after vinblastine application to the ganglion. There appear to be variable numbers of nerves in the irises ranging from no nerves to completely normal plexuses (Table 1). However it is of interest that at 47 days, in rats with nerve-depleted irises, there was a variable number of nerves in the submaxillary gland. It is therefore likely that after 47 days reinnervation was taking place in the submaxillary gland. The presence of vascular nerves at a time when no or few acinar nerves are observed, suggests that the course of reinnervation is along the vasculature. The appearance of large non-terminal axons, which contain varicose fibers, further supports the contention that an ingrowth of adrenergic nerves into the submaxillary gland is occurring at this time. Reinnervation of the submaxillary gland may precede the iris because of the shorter length of axons to the gland.

REFERENCES

AXELROD, J. (1972) Dopamine-β-hydroxylase: regulation of its synthesis and release from nerve terminals. *Pharmac. Rev.* **24**, 233–243.

BENSCH, K. G., MARANTZ, R., WISNIEWSKI, H., and SHELANSKI, M. (1969) Induction *in vitro* of microtubular crystals by vinca alkaloids. *Science* **165**, 495–496.

BJÖRKLUND, A., CEGRELL, L., FALCK, B., RITZEN, M., and ROSENGREN, E. (1970) Dopamine-containing cells in sympathetic ganglia. *Acta physiol. scand.* **78**, 334–338.

CHENEY, D. L., HANIN, I., MASSARELLI, R., TRABUCCHI, M., and COSTA, E. (1973) Vinblastine and vincristine: a study of their action on tissue concentrations of epinephrine, norepinephrine and acetylcholine. *Neuropharmacology* **12**, 233–238.

DAHLSTRÖM, A. (1965) Observations on the accumulation of noradrenaline in the proximal and distal parts of peripheral adrenergic nerves after compression. *J. Anat.* **99**, 677–689.

DAHLSTRÖM, A. (1968) Effect of colchicine on transport of amine storage granules in sympathetic nerves of the rat. *Eur. J. Pharmac.* **5**, 111–113.

DAHLSTRÖM, A. (1970) Effect of mitosis inhibitors on the transport of amine storage granules in monoaminergic neurons in the rat. *Acta physiol. scand.*, Suppl. 357, 6.

DAHLSTRÖM, A. (1972) The axonal transport of monoamine oxidases. *Adv. Biochem. Psychopharmac.* **5**, 293–305.

DAHLSTRÖM, A., and FUXE, K. (1964) A method for the demonstration of adrenergic nerve fibers in peripheral nerves. *Z. Zellforsch.* **2**, 602–607.

FALCK, B. (1962) Observations on the possibilities of the cellular localization of monoamines by a fluorescence method. *Acta physiol. scand.* **56** Suppl. 197, 1–25.

FALCK, B., HILLARP, N. A., THIEME, G., and TORP, A. (1962) Fluorescence of catecholamines and related compounds with formaldehyde. *J. Histochem. Cytochem.* **10**, 348–354.

FUXE, K., GOLDSTEIN, M., HÖKFELT, T., and JOH, T. H. (1970) Immunohistochemical localization of dopamine-β-hydroxylase in the peripheral and central nervous systems. *Res. Communs. Chem. Pathol. Pharmac.* **1**, 627.

GOLDMAN, H., and JACOBOWITZ D. (1971) Correlation of norepinephrine content with observations of adrenergic nerves after a single dose of 6-hydroxydopamine in the rat. *J. Pharmac. Exp. Ther.* **176**, 119–133.

HANBAUER I. (1972) Effect of local application of colchicine or vinblastine on the uptake of ³H-norepinephrine by rat superior cervical ganglion. *Fed. Proc.* **31**, 1982.

HÖKFELT, T., and DAHLSTRÖM, A. (1971) Effects of two mitosis inhibitors (colchicine and vinblastine) on the distribution and axonal transport of noradrenaline storage particles, studied by fluorescence and electron microscopy. *Z. Zellforsch.* **119**, 460–482.

JACOBOWITZ, D. (1970) Catecholamine fluorescence studies of adrenergic neurons and chromaffin cells in sympathetic ganglia. *Fed. Proc.* **29**, 1929–1944.

JACOBOWITZ, D. M., and GREENE, L. A. (1974) Histofluorescence study of chromaffin cells in dissociated cell cultures of chick embryo sympathetic ganglia. *J. Neurobiol.* (in press).

JACOBOWITZ, D., and WOODWARD, J. K. (1968) Adrenergic neurons in the cat superior cervical ganglion and cervical sympathetic nerve trunk. A histochemical study. *J. Pharmac. Exp. Ther.* **162**, 213–226.

KEBABIAN, J. W., and GREENGARD, P. (1971) Dopamine-sensitive adenyl cyclase: Possible role in synaptic transmission. *Science* **174**, 1346–1349.

KEEN, P., and LIVINGSTONE, A. (1970) Decline of tissue noradrenaline under the influence of a mitotic inhibitor. *Nature (Lond.)* **227**, 967–968.

KOELLE, G. B. (1955) Histochemical identification of acetylcholinesterase in cholinergic, adrenergic and sensory neurons. *J. Pharmac. Exp. Ther.* **114**, 167–184.

KOPIN, I. J., and SILBERSTEIN, S. D. (1972) Axons of sympathetic neurons: transport of enzymes *in vivo* and properties of axonal sprouts *in vitro*. *Pharmac. Rev.* **24**, 245–254.

LAMPRECHT, F., WEISE, V. K., and KOPIN, I. J. (1972) Effect of colchicine and vinblastine on the tyrosine hydroxylase and dopamine-β-hydroxylase content of the rat superior cervical ganglion and salivary gland. *Fed. Proc.* **31**, 1860.

LEVI-MONTALCINI, R., and ANGELETTI, P. V. (1968) Nerve growth factor. *Physiol. Rev.* **48**, 534–569.

MALAWISTA, S. E., SATO, H. H., and BENSCH, K. G. (1968) Vinblastine and griseofulvin reversibly disrupt the living mitotic spindle. *Science* **160**, 770–772.

MARANTZ, R., VENTILLA, M., and SHELANSKI, M. (1969) Vinblastine-induced precipitation of microtubule protein. *Science* **165**, 498–499.

MARMONT, A., and DAMASIO, E. (1967) The effect of two alkaloids derived from vinca razeor on the malignant cells of Hodgkin's disease, lymphosarcoma and acute leukemia *in vivo. Blood* **29**, 1–21.

MATTHEWS, M. R., and RAISMAN, G. (1972) A light and electron microscopic study of the cellular response to axonal injury in the superior cervical ganglion of the rat. *Proc. R. Soc. Lond.* **181**, 43–79.

MOLINOFF, P. B., WEINSHILBOUM, R. M., and AXELROD, J. (1971) A sensitive enzymatic assay for dopamine β-hydroxylase. *J. Pharmac. Exp. Ther.* **178**, 425–431.

MOORE, R. Y., BJÖRKLUND, A., and STENEVI, U. (1971) Plastic changes in the adrenergic innervation of the rat septal area in response to denervation. *Brain Res.* **33**, 13–36.

NOBLE, R. L., BEER, C. T., and CUTTS, J. H. (1958) Role of chance observations in chemotherapy. *Ann. N Y Acad. Sci.* **76**, 882–894.

OLSON, L., and MALMFORS, T. (1970) Growth characteristics of adrenergic nerves in the adult rat. *Acta physiol. scand.* **63** Suppl. 238, 1–112.

RAISMAN, G. (1969a) A comparison of the mode of termination of the hippocampal and hypothalamic afferents to the septal nuclei as revealed by electron microscopy of degeneration. *Expl. Brain Res.* **7**, 317–343.

RAISMAN, G. (1969b) Neuronal plasticity in the septal nuclei of the adult rat. *Brain Res.* **14**, 25–48.

SCHMITT, F. O. (1968) The molecular biology of neuronal fibrous proteins. *Neurosci. Res. Prog. Bull.* **6**, 119–144.

SCHRIER, B. K., and SCHUSTER, L. (1967) A simplified radiochemical assay for choline acetyltransferase. *J. Neurochem.* **14**, 977–985.

SHIMAN, R., AKINO, M., and KAUFMAN, S. (1971) Solubilization and partial purification of tyrosine hydroxylase from bovine adrenal medulla. *J. Biol. Chem.* **246**, 1330–1340.

SILBERSTEIN, S. D., JOHNSON, D. G., JACOBOWITZ, D. M., and KOPIN, I. J. (1971) Sympathetic reinnervation of the rat iris in organ culture. *Proc. Natn. Acad. Sci. USA* **68**, 1121–1124.

TRIFARO, J. M., COLLIER, B., LASTOWECKA, A., and STERN, D. (1972) Inhibition by colchicine and by vinblastine of acetylcholine-induced catecholamine release from the adrenal gland: an anticholinergic action, not an effect on microtubules. *Molec. Pharmac.* **8**, 264–267.

TSUKAHARA, S., JACOBOWITZ, D., and LATIES, A. M. (1972) Cholinergic reinnervation of the iris transplants to the anterior chamber of the eye. *Am. J. Ophthalmol.* **73**, 394–399.

NERVE GROWTH SPECIFICITY AND REGULATION AS REVEALED BY INTRAOCULAR BRAIN TISSUE TRANSPLANTS

LARS OLSON AND ÅKE SEIGER

Department of Histology, Karolinska Institutet, S-104 01 Stockholm, Sweden

INTRODUCTION

The central monoamine neurons have a remarkable growth potential. They develop early, often innervate large areas, and in most cases respond to axotomy by pronounced regenerative growth also in the mature animal. In order to learn more about the qualitative and quantitative aspects of monoamine nerve growth, about factors that regulate growth and about growth specificity, we are presently using the technique of intraocular brain tissue transplantation.

In this respect we describe the intraocular transplantation technique and the possibilities for studying nerve growth regulation in general that it offers. Evidence will be presented for a homotypical and functional organization of transplanted brain areas. Immature central dopamine (DA), noradrenaline (NA), and 5-hydroxytryptamine (5-HT) neurons all survive transplantation well, and innervate the transplant as well as the sympathetically denervated host iris.

THE INTRAOCULAR TRANSPLANTATION TECHNIQUE

The anterior chamber of the eye has been used as a convenient site for transplantation for a multitude of purposes during the last 50 years. Earlier we have used the technique in qualitative and quantitative studies of the growth characteristics of sympathetic adrenergic nerves (Malmfors and Olson, 1967; Olson and Malmfors, 1970) to study the production of nerve fibers by adrenal chromaffine cells (Olson, 1970) and for studies of the influence of prolactin on DA turnover in the median eminence using anterior pituitary transplants (Olson *et al.*, 1972). For a detailed description of the technical procedure in general, see Olson and Malmfors (1970) (Fig. 1).

Transplantation of brain tissue to the anterior chamber offers a good alternative to the commonly used *in vitro* culture procedures, and it has several specific advantages. When the

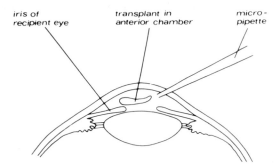

FIG. 1. Schematic drawing showing the way of administrating small brain tissue pieces to the anterior chamber of the eye. The transplant is injected into the recipient eye with the micropipette through a slit in the cornea. For details, see Olson and Malmfors (1970).

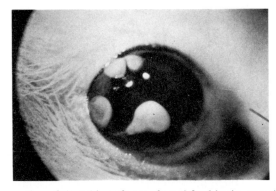

FIG. 2. *In vivo* observation of the taking of transplanted fetal brain stem tissue. Microphotograph of the eye through a dissection microscope. Four well-demarcated ovoid transplants can be seen in this eye.

technique is used with rats it is fast, simple, and gives highly reproducible and constant results (Olson and Seiger, 1972a, 1973a, b; Ljungdahl *et al.*, 1973; Hoffer *et al.*, 1974; Farnebo *et al.*, in preparation).

In brief, the technique consists of preparing small pieces of brain tissue, preferably from fetal rats, and injecting them into the anterior eye chamber of adult recipients through a slit in the cornea by means of a modified pasteur pipette under sterile conditions.

Using fetal brain tissue, the taking of the transplants is very good. They become attached to and rapidly vascularized from the anterior surface of the host iris, which has no epithelial coverage. During the avascular phase the small brain tissue pieces (approximately 1–2 mm³) are supported by the aqueous humor which normally supports vascular tissues such as the cornea and lens. Following vascularization, the transplants rapidly develop and often grow considerably in size. After an initial delay of possibly a few days because of the operation, the embryonic tissues seem to mature in the eye at an approximately normal rate. The end result may be a large (10–30 mm³), partly well organized, well vascularized smoothly outlined piece of brain tissue that will remain in good condition intraocularly for at least many months (longest postoperative time studied, 8 months).

The taking of the transplant, its growth, and vascularization can be monitored *in vivo* by direct microscopical observation through the cornea (Fig. 2).

Three types of transplantations have been studied. The first group consists of transplants containing monoamine nerve cell bodies. Knowing in detail the time of birth and further prenatal development of the 22 different monoamine nerve cell groups (Olson and Seiger, 1972b; Seiger and Olson, 1973), it is possible to obtain, by microscopic dissection, small tissue pieces containing DA, NA, and 5-HT neuroblasts separately or in various combinations and from different developmental stages. These dissections have been described elsewhere (Olson and Seiger, 1972a). The second group consists of transplants from early embryos including areas where monoamine neurons would normally develop at later stages. The first and second group of transplantations were performed into eyes that were simultaneously sympathetically denervated by extirpation of the superior cervical ganglion (SCG).

The third group of transplantations consists of areas that do not contain any monoamine neuroblasts. This group so far includes cerebral and cerebellar cortex, the caudate nucleus, and the spinal cord. In this case the host eyes were not sympathetically denervated.

CENTRAL MONOAMINE NEURONS IN THE EYE

After various postoperative times the transplants were carefully dissected free from their host irides, frozen, and freeze-dried (Olson and Ungerstedt, 1970), while the host irides were prepared as whole mounts (Falck, 1962; Malmfors, 1965) and air-dried. All tissues were then further processed for fluorescence microscopy of monoamines according to Falck and Hillarp (Falck *et al.*, 1962; see also Corrodi and Jonsson, 1967).

All the three types of monoamine neurons, that is DA neuroblasts from the developing substantia nigra, NA neuroblasts from, e.g., the developing locus coeruleus area, and 5-HT neuroblasts from the raphe systems survived and proliferated in the transplants. In the second set of experiments, using early embryonic tissues, monoamine neurons did develop in the transplants. A serious complication in this type of experiment was the concomitant development of nonneuronal tissues such as cartilage, bone, skin, giving rise to transplants that soon became too large for the anterior chamber.

Using the group-one type of monoamine neuroblast-containing transplants from the brain stem more or less homotypical innervation patterns were found. After a month or more *in oculo*, clusters of mature multipolar monoamine nerve cell bodies were found that gave rise to varicose nerve terminals innervating other areas of the transplant containing groups of nonfluorescent neurons (Fig. 7a). When NA and 5-HT neurons or DA and 5-HT neurons were present together, they tended to form separate groups of cell bodies while their terminal ramifications were closely intermingled, often seemingly innervating the same cells in the transplants.

A most interesting feature of the central monoamine neurons was their pronounced ability to reinnervate the sympathetically denervated host iris. From the site of attachment of the transplants, heavy bundles of fluorescent axons radiated out over the surface of the iris just like adrenergic nerves fan out over the iris from a transplant of an adrenergic ganglion (Olson and Malmfors, 1970). DA, NA, and 5-HT fibers were all able to form varicose plexuses of nerve terminals similar in morphology and location to the normally present sympathetic ground plexus (see Olson and Seiger, 1972a) (Figs. 3–6). Thus the same group of, e.g., NA neuroblasts were able to give rise to thin, moderately fluorescent simple running varicose fibers of CNS type in the transplant and thicker fibers with larger, more strongly fluorescent varicosities and often running two or more together in bundles, i.e.

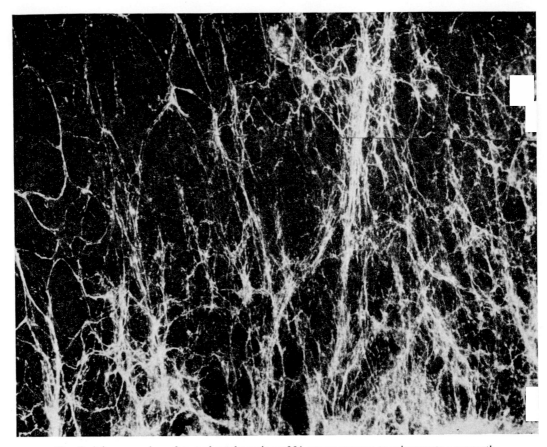

Fig. 3. A large number of central partly varicose NA axons are seen to reinnervate a sympathectomized host iris near the site of attachment of the transplant in a plexus-like manner. The
brain tissue was obtained from a 29–30 mm fetus. Pretreatment with MAO inhibitor. Postoperative time: 23 days. Montage of fluorescence microphotographs of an iris whole mount
preparation. (×165.)

iris-like in the host iris (Fig. 7b). Catecholamine and 5-HT fibers readily innervate the iris
together, sharing the same tracks on the iris. Thus, also DA neurons sometimes giving the
typically diffuse dense innervation pattern of the transplants gave rise to iris-like fibers on
the host iris. Blood vessels became reinnervated, with the nerves located at the normal
position at the medioadventitial border.

The overall impression of the iris reinnervation is thus that the fluorescence morphology
of the individual fibers as well as the pattern of innervation is determined by the iris and
organotypical. The ingrowing fibers adapt to a pattern preserved in the sympathetically
denervated host iris, perhaps in the Schwann cell plexus, without the fibers losing their
transmitter identities.

Another, and maybe even more striking example of the ability of the iris to modulate
heterotypic sources of amine storing cells to suit its own needs, is the transformation of
chromaffin adrenal medullary cells that occurs following transplantation to sympathetically denervated eyes (Olson, 1970). Here the mature chromaffin cells elongate and produce

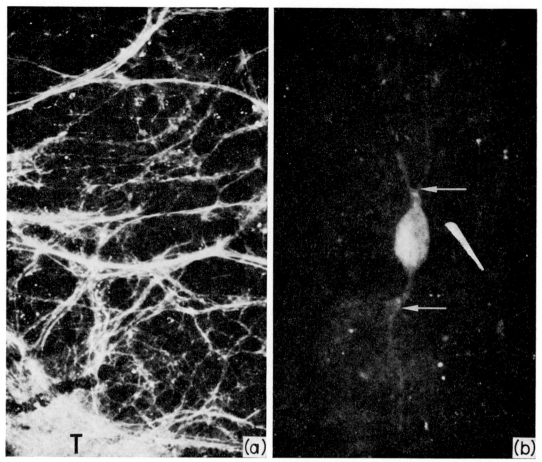

FIG. 4. Central yellow fluorescent 5-HT neurons on sympathectomized host irides. The brain stem tissue was taken from 33 to 35 mm fetuses. Pretreatment with MAO inhibitor. Fluorescence microphotographs of iris whole mount preparations. (a) A dense irregular plexus of nonterminal 5-HT axons intermingled with weakly fluorescent varicose terminal plexuses can be seen near the site of attachment of the transplant (T). Postoperative time: 6 months 1 week. ($\times 130$.) (b) One single bipolar 5-HT neuron which seems to have migrated out on the iris and attached to it. Note the branching of the two main processes (arrows). Postoperative time: 23 days. ($\times 295$.)

processes which in their most proximal ends still have the intense almost yellow fluorescence typical of adrenal medullary cells while their distal parts become indistinguishable in the fluorescence microscope from normal varicose sympathetic fibers and reinnervates the iris.

From a qualitative point of view the transmitter mechanisms of the newly formed nerves of central origin on the iris seem to be normal. They have a normal storage of amines and they can take up, store, and release exogenous amines upon electrical field stimulation (Farnebo *et al.*, in preparation). From preliminary experiments with tyrosine hydroxylase inhibition it would seem, however, as if the rate of amine depletion, i.e. the impulse activity in the transplanted neurons was low. The quantitative aspects of this growth have so far not been studied in detail. The amount of nerves increases with time, especially during the first month *in oculo*, and a better yield of nerves seems to be obtained using more immature

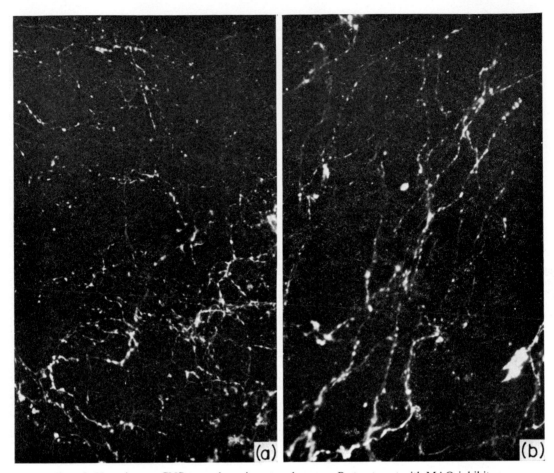

FIG. 5. Homologous CNS transplants in rat and mouse. Pretreatment with MAO inhibitor. Fluorescence microphotographs of whole mount preparations. (a) Outgrowth of a varicose nerve plexus on an albino rat iris by NA neurons from a 33–35 mm albino rat fetus. Post-operative time: 23 days. (×130.) (b) Varicose nerves on an albino mouse iris derived from NA neurons of a 16–17 mm albino mouse fetus. Postoperative time: 48 days. (×330.)

transplants. The reinnervated area of the iris seldom exceeds 25–50% of the total area. It is to be noted, however, that also monoamine neurons from newborn and even adult animals are able to reinnervate the iris to a certain extent (Fig. 6a, b).

From the evidence so far obtained we think it is possible to extend now to the CNS monoamine neurons some conclusions regarding specificity of growth that was earlier obtained in our studies of growing adrenergic neurons (Olson and Malmfors, 1970). Thus there seems to be a *general lack of specificity* between different monoamine neurons towards various receptor areas, since any type of central or peripheral monoamine neuron can reinnervate a sympathetically denervated iris. Regardless of the neuronal input, the innervation pattern is determined by the receptor organ.

The central monoamine neurons have a very widespread distribution normally. Thus central NA fibers not only innervate neurons in extremely large areas of the brain, but seem to innervate also secretory-like tissues such as the ependymal lining (Hartman, 1973;

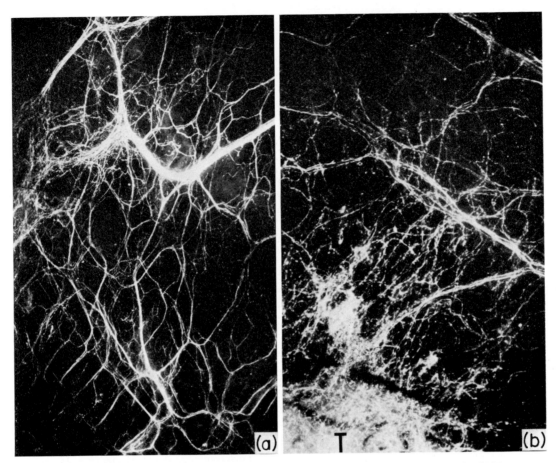

FIG. 6. Abundant outgrowth on sympathectomized host irides of locus coeruleus-derived NA plexuses. The brain stem pieces were taken from born animals. Pretreatment with MAO inhibitor. Iris whole mount preparations. Postoperative time: 2½ months. (a) A plexus of mostly nonterminal NA axons running together in small bundles from coeruleus neurons which were 1-day-old at the time of transplantation. Montage of fluorescence microphotographs (×50.) (b) A varicose irregular terminal plexus of NA nerves from 3-day-old coeruleus neurons near the site of attachment of the transplant (T). Fluorescence microphotograph. (×130.)

Olson *et al.*, 1973a) and smooth muscle of intracerebral blood vessels (Hartman, 1973). Moreover, central NA fibers normally seem to leave the CNS through the ventral nerve roots of the spinal cord (Dahlström and Fuxe, 1965) and through the cranial nerves (Seiger and Olson, 1973; Olson *et al.*, 1973b). Many CNS monoamine neurons thus seem to have a general programming to fill up receptor areas which may explain the readiness by which the iris becomes reinnervated. In this respect, the monoamine neurons seem to be the absolute opposite to the highly specified neurons of the retino-tectal projection with an almost cell to cell specificity.

Our experiments, together with other experimental approaches presently explored, demonstrate a remarkable growth potential of the monoamine neurons, both immature and mature, and both in the form of collateral sprouting and axon regeneration (Björklund *et al.*, 1971; Nygren *et al.*, 1971; Björklund and Stenevi, 1971; Katzman *et al.*, 1971; Björklund

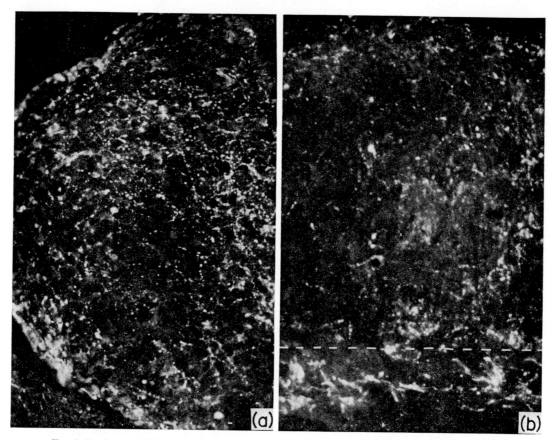

FIG. 7. Brain stem "NA-transplants", removed from their sympathectomized host irides and sectioned. Fluorescence microphotographs. ($\times$ 195.) (a) A transplant from a 35 mm fetus. In this "brain stem'"a large number of negative neurons can be observed, most of which are richly innervated by NA nerve terminals. Postoperative time: 12 days. (b) A transplant from a 40 mm fetus, well innervated by fluorescent NA nerve terminals and still attached to a part of its sympathectomized host iris. Note the marked difference in nerve morphology between the small NA nerve terminals within the transplant tissue (above), and the thick axons in the iris tissue (below) which of course are derived from the same central NA neurons in the transplant. No fluorescent cell body can be seen in this section. The borderline between the transplant and the iris is indicated by a darker line. Postoperative time: 4 months 1 week.

et al., 1973; Baumgarten *et al.*, 1973; Fuxe *et al.*, 1973, this volume; Nobin *et al.*, 1973). The fact that the central monoamine neurons so easily produce new nerve terminals under a variety of experimental conditions may suggest that they do so also under normal conditions, possibly following more suitable environmental stimuli.

TRANSPLANTS WITHOUT MONOAMINE NEURONS

Several aspects of this third group of transplants are under study. Using fluorescence microscopy one can study whether the sympathetic adrenergic fibers of the host iris are able to innervate the developing transplant. This may be the case, although the ingrowth of mature sympathetic nerves in the immature CNS transplants seems to be more restricted than the reverse phenomenon described above. The blood vessels of transplants of cerebral and cerebellar cortices, spinal cord, or caudate nucleus become well innervated.

Cerebellar transplants provide a good opportunity to study transplant organization at the light and electron microscopic level because of the strict and well known normal development and adult organization of the cerebellum. Using transplants from, e.g., 16-day-old fetuses, the transplants can be shown to develop *in oculo* to reach a mature stage with well organized areas of molecular cells, larger Purkinje cells, and granule cells. Folia are, however, mostly missing, and the organization is therefore chaotic at the macroscopic level (Ljungdahl *et al.*, 1973; Hoffer *et al.*, 1973). The functional properties of the cerebellar transplants are being studied using two techniques. With autoradiography an uptake of ^{3}H-GABA has been demonstrated in stellate cells, basket cells, Golgi cells, and a small population of Purkinje cells apart from certain glial cells (Ljungdahl *et al.*, 1973). Using extracellular recording electrodes *in oculo*, the spontaneous electrical activity of the cerebellar transplants is analyzed. It seems as if the discharge pattern of the transplanted Purkinje cells is almost undistinguishable from their normal pattern of discharge *in situ*.

Studies similar to those performed on the cerebellar transplants are under way using transplants of the caudate nucleus and spinal cord, two areas that also, at the light microscopical level, develop a fairly homotypical organization in spite of the massive lack of input.

CONCLUSION

In conclusion, we find intraocular brain tissue transplantations a most useful experimental model for a number of different purposes to complement other available methods of experimental neurosurgery and tissue culture. Defined areas of the developing CNS can be isolated from normal input and output connections and its further development studied. Rapid vascularization permits a good taking and growth of the transplants. No adverse immunological reactions have been observed using inbred rats. Survival and proliferation of central monoamine neurons, innervating the transplant tissue as well as the sympathetically denervated host iris, have been demonstrated using this model.

ACKNOWLEDGEMENTS

This work was supported by grants from the Swedish Medical Research Council (04X-3185), Karolinska Institutets Fonder, and Magnus Bergvalls Stiftelse. We thank Miss Monica Eliasson, Mrs. Barbro Norstedt, and Miss Ingrid Strömberg for skilful technical assistance. The generous gifts of Nialamide, Pfizer, and Pargyline, Abbott, are gratefully acknowledged.

REFERENCES

BAUMGARTEN, H. G., LACHENMAYER, L., BJÖRKLUND, A., NOBIN, A., and ROSENGREN, E. (1973) Long-term recovery of serotonin concentrations in the rat CNS following 5,6-dihydroxytryptamine. *Life Sci.* **12**, 357–364.

BJÖRKLUND, A., and STENEVI, U. (1971) Growth of central catecholamine neurons into smooth muscle grafts in the rat mesencephalon. *Brain Res.* **31**, 1–20.

BJÖRKLUND, A., KATZMAN, R., STENEVI, U., and WEST, K. A. (1971) Development and growth of axonal sprouts from noradrenaline and 5-hydroxy-tryptamine neurones in the rat spinal cord. *Brain Res.* **31**, 21–33.

BJÖRKLUND, A., NOBIN, A., and STENEVI, U. (1973) Regeneration of central serotonin neurons after axonal degeneration induced by 5,6-dihydroxy-tryptamine. *Brain Res.* **50**, 214–220.

CORRODI, H., and JONSSON, G. (1967) The formaldehyde fluorescence method for the histochemical demonstration of biogenic monoamines. A review on the methodology. *J. Histochem. Cytochem.* **15**, 65–78.

DAHLSTRÖM, A., and FUXE, K. (1965) Evidence for the existence of an outflow of noradrenaline nerve fibers in the ventral roots of the rat spinal cord. *Experientia* **21**, 409.

FALCK, B. (1962) Observations on the possibilities of the cellular localization of monoamines by a fluorescence method. *Acta physiol. scand.* **56**, Suppl. 197, 1–26.

FALCK, B., HILLARP, N.-Å., THIEME, G., and TORP, A. (1962) Fluorescence of catecholamines and related compounds condensed with formaldehyde. *J. Histochem. Cytochem.* **10**, 348–354.

FUXE, K., JONSSON, G., NYGREN, L.-G., and OLSON, L. (1974) Studies on central 5-HT neurons using dihydroxytryptamines: evidence for regeneration of bulbospinal 5-HT axons and terminals (in this volume).

HARTMAN, B. (1973) The innervation of cerebral blood vessels by central noradrenergic neurons. Abstract of paper read at the III Int. Catecholamin Symp., Strasbourg, May 1973.

HOFFER, B., SEIGER, A., LJUNGBERG, T., and OLSON, L. (1974) Electrophysiological and cytological studies of neonatal brain homografts in the anterior chamber of the eye: Maturation of cerebellar cortex *in oculo*. (to be published).

KATZMAN, R., BJÖRKLUND, A., OWMAN, CH., and WEST, K. A. (1971) Evidence for regenerative axon sprouting of central catecholamine neurons in the rat mesencephalon following electrolytic lesions. *Brain Res.* **25**, 579–596.

LJUNGDAHL, Å., SEIGER, Å., HÖKFELT, T., and OLSON, L. (1973) ^{3}H-GABA uptake in growing cerebellar tissue: autoradiography of intraocular transplants. *Brain Res.* **61**, 379–384.

MALMFORS, T. (1965) Studies on adrenergic nerves: the use of rat and mouse iris for direct observations on their physiology and pharmacology at cellular and subcellular levels. *Acta physiol. scand.* Suppl. 248, 1–93.

MALMFORS, T., and OLSON, L. (1967) Adrenergic reinnervation of anterior chamber transplants. *Acta physiol. scand.* **71**, 401–402.

NOBIN, A., BAUMGARTEN, H. G., BJÖRKLUND, A., LACHENMAYER, L., and STENEVI, U. (1973) Axonal degeneration and regeneration of the bulbospinal indolamine neurons after 5,6-dihydroxytryptamine treatment. *Brain Res.* **56**, 1–24.

NYGREN, L.-G., OLSON, L., and SEIGER, Å. (1971) Regeneration of monoamine-containing axons in the developing and adult spinal cord of the rat following intraspinal 6-OH-dopamine injections or transection. *Histochemie* **28**, 1–15.

OLSON, L. (1970) Fluorescence histochemical evidence for axonal growth and secretion from transplanted adrenal medullary tissue. *Histochemie* **22**, 1–7.

OLSON, L., and MALMFORS, T. (1970) Growth characteristics of adrenergic nerves in the adult rat: fluorescence histochemical and ^{3}H-noradrenaline uptake studies using tissue transplantations to the anterior chamber of the eye. *Acta physiol. scand.*, Suppl. 348, 1–112.

OLSON, L., and UNGERSTEDT, U. (1970) A simple high capacity freeze-drier for histochemical use. *Histochemie* **22**, 8–19.

OLSON, L., and SEIGER, Å. (1972a) Brain tissue transplanted to the anterior chamber of the eye: 1, Fluorescence histochemistry of immature catecholamine and 5-hydroxytryptamine neurons reinnervating the rat iris. *Z. Zellforsch.* **135**, 175–194.

OLSON, L., and SEIGER, Å. (1972b) Early prenatal ontogeny of central monamine neurons in the rat: fluorescence histochemical observations. *Z. Anat. EntwGesch.* **137**, 301–316.

OLSON, L., and SEIGER, Å. (1973a) Fluorescence histochemistry of immature central noradrenaline-, dopamine- and 5-hydroxytryptamine-containing neurons transplanted to the anterior chamber of the rat eye. In: *Fluorescence Histochemistry of Biogenic Amines* (M. Fujiwara, ed.), Igako Shoin Ltd., Tokyo.

OLSON, L., and SEIGER, Å. (1973b) Development and growth of immature neurons in rat and man *in situ* and following intraocular transplantation in the rat. *Brain Res.* **62**, 353–360.

OLSON, L., FUXE, K., and HÖKFELT, T. (1972) The effect of pituitary transplants on the tubero-infundibular dopamine neurons in various endocrine states. *Acta endocrinol.* **17**, 233–244.

OLSON, L., NYSTRÖM, B., and SEIGER, Å. (1973a) Monoamine fluorescence histochemistry of human post mortem brain. *Brain Res.* **63**, 231–247.

OLSON, L., BOREUS, L. O., and SEIGER, Å. (1973b) Histochemical demonstration and mapping of 5-hydroxytryptamine- and catecholamine-containing neuron systems in the human fetal brain. *Z. Anat. EntwGesch.* **139**, 259–282.

SEIGER, Å., and OLSON, L. (1973) Late prenatal ontogeny of central monoamine neurons in the rat: fluorescence histochemical observations. *Z. Anat. EntwGesch.* **140**, 281–318.

DEGENERATION AND ORIENTED GROWTH OF AUTONOMIC NERVES IN RELATION TO SMOOTH MUSCLE IN JOINT TISSUE CULTURES AND ANTERIOR EYE CHAMBER TRANSPLANTS

G. Burnstock

Department of Zoology, University of Melbourne, Parkville, Victoria 3052, *Australia*

SUMMARY

The growth, degeneration, and regeneration of sympathetic nerves in a variety of experimental situations is discussed. In both normal development of smooth muscle and in anterior eye chamber transplants, varicose adrenergic nerves exhibiting characteristic fluorescence and ultrastructure invade the muscle early although functional transmission may not occur until a few days later. The density of innervation reached in transplants of a particular tissue is comparable to that seen *in situ*, and continues to increase in both situations up to at least 6 months. Only nerves of the type previously supplying the tissue reinnervate transplants. In tissue culture, sympathetic nerves grow preferentially over distances of up to 2 mm towards explants of normally densely innervated tissues (vas deferens and atrium) in competition with explants of normally sparsely innervated tissues (uterus, ureter, lung, kidney). It is suggested that NGF produced by the explants is the chemical involved in this "attraction" process. No "attraction" from a distance of sympathetic nerves to single smooth or cardiac muscle cells occurs, but random contact leads to close, extensive, and long-lasting associations; in contrast, contact with fibroblasts is always transitory. Questions have been posed regarding the membrane "recognition" mechanism. Finally, the retraction of sympathetic nerves induced by guanethidine is described for both *in situ* and *in vitro* situations.

INTRODUCTION

Our laboratory in Melbourne has developed a number of experimental approaches to study autonomic nerve growth, degeneration, and regeneration, with particular emphasis on the relation between nerves and smooth or cardiac muscle effectors.

These processes have been examined in the following situations:

(1) during normal development;
(2) in anterior eye-chamber transplants;
(3) in joint tissue cultures;
(4) following chronic treatment of the animal with drugs and hormones.

This work is the result of collaborations with some outstanding colleagues, including Akio Yamauchi, Julia Read, Bren Gannon, John Furness, John McLean, Terry Bennett, Torbjorn Malmfors, Jim Cobb, Gordon Campbell, Sheila Gillard, Yasuo Uehara, Gerda Mark, Takashi Iwayama, Don Rogers, Barbara Evans, John Heath, Olavi and Liisa Eränkö, Julie Chamley, and Caryl Hill.

Before concentrating on our most recent studies of nerve growth in joint tissue cultures, a brief description of the results of our earlier studies of nerves during normal development and in anterior eye-chamber transplants will be given, since these raised some interesting questions.

AUTONOMIC NERVE GROWTH IN NORMAL DEVELOPMENT

In a series of multidisciplinary studies of the postnatal development of the mouse vas deferens (Yamauchi and Burnstock, 1969a, b; Furness *et al.*, 1970), it was shown that the adrenergic nerves which are present at about 12 days are mature on the basis of their varicose fluorescent appearance and that the proportion of various intra-axonal vesicle types remains constant after this stage. However, the *density* of innervation, in terms of both the number of axons per 100 muscle cells seen in section and the number of close (200 Å) neuromuscular junctions, continues to increase up to at least 6 months, even though the mouse becomes pubescent at 3 months (Table 1). Excitatory junction potentials could not be recorded in smooth muscle cells until 18 days after birth; thus there appears to be a

TABLE 1. DEVELOPMENT OF INNERVATION IN THE MOUSE VAS DEFERENS
(adapted by Burnstock, 1970, from Yamauchi and Burnstock, 1969b)

Age of specimens	Number of axons per 100 muscle cells	Number of close (200 Å) neuromuscular contacts per 100 muscle cells	Percentage of different vesicle types found in profiles through varicose regions of noradrenergic nerves		
			Small granular vesicles	Large granular vesicles	Agranular vesicles
1 day	15	1	37	10	53
5 days	63	17	51	8	41
10 days	80	30	65	9	27
15 days	71	12[a]	81	4	15
20 days	87	19[a]	81	4	14
25 days	99	25[a]	82	3	15
3 months	112	32	84	4	12
6 months	121	50	85	3	12

[a] These low figures can probably be explained in terms of the increase in the size of muscle cells at this stage (Yamauchi and Burnstock, 1969a).

delay between the establishment of morphologically mature axons and neuromuscular junctions and the onset of functional neuromuscular transmission. This apparent phasing of structure and function has also been described in the development of synapses in the human foetal gut (Read and Burnstock, 1970), and in the regeneration of neuromuscular junctions in anterior eye-chamber transplants of vas deferens (see below).

DEGENERATION, GROWTH, AND REGENERATION OF NERVES IN ANTERIOR EYE-CHAMBER TRANSPLANTS

The anterior eye-chamber transplantation technique (see Olson and Malmfors, 1970) has been used in our laboratory to study the cellular changes which occur during reinnervation of transplanted vas deferens (Malmfors *et al.*, 1971; Campbell *et al.*, 1971) and taenia coli (Burnstock *et al.*, 1971b; Rogers, 1972). The results of these studies have raised several interesting questions which have been examined further with tissue culture methods (see below). All the severed postganglionic nerve fibres in the transplants degenerate within two days following the operation. The nerves which appear in the transplant after 1–3 weeks consist of sympathetic nerves arising from the superior cervical ganglion and parasympathetic nerves from the ciliary ganglion, demonstrating that outgrowth of autonomic nerves is not restricted to the organs they normally innervate.

While the individual nerve fibres which penetrate transplants of vas deferens reach structural maturity very early, the density of innervation continues to increase up to at least 6 months (Table 2). Thus the pattern of ingrowth of nerves into the transplants is comparable to that observed for growing sympathetic nerves during normal development of the vas deferens. Since muscle effector bundle formation in transplants occurs at about the same time as varicose adrenergic nerves penetrate into the muscle layer, the possibility was raised that nerves might influence muscle differentiation and aggregation. This possibility has been supported in part by recent tissue culture experiments: sympathetic nerves delay dedifferentiation and consequently division of cultured muscle; while they are not necessary for muscle bundle formation, they accelerate both bundle and nexus formation (Chamley *et al.*, 1974).

TABLE 2. SUMMARY OF THE MORPHOLOGICAL AND FUNCTIONAL CHANGES IN THE VAS DEFERENS FOLLOWING TRANSPLANTATION TO THE ANTERIOR CHAMBER OF THE EYE

A rough quantitation of particular features is indicated by the height of the shaded areas. The density of innervation and the amplitude of contractions in control preparations are represented by broken lines. Note the following major phases: (1) initial degeneration of nerves and muscles; (2) vascularization and regeneration of muscle; (3) reinnervation and muscle-bundle formation; (4) restitution of functional transmission. (Courtesy of Malmfors *et al.*, 1971.)

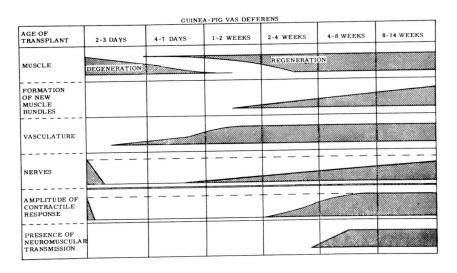

Experiments with taenia coli transplants have shown that both cholinergic and "purinergic" neurons (Burnstock, 1972) survive without central connections for at least 4 weeks. During the first few days following transplantation the processes of the ganglion cells appear to retract; however nerve-mediated cholinergic and purinergic responses reappear at about 3 days, presumably coinciding with outgrowth of axons from the ganglia.

Adrenergic and cholinergic nerves reinnervate vas deferens transplants, while purinergic as well as cholinergic and adrenergic nerves reinnervate ganglion-free transplants of taenia coli. Similarly, in recent experiments (Bell, personal communication), it was shown that reinnervation of rat femoral artery transplants (normally supplied only by adrenergic fibres) is limited to adrenergic nerves, whereas guinea-pig uterine artery transplants are reinnervated by both adrenergic and cholinergic nerves, which are their normal innervation components. These results confirm earlier claims (Langley and Anderson, 1904) that denervated smooth muscle will only receive growing nerve fibres of the types previously supplying it. However, preliminary experiments suggest that while the overall *density and type* of reinnervation is determined by the vas deferens transplant, the *proportion* of adrenergic to cholinergic excitatory fibres may vary depending on the accessibility of the different nerve types.

Finally, the question of whether the ingrowing autonomic nerves influence the distribution of receptors developed on the target effector muscle is raised. Reinnervation of vas deferens leads to excitatory adrenergic control of the muscle, which is the normal response in this tissue, while adrenergic reinnervation of taenia coli results in the normal inhibitory response.

ORIENTED GROWTH OF SYMPATHETIC NERVES IN TISSUE CULTURE

(1) SYMPATHETIC NEURONS ALONE

Two types of neurons can be identified in cultures of sympathetic ganglia of rat and guinea-pig (Chamley *et al.*, 1972): type I neurons are in the minority, migrate into the outgrowth, and may represent immature, retarded, or abnormal cells; type II neurons are in the majority, do not show migratory activity, and appear to correspond to those seen *in situ* (see also Murray, 1965). Processes of cultured sympathetic neurons are varicose and show fluorescence histochemical and ultrastructural features characteristic of adrenergic nerves growing or regenerating *in situ* (Fig. 1) (Burnstock and Iwayama, 1971). Nerve growth factor (NGF) generally increases the size, growth rate, and noradrenaline levels of cultured sympathetic neurons (see also Levi-Montalcini and Angeletti, 1968).

(2) SYMPATHETIC NERVES IN RELATION TO EXPLANTS OF SMOOTH AND HEART MUSCLE

When sympathetic ganglia from midterm foetal to 2-day-old rats are grown in modified Rose chambers between explants of normally densely innervated tissue (e.g. vas deferens and atrium) and normally sparsely innervated tissue (e.g. kidney medulla, uterus, ureter, and lung), nerve fibres grow preferentially towards the normally densely innervated tissues over distances of up to 2 mm (Fig. 2) (Chamley *et al.*, 1973b). These results are consistent with the concept of attraction by a specific chemical substance (Cajal, 1928). It is suggested that NGF is the chemical involved. NGF introduced into the culture chamber produces comparable increases in size of sympathetic neurons and in amount of nerve fibre growth

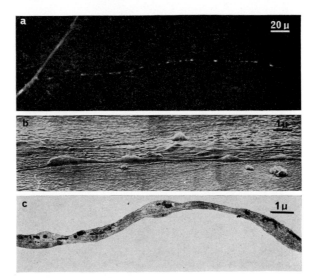

FIG. 1. Sympathetic nerves in tissue culture. (a) Fluorescence histochemical localization of catecholamines in a single varicose fibre from newborn guinea-pig sympathetic chain, 16 days *in vitro*. (Courtesy of Chamley *et al.*, 1972.) (b) Scanning electronmicrograph of varicosities in a single nerve fibre growing in a culture of newborn guinea-pig sympathetic ganglia. (Courtesy of Chamley, in Burnstock, 1974). (c) Transmission electronmicrograph of a longitudinal section through a single axon from cultures of 5-day-old rat sympathetic chain, 21 days *in vitro*. (Courtesy of Chamley *et al.*, 1972.)

comparable to those seen in the presence of developing vas deferens or atrium. The NGF level in vas deferens from 5-week-old mice was shown recently with radio-immunoassay methods to be high relative to the levels found in normally sparsely innervated tissues (Johnson *et al.*, 1971, 1972). Transplanted NGF-producing sarcomas become densely penetrated by sympathetic nerve fibres *in vivo* (Levi-Montalcini and Hamberger, 1953). It should be noted here that recent experiments on other systems by workers in other laboratories suggest that cyclic AMP may also be involved in the stimulation of nerve fibre growth (Aloe and Levi-Montalcini, 1972; Lenz, 1972) and perhaps related to the action of NGF (Roisen *et al.*, 1972; Haas *et al.*, 1972; Hier *et al.*, 1972).

(3) SYMPATHETIC NERVES IN RELATION TO SINGLE MUSCLE CELLS

When muscle cells from the vas deferens and atrium are separated enzymatically with trypsin and collagenase and introduced into the culture chamber, no "attraction" of sympathetic nerve fibres from a distance occurs (Mark *et al.*, 1973; Chamley *et al.*, 1973a). However, random contact with a muscle cell often leads to close, extensive, and long-lasting associations (Figs. 3 and 4). In contrast, contact with fibroblasts is always transitory. When nerve fibres come into contact with any tissue or tissue debris, there is a period of halted growth for about 50 min during which time continual palpation of the tissue occurs (see also Nakai and Kawasaki, 1959). However, after this period, the rate of nerve-fibre growth over individual muscle cells is faster than over fibroblasts, which in turn is faster than over the collagen-coated surface of the coverslip (Table 3). Furthermore, palpation by a nerve-fibre growth cone increases the rate of spontaneous contraction of a muscle cell, the extent of the increase being dependent on the number of nerve fibres involved (Table 4). Multiple

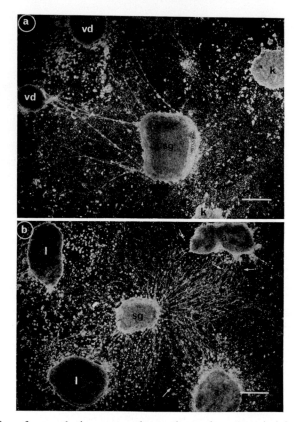

FIG. 2. Interaction of sympathetic nerves and smooth muscle explants in joint tissue cultures.
(a) Nerve-fibre growth from a sympathetic ganglion explant (sg) to explants of vas deferens
(vd) and kidney (k). Five-day-old rat, 5 days *in vitro*. At all stages of growth, nerve fibres grow
to vas deferens explants in marked preference to kidney explants. Scale 400 μ. 1 units NGF/ml.
(b) Nerve-fibre growth from a sympathetic ganglion explant (sg) to explants of lung (l) and
atrium (a). Five-day-old rat, 5 days *in vitro*. At all times a greater number of nerve fibres grow
on the side of the sympathetic ganglion explant nearer the atrium explants. The nerve fibre
growth to the atrium explants appeared to be "directed", many fibres changing course to
penetrate atrium explants (arrows). Nerve fibre growth to lung explants always appeared
random. Scale 400 μ. (Courtesy of Chamley *et al.*, 1973b.)

innervation of a smooth muscle cell occurs only if several nerve fibres reach the cell at about
the same time, but not if there is a close nerve–muscle association already established.

Thus it would appear that, while NGF may determine the number of nerve fibres that
grow to an autonomic effector organ, the final density of innervation is controlled by the
individual cells after contact has been made. A question that remains to be solved is the
nature of this contact interaction between nerve and muscle. What is the mechanism
whereby, after an initial palpation period, the nerve "recognizes" the muscle cells as
distinct from the fibroblast and forms a close, extensive, and long-lasting contact with it?
Does the muscle membrane have some genetically determined surface characteristics which
interact with nerve membranes? Or is a substance released by the nerve on contact that
results in a sequence of changes in the muscle (but not the fibroblast) during the 50 min
palpation period which leads to specific interaction and long-term association? What is the

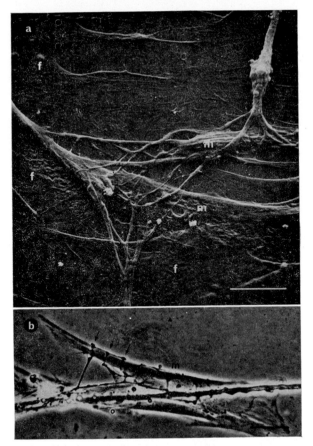

Fig. 3. (a) Close and extensive associations between nerve fibres and two smooth muscle cells (m) as observed with scanning electronmicroscopy. Note that the nerve fibres do not form associations with the background fibroblasts (f). Newborn guinea-pig sympathetic chain 14 days *in vitro*, vas deferens 7 days *in vitro*. 1 unit NGF/ml. Horizontal marker 25 μ. (b) Complex relationship between nerve fibres and a smooth muscle cell (m) seen under a phase-contrast microscope. Note many areas of close contact, often with varicosities (arrows). Newborn guinea-pig sympathetic chain 14 days *in vitro*, vas deferens 7 days *in vitro*. 1 unit NGF/ml. (×740.) Horizontal marker 25 μ. (Courtesy of Chamley *et al.*, 1973a.)

mechanism whereby nerve fibres are "rejected" by muscle cells that have previously formed long-term associations with another fibre or fibres?

SYMPATHETIC NERVE RETRACTION AND DEGENERATION WITH GUANETHIDINE

In this last section, the action of one drug, namely guanethidine, on the growth and degeneration of sympathetic nerves has been selected for consideration.

Chronic injection of rats with guanethidine produces long-term damage selectively to adrenergic neurons and particularly to the "short" adrenergic neurons that supply the male reproductive system (Gannon *et al.*, 1971; Heath *et al.*, 1972; Evans *et al.*, 1972). Treatment with high doses produces near-complete sympathectomy in rats (Burnstock *et al.*, 1971a).

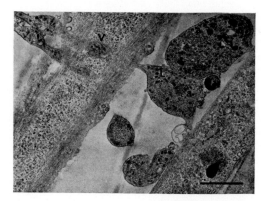

FIG. 4. Transmission electron micrograph of a number of axons in relation to an undifferenti-ated muscle cell in joint cultures of newborn guinea-pig sympathetic chain 12 days *in vitro*, vas deferens 5 days *in vitro*. The varicosities contain both large granular vesicles (L) and small agranular vesicles (a). Note the section of a varicosity (v) in the undifferentiated muscle cell, indicating that it lies within a groove on the surface of the cell. No NGF. Horizontal marker 1 μ. (Courtesy of Chamley *et al.*, 1973a.)

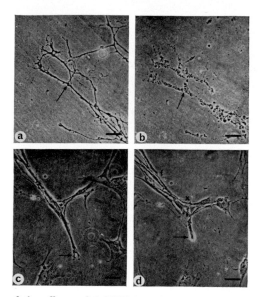

FIG. 5. Comparison of the effects of 6-OH-DA and guanethidine on cultured sympathetic nerves. (a), (b) Phase-contrast photomicrographs illustrating 6-OH-DA-induced *fragment-ation* of nerve fibres and subsequent regeneration in chick embryo sympathetic ganglion cultures. (a) Three hours after exposure to 20 mg/l 6-OH-DA. Note that growth cones and fibres are still intact and healthy. (b) Same field as (a) after a further 17 h exposure to 20 mg/l 6-OH-DA. The fibres have fragmented and a "ghost" fibre of the resulting debris remains. Horizontal bar 20 μ. (c), (d) Phase-contrast photomicrographs of nerve fibre retraction produced by guanethidine sulphate in newborn rat sympathetic ganglion cultures. (c) Terminal nerve fibres and growth cones before addition of guanethidine. The nerve fibre bundle (f) bifurcates at x, one branch terminating in growth cones (arrow). (d) Same field as (c) after 1.5 h exposure to 100 mg/l guanethidine sulphate. The growth cones and terminal fibres have retracted back towards the point where the bundle bifurcates. The halo around these retracted fibres (arrow) is caused by the thickness of the tissue. Horizontal bar 30 μ. (Courtesy of Hill *et al.*, 1973.)

TABLE 3. TEN SEPARATE EXPERIMENTS IN DIFFERENT CULTURES MEASURING THE RATE OF GROWTH (μ/MINUTE) OF A NERVE FIBRE OVER COLLAGEN, A FIBROBLAST AND A MUSCLE CELL

Each horizontal line represents one experiment. In each experiment the growth over each of the three surfaces was divided into intervals of 20 min of actual filming time (or part thereof). As there was little or no variation between the intervals the values were averaged to give the mean growth rate over the particular surface. The total period of time over which the rate was measured for each surface varied from 1 h 30 min to 2 h 50 min. (From Chamley et al., 1973a.)

	Collagen	Fibroblast		Muscle	
	(μ/min)	(μ/min)	% increase over collagen	(μ/min)	% increase over collagen
No NGF	0.24	0.30	25	0.36	50
	0.26	0.32	23	0.37	42
	0.21	0.26	24	0.31	48
	0.22	0.27	23	0.35	59
	0.26	0.31	19	0.37	42
NGF	0.27	0.35	30	0.42	55
	0.29	0.39	38	0.46	56
	0.28	0.35	25	0.48	71
	0.27	0.36	33	0.45	66
	0.29	0.37	28	0.45	55

TABLE 4. CONTRACTION RATE (CONTRACTIONS PER MINUTE) OF EIGHT SMOOTH MUSCLE CELLS BEFORE, DURING AND AFTER PALPATION BY NERVE GROWTH CONES

In this case the palpation included both the period when nerve growth was halted and when the cone moved along the cell during growth. The total palpation of each muscle cell took between 2 h 5 min and 3 h 36 min. It was divided into intervals of 20 min of actual filming time (or part thereof) and the contractions counted. As there was little or no variation between the intervals, the values were averaged to give the mean rate of contraction. Similarly, the number of contractions before and after the growth cone palpated the muscle cells was counted in several 20 min intervals, and as there was little or no variation between these values, means of the figures were obtained. Each horizontal line represents one experiment. (From Chamley et al., 1973a.)

	Mean rate of muscle contraction (per min)			
	Before palpation	During palpation	% increase	After palpation
No NGF	1.7	3.2	88	1.8
	1.5	3.0	100	2.0
	0.5	0.8	66	—
	1.0	1.8	80	1.2
NGF	1.5	3.0	100	1.4
	3.3	5.0	82	3.8
	1.6	2.3	44	1.5
	2.3	4.1	78	2.6

In our recent experiments we have been examining the mechanism of action of guanethidine in producing these effects, including the use of tissue cultures (Hill et al., 1973; Heath et al., 1974). While it has been known for some time that the initial action of guanethidine is to damage the mitochondria (Jensen-Holm and Juul, 1971; Heath et al., 1972), it has been possible to show with time-lapse cinematography of cultured neurons that guanethidine causes *retraction* of the axons (Fig. 5b). This appears to be associated with inhibition of anterograde flow of material in the terminal varicose nerves, even while the growth cone shows near-normal palpation activity (Hill, personal communication). Axon retraction following guanethidine administration has been confirmed in studies of the vas deferens *in situ*, where loss in fibre numbers occurs but no degenerating nerves are seen (Heath *et al.*, 1974), and is in contrast to the action of 6-hydroxydopamine, which causes *fragmentation* (Fig. 5d) and degeneration of terminal varicose nerves both in culture (Hill *et al.*, 1973) and *in situ* (see Malmfors and Thoenen, 1971).

ACKNOWLEDGEMENTS

The work described in this paper was supported by grants from the National Heart Foundation of Australia and the Australian Research Grants Committee.

REFERENCES

ALOE, L., and LEVI-MONTALCINI, R. (1972) *In vitro* analysis of the frontal and ingluvial ganglia from nymphal specimens of the cockroach *Periplaneta. Brain Res.* **44,** 147–163.

BURNSTOCK, .G. (1970) Structure of smooth muscle and its innervation. In *Smooth Muscle* (Edith Bülbring, Alison Brading, Alan Jones, and Tadeo Tomita, eds.), Edward Arnold, London, pp. 1–69.

BURNSTOCK, G. (1972) Purinergic nerves. *Pharmac. Rev.* **24,** 509–581.

BURNSTOCK, G. (1974) Electronmicroscopy: vesicles, synaptic gaps, pharmacological agents. In *Methods in Pharmacology*, vol. 3, *Smooth Muscle* (E. E. Daniel and D. M. Paton, eds.), Appleton–Century–Crofts, Edmonton (in press).

BURNSTOCK, G., and IWAYAMA, T. (1971) Fine structural identification of autonomic nerves and their relation to smooth muscle. *Progress in Brain Research,* **34,** 389-404, *Histochemistry of Nervous Transmission,* Elsevier, Amsterdam.

BURNSTOCK, G., EVANS, B., GANNON, B. J., HEATH, J. W., and JAMES, V. (1971a) A new method of destroying adrenergic nerves in adult animals using guanethidine. *Br. J. Pharmac.* **43,** 295–301.

BURNSTOCK, G., GANNON, B. J., MALMFORS, T., and ROGERS, D. C. (1971b) Changes in the physiology and fine structure of the taenia of the guinea-pig caecum following transplantation into the anterior eye chamber. *J. Physiol.* **219,** 139–154.

CAJAL, S. R. Y. (1928) *Degeneration and Regeneration of the Nervous System*, vols. 1 and 2, Hafner, London, and New York.

CAMPBELL, G. R., UEHARA, Y., MALMFORS, T., and BURNSTOCK, G. (1971) Degeneration and regeneration of smooth muscle transplants in the anterior eye chamber: an ultrastructural study. *Z. Zellforsch.* **117,** 155–175.

CHAMLEY, J. H., MARK, G. E., CAMPBELL, G. R., and BURNSTOCK, G. (1972) Sympathetic ganglia in culture: I, Neurons. *Z. Zellforsch.* **135,** 287–314.

CHAMLEY, J. H., CAMPBELL, G. R., and BURNSTOCK, G. (1973a) An analysis of the interactions between sympathetic nerve fibres and smooth muscle cells in tissue culture. *Devel. Biol.* **33,** 341–361.

CHAMLEY, J., GOLLER, I., and BURNSTOCK, G. (1973b) Sympathetic nerve fibre growth to explants of autonomic effector organs in tissue culture. *Devel. Biol.* **31,** 362–379.

CHAMLEY, J., CAMPBELL, G. R., and BURNSTOCK, G. (1974) Dedifferentiation, and bundle formation of smooth muscle cells in tissue culture: the influence of cell number and nerve fibres. *J. Embryol. exp. Morph.* (in press).

EVANS, B., GANNON, B. J., HEATH, J. R., and BURNSTOCK, G. (1972) Long lasting damage to the internal male genital organs and their adrenergic innervation in rats following chronic treatment with the antihypertensive drug guanethidine. *Fertil. Steril.* **23,** 657–667.

FURNESS, J. B., McLEAN, J. R., and BURNSTOCK, G. (1970) Distribution of adrenergic nerves and changes in neuro-muscular transmission in the mouse vas deferens during postnatal development. *Devel. Biol.* **21,** 491–505.

GANNON, B. J., IWAYAMA, T., BURNSTOCK, G., GERKENS, J., and MASHFORD, M. L. (1971) Prolonged effects of chronic guanethidine treatment on the sympathetic innervation of the genitalia of male rats. *Med. J. Aust.* **2,** 207–208.

HAAS, D. C., HIER, D. B., ARNASON, B. G. W., and YOUNG, M. (1972) On a possible relationship of cyclic AMP to the mechanism of action of nerve growth factor. *Proc. Soc. Exp. Biol. Med.* **140,** 45–47.

HEATH, J. W., EVANS, B., GANNON, B. J., BURNSTOCK, G., and JAMES, V. (1972) Degeneration of adrenergic nerves following guanethidine treatment: an ultrastructural study. *Virchows Arch.,* Abt. B, Zellpath. **11,** 182–197.

HEATH, J. W., EVANS, B. K., and BURNSTOCK, G. (1974) Axon retraction following guanethidine treatment: studies of sympathetic neurons *in vivo*. *Cell. Tiss. Res.* (in press).

HEATH, J. W., HILL, C. E., and BURNSTOCK, G. (1974) Axon retraction following guanethidine treatment. Studies of sympathetic neurons in tissue culture. *J. Neurocytol.* (in press).

HIER, D. B., ARNASON, B. G. W., and YOUNG, M. (1972) Studies on the mechanism of action of nerve growth factor. *Proc. Natn. Acad. Sci. USA* **69**, 2268–2272.

HILL, C., MARK, G., ERÄNKÖ, O., ERÄNKÖ, L., and BURNSTOCK, G. (1973) The use of tissue culture to examine the action of guanethidine and 6-hydroxydopamine. *Eur. J. Pharmac.* **23**, 162–174

JENSEN-HOLM, J., and JUUL, P. (1971) Ultrastructural changes in the rat superior cervical ganglion following prolonged guanethidine administration. *Acta pharmac. tox.* **30**, 308–320.

JOHNSON, D. G., GORDON, P., and KOPIN, I. J. (1971) A sensitive radioimmunoassay for 7 S nerve growth factor antigens in serum and tissues. *J. Neurochem.* **18**, 2355–2362.

JOHNSON, D. G., SILBERSTEIN, S. D., HANBAUER, I., and KOPIN, I. J. (1972) The role of nerve growth factor in the ramification of sympathetic nerve fibres into the rat iris in organ culture. *J. Neurochem.* **19**, 2025–2029.

LANGLEY, J. N., and ANDERSON, H. K. (1904) The union of different kinds of nerve fibres. *J. Physiol. Lond.* **31**, 365–391.

LENZ, T. L. (1972) A role of cyclic AMP in a neurotrophic process. *Nature New Biol.* **238**, 154–155.

LEVI-MONTALCINI, R., and HAMBERGER, V. (1953) A diffusible agent of mouse sarcoma, producing hyperplasia of sympathetic ganglia and hyperneurotization of viscera in the chick embryo. *J. Exp. Zool.* **123**, 233–288.

LEVI-MONTALCINI, R., and ANGELETTI, P. U. (1968) Nerve growth factor. *Physiol. Rev.* **48**, 534–569.

MALMFORS, T., and THOENEN, H. (eds.) (1971) 6-*Hydroxydopamine and Catecholamine Neurons*. North-Holland, Amsterdam and London.

MALMFORS, T., FURNESS, J. B., CAMPBELL, G. R., and BURNSTOCK, G. (1971) Reinnervation of smooth muscle of the vas deferens transplanted into the anterior chamber of the eye. *J. Neurobiol.* **2**, 193–207.

MARK, G., CHAMLEY, J., and BURNSTOCK, G. (1973) Interactions between autonomic nerves and smooth and cardiac muscle cells in tissue culture. *Devel. Biol.* **32**, 194–200.

MURRAY, M. R. (1965) Nervous tissues *in vitro*. In *Cells and Tissues in Culture: Methods, Biology and Physiology* (E. N. Willmer, ed.), Academic Press, London and New York, vol. 2 pp. 373–455.

NAKAI, J., and KAWASAKI, Y. (1959) Studies on the mechanism determining the course of nerve fibres in tissue culture: I, The reaction of the growth cone to various obstructions. *Z. Zellforsch. mikrosk. Anat.* **51**, 108–122.

OLSON, L., and MALMFORS, T. (1970) Characteristics of adrenergic nerves in the adult rat: fluorescence histochemical and H³-noradrenaline uptake studies using tissue transplantations to the anterior chamber of the eye. *Acta physiol. scand.*, Suppl. 348, 1–112.

READ, J. B., and BURNSTOCK, G. (1970) Development of the adrenergic innervation and chromaffin cells in the human fetal gut. *Devel. Biol.* **22**, 513–534.

ROGERS, D. C. (1972) Cell contacts and smooth muscle bundle formation in tissue transplants into the anterior eye chamber. *Z. Zellforsch.* **133**, 113–124.

ROISEN, F. J., MURPHY, R. A., and BRADEN, W. G. (1972) Neurite development *in vitro*: I, The effects of adenosine 3′,5′,cyclic monophosphate (cyclic AMP). *J. Neurobiol.* **3**, 347–368.

YAMAUCHI, A., and BURNSTOCK, G. (1969a) Post-natal development of smooth muscle cells in the mouse vas deferens: a fine structural study. *J. Anat. Lond.* **104**, 1–15.

YAMAUCHI, A., and BURNSTOCK, G. (1969b) Post-natal development of the innervation of the mouse vas deferens: a fine structural study. *J. Anat. Lond.* **104**, 17–32.

ELECTROPHYSIOLOGICAL AND HISTOCHEMICAL PROPERTIES OF FETAL HUMAN SPINAL CORD IN TISSUE CULTURE

L. Hösli, E. Hösli, and P. F. Andrès

Department of Neurophysiology, Neurological Clinic of the University of Basle,
Socinstrasse 55, 4051 Basle, Switzerland

SUMMARY

A study was made of histochemical and electrophysiological properties of fetal human spinal cord in tissue culture. The observations that neurons in spinal cord cultures and sections prepared from older fetuses (12–18 weeks *in utero*) had a higher acetylcholinesterase (AChE) content than neurons in cultures from younger fetuses (8 weeks *in utero*) suggest that there is a correlation between the AChE content and functional development.

Microelectrode studies demonstrating that glycine hyperpolarizes human spinal neurons and that glutamate causes a depolarization, suggest that neurons of cultured human spinal cord have receptors similar to those of cultured rat spinal cord and those of cat spinal motoneurones *in situ*. An increase of extracellular potassium concentration reversibly depolarized the cell membrane of rat and human spinal neurons as well as of glial cells. These investigations show that the technique of tissue culture is a unique possibility to investigate electrophysiological and pharmacological properties of single neurons and glial cells under direct visual control and to study effects of alterations in the extra-cellular ionic environment as well as the action of neurotransmitters on the membrane potential of single cells of the human central nervous system.

The autoradiographic investigations demonstrating that ^{3}H-glycine and L-^{3}H-glutamic acid are taken up in neurons and glial cells of cultures of fetal human spinal cord indicate that the technique of tissue culture is also a good model to study the cellular localization of the uptake of putative neurotransmitters into human central nervous tissue.

INTRODUCTION

It has been shown by several authors that central nervous tissue grown in cultures retain similar morphological properties to those *in situ* (for ref. see Murray, 1965). The majority of investigations on nervous tissue cultures have been made with tissue prepared from various animals (chick, rat, mouse, kitten) and only few studies have been performed on cultures of human central nervous tissue (Hogue, 1947; Okamoto, 1958; Lapham and Markesbery, 1971; Hösli *et al.*, 1973a). Peterson *et al.* (1965) have done an extensive study on the differentiation and prolonged maintenance of organized explants of fetal human spinal cord correlating morphological development with the onset of bioelectric activity in these cultures.

From studies by Windle and Fitzgerald (1937) it is suggested that the reflex arc in human spinal cord is completed during the eighth week *in utero*. Furthermore, Youngstrom (1941), using bioassays, has shown that there is a rapid increase in acetylcholinesterase (AChE) activity in fetal human spinal cord between 8–17 weeks *in utero* suggesting a correlation between AChE content and functional development. In the present paper a histochemical study was made of the presence of AChE in neurons of fetal human spinal cord *in situ* and in tissue culture at different stages of development (8–18 weeks *in utero*).

Autoradiographic investigations on the uptake of the suspected transmitters glycine and glutamate into cultures of rat brain stem (Hösli and Hösli, 1972) and spinal cord (Hösli *et al.*, 1972a, 1973b) have shown that nervous tissue cultures are a good model to study the cellular and fine structural localization of the uptake of neurotransmitters. We were interested to investigate the cellular localization of the uptake of ^{3}H-glycine and L-^{3}H-glutamic acid into cultures of fetal human spinal cord using autoradiographic techniques.

The technique of tissue culture also offers a unique possibility to study electrophysiological and pharmacological properties of single neurons and glial cells of the human central nervous system by means of microelectrodes under direct microscopic control and to correlate morphological observations with electrophysiological results. Furthermore, tissue culture techniques also provide a useful model to study the effects of alterations in extracellular ion concentrations and the action of neurotransmitters on the membrane potential of single cells. In the present paper we have studied the influence of an increase of the extracellular potassium concentration and the effects of glycine and glutamate on the membrane potential of cultured neurons of fetal human spinal cord.

A comparison was made of the results obtained from cultured human spinal cord and those of animal spinal cord both *in situ* and in tissue culture.

I. MORPHOLOGICAL AND HISTOCHEMICAL STUDIES

(a) OUTGROWTH PATTERN AND GENERAL PROPERTIES OF CULTURES

Although the outgrowth pattern and neuronal organization of rat and mouse spinal cord in tissue cultures have been investigated extensively by many authors (Bunge *et al.*, 1965; Murray, 1965; Peterson *et al.*, 1965; Sobkowicz *et al.*, 1968; Wolff *et al.*, 1971), there are only few studies on cultures of fetal human spinal cord (Peterson *et al.*, 1965; Hösli *et al.*, 1973a).

In the present study cultures were prepared from spinal cord of human fetuses (8–18 weeks *in utero*) and cultivated for 8–56 days on collagen-coated coverslips in the Maximov assembly (Peterson *et al.*, 1965; Hösli and Hösli, 1971; Hösli *et al.*, 1973a). The outgrowth and development of the cultures were observed daily on a Zeiss reverse microscope by phase-contrast and light-microscopic optics.

As described previously, the majority of neurons and glial cells in cultures of fetal human spinal cord were more differentiated than those from cultures of cerebellum and cortex (Hösli *et al.*, 1973a). During the first week the outgrowth from the explant consists chiefly of flattened mesenchymatous cells of possible pial/vascular origin and of oligodendrocyte-like cells. Bundles of neurites accompanied by glial cells grow out from the explant (Fig. 1B). Most of the neurons usually remain in the beveled and dense zones of the cultures although healthy neurons are sometimes found in the outgrowth zones (Fig. 1A, C, and 3A).

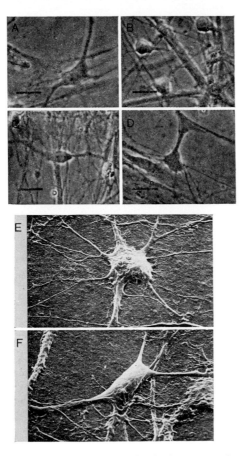

FIG. 1. A-D: Phase-contrast pictures. A, Neuron lying in the outgrowth zone of a human spinal cord culture (8 days *in vitro*, fetus 18 weeks *in utero*). Bar: 20 μm. B, Glial cells and bundles of outgrowing neurites in cultured human spinal cord (18 days *in vitro*; fetus 12 weeks *in utero*). Bar 20 μm. C, Bipolar neuron lying in the outgrowth zone approximately 100–200 μm away from the explant. Human spinal cord culture (18 days *in vitro*; fetus 12 weeks *in utero*). Bar: 20 μm. D, Astrocyte which seems to make contact with mesenchymatous cells located in the marginal zone of a human spinal cord culture (8 days *in vitro*; fetus 18 weeks *in utero*). Bar: 20 μm. E, F: Scanning electron microscopic pictures (kindly provided by Dr. F. Spinelli, Ciba-Geigy Ltd. Basel). E, Astrocyte lying in the outgrowth zone of a human spinal cord culture (10 days *in vitro*; fetus 18 weeks *in utero*). F, Neuron in the outgrowth zone of a 10-day-old spinal cord culture (human fetus 18 weeks *in utero*). Magnification for E and F: ×2400.

(b) CYTOLOGICAL PROPERTIES OF THE VARIOUS CELL TYPES

The identification of the various cell types was made by their morphological appearance using phase-contrast microscopy and by Nissl staining.

In the marginal zones spindle shaped/discus-like cells were observed with round or oval nuclei generally containing multiple nucleoli. These cells derive presumably from connective tissue of the blood vessels and from unremoved parts of the meninges. The glial cells show many morphological features of protoplasmic astrocytes, but also fibrillar astrocytes were observed (Wolff *et al.*, 1971). The cell bodies of the astrocytes vary considerably in size and shape. The nuclei were generally oval or round with 2–3 nucleoli (Fig. 1D). The cytoplasm of the cell body often contains granular inclusions and usually appears pale in phase contrast microscopy. Numerous processes arise from the perikarya often forming a dense network in the outgrowth zone. The cell bodies of oligodendrocytes are much smaller than those of astrocytes and the cytoplasm is very dense with a hardly visible nucleus. The neurons were identified by their size, shape, and nuclear morphology as well as by their location in the culture. The majority of neurons remain in or at the edge of the explant, those at the edge being surrounded by astrocytes and their processes. Figures 1A and c illustrate neurons lying in the outgrowth zone approximately 100–200 μm away from the explant. These neurons have a well-defined nuclear membrane with a prominent nucleolus and several thick dendrites. The axon, which is usually much thinner than the dendrites and arises more abruptly from the cell body, cannot be clearly identified in these cells. After staining with toluidine blue, the neurons lying in the dense and beveled zones of the cultures revealed abundant Nissl substance whereas neurons which have migrated to the outgrowth zone contained less Nissl bodies. Many of these cytological features have also been observed in electronmicroscopic studies (Wolff *et al.*, 1971; Wolff *et al.*, unpublished observations).

(c) ONTOGENESIS OF AChE ACTIVITY IN SPINAL CORD *IN SITU* AND IN TISSUE CULTURE

A study was made of the AChE activity in cultured spinal cord prepared from human fetuses at different ages *in utero* (8–18 weeks) in order to investigate if there are differences in AChE content at various stages of development. The method of Karnovsky and Roots (1964) modified by El Badawi and Schenk (1967) was used to demonstrate the presence of AChE. Iso-OMPA (tetraisopropyl pyrophosphoramide) was added to the incubation medium to inhibit non-specific cholinesterase activity (for details see also Hösli and Hösli, 1971; Hösli *et al.*, 1973a).

In almost all the spinal cord cultures (8–22 days *in vitro*) AChE-containing neurons were observed. Although the AChE content varied considerably between individual cells, it was found that neurons lying in the dense and beveled zones of the cultures usually showed a higher AChE activity than neurons located in the outgrowth zones. Similar observations have been made in cultures of rat spinal cord (Hösli and Hösli, 1971). It was also observed that neurons in cultures prepared from young fetuses (8 weeks *in utero*) usually had a lower AChE content than cultured neurons obtained from spinal cord of older fetuses (12–18 weeks *in utero*). Figure 2A illustrates a large spinal neuron of a fetus of 8 weeks *in utero* showing a much lower AChE activity than the neuron in Figure 2B which is from a spinal cord culture obtained from a fetus of 12 weeks *in utero*. The enzyme was unevenly distributed in the cytoplasm of the perikaryon and sometimes also of the dendrites. The axons were only faintly stained. Several neurons did not stain for AChE. Glial cells usually contained no AChE.

Some studies were also performed on sections of human spinal cord obtained from fetuses of 8 and 18 weeks *in utero*. In these sections groups of large AChE-containing neurons mainly located in the ventral horns were observed. The neurons of the sections from the 18-week-old fetus revealed a considerably higher AChE activity (Fig. 2D) than those in the sections of the 8-week-old fetus (not illustrated). Similar observations were made by Duckett and Pearse (1969) in an extensive study on the developing human spinal cord.

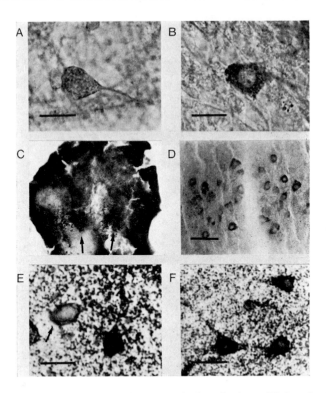

FIG. 2. A, Neuron with low AChE activity in a spinal cord culture (18 days *in vitro*) from a human fetus, 8 weeks *in utero*. Bar: 20 μm. B, Spinal neuron of a culture (15 days *in vitro*) from a human fetus of 12 weeks *in utero* showing a higher AChE content. Bar: 20 μm. C, Explant of a spinal cord culture (22 days *in vitro*) of a human fetus 17 weeks *in utero* with two groups of AChE-containing neurones (arrows). (×55.) D, Spinal cord section of an 18-week-old human fetus. Groups of large AChE-containing neurons lying in the ventral horns. Bar: 30 μm. E, Autoradiograph of an 18-day-old spinal cord culture (human fetus, 12 weeks *in utero*) after incubation with ^{3}H-glycine, 10^{-6} M for 5 min. One neuron shows a strong accumulation of grains whereas the other cell (arrow) seems to be free of label. Bar: 20 μm. F, Spinal cord culture of a 12-week-old human fetus (18 days *in vitro*) incubated with L-^{3}H-glutamic acid, 10^{-6} M, for 5 min. Neurons showing an intense autoradiographic reaction over the cell bodies and processes. Bar: 20 μm.

Groups of large intensely stained neurons were also observed in spinal cord cultures prepared from fetuses of 17 and 18 weeks *in utero*, suggesting an organotypic organization of these cultures (Fig. 2c).

Our findings that the AChE content is much higher in neurons of spinal cord cultures and sections prepared from older fetuses (12–18 weeks *in utero*) than from younger ones (8 weeks *in utero*) are consistent with pharmacological studies by Youngstrom (1941) on fetal human spinal cord *in situ* demonstrating a rapid increase of AChE activity between 8–17 weeks *in utero*.

As was already observed in rat spinal cord cultures (Hösli and Hösli, 1971) our results suggest that neurons of fetal human spinal cord in tissue culture have similar histochemical properties to neurons of fetal human spinal cord *in situ* (Duckett and Pearse, 1969).

(d) AUTORADIOGRAPHIC STUDIES ON THE UPTAKE OF ^{3}H-GLYCINE AND L-^{3}H-GLUTAMIC ACID

In recent years evidence has accumulated that uptake may be an important mechanism for terminating the action of neurotransmitters such as monoamines and amino acids (Iversen, 1967; Iversen and Neal, 1968; Neal, 1971). Specific uptake mechanisms for several transmitter substances into various regions of the central nervous system were demonstrated by several authors (for ref. see Snyder *et al.*, 1970). It has been shown that the putative transmitters glycine and glutamate are taken up by a high affinity transport system into slices and synaptosomes of rat spinal cord (Snyder *et al.*, 1970; Johnston and Iversen, 1971; Hammerschlag and Weinstein, 1972; Logan and Snyder, 1972). Although few studies on the cellular and fine structural localization of the uptake of glycine and glutamate into rat central nervous tissue have been made (Matus and Dennison, 1971; Hökfelt and Ljungdahl, 1971, 1972; Iversen and Bloom, 1972; Hösli and Hösli, 1972; Hösli *et al.*, 1972a, 1973b) there is no information to our knowledge available on the cellular localization of the uptake of these amino acids into human central nervous system.

In the present investigation we have studied the localization of the uptake of glycine and glutamate into cultures of fetal human spinal cord using autoradiographic techniques.

The cultures were incubated with either ^{3}H-glycine or L-^{3}H-glutamic acid (10^{-6} M, specific activity: 4.7 C/mM and 20.4 C/mM respectively, New England Nuclear Corp.) in Hanks solution for 1–5 min, rinsed in Tyrode solution, fixed in Susa, and dehydrated. The air-dried cultures were mounted on object slides covered with Ilford L4 emulsion by the loop technique and developed after 2 weeks (for details see Hösli and Hösli, 1972). As has been described previously in rat spinal cord cultures (Hösli *et al.*, 1972a, 1973b), ^{3}H-glycine and L-^{3}H-glutamic acid have also been taken up in a large number of neurons and glial cells in cultures of human spinal cord. The accumulation of grains was observed to cover the cell body and processes of neurons as well as of glial cells. Figure 2E illustrates a light microscopic autoradiograph of two neurons from a fetal human spinal cord culture after incubation with ^{3}H-glycine (10^{-6} M) for 5 min. One neuron reveals an intense autoradiographic reaction whereas the other cell seems to be free of label. Figure 2F shows intensely labeled neurons of a 15-day-old spinal cord culture after incubation with L-^{3}H-glutamic acid (10^{-6} M) for 5 min.

The activity of the amino acids varied considerably between individual neurons whereas glial cells showed a more even distribution of grains. Preliminary investigations have shown that ^{3}H-glycine and L-^{3}H-glutamic acid were also taken up by neurons and glial cells in cultures of fetal human brain stem.

Our autoradiographic studies show that fetal human spinal cord in tissue culture reveals a similar uptake pattern for glycine and glutamate as cultures of rat spinal cord and that the technique of tissue culture also provides a good model to study the uptake of neurotransmitters into human central nervous system.

II. ELECTROPHYSIOLOGICAL STUDIES

(a) MEMBRANE POTENTIALS

For the electrophysiological experiments the cultures were placed in a perfusion chamber (Andrès and Hösli, 1972) which was mounted on a reverse microscope. Microelectrodes (3 M KCl, 1 M K-acetate, and 1 M K-citrate) were introduced into the cultures by a Leitz

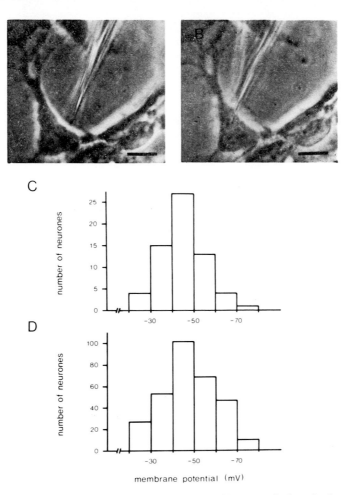

FIG. 3. A, B, Phase-contrast pictures of a neuron of a fetal human spinal cord culture (8 days *in vitro*; fetus 11 weeks *in utero*). A, before, and B, after, impalement with the microelectrode. Bar: 10 μm. C, D, Histograms showing the distribution of membrane potentials of 64 human spinal neurons (C) and 308 rat spinal neurons (D) in tissue culture.

micromanipulator under direct visual control. The technique is described in detail in previous publications (Hösli *et al.*, 1971, 1972c). Intracellular microelectrode recordings were made from neurons (Fig. 3A, B) and glial cells in the dense zones of the explant as well as in the zones of migration of cultures of fetal human spinal cord (8–56 days *in vitro*, fetuses 8–18 weeks *in utero*). As was observed previously in cultures of rat spinal cord (Hösli *et al.*, 1971, 1972c), it was often difficult to impale cells and to maintain stable membrane potentials over a longer period of time. In most cells the membrane potential decayed within several seconds after impalement. However, in a small number of cells stable membrane potentials could be recorded for up to 30 min. After penetration with the microelectrode we often observed morphological changes of the cells which were usually accompanied by a fall in membrane potentials (Hösli *et al.*, 1971, 1972c). The membrane potentials of 64 human spinal neurons ranged from -25 mV to -74 mV with an average of -44.2 ± 9.8 mV. The frequency distribution of membrane potentials of these neurons is illustrated in Fig. 3c. A comparison of this histogram with that in Fig. 3D which was obtained from 308 neurons of rat spinal cord cultures shows a similar distribution pattern with a mean value of −45.4 ± 12.7 mV. The relatively wide scatter of membrane potentials might be due to differences in the morphology of the cultures (outgrowth pattern, collagen layers), to different ways of penetrating the cell membrane and to slight differences in microelectrode properties. Using the same recording electrode we have observed considerable differences in membrane potentials between individual cells in the same culture but even more between different cultures, although the impaled cells had a similar morphological appearance. Microelectrode recordings were also made from cells which were identified by their morphological appearance as astrocytes. The membrane potentials ranged from −32 mV to −80 mV. Seven out of seventeen cells had membrane potentials between −68 and −80 mV. In three cells we were able to record stable membrane potentials of −80 mV for several minutes. These values were higher than those recorded from neurons which were usually less than −70 mV (Fig. 3c).

It has also been shown in other mammals (Krnjević and Schwartz, 1967; Grossman and Hampton, 1968; Dennis and Gerschenfeld, 1969) and in the leech (Nicholls and Kuffler, 1964) that neuroglial cells usually have higher membrane potentials than neurons, although Trachtenberg *et al.* (1972) recorded only very low resting potentials (average −7.7 mV) from cultured glial cells of fetal human cortex.

As we have reported in cultures of rat spinal cord (Hösli *et al.*, 1972b), we occasionally observed spontaneous discharges of action potentials from a few neurons of human spinal cord.

(b) EFFECTS OF AN INCREASE OF THE EXTRACELLULAR POTASSIUM CONCENTRATION ON THE MEMBRANE POTENTIAL

It has been shown by several authors (Huxley and Stämpfli, 1951; Hodgkin and Keynes, 1955; Adrian, 1956; Nicholls and Kuffler, 1964) that the membrane potential of excitable cells can be altered by changes in extracellular potassium concentrations, e.g. an increase of the external potassium concentration causes a marked depolarization of the cell membrane.

The effect of an increase in extracellular potassium concentration on the membrane potential was studied on nine neurons and three glial cells in cultures of fetal human spinal cord (for details about method, see Hösli *et al.*, 1972c). As was observed in neurons of rat spinal cord cultures (Fig. 4B), an increase of the potassium concentration from 5 mM (normal bathing fluid) to 50 mM caused a marked depolarization of the cell membrane of human spinal neurons (Fig. 4A). This depolarization was reversible after changing to normal bathing fluid (5 mM). A similar action of an increase of potassium in the bathing fluid was observed on the membrane potential of three glial cells (Fig. 4C). Studies by Nicholls and Kuffler (1964) which related the change of membrane potentials in glial cells and the relative K^+-concentration in the bathing fluid suggest that glial cells behave like a K^+-electrode over a wide range of extracellular K^+-concentrations.

(c) ACTION OF GLYCINE AND GLUTAMATE ON THE MEMBRANE POTENTIAL

There is strong electrophysiological evidence for glycine and glutamate to function as transmitter substances in the mammalian spinal cord. Glutamate depolarizes the membrane

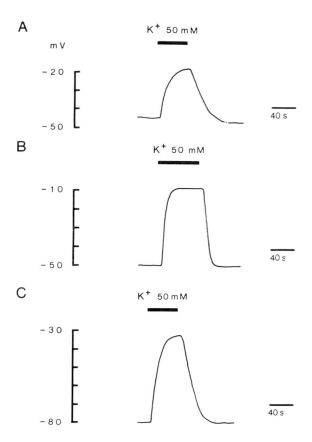

FIG. 4. Effects of an increase of the extracellular potassium concentration on the membrane potential. A, Neuron of fetal human spinal cord (15 days *in vitro*; fetus 11 weeks *in utero*). B, Rat spinal neuron (35 days *in vitro*). C, Glial cell of a human spinal cord culture (15 days *in vitro*; fetus 11 weeks *in utero*). Duration of perfusion with 50 mM potassium (K⁺ 50 mM) is indicated by bar above tracings. Ordinate: membrane potential in mV. Time: bar represents 40 s.

of cat spinal motoneurons *in situ* (Curtis *et al.*, 1972) and of rat spinal neurons in tissue culture (Hösli *et al.*, 1973b), whereas glycine causes a hyperpolarization associated with an increase in membrane conductance (Curtis *et al.*, 1968; Werman *et al.*, 1968; Hösli *et al.*, 1971, 1973b). In the present investigation we studied the action of glycine and glutamate on neurons of cultures of fetal human spinal cord. Glutamate (10^{-4} M) added to the bathing fluid (for details, see Hösli *et al.*, 1973b) caused a depolarization of the cell membrane (Fig. 5B) similar to that observed in cultured neurons of rat spinal cord (Fig. 5A) whereas glycine administered with the same concentration hyperpolarized the cell membrane of another human spinal neuron (Fig. 5C). Similar observations of the action of glutamate and glycine have been made on eight and five other human spinal neurons respectively.

Our microelectrode studies suggest that neurons of fetal human spinal cord grown in culture have similar electrophysiological and pharmacological properties to those of cultured rat spinal cord and those of cat spinal neurons *in situ*.

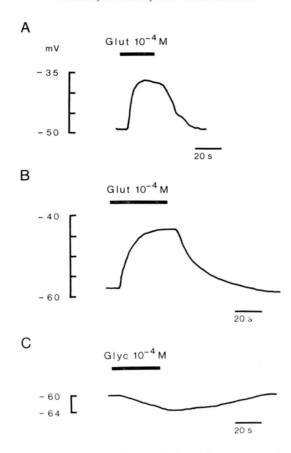

FIG. 5. Depolarization by glutamate (Glut 10^{-4} M) and hyperpolarization by glycine (Glyc 10^{-4} M) of spinal neurons in tissue culture. A, Neuron of a human fetus (11 weeks *in utero*; 12 days *in vitro*). B, Rat spinal neuron (16 days *in vitro*). C, Human spinal neuron (15 days *in vitro*; fetus 11 weeks *in utero*). Duration of perfusion with the amino acids is indicated by horizontal bar above tracings. Ordinate: membrane potential in mV. Time: bar represents 20 s.

ACKNOWLEDGEMENTS

We are grateful to Prof. J. R. Wolff, Max Planck Institut für Biophysikalische Chemie, Göttingen, for his valuable comments on the manuscript, to Dr. Ph. Heitz, Pathological Institute, University of Basel, for helpful technical advice and for preparing the spinal cord sections, and to Dr. F. Spinelli, Ciba-Geigy Ltd., Basel, for the scanning electron micrographs (Fig. 1E, F). We should also like to thank Miss D. Poms for typing the manuscript.

REFERENCES

ADRIAN, R. H. (1956) The effect of internal and external potassium concentration on the membrane potential of frog muscle. *J. Physiol. Lond.* **133**, 631–658.

ANDRÈS, P. F., and HÖSLI, L. (1972) Eine Perfusionskammer für in vitro Versuche unter mikroskopischer Kontrolle. *Microscopica acta* **73**, 38–44.

BUNGE, R. P., BUNGE, M. B., and PETERSON, E. R. (1965) An electron microscope study of cultured rat spinal cord. *J. Cell Biol.* **24**, 163–191.

CRAIN, S. M. (1966) Development of "organotypic" bioelectric activities in central nervous tissues during maturation in culture. *Int. Rev. Neurobiol.* **9**, 1–43.

CURTIS, D. R., HÖSLI, L., JOHNSTON, G. A. R., and JOHNSTON, I. H. (1968) The hyperpolarization of spinal motoneurones by glycine and related amino acids. *Expl. Brain Res.* **5**, 235–258.

CURTIS, D. R., DUGGAN, A. W., FELIX, D., JOHNSTON, G. A. R., TEBĒCIS, A. K., and WATKINS, J. C. (1972) Excitation of mammalian central neurones by acidic amino acids. *Brain Res.* **41**, 283–301.

DENNIS, M. J., and GERSCHENFELD, H. M. (1969) Some physiological properties of identified mammalian neuroglial cells. *J. Physiol. Lond.* **203**, 211–222.

DUCKETT, S., and PEARSE, A. G. E. (1969) Histoenzymology of the developing human spinal cord. *Anat. Rec.* **163**, 59–66.

EL BADAWI, A., and SCHENK, E. A. (1967) Histochemical methods for separate, consecutive and simultaneous demonstration of acetylcholinesterase and norepinephrine in cryostat sections. *J. Histochem. Cytochem.* **15**, 580–588.

GROSSMAN, R. G., and HAMPTON, T. (1968) Depolarization of cortical glial cells during electrocortical activity. *Brain Res.* **11**, 316–324.

HAMMERSCHLAG, R., and WEINSTEIN, D. (1972) Glutamic acid and primary afferent transmission. In *Studies of Neurotransmitters at the Synaptic Level, Advances in Biochemical Psychopharmacology*, vol. 6 (E. Costa, L. L. Iversen, and R. Paoletti, eds.), Raven Press, New York, pp. 165–180.

HODGKIN, A. L., and KEYNES, R. D. (1955) The potassium permeability of a giant nerve fibre. *J. Physiol. Lond.* **128**, 61–88.

HOGUE, M. J. (1947) Human fetal brain cells in tissue cultures: their identification and motility. *J. Exp. Zool.* **106**, 85–108.

HÖKFELT, T., and LJUNGDAHL, Å. (1971) Light and electron microscopic autoradiography on spinal cord slices after incubation with labeled glycine. *Brain Res.* **32**, 189–194.

HÖKFELT, T., and LJUNGDAHL, Å. (1972) Application of cytochemical techniques to the study of suspected transmitter substances in the nervous system. In *Studies of Neurotransmitters at the Synaptic Level, Advances in Biochemical Psychopharmacology*, vol. 6, (E. Costa, L. L. Iversen, and R. Paoletti, eds.), Raven Press, New York, pp. 1–35.

HÖSLI, E., and HÖSLI, L. (1971) Acetylcholinesterase in cultured rat spinal cord. *Brain Res.* **30**, 193–197.

HÖSLI, L., and HÖSLI, E. (1972) Autoradiographic localization of the uptake of glycine in cultures of rat medulla oblongata. *Brain Res.* **45**, 612–616.

HÖSLI, L., ANDRÈS, P. F., and HÖSLI, E. (1971) Effects of glycine on spinal neurones grown in tissue culture. *Brain Res.* **34**, 399–402.

HÖSLI, E., LJUNGDAHL, Å., HÖKFELT, T., and HÖSLI, L. (1972a) Spinal cord tissue cultures—a model for autoradiographic studies on uptake of putative neurotransmitters such as glycine and GABA. *Experientia* **28**, 1342–1344.

HÖSLI, L., ANDRÈS, P. F., and HÖSLI, E. (1972b) Electrophysiological properties of spinal neurones in tissue culture. *Experientia* **28**, 728.

HÖSLI, L., ANDRÈS, P. F., and HÖSLI, E. (1972c) Effects of potassium on the membrane potential of spinal neurones in tissue culture. *Pflügers Arch.* **333**, 362–365.

HÖSLI, L., ANDRÈS, P. F., and HÖSLI, E. (1972d) Electrophysiological and pharmacological studies of cultured human and rat central nervous tissue. *Pflügers Arch.* **335**, Suppl. R 80.

HÖSLI, L., HÖSLI, E., and ANDRÈS, P. F. (1973a) Light microscopic and electrophysiological studies of cultured human central nervous tissue. *Eur. Neurol.* **9**, 121–130.

HÖSLI, L., HÖSLI, E., and ANDRÈS, P. F. (1973b) Nervous tissue cultures—a model to study action and uptake of putative neurotransmitters such as amino acids. *Brain Res.* **62**, 597–602.

HUXLEY, A. F., and STÄMPFLI, R. (1951) Effect of potassium and sodium on resting and action potentials of single myelinated nerve fibres. *J. Physiol. Lond.* **112**, 496–508.

IVERSEN, L. L. (1967) *The Uptake and Storage of Noradrenaline in Sympathetic Nerves*, Cambridge University Press, p. 253.

IVERSEN, L. L., and BLOOM, F. E. (1972) Studies of the uptake of ^{3}H-GABA and (^{3}H) glycine in slices and homogenates of rat brain and spinal cord by electron microscopic autoradiography. *Brain Res.* **41**, 131–143.

IVERSEN, L. L., and NEAL, M. J. (1968) The uptake of (^{3}H) GABA by slices of rat cerebral cortex. *J. Neurochem.* **15**, 1141–1149.

JOHNSTON, G. A. R., and IVERSEN, L. L. (1971) Glycine uptake in rat central nervous system slices and homogenates: evidence for different uptake systems in spinal cord and cerebral cortex. *J. Neurochem.* **18**, 1951–1961.

KARNOVSKY, M. J., and ROOTS, L. (1964) A "direct-coloring" thiocholine method for cholinesterase. *J. Histochem. Cytochem.* **12**, 219–221.

KRNJEVIĆ, K., and SCHWARTZ, S. (1967) Some properties of unresponsive cells in the cerebral cortex. *Expl. Brain Res.* **3**, 306–319.

LAPHAM, L. W., and MARKESBERY, W. R. (1971) Human fetal cerebellar cortex: Organization and maturation of cells *in vitro*. *Science* **173**, 829–832.

LOGAN, W. J., and SNYDER, S. H. (1972) High affinity uptake systems for glycine, glutamic and aspartic acids in synaptosomes of rat central nervous tissues. *Brain Res.* **42**, 413–431.

MATUS, A. I., and DENNISON, M. E. (1971) Autoradiographic localisation of tritiated glycine at "flat-vesicle" synapses in spinal cord. *Brain Res.* **32**, 195–197.

MURRAY, M. R. (1965) Nervous tissues *in vitro*. In *Cells and Tissues in Culture, Methods, Biology and Physiology* (Willmer, E. N. ed.), Academic Press, vol. 2, pp. 373–455.

NEAL, M. J. (1971) The uptake of (^{14}C) glycine by slices of mammalian spinal cord. *J. Physiol. Lond.* **215**, 103–117.

NICHOLLS, J. G., and KUFFLER, S. W. (1964) Extracellular space as a pathway for exchange between blood and neurons in the central nervous system of the leech: ionic composition of glial cells and neurons. *J. Neurophysiol.* **27**, 645–671.

OKAMOTO, M. (1958) Observations on neurons and neuroglia from the area of the reticular formation in tissue culture. *Z. Zellforsch.* **47**, 269–287.

PETERSON, E. R., CRAIN, S. M., and MURRAY, M. R. (1965) Differentiation and prolonged maintenance of bioelectrically active spinal cord cultures (rat, chick and human). *Z. Zellforsch.* **66**, 130–154.

SNYDER, S. H., KUHAR, M. J., GREEN, A. I., COYLE, J. T. and SHASKAN, E. G. (1970) Uptake and subcellular localization of neurotransmitters in the brain. *Int. Rev. Neurobiol.* **13**, 127–159.

SOBKOWICZ, H. M., GUILLERY, R. W., and BORNSTEIN, M. B. (1968) Neuronal organization in long term cultures of the spinal cord of the fetal mouse. *J. Comp. Neurol.* **132**, 365–396.

TRACHTENBERG, M. C., KORNBLITH, P. L., and HÄUPTLI, J. (1972) Biophysical properties of cultured human glial cells. *Brain Res.* **38**, 279–298.

WERMAN, R., DAVIDOFF, R. A., and APRISON, M. H. (1968) Inhibitory action of glycine on spinal neurons in the cat. *J. Neurophysiol.* **31**, 81–95.

WINDLE, W. F., and FITZGERALD, J. E. (1937) Development of the spinal reflex mechanism in human embryos. *J. Comp. Neurol.* **67**, 493–509.

WOLFF, J. R., HÖSLI, E., and HÖSLI, L. (1971) Basement membrane material and glial cells in spinal cord cultures of newborn rats. *Brain Res.* **32**, 198–202.

YOUNGSTROM, K. A. (1941) Acetylcholine esterase concentration during the development of the human fetus. *J. Neurophysiol.* **4**, 473–477.

RECEPTOR CHANGES IN RELATION TO DEGENERATION AND DEVELOPMENT OF NEURONS AND DRUG TREATMENT

SESSION I

Chairman: S. THESLEFF

AUTONOMIC NEURO-RECEPTOR MECHANISMS IN BRAIN VESSELS

Ch. Owman, L. Edvinsson, and K. C. Nielsen

Departments of Histology and Neurosurgery A, University of Lund, Lund, Sweden

SUMMARY

Intracranial vessels are well innervated by both adrenergic and cholinergic nerves. The vessels possess adrenergic and cholinergic receptors. A strong vasomotor response can be provoked by various amines, and noradrenaline in the perivascular nerve plexus can be released from the axons in amounts sufficient to induce strong local vasoconstriction. The close relationship between adjacent perivascular cholinergic and adrenergic nerve terminals, also in the effector area, suggests axonal interaction. It is proposed that the autonomic innervation of brain vessels participates in the control not only of the cerebral circulation but also of associated intracranial pressure phenomena.

INTRODUCTION

Problems concerning the existence of autonomic receptors in the smooth musculature of pial and intracerebral vessels have usually been linked together with the question of an autonomic innervation of these brain vessels, although there are examples of vascular areas that possess autonomic receptors but are devoid of nerve supply (see Owman *et al.*, 1973). Morphological evidence for the presence of nerves associated with the brain circulation has been presented through many years, but the histological methods applied have been non-specific and therefore usually non-selective, and they have seldom been accompanied with conformative denervation experiments. A number of these and related aspects have recently been reviewed by, e.g. Rosenblum (1965, 1971), Nelson and Rennels (1970a), and Purves (1972). Although Forbes and Wolff (1928) obtained convincing early evidence that electric stimulation of nerves in the neck region elicits a vasomotor reaction, the relatively slight effect of nerve stimulation on cerebrovascular calibre and/or flow, compared with the action of vasomotor nerves in other organs, has been taken as a strong indication for the lack of neural control of the brain circulation. Unfortunately, the interpretation of certain negative electronmicroscopic findings has assisted many investigators in their doubt about the involvement of a neurogenic mechanism: thus Pease and Molinari (1960) concluded that the smooth musculature of pial blood vessels is without innervation because no

535

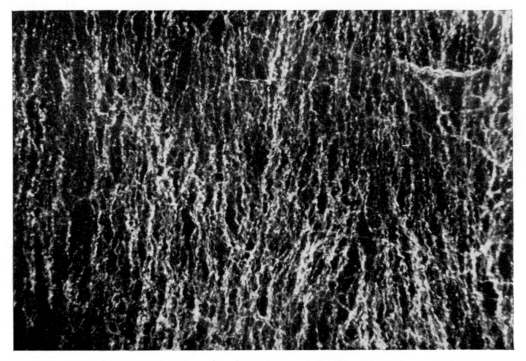

FIG. 1. Fluorescence photomicrograph of stretch-preparation of cat's anterior cerebral artery which has been cut open longitudinally and mounted flat on the microscope slide followed by formaldehyde gas treatment under dry conditions. A very dense plexus of green-fluorescent adrenergic nerves is seen in the wall of the artery. ($\times$180.)

nerves penetrated into the tunica media from the adventitia, and Samarasinghe (1965) could only detect nerve fibres around the larger extracerebral arteries. More recent observations on several types of vascular beds have demonstrated that the penetration of nerves into the tunica media is *not* a prerequisite for a vasomotor innervation and, furthermore, that smaller extra- as well as intracerebral vessels (arterioles) in fact *are* supplied with autonomic nerve fibres.

ADRENERGIC INNERVATION

The Falck–Hillarp fluorescence method for the histochemical demonstration of noradrenaline (Björklund *et al.*, 1972) has proved to be a highly specific and sensitive neuroanatomical technique for the localization and mapping of sympathetic nerves. Using this method, Falck *et al.* (1965) were able to establish beyond doubt that pial arteries are accompanied by adrenergic nerves which arise from the superior cervical sympathetic ganglia. In some pial vascular areas (Nielsen and Owman, 1967) the adrenergic nerve plexus is more dense (Fig. 1) than in any other region of the body, including the mesenteric circulation (Falck, 1962). Fluorescent nerve terminals were also found to accompany or enclose arterioles, both in the extracerebral (Fig. 2a) and the intracerebral vascular beds (Fig. 2b). The arteriolar nerve plexus is not particularly dense, which, however, does not necessarily imply that the innervation is scarce: the number of nerves may well be sufficient to supply the

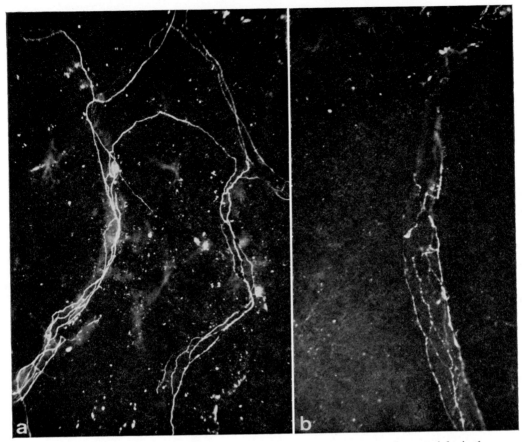

FIG. 2. Fluorescence photomicrograph of adrenergic nerve fibres accompanying arterioles in the cat's brain. (a) Pial arteriole. Granular material in the leptomeningeal tissue is autofluorescent. (×125.) (b) Intracerebral arteriole branching into the brain from the pial arteries visible in the upper left margin of the picture. (×250.)

relatively small volume of musculature present in the wall of the arteriole. It is notable that also the intracranial veins receive a substantial amount of adrenergic nerve terminals. This vascular innervation pattern of the brain has since been confirmed in numerous studies on a variety of mammals, including man (for references, see Edvinsson et al., 1972a).

It has recently been proposed, on the basis of immunohistochemical localization of dopamine-β-hydroxylase, that intracerebral arteries are innervated also by adrenergic fibres which are non-sympathetic, originating from an intracerebral source, probably the locus coeruleus (Hartman et al., 1972; Hartman and Udenfriend, 1972). A close relation of single adrenergic nerve terminals to the wall of many small intracerebral vessels (Fig. 3) has been confirmed (Edvinsson et al., 1973a) by formaldehyde histochemistry carried out on Vibratome sections (Hökfelt and Ljungdahl, 1972) from mesencephalon. The neurovascular arrangement resembles that observed with the formaldehyde technique also by Csillik et al. (1971) in the hypothalamus. However, the significance of the findings is difficult to evaluate as it is not yet established whether—in an ultrastructural and functional sense—this close topographical relationship reflects a true innervation of certain

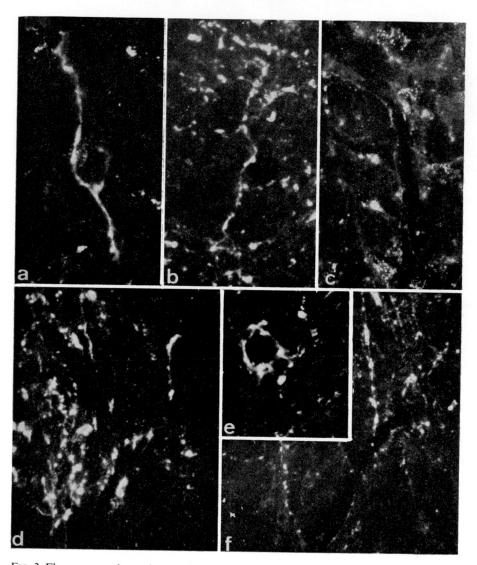

Fig. 3. Fluorescence photomicrographs of Vibratome sections from rat brain stem showing examples of close relationships between central catecholamine fibres and small intracerebral blood vessels. (a) and (b) When axons override the vessel they issue small branches forming a loop around its wall; (c) and (d) fluorescent nerve terminals run along vessels for a considerable distance; (e) several terminals enclose a vessel; and (f) two axons with well visible varicosities approach a vessel, the right nerve crossing the vessel to continue downwards to the left along its right side. (×325.)

brain vessels by intracerebral, non-sympathetic adrenergic nerves. An interesting result that should be mentioned in this context is that the regenerative sprouting of dopamine axons, which can be induced by lesions in the mesencephalon, also includes a massive growth of nerves into the walls of brain vessels previously deprived of their noradrenaline innervation by sympathectomy (Katzman et al., 1971).

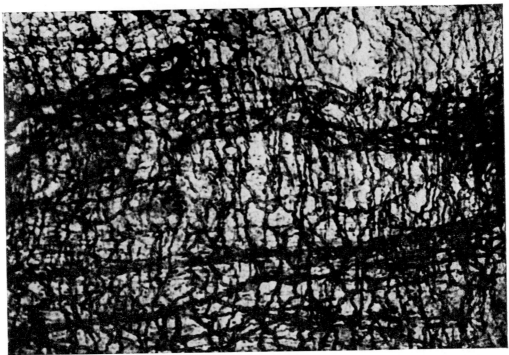

FIG. 4. Stretch-preparation of cat's anterior cerebral artery prepared as described in Fig. 1 and incubated fresh during 4 h in a buffer containing acetylthiocholine, after preincubation with the cholinesterase inhibitor Mipafox. A dense plexus of acetylcholinesterase-containing cholinergic nerve fibres is present in the arterial wall. (×180.)

CHOLINERGIC INNERVATION

The histochemical cholinesterase technique, in combination with appropriate enzyme inhibition (Holmstedt, 1957; Koelle, 1963), is at present the most reliable technique for demonstration of cholinergic nerves at the level of optical microscopy. It has been applied to localize acetylcholinesterase-containing nerves, and we have tried to correlate their distribution with the adrenergic innervation in the brain circulation. Confirming the observations by Plechkova *et al.* (1969) and Motavkin and Dovbish (1971), a rich supply of cholinergic nerves (Fig. 4) was found around the pial vessels (Edvinsson *et al.*, 1972a); fibres also entered the brain together with the intracerebral vascular branches (Motavkin and Dovbish, 1971). This dual adrenergic/cholinergic vascular supply is a common phenomenon (Schenk and el Badawi, 1968), although there are exceptions: most vessels in, for example, the mesenterial circulation seem to receive only adrenergic fibres. In the brain vessels the regional distribution of the cholinesterase-containing nerve plexuses closely resembled those of adrenergic nerves (cf. Fig. 1). This gave us reason to analyze the arrangement in some more detail (Edvinsson *et al.*, 1972a). When mild formaldehyde gas treatment was first applied to whole mounts of pial vessels (for demonstration of adrenergic nerves) and, after photography, was followed by extended incubation in the presence of acetylthiocholine and Mipafox (to show cholinergic nerves), re-photography revealed that the two systems of fibres usually ran side by side in the strands of the autonomic nerve plexuses

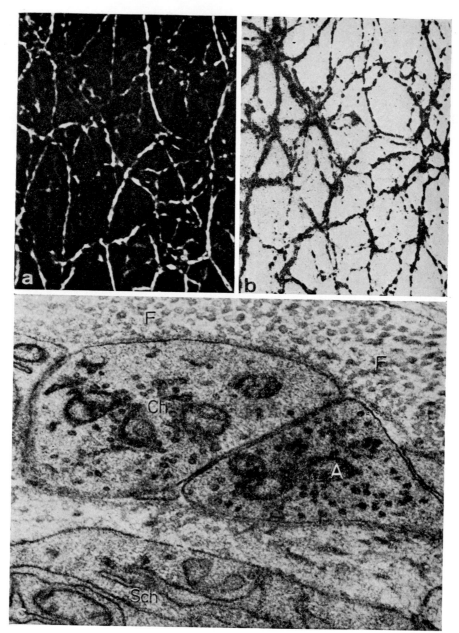

FIG. 5. Cat's posterior cerebral artery, stretch-preparation first treated (a) with formaldehyde gas at 37°C for 20 min for visualization of noradrenaline and subsequently, (b) incubated during 10 h for staining of acetylcholinesterase. There is a close correspondence between the adrenergic and cholinergic nerve plexuses. (×230.) (c) Electron micrograph of the cat's anterior cerebral artery after potassium permanganate fixation. Cholinergic nerve varicosity (Ch) containing electron-lucent synaptic vesicles and mitochondria located in close apposition to an adrenergic varicosity (A) containing mitochondria and electron-dense synaptic vesicles. Adventitial cholagenous fibres (F) and Schwann cell (Sch.) (×60,000.)

(Fig. 5a, b). This close relationship between adrenergic and cholinergic terminals could be confirmed by electronmicroscopy which, moreover, showed that the axonal membranes from adjacent varicosities sometimes were separated only by a 250 Å distance (Fig. 5c), thus offering a structural possibility for a functional interaction between the two systems of nerves of the kind referred to by Ehinger *et al.* (1970).

Denervation experiments have established that all cerebral adrenergic nerves arise in the superior cervical ganglia. Excision of these ganglia does not overtly affect the number of cholinesterase-containing nerves. The conditions under which the acetylcholinesterase reaction developed indicated that the cholinergic nerves are parasympathetic rather than sensory. The parasympathetic fibres have been found to run, via the facial nerve, in the greater superficial petrosal nerve (Chorobski and Penfield, 1932; see also Nelson and Rennels, 1970a; Edvinsson *et al.*, 1972a).

ULTRASTRUCTURAL ASPECTS

Both the adrenergic and cholinergic nerve terminals, running in the adventitia, reach the superficial layer of the smooth muscle cells in the tunica media of the pial arteries (Fig. 6) and approach the cell membrane with a distance of about 1000 Å (Sato, 1966; Hagen and Wittkowski, 1969; Iwayama *et al.*, 1970; Nelson and Rennels, 1970a, b; Nielsen *et al.*, 1971a). The terminals were sometimes found to lie in a shallow trough of the smooth muscle cell, but they never penetrated further in between the muscle cells of the media. The neuro-muscular contacts thus have the same appearance as in those vascular areas where a functioning autonomic innervation has been proven (for references, see Nelson and Rennels, 1970a; Nielsen *et al.*, 1971a). Pease and Molinari (1960) were the first to present a structural basis, such as evidenced by the special organization of myofibrillar attachments within the smooth muscle cells and the shared basement membrane or even direct contacts between neighbouring cells, for a myogenic (mechanical and/or electrotonic) propagation of con-traction in the brain vessel wall following stimulation of the innervated smooth muscle cells at the surface of tunica media. Unfortunately, their observations preceded the functional analysis of mechanisms underlying excitation spread in smooth musculature (see Barr *et al.*, 1968) and were actually misinterpreted as lack of innervation. It should be mentioned in this context that close appositions between the membranes of the adrenergic and cholin-ergic axons also occur in the terminal neuroeffector area (Edvinsson *et al.*, 1972a) as illustrated in Fig. 6.

VASCULAR RECEPTOR MECHANISMS

We have used the findings of an ample adrenergic and cholinergic nerve supply to brain vessels, including arterioles, and the fact that the nerves fulfil structural criteria for a true autonomic vasomotor innervation, as a basis for functional studies. Attempts have first been made to define the autonomic receptor mechanisms involved and then to elucidate the ability of extra- and intracerebral vessels to influence the hemodynamics in the brain following experimental interference with the sympathetic nerves, alone or in combination with administration of sympatho/parasympathomimetic drugs.

In spite of an overwhelming interest in the mechanisms influencing and controlling cerebral blood circulation, only comparatively few reports have been concerned with investigations of basic properties of the smooth musculature in intracranial vessels. By the

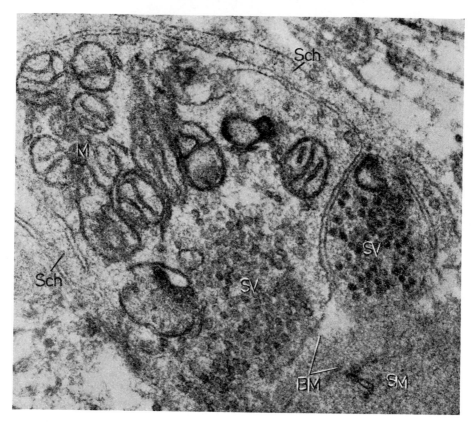

Fig. 6. Electron micrograph of the cat's anterior cerebral artery after potassium permanganate fixation. Large cholinergic terminal with an accumulation of mitochondria (M) and electron-lucent synaptic vesicles (SV) in close contact with an adrenergic terminal (right) containing numerous electron-dense synaptic vesicles (SV), both partly surrounded by Schwann cell cyto-plasm (Sch.). The "naked" parts of the terminals are located 1100 Å from the membrane of the smooth muscle cell (SM) and separated from this only by the fused basement membranes (BM). (×60 000.)

use of simple models it has been possible to clarify the receptor mechanisms implicated in the mechanical reactivity of several other vessels, e.g. aorta and the coronary, renal, and mesenteric arteries. Besides direct examination of changes in the vessel diameter *in vivo*, the methods have involved the recording either of tension in the vessel wall, or of vascular resistance in terms of altered flow or pressure in perfused blood vessels.

It is understandable that the failure of helical strips from cerebral resistance vessels (200–300 μ in diameter) to respond mechanically in the presence of catecholamines or acetylcholine (Bohr *et al.*, 1961), reported at a time when electronmicroscopists interpreted their data as evidence for a lack of direct innervation of cerebral arteries, for a long time supported many investigators in their doubt about a neurogenic control of the brain circulation. If, however, intact pial arteries (diameter about 300 μ) are mounted in a rigid, and therefore sensitive, *in vitro* system for registration of circular contractions, a strong response can be obtained with several amines, including catecholamines and acetylcholine (Nielsen and Owman, 1970, 1971). Drug-induced constriction can also be elicited in smaller

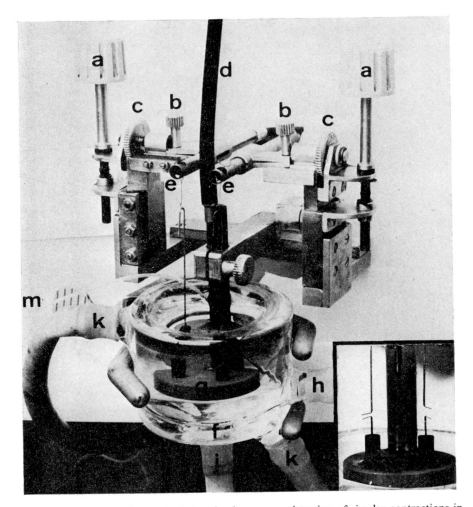

Fig. 7. Arrangement of organ bath for simultaneous registration of circular contractions in two blood vessels. (a) Screw device for vertical fine-adjustment of transducers, (b) screw for fixation of transducer, (c) screw for horizontal adjustment of transducer, (e) pen-formed force-displacement transducers from which an L-formed steel holder is hanging into the bath, forming the upper fixation of the vessel (see inset), (f) mantled organ bath in which base-plate (g) is fixed to form the lower fixation of the vessel (see inset), (h) inlet for pre-warmed buffer solution, (j) outlet for washout of the buffer in the bath, which is warmed by water circulating via (k), (m) small tubing for aeration of buffer solution. Inset: each vessel in the bath is suspended horizontally between the two L-formed holders, the lower fixed in the base-plate and the upper hanging from the transducer.

cerebral arteries (down to 50 μ in diameter) as evidenced by changes in pressure and flow of perfused isolated vessels (Politoff and Macri, 1966; Uchida *et al.*, 1967). Our *in vitro* technique has been used in attempts to define the various types of amine receptors mediating motor activity in cerebral arteries. The experimental set-up (Fig. 7) was designed for simultaneous testing of two vessels in the same organ bath, thus allowing comparison between treated (denervation, drugs, etc.) and non-treated vessels, or between different types of vessels, e.g. intracranial and extracranial vessels.

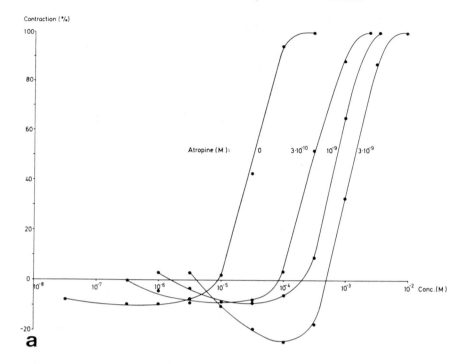

a

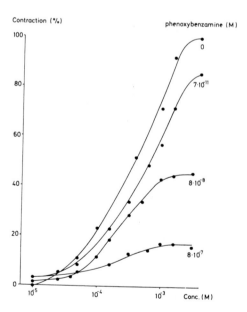

b

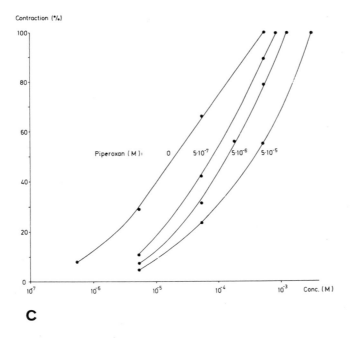

c

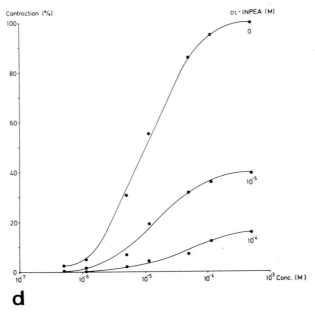

d

FIG. 8. Contractile response of isolated cat's middle cerebral artery suspended in the organ bath illustrated in Fig. 7, (a) Effect of acetylcholine and inhibition by atropine. (b) Effect of noradrenaline and inhibition by phenoxybenzamine. (c) Effect of phenylephrine and inhibition by piperoxan. (d) Effect of isoprenaline and inhibition by DL-INPEA.

Pial arteries (from cat and man) appear to be most sensitive to 5-HT, which also produces a strong contraction (up to 800 dyn). The effect is inhibited by methysergide in a non-competitive manner. Histamine has a dual action on the intracranial arteries: at lower concentrations (below approximately 10^{-5} M in the organ bath) it produces a dilation which can be registered under resting conditions as well as after the vessel has been given an active tension by previous administration of 5-HT. This relaxation by histamine is inhibited in a competitive manner by burimamide and is thus mediated mainly through H_2 receptors (Black et al., 1972). At higher histamine concentrations the pial arteries contract, and the response is antagonized by the H_1 receptor blocking agents, mepyramine or chlorpheniramine. It is notable that in extracranial arteries (such as small branches from the temporal artery) tested in the same bath along with the pial artery, histamine only produces a contraction through an effect on H_1 receptors, even in doses that dilate the intracranial vessels. Also acetylcholine exerts a dual effect on the intracranial arteries (Fig. 8a), although the contractile response (up to 800 dyn) by far exceeds the magnitude of the dilatory action. Atropine produces a competitive inhibition of both the dilation and contraction (Fig. 8a). Postganglionic sympathetic denervation of the artery had no overt effect on the acetylcholine response; if anything, the dilatory response was slightly reduced.

Various catecholamines were studied on isolated pial arteries (sympathectomized to abolish neuronal amine uptake) in order to define the types of adrenergic receptors involved. All tested compounds contracted the vessels from the resting level, the relative potencies being in the order of adrenaline > noradrenaline > phenylephrine > isoprenaline. The α-receptor antagonist, phenoxybenzamine, inhibited the noradrenaline-induced response (Fig. 8b). The effects of phenylephrine (Fig. 8c) and adrenaline were antagonized in a competitive manner in the presence of another α-adrenergic blocking agent, piperoxan. This agrees with observations under in vivo conditions in which α-blocking compounds counteract induced constriction of intracranial vessels (Lende, 1960; Flamm et al., 1972; Edvinsson et al., 1973d) and cause marked vasodilation relative to normal vascular tone (Wahl et al., 1971/2). There is now reason to believe that the above-mentioned contraction induced by isoprenaline is not mediated by β-receptors since the doses needed to produce the effect were quite large (above 10^{-6} M). This is supported by findings from a more detailed analysis of the blocking effects of propranolol and INPEA, which showed inhibition of the isoprenaline-induced contraction only in high concentrations, and the action was non-competitive. Moreover, the β-agonist terbutaline had no contractile effect on the resting vessel. If, on the other hand, an active constriction of the vessel was induced beforehand (by, e.g., 5-HT), a dilation could be obtained both with terbutaline and isoprenaline (at considerably lower dose levels than those producing a contraction). Recent studies in which local cerebral blood flow has been recorded in conscious animals by chronically implanted thermoprobes corroborate the presence of dilatory adrenergic receptors (Seylaz et al., 1973). However, there appears to be a regional heterogeneity in that isoprenaline increased flow (effect blocked by propranolol) in the caudate nucleus but not in the lateral geniculate body (where flow sometimes even showed a slight decrease). A notable observation that may be of relevance in this connection was that the vascular adrenergic nerve supply seemed to be more pronounced in the former structure.

Against this background it is probable that the vasodilatory effect seen by certain β-blockers (Falck et al., 1968; Rosenblum, 1969; Wahl et al., 1971/2) has been due to unspecific actions rather than a true β-receptor antagonism.

TYRAMINE RESPONSE *IN VITRO*

Although the pial arteries were found to possess structural prerequisites for a true autonomic innervation and responded to certain vasoactive amines, the question was still open whether activation of the adrenergic nerves in fact was able to produce a contractile response which would be a minimum requirement for a physiological role in the vasomotor regulation of the arteries. In order to find indications of whether the perivascular adrenergic nerves can release endogenous noradrenaline in amounts sufficient to bring about a local vascular response, the effect of tyramine was tested on isolated pial arteries (Nielsen *et al.*, 1971b). Tyramine exerts its specific sympathomimetic action through an uptake into the nerve followed by displacement of the noradrenaline transmitter (Burn and Rand, 1958; Langer *et al.*, 1967). Small segments from the proximal portion of the cat's middle cerebral artery were mounted in the previously described organ bath for registration of circular contractions.

Figure 9a illustrates a typical cumulative log dose–response curve showing the response to tyramine in a preparation from a normal, untreated cat. In arteries from animals whose sympathetic nerves had been depleted of their noradrenaline content by reserpine (5 mg/kg intraperitoneally the day before sacrifice), a contraction was not obtained until a tyramine concentration in the bath of about 10^{-4} M was reached, and the intensity of the contraction was then very low (Fig. 9a). A similar marked reduction in the tyramine response was seen with arteries from animals that had been sympathectomized by removal of the superior cervical ganglion 1 week prior to the experiment (Fig. 9b). The findings from the vessels with an intact adrenergic innervation show that tyramine can induce a vascular contraction through the release of transmitter from the noradrenaline-containing sympathetic nerves present in the wall of the vascular preparation. At tyramine concentrations in the bath above approximately 10^{-4} M, however, a contractile response which did not require the local presence of the adrenergic transmitter became evident. This effect corresponds to the direct, unspecific sympathomimetic action of tyramine. Three weeks after ganglionectomy, the response of the sympathectomized arteries to tyramine was almost comparable to that obtained with the non-denervated control arteries (Fig. 9c) owing to the progressive development of denervation supersensitivity to this unspecific sympathomimetic effect of tyramine (Trendelenburg, 1963; Langer *et al.*, 1967).

Although tyramine had lost its specific sympathomimetic action on arteries from reserpinized animals, a normal contractile response could still be induced with noradrenaline. When the noradrenaline was washed out from the bath 15 min later, the vessel relaxed to its original tension. After this noradrenaline exposure of the vessel from a reserpine-treated animal, tyramine was again able to induce a contraction that was of the same magnitude as for a vessel from a non-reserpinized animal. This indicates that tyramine now acted through the release of exogenous noradrenaline, which had been taken up into the nerve terminals and replaced the endogenous noradrenaline previously depleted from the nerves by reserpine. This assumption was confirmed by the addition of cocaine (10^{-4} M) to the bath 10 min before noradrenaline. Under these conditions, noradrenaline was not able to restore the tyramine-induced contraction in the reserpinized vessel, obviously due to cocaine blockade of the neural uptake mechanism for exogenous noradrenaline into the adrenergic nerves (Hertting, 1965).

The results have offered strong evidence to support the view that the adrenergic nerve plexus around the pial arteries contributes to a true innervation apparatus, and that nor-

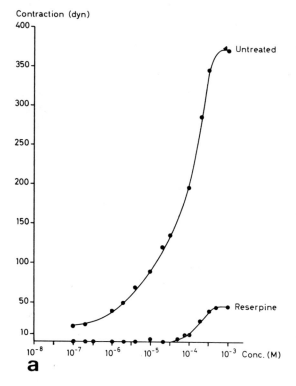

a

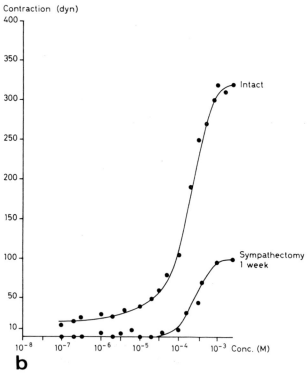

b

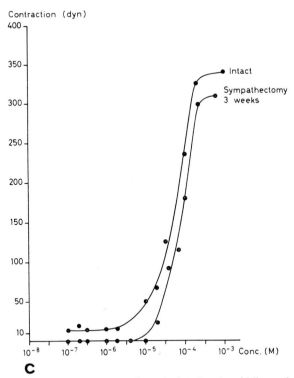

C

FIG. 9. Cumulative dose–response curves from isolated cat's middle cerebral artery *in vitro* showing tyramine-induced contraction. (a) The tyramine effect is markedly reduced in artery from an animal pretreated with reserpine. (b) The tyramine effect is markedly reduced in artery taken from the side sympathectomized by excision of the superior cervical ganglion 1 week before testing. (c) If sympathectomy has been performed 3 weeks before testing, the tyramine-induced response on the sympathectomized side is similar to that obtained on the intact side.

adrenaline can induce a contraction of the vascular smooth muscle through a local release from these nerves.

EFFECTS OF SYMPATHETIC DENERVATION

Soon after our histochemical findings of an ample sympathetic supply of the pial vessels, attempts were made to elucidate their functional role in a vasomotor action on the pial circulation through which the brain receives its blood supply. The first experiments were designed with the idea that the vasomotor effects could be expected to be particularly well revealed under conditions when the vasomotor control mechanism had been challenged by extreme loading. Hyperventilation during hypothermia (Falck *et al.*, 1968) is a situation known to produce marked pial vasoconstriction and signs of cerebral hypoxia. Cats were anaesthetized with nembutal and the trachea was exposed and cannulated. The left superior cervical sympathetic ganglion was carefully freed through the neck incision over the trachea, and a ligature loop was loosely tied around the sympathetic trunk immediately cranial to the ganglia. The ends of the loop were drawn through the wound, which was closed by clips. The animals were cooled by submersion in an ice-water bath (about 7°C),

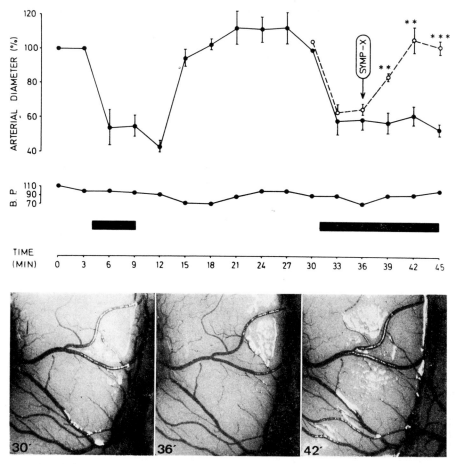

Fig. 10. Relative changes in mean pial arterial diameter (SEM) and arterial blood pressure (BP in mmHg) of five cats at 27°C rectal temperature. The arterial diameter was reduced by hyperventilation (black horizontal bars) performed at two different time periods but otherwise identically. Arterial diameter in the right craniotomy: ●——●, in the left craniotomy: ○ -- ○. Immediately after left-sided transection of the sympathetic trunk just above the superior cervical ganglion (SYMP-X), the arteries on the ipsilateral side dilated (differences between means on SYMP-X side and on normal side compared according to Student's t-test: **$0.001 < p < 0.01$, ***$p < 0.001$). Below: photographs from pial vessels in the left craniotomy in one of the cats at three different times during the experiment. (×20).

and cooling was controlled so that the body temperature stabilized at approximately 27°C. The animals were first allowed to breathe spontaneously. Craniotomies (15 × 15 mm size) were made on the convexity over the parietal lobe symmetrically on both sides. As soon as the dura had been opened, the pia-arachnoid was constantly irrigated with Krebs–Ringer solution at room temperature. The pial vessels were examined continuously in an operation microscope and photographed at 16 × objective ($f = 200$) magnification every 3 min during the course of the experiments. On the magnified photographs the outer diameter was measured in pial arteries with a size of 40–130 μ, i.e. arteries known to receive adrenergic nerve terminals (Nielsen and Owman, 1967). Hyperventilation with air was induced with a pump respirator (connected to the endotracheal cannula via a T-tube) during 5 min, resulting in a pial vasoconstriction to an extent by which the diameter of the measured arteries was reduced by 35–40% (Fig. 10). After interruption of the hyperventilation, the animals were allowed to breathe spontaneously and the pial arteries dilated to the initial diameter. This gave an estimate of the extent of the pial vasoconstriction (measured in the right side craniotomy) produced with the pump frequency and volume used. After the animals had been allowed to respirate spontaneously several minutes they were again exposed to hyperventilation with the standard volume and frequency employed in this series, but uninterrupted for 14 min. In these experiments the effects on the pial arteries were compared in the craniotomies on both sides. Hyperventilation produced the expected reduction in the arterial diameter (Fig. 10). Five minutes after beginning of hyperventilation, the left cervical sympathetic trunk was divided by traction of the loop previously tied above the superior cervical ganglion (left-sided postganglionic sympathectomy). On this left side the pial arterial vasoconstriction started to release, and within 6 min after sympathectomy, the arteries had dilated to normal size (Fig. 10). On the non-sympathectomized right side, the pial arteries remained markedly constricted. The finding that acute sympathectomy released the vasoconstriction induced by hyperventilation agreed with the anticipated vasoconstrictor property of the pial sympathetic nerves and with our hypothesis that a lost sympathetic control of these vessels should be particularly well demonstrable under conditions when they are already constricted.

Also the specialized vascular regions comprising the choroid plexuses have recently been found to receive both adrenergic (Fig. 11) and cholinergic nerves (Edvinsson et al., 1973b, e), and there is reason to believe that the adrenergic innervation inhibits cerebrospinal fluid production in the plexuses as evidenced by the effect of sympathetic denervation on their carbonic anhydrase activity (Edvinsson et al., 1971a). In our further studies on the neuro-receptor mechanisms in the brain vessels, two types of experimental models have been utilized: measurements of cerebral blood volume (CBV) in mice (Edvinsson et al., 1973d) determined by dilution of a non-diffusible radioactive tracer (RIHSA), and continuous recordings of intracranial pressure (which is primarily maintained and regulated through combined effects on CBV and cerebrospinal fluid circulation) obtained via a cannula implanted into one of the lateral ventricles of conscious rabbits (Owman and West, 1970).

In accordance with previous observations on isolated pial arteries in vitro (Nielsen et al., 1971b), systemic administration of tyramine lowered CBV (cerebral vasoconstriction), and the effect was markedly reduced after cranial sympathectomy (Edvinsson et al., 1972b). Accordingly, bilateral electrical stimulation of the sympathetic trunks in the neck produced a significant reduction in CBV. This vasoconstriction was blocked by previous treatment of the animals with the α-receptor antagonist, phenoxybenzamine (Edvinsson et al., 1973d). The findings are in good agreement with the marked pial vasodilation that we previously had observed in hyperventilated, hypothermic cats as a consequence of acute transection of the preganglionic sympathetic nerves to the head (Fig. 10). In contrast to the effects of tyramine administration or sympathetic stimulation, systemic injection of noradrenaline did not overtly change CBV. This failure to detect a cerebrovascular response to noradrenaline agrees with several other reports and could have a variety of explanations: the changes may be too small to be revealed by the technique used; the total vasomotor events in the body may mask those occurring in the brain; the access of circulating noradrenaline may be efficiently inactivated by an uptake into the rich plexuses of brain vascular adrenergic nerves before it reaches the receptors. Attempts were therefore made to get the experimental model more sensitive. The mice were bilaterally ganglionectomized at various time intervals

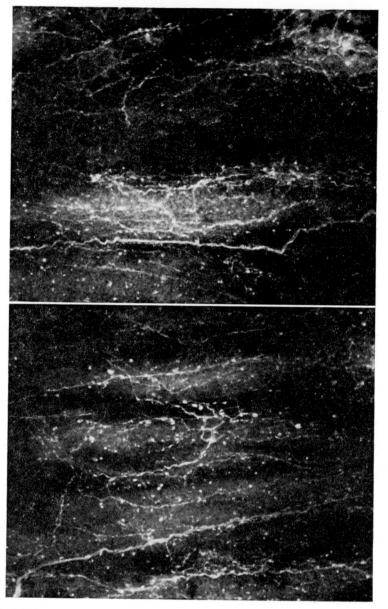

FIG. 11. Whole-mount on microscope slide of choroid plexus from 3rd ventricle of rabbit. Drying of the preparation has been followed by formaldehyde gas treatment. Picture is composed of two adjacent fields. The plexus is supplied by a dense network of delicate green-fluorescent adrenergic nerve fibres. Autofluorescent cells and granulars are also present. ($\times 100$.)

before the injection (Fig. 12) in order to obtain a state of denervation supersensitivity of the cerebrovascular adrenergic receptors to circulating (administered) noradrenaline (Langer et al., 1967). Twelve hours after sympathectomy, noradrenaline still failed to alter CBV (receptors not yet supersensitive enough). On the other hand, it did lower CBV at 24 h and particularly at 48 h, when receptor supersensitivity is known to have reached a pronounced

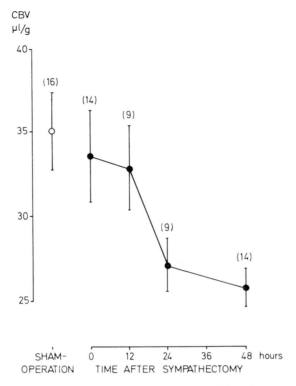

FIG. 12. Changes in CBV on mice measured by dilution of non-diffusible radioactive tracer. The CBV determined 2 min after intravenous injection of 5 μg/kg of noradrenaline does not differ in sham-operated animals compared with non-operated animals (time 0) or animals sympathectomized 12 h previously. However, the same schema of noradrenaline significantly reduces CBV when tested 24 or 48 h after sympathectomy.

degree (Langer *et al.*, 1967). The results show that the cerebral vessels indeed can respond to exogenous noradrenaline. Furthermore, they illustrate that a failure to register a vasomotor effect of this amine may be due only to quantitative factors, and thus cannot be used as an argument against reactivity of the brain circulation to administered noradrenaline and, of course, not as an argument against a neurogenic control.

Although sympathetic denervation of the brain is easily performed as the sympathetic nerves run in the paravertebral trunks of the neck, conflicting results from denervation experiments have been another reason for denying a sympathetic nervous influence on the cerebral blood circulation. At least two explanations for these conflicting results can be offered. One is that only little attention has been paid to whether the denervation has been preganglionic or postganglionic, partly because of incomplete knowledge about the origin of the cerebrovascular sympathetic nerves. It has now been clarified that the sympathetic fibres to the brain vessels originate in the superior cervical ganglia, and that each ganglion has a unilateral contribution (Nielsen and Owman, 1967). Another reason is that the effects of surgical interference with the sympathetic nerves have been analysed after widely varying time periods. Thus such mechanisms as degeneration release of the transmitter and denervation supersensitivity of the vascular receptors have not been taken into account.

As a basis for our studies on the influence of sympathectomy on cerebral hemodynamics

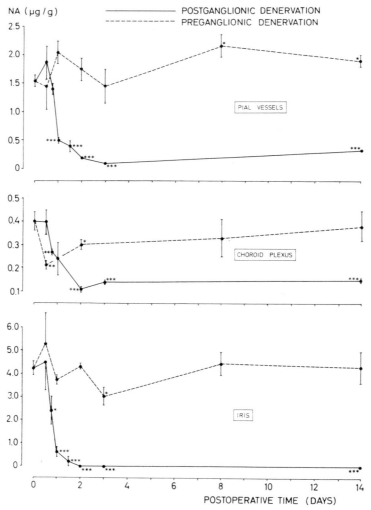

FIG. 13. Organ concentration of noradrenaline (μg/g wet weight) determined fluorometrically at various periods after postganglionic denervation (bilateral removal of superior cervical sympathetic ganglia) or preganglionic denervation (decentralization). Organs from three animals were pooled for each determination. Each point gives the mean ($\pm$ SEM) of four determinations (pial vessels time 0: 10 determinations). Differences between non-operated (postoperative time 0 days) and operated animals according to Student's t-test: *$0.01 < p < 0.05$, **$0.001 < p < 0.01$, and ***$p < 0.001$.

—measured in terms of changes in CBV and ventricular fluid pressure (VFP)—alterations in chemically determined noradrenaline levels were followed in various sympathetically innervated structures, including the pial vascular system and the choroid plexus, at various stages after preganglionic (decentralization) or postganglionic (ganglionectomy) sympathetic denervation (Edvinsson *et al.*, 1972c). The findings are illustrated in Fig. 13, and are in good agreement with changes in formaldehyde-induced noradrenaline fluorescence of the postganglionic adrenergic nerves after the operations. Histochemical and chemical studies following administration of noradrenaline have shown that the mechanisms for uptake and retention of the amine still operate shortly after ganglionectomy, but are then deteriorated with approximately the same speed as the disappearance of the endogenous transmitter (Malmfors and Sachs, 1965; Sears and Gillis, 1967; Sedvall, 1969). At the same time there is an increase in the release of noradrenaline from the nerves (Sears and Gillis, 1967). The measured tendency to a delay in noradrenaline reduction of the choroid plexus, compared with that found for the pial vessels and iris, could be explained by a slower loss of the amine from the former tissue after the postganglionic denervation.

On the basis of chemical and histochemical investigations it is generally accepted that preganglionic sympathetic denervation (decentralization) does not alter the organ content of noradrenaline (Rehn, 1958; Falck, 1962). From the data in Fig. 13 it can be seen that it is not possible to make a generalization of the phenomenon; the results obviously depend on the organ studied and at which time after denervation the chemical determinations have been done. Thus in the choroid plexus, a 50% reduction in the noradrenaline concentration was registered 12 h after the decentralization followed by a slow normalization of the amine level. In the iris a similar tendency was seen, although the reduction occurred 2 days later. In the pial vessels, on the other hand, the transmitter concentration shows a post-operative increase, so that a week after decentralization the amine level was 40% higher than in non-operated controls. The noradrenaline level measured in the postsynaptic sympathetic neuron after deprivation of its afferent innervation appears to be a function of two counteracting mechanisms in the neuron: a diminished physiological activity and a lowered noradrenaline synthesis (Sedvall, 1969). The net neuronal concentration of nora-drenaline in a given neuron after decentralization will therefore depend on the relative alteration in its activity (rate of noradrenaline release) and its rate of noradrenaline form-ation. It is possible that the observed heterogeneity in the tissue content of noradrenaline after decentralization reflects a different rate of functional turnover of the transmitter, which might imply that different types of sympathetic neurons are present in one and the same ganglion.

Following bilateral sympathetic denervation of the brain vascular system, it was possible to register marked alterations in cerebral hemodynamics (Fig. 14) reflected in terms of changes in CBV (Edvinsson et al., 1973d) and VFP (Edvinsson et al., 1971b, 1972d). Thus shortly after excision of the superior cervical ganglia (postganglionic sympathectomy), there was a significant fall in both parameters studied. This has been interpreted as a cerebral vasoconstriction due to increased activation of the vascular receptors when the stored transmitter is leaking out from the degenerating sympathetic nerve terminals (see Lundberg, 1970). Following this fall the CBV increased markedly to levels well above that of the controls, and there was a concomitant marked elevation in VFP. The changes are consistent with a vasodilation, probably in combination with an increase in the production of cere-brospinal fluid from the choroid plexuses when noradrenaline has disappeared from the degenerating postganglionic sympathetic nerves (cf. Fig. 13). Several days after ganglion-ectomy, both CBV and VFP returned to normal or even subnormal values. This is well explainable by the postoperative development of denervation supersensitivity of the adrenergic receptors (in blood vessels of the brain as well as of the choroid plexus, and perhaps also in the plexus epithelium) to circulating catecholamines, which will lead to an increase in the cerebrovascular tone and possibly also to a decrease in the rate of formation of cerebrospinal fluid.

Preganglionic denervation was accomplished by bilateral division of the sympathetic trunks just caudal to the superior cervical ganglia. The preganglionic nerves are known to lose their ability to synthetize acetylcholine within 3 days of degeneration, and the neuronal

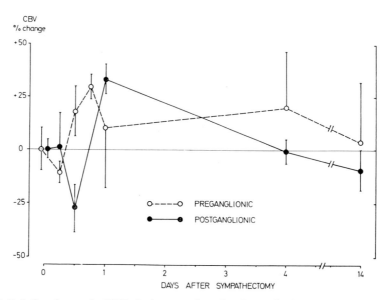

FIG. 14. Relative changes in CBV of mice at various time intervals after pre- or postganglionic sympathetic denervation. The zero-level (non-operated animals) is indicated. Mean $\pm$ SEM, n = 6. Student's t-test for postganglionic operations: time 0 vs. time 12 h, $p < 0.05$; time 0 vs. time 24 h, $p < 0.02$; time 12 h vs. time 24 h, $p < 0.001$. Preganglionic operations: time 0 vs. time 18 h, $p < 0.01$.

content of the amine is markedly reduced (McIntosh, 1938; Feldberg, 1943). This coincides with the impairment and subsequent abolishment of synaptic transmission in the sympathetic ganglia (Coppé and Bacq, 1938; McIntosh, 1938). Provided the brain vessels are under the influence of a continuous sympathetic tone, decentralization could be expected to result in a certain degree of vasodilation. This agrees with our findings of a trend to increased CBV after preganglionic denervation. Moreover, the VFP was significantly increased during most of the postoperative observation time, which thus might be explained by a vasodilatory tendency in the brain vessels combined with an increase in the production of cerebrospinal fluid following deprivation of sympathetic inhibition. Two weeks after the operation, the CBV as well as the VFP showed fairly normal levels, conceivably due to the counteracting effect of a decentralization supersensitivity of the adrenergic receptors (Langer *et al.*, 1967).

CONCLUDING REMARKS

The denervation experiments have emphasized the importance of an exact knowledge of the time interval that elapses after the operation until the vascular reactions in the brain are being analyzed. The experiments have also called attention to the expected, but often overlooked, difference in the vasomotor effects after preganglionic compared to postganglionic interference with the sympathetic nerves. Against the background of our results, together with related findings by others, the question is no longer *if* cerebral vessels are under neurogenic influence, but rather *how* this influence by autonomic nerves operates in a physiological control function of the cerebral blood circulation. There is thus no reason for those workers who deny the importance of neurogenic stimuli to, as Rosenblum (1971) has put it, "believe that positive results are artifacts of the experimental situation, caused by variables not controlled by the investigators". It is important to realize that in several respects the intracranial vascular system is in a unique situation, so that it can be expected to present physiological features different from those documented from studies on other vascular systems. For example. the brain is enclosed in a rigid compartment which limits the physiological possibilities for an increase in volume of its vascular bed; owing to the presence of a blood–brain barrier, circulating compounds may not have an immediate access to the vascular receptors; the venous system (also innervated by autonomic nerves) has a different construction compared to peripheral veins; in the brain, also vessels with a calibre corresponding to that of conducting arteries receive an autonomic innervation, and this is in some areas

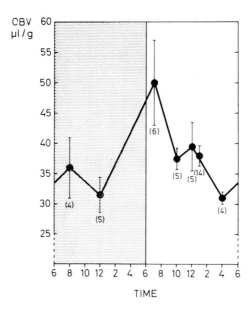

FIG. 15. Determinations of CBV in mice killed throughout the last 24 h cycle of a 12 h darkness/12 h light schedule maintained during 2 weeks. Diurnal changes in cerebral hemodynamics. Mean values ± SEM, number of animals within parentheses.

better developed than in any other vascular system of the body; and, there is, furthermore, recent evidence (Edvinsson *et al.*, 1973c) that cerebral hemodynamics show circadian rhythmicity (Fig. 15).

It is a well-established fact that marked changes in cerebral blood flow (and volume) are produced by alterations in arterial carbon dioxide tension and extracellular pH. *These chemical mechanisms do not, of course, exclude the existence also of a neurogenic control*; the two control mechanisms may even interact or exert their actions on a common vascular receptor. One suggestion for an example of a control function which could involve both mechanisms during a situation that requires increased blood flow to the brain might operate by a simultaneous increase in sympathetic tone of the innervated cerebral arteries in order to limit the intracranial blood supply to amounts necessary to satisfy a local demand for chemically mediated increase in flow without producing a simultaneous elevation of intracranial pressure through a generalized increase in cerebral blood volume. The consequence of this would be that a measured increase in cerebral blood flow does not immediately reflect a vasodilation but may be the result of a combined vasoconstriction and dilation, the same applying when a decrease in cerebral blood flow is found. It is obvious that measurements of flow only present the net hemodynamic consequences of several types of control mechanisms. This can explain the difficulties in obtaining direct experimental evidence for the neurogenic influence. It is consistent with our findings, including those from studies of the intracranial pressure, that the autoregulation of cerebral perfusion in the presence of varying perfusion pressure is maintained by the autonomic nervous system.

ACKNOWLEDGEMENT

This work was supported by grant No. 04X–732 from the Swedish Medical Research Council.

REFERENCES

BARR, L., BERGER, W., and DEWEY, M. M. (1968) Electrical transmission at the nexus between smooth muscle cells. *J. Gen. Physiol.* **51**, 347–368.

BJÖRKLUND, A., FALCK, B., and OWMAN, CH. (1972) Fluorescence microscopic and microspectro-fluorometric techniques for the cellular localization and characterization of biogenic amines. In *Methods of Investigative and Diagnostic Endocrinology* (S. A. Berson, ed.), vol. 1, *The Thyroid and Biogenic Amines*, (J. E. Rall and I. J. Kopin, eds.), North-Holland, Amsterdam, pp. 318–368.

BLACK, J. W., DUNCAN, W. A. M., DURANT, C. J., GANELLIN, C. R., and PARSONS, E. M. (1972) Definition and antagonism of histamine H_2-receptors. *Nature*, **236**, 385–390.

BOHR, D. F., GOULET, P. L., and TAQUINI, A. C. (1961) Direct tension recording from smooth muscle of resistance vessels from various organs. *Angiology* **12**, 478–485.

BURN, J. H., and RAND, M. J. (1958) The action of sympathomimetic amines in animals treated with reserpine. *J. Physiol. Lond.* **144**, 314–336.

CHOROBSKI, J., and PENFIELD, W. (1932) Cerebral vasodilator nerves and their pathway from the medulla oblongata. *Archs. Neurol. Psychiat.* **28**, 1257–1289.

COPPÉ, G., and BACQ, Z. M. (1938) Dégénérescence, conduction et transmission synaptique dans le sympathique cervical. *Arch. int. Physiol.* **47**, 312–320.

CSILLIK, B., JANCSÓ, G., TÓTH, L., KOZMA, M., KÁLMÁN, G., and KARXSU, S. (1971) Adrenergic innervation of hypothalamic blood vessels: a contribution to the problem of central thermodetectors. *Acta anat.* **80**, 142–151.

EDVINSSON, L., HÅKANSON, R., OWMAN, CH., and WEST, K. A. (1971a) Sympathetic influence on carbanhydrase activity in choroid plexus. *Exp. Cell Res.* **67**, 245.

EDVINSSON, L., OWMAN, CH., and WEST, K. A. (1971b) Changes in continuously recorded intracranial pressure of conscious rabbits at different time-periods after superior cervical sympathectomy. *Acta physiol. scand.* **83**, 42–50.

EDVINSSON, L., NIELSEN, K. C., OWMAN, CH., and SPORRONG, B. (1972a) Cholinergic mechanisms in pial vessels. Histochemistry, electron microscopy and pharmacology. *Z. Zellforsch.* **134**, 311–325.

EDVINSSON, L., NIELSEN, K. C., OWMAN, CH., and WEST, K. A. (1972b) Sympathetic neural influence on norepinephrine vasoconstriction in brain vessels. *Archs. Neurol.* **27**, 492–495.

EDVINSSON, L., OWMAN, CH., ROSENGREN, E., and WEST, K. A. (1972c) Concentration of noradrenaline in pial vessels, choroid plexus and iris during two weeks after sympathetic ganglionectomy or decentralization. *Acta physiol. scand.* **85**, 201–206.

EDVINSSON, L., OWMAN, CH., and WEST, K. A. (1972d) Intracranial pressure in conscious rabbits after decentralization of the superior cervical sympathetic ganglia. *Acta physiol. scand.* **85**, 193–200.

EDVINSSON, L., LINDVALL, M., NIELSEN, K. C., and OWMAN, CH. (1973a) Are brain vessels innervated also by central (non-sympathetic) adrenergic neurons? *Brain Res.* **63**, 496–499.

EDVINSSON, L., NIELSEN, K. C., and OWMAN, CH. (1973b) Cholinergic innervation of rabbit and cat choroid plexus. *Brain Res.* **63**, 500–503.

EDVINSSON, L., NIELSEN, K. C., and OWMAN, CH. (1973c) Diurnal rhythm in cerebral blood volume of mice. *Experientia* **29**, 432–433.

EDVINSSON, L., NIELSEN, K. C., OWMAN, CH., and WEST, K. A. (1973d) Evidence of vasoconstrictor sympathetic nerves in brain vessels of mice. *Neurology* **23**, 73–77.

EDVINSSON, L., NIELSEN, K. C., OWMAN, CH., and WEST, K. A. (1973e) Adrenergic innervation of mammalian choroid plexus. *Am. J. Anat.*, in press.

EHINGER, B., FALCK, B., and SPORRONG, B. (1970) Possible axo-axonal synapses between peripheral adrenergic and cholinergic nerve terminals. *Z. Zellforsch.* **107**, 508–521.

FALCK, B. (1962) Observations on the possibilities of the cellular localization of monoamines by a fluorescence method. *Acta physiol. scand.* **56**, Suppl. 197, 1–25.

FALCK, B., MCHEDLISHVILI, G. I., and OWMAN, CH. (1965) Histochemical demonstration of adrenergic nerves in cortex-pia of rabbit. *Acta pharmac. tox.* **23**, 133–142.

FALCK, B., NIELSEN, K. C., and OWMAN, CH. (1968) Adrenergic innervation of the pial circulation. *Scand. J. Clin. Lab. Invest.*, Suppl. **102**, 96–98.

FELDBERG, W. (1943) Synthesis of acetylcholine in sympathetic ganglia and cholinergic nerves. *J. Physiol. Lond.* **101**, 432–445.

FLAMM, E. S., YASARGIL, M. G., and RANSOHOFF II, J. (1972) Alteration of experimental cerebral vasospasm by adrenergic blockade. *J. Neurosurg.* **37**, 294–301.

FORBES, H. S., and WOLFF, H. G. (1928) Cerebral circulation: III, The vasomotor control of cerebral vessels. *Archs. Neurol. Psychiat.* **19**, 1057–1080.

HAGEN, E., and WITTKOWSKI, W. (1969) Licht- und elektronmikroskopische Untersuchungen zur Innervation der Piagefässe. *Z. Zellforsch.* **95**, 429–444.

HARTMAN, B. K., and UDENFRIEND, S. (1972) The application of immunological techniques to the study of enzymes regulating catecholamine synthesis and degradation. *Pharmac. Rev.* **24**, 311–330.

HARTMAN, B. K., ZIDE, D., and UDENFRIEND, S. (1972) The use of dopamine β-hydroxylase as a marker for the central noradrenergic nervous system in rat brain. *Proc. Natn. Acad. Sci. USA* **69**, 2722–2726.

HERTTING, G. (1965) Effect of drugs and sympathetic denervation on noradrenaline uptake and binding in animal tissues. In *Pharmacology of Cholinergic and Adrenergic Transmission.* (G. B. Koelle, W. W. Douglas, and A. Carlsson, eds.), Pergamon Press and Czechoslovak Medical Press, Oxford and Praha, pp. 277–289.

HÖKFELT, T., and LJUNGDAHL, A. (1972) Modification of the Falck–Hillarp formaldehyde fluorescence method using the Vibratome®: simple, rapid and sensitive localization of catecholamines in sections of unfixed or formalin fixed brain tissue. *Histochemie* **29**, 325–339.

HOLMSTEDT, B. (1957) A modification of the thiocholine method for the determination of cholinesterase: II, Histochemical application. *Acta physiol. scand.* **40**, 331–357.

IWAYAMA, T., FURNESS, J. B., and BURNSTOCK, G. (1970) Dual adrenergic and cholinergic innervation of the cerebral arteries of the rat: an ultrastructural study. *Circ. Res.* **26**, 635–646.

KATZMAN, R., BJÖRKLUND, A., OWMAN, CH., STENEVI, U., and WEST, K. A. (1971) Evidence for regenerative axon sprouting of central catecholamine neurons in the rat mesencephalon following electrolytic lesions. *Brain Res.* **25**, 579–596.

KOELLE, G. B. (1963) Cytological distributions and physiological functions of cholinesterases. In *Cholinesterases and Anticholinesterase Agents* (G. B. Koelle, ed.), Heffter-Heubner, *Handbuch der experimentellen Pharmakologie*, Suppl. 15, Springer-Verlag, Berlin and Heidelberg.

LANGER, S. Z., DRASKOCZY, P. R., and TRENDELENBURG, U. (1967) Time course of the development of supersensitivity to various amines in the nictitating membrane of the pithed cat after denervation or decentralization. *J. Pharmac. Exp. Ther.* **157**, 255–273.

LENDE, R. A. (1960) Local spasm in cerebral arteries. *J. Neurosurg.* **17**, 90–113.

LUNDBERG, D. (1970) Some aspects of the pharmacology of the degeneration contraction of rat periorbital smooth muscle after sympathetic denervation. *Acta Univ. Uppsal.* **79**, 1–10.

MCINTOSH, F. C. (1938) L'effet de la section des fibres préganglionnaires sur la teneur en acétylcholine du ganglion sympathique. *Archs. int. Physiol.* **48**, 321–324.

MALMFORS, T., and SACHS, CH. (1965) Direct studies on the disappearance of the transmitter and changes in the uptake–storage mechanisms of degenerating adrenergic nerves. *Acta physiol. scand.* **64**, 211–223.

MOTAVKIN, P. A., and DOVBISH, T. V. (1971) Histochemical characteristics of acetyl-cholinesterase of the nerves innervating the brain vessels. *Acta morph. hung.* **19**, 159–173.

NELSON, E. and RENNELS, M. (1970a) Innervation of intracranial arteries. *Brain* **93**, 475–490.

NELSON, E., and RENNELS, M. (1970b) Neuromuscular contacts in intracranial arteries of the cat. *Science* **167**, 301–302.

NIELSEN, K. C., and OWMAN, CH. (1967) Adrenergic innervation of pial arteries related to the circle of Willis in the cat. *Brain Res.* **6**, 773–776.

NIELSEN, K. C., and OWMAN, CH. (1970) Contractile response and amine receptor mechanisms in isolated pial arteries. *Acta neurol. scand.* **46**, 626–627.

NIELSEN, K. C., and OWMAN, CH. (1971) Contractile response and amine receptor mechanisms in isolated middle cerebral artery of the cat. *Brain Res.* **27**, 33–42.

NIELSEN, K. C., OWMAN, CH., and SPORRONG, B. (1971a) Ultrastructure of the autonomic innervation apparatus in the main pial arteries of rats and cats. *Brain Res.* **27**, 25–32.

NIELSEN, K. C., OWMAN, CH., and SPORRONG, B. (1971b) Sympathetic nervous control of pial arteries: tyramine-induced contraction of the isolated middle cerebral artery of the cat. In *Brain and Blood Flow* (R. W. Ross Russell, ed.), Pitman, London, pp. 244–247.

OWMAN, CH., and WEST, K. A. (1970) Effect of superior cervical sympathectomy on experimentally induced intracranial hypertension. *Brain Res.* **18**, 469–476.

OWMAN, CH., ARONSON, S., GENNSER, G., and SJÖBERG, N.-O. (1973) Histochemical and pharmacological evidence of amine mechanisms in human fetal vascular shunts. In *Fetal Pharmacology* (L. Boréus, ed.), Raven Press, New York, pp. 179–191.

PEASE, D. C. and MOLINARI, S. (1960) Electron microscopy of muscular arteries; pial vessels of the cat and monkey. *J. Ultrastruct. Res.* **3**, 447–468.

PLECHKOVA, E. K., MCHEDLISHVILI, G. I., LAVRENTIEVA, N. B., and NIKOLAISHVILI, L. S. (1969) On the cholinergic mechanism responsible for the functional dilation of the arteries supplying the cerebral cortex. In *Correlation of Blood Supply with Metabolism and Function* (G. I. Mchedlishvili, ed.), Met-sniereba Publishing House, Tbilisi, pp. 172–178.

POLITOFF, A., and MACRI, F. (1966) Pharmacologic differences between isolated, perfused arteries of the choroid plexus and of the brain parenchyma. *Int. J. Neuropharmac.* **5**, 155–162.

PURVES, M. J. (1972) *The Physiology of the Cerebral Circulation*, Cambridge University Press, Cambridge, pp. 1–420.

REHN, N. O. (1958) Effect of decentralization on the content of catecholamines in the spleen and kidney of the cat. *Acta physiol. scand.* **42**, 309–312.

ROSENBLUM, W. I. (1965) Cerebral microcirculation: a review emphasizing the interrelationship of local blood flow and neuronal function. *Angiology* **16**, 485–507.

ROSENBLUM, W. I. (1969) Cerebral arteriolar spasm inhibited by β-blocking agents. *Archs. Neurol. Chicago* **21**, 296–302.

ROSENBLUM, W. I. (1971) Neurogenic control of cerebral circulation. *Stroke* **2**, 429–439.

SAMARASINGHE, D. D. (1965) The innervation of the cerebral arteries in the rat: an electron microscope study. *J. Anat.* **99**, 815–828.

SAMORAJSKI, T., and MARKS, B. H. (1962) Localization of tritiated norepinephrine in mouse brain. *J. Histochem. Cytochem.* **10**, 392–399.

SATO, S. (1966) An electron microscopic study on the innervation of the intracranial artery of the rat. *Am. J. Anat.* **118**, 873–890.

SCHENK, E. A. and EL BADAWI, A. (1968) Dual innervation of arteries and arterioles: histochemical study. *Z. Zellforsch.* **91**, 170–177.

SEARS, M. L., and GILLIS, C. N. (1967) Mydriasis and the increase in outflow of aqueous humor from the rabbit eye after cervical ganglionectomy in relation to the release of norepinephrine from the iris. *Biochem. Pharmac.* **16**, 777–782.

SEDVALL, G. C. (1969) Effect of nerve stimulation on accumulation and disappearance of catecholamines formed from radioactive precursors *in vivo*. In *Metabolism of Amines in the Brain* (G. Hooper, ed.), Macmillan, New York, pp. 23–28.

SEYLAZ, J., AUBINEAU, P., EDVINSSON, L., MAMO, H., NIELSEN, K. C., OWMAN, CH., and SERCOMBE, R. (1973) Regional differences in beta-adrenergic effects on local cerebral blood flow and in sympathetic vascular innervation. *Stroke* **4**, 369–370.

TRENDELENBURG, U. (1963) Time course of changes in sensitivity after denervation of the nictitating membrane of the spinal cat. *J. Pharmac. Exp. Ther.* **142**, 335–342.

UCHIDA, E., BOHR, D. F., and HOOBLER, S. W. (1967) A method for studying isolated resistance vessels from rabbit mesentery and brain and their responses to drugs. *Circulation Res.* **21**, 525–536.

WAHL, M., KUSCHINSKY, W., BOSSE, O., OLESEN, J., LASSEN, N. A., INGVAR, D. H., and THURAU, K. (1971/2) Adrenergic control of cerebral vascular resistance: a micropuncture study. *Eur. Neurol.* **6**, 185–189.

PHARMACOLOGICAL APPROACHES TO MONOAMINE RECEPTORS DURING BRAIN DEVELOPMENT

PER LUNDBORG AND CAROL KELLOGG

Department of Pharmacology, University of Göteborg, Göteborg, Sweden and
Department of Psychology, University of Rochester, Rochester, New York 14627, USA

SUMMARY

Using biochemical, pharmacological, and behavioral methods, we have initiated studies on the ontogeny of functional catecholamine neurons in the brain. Studies in both rats and rabbits have suggested that receptors sensitive to dopamine develop over the first week or two of postnatal life. This period may represent a critical period for the development of these receptors in that chronic pharmacologic interference during the maturation of these receptors produces aberrant motor development. This evidence was interpreted to suggest that the drugs used interfered with dopamine receptor maturation and/or maturation of feedback control mechanisms in the synapse. Further, the evidence collected to date indicate that physiologically functional noradrenaline-containing neurons develop earlier than do dopamine-containing neurons. The differential rate of development of these neurons provides for a potential imbalance of released transmitter which may be of considerable significance. The studies we have presented have assisted in determining when the morphologic and enzymatic development of catecholamine pathways become integrated into functioning catecholamine neurons.

INTRODUCTION

The mechanisms for the synthesis, release, and inactivation of catecholamine (CA) in the brain as well as mechanisms for the control of these processes have been extensively investigated in the adult animal and many functional implications involving these neurotransmitters have been suggested. However, until very recently, the ontogeny of these mechanisms have not been thoroughly investigated. The information that could be acquired from such studies as pertains to the interaction of neurotransmitters, the relation of CA to various pathologic states in infancy and childhood, and the effect that psychotropic agents interacting with the CA neurons in the brain may exert on the ontogeny of these systems deems it of considerable interest to gain an understanding of the ontogeny of the CA.

We have chosen to examine the functional maturation of noradrenaline (NA) and dopamine (DA) terminals in the brain, i.e. when does the morphologic and enzymatic development become integrated into a fully functioning CA system as has been described

561

in the adult brain. Towards this end we have utilized pharmacologic, behavioral, and bio-chemical methods of studying a dynamic process.

ACCUMULATION OF HOMOVANILIC ACID (HVA) IN THE BRAIN IN RESPONSE TO HALOPERIDOL TREATMENT OF DEVELOPING RABBITS

The neuroleptic drug haloperidol is known to block CA receptors in the brain. When used in low doses it acts almost exclusively as a DA receptor blocking agent (Andén et al., 1970a) and it has been suggested that such an inhibition of the CA receptors of the effector cells may result in an increased release of the transmitter from the neurons with a com-pensatory stimulation of the CA synthesis. Such an increase in release of DA results in an increase in the amount of DA metabolites in brain (Andén et al., 1964; Roos, 1965). The major metabolite of DA is HVA, which is formed from dihydroxyphenyl acetic acid after attack by the enzyme catechol-O-methyl transferase. Applying these observations to the problem of analyzing development of functional nerve terminals suggested that the amount of HVA formed after administration of haloperidol could give information concerning the ontogenic development of DA receptors in the brain (Kellogg et al., 1972).

In the study, albino rabbits of the same strain were used. Prenatally the mothers were given haloperidol (0.2 mg/kg) intravenously into an ear vein on day 24, 26, 28, or 29 of gestation. Control animals were given 5.5% glucose only. The pregnant animals were killed 4 h after injection; the fetuses were removed by caesarian section and were killed by decapitation. Postnatally the animals were utilized either 3 or 4 h after birth or at 4, 7, 14, 21, and 28 days of age. Within each litter the animals were divided into haloperidol-treated (0.2 mg/kg) and glucose-treated groups. They were all injected subcutaneously in the back. Also these animals were killed 4 h after injection and the brains were analyzed for DA, HVA, or 5-hydroxyindoleacetic acid (5-HIAA).

The fetal brain levels of HVA were almost unmeasurable until at 28 days of gestation. At this age the foetal brain levels of HVA were the same in treated and control animals. However, on the twenty-ninth day there was a significant difference ($p < 0.001$) between controls and haloperidol-treated animals (Fig. 1).

Postnatally the HVA level in the brain of newborn animals was 0.119 ± 0.008 μg/g. A gradual increase in the level of HVA in control animals was observed up to 3–4 weeks of age, reaching a level of 0.265 μg/g. Haloperidol caused an increase in HVA levels at all postnatal ages with the magnitude of the increase more pronounced at 3–4 weeks of age than in the newborn animals. Analysis of the individual regression coefficients, calculated for the data of each curve, indicated that the curves were significantly different from zero ($p < 0.001$) and significantly different from each other ($p < 0.001$).

The pronounced increase in HVA levels observed in adult animals after haloperidol treatment is thought to be related to an increase in release of DA from the nerve endings with a subsequent metabolism of the amine. Such a release could be looked upon as a compensatory mechanism induced by the interference of haloperidol with the receptors on the effector cell. In the present study, a gradual increase in the magnitude of the HVA response in the brain induced by haloperidol treatment was observed to occur from birth to 4 weeks of age.

Various factors could be responsible for the age-dependent response to haloperidol, including ontogeny of the mechanisms of excretion of acid metabolites from the brain, changes in turnover rate of DA with age, and changes in the metabolism of DA. However, the most probable explanation for the findings would appear to be related to DA receptor-blocking activity of haloperidol. If the central DA receptors on the effector cells develop slowly with age, or if an important link in the feedback control is not fully developed at birth, an increased response to haloperidol treatment would be expected to occur with an increase in age.

If the DA receptors are developing during the first period of rabbit postnatal life, an interesting hypothesis would be to consider this period as a "vulnerable period" with respect to the DA receptors. To test this hypothesis the possible interference by a DA receptor-blocking agent on the maturation of monoaminergic pathways of the brain was studied (Lundborg, 1972). Ten albino female rabbits were used for the study. At parturition, five mothers were randomly chosen as experimental animals and the other five as controls.

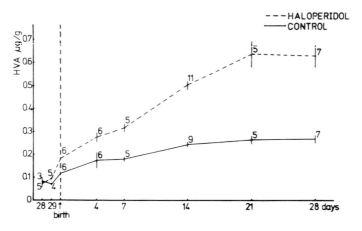

FIG. 1. Levels of homovanilic acid (HVA, $\mu g/g$) in the brains of rabbits at various pre- and postnatal ages. Control animals were treated with saline, and experimentals were given halo-peridol (0.2 mg/kg). Prenatally both drug and saline were given intravenously to the mother, and the foetuses were delivered by caesarian section. Postnatally the animals were injected subcutaneously in the back. All animals were killed 4 h after injection. Data expressed as means $\pm$ SEM.

From the day after birth (day 1) and for a period of 7 days, the experimental animals were given haloperidol, 1 mg/kg/day, in the daily supply of drinking water. The magnitude of response, noted as an increase in brain HVA, after this oral dose corresponds fairly well to 0.2 mg/kg given subcutaneously. Control animals received only the drug vehicle. After the 7-day period of drug treatment, all animals were given water *ad libitum*.

No behavioral difference could be observed between treated and untreated mothers during or after haloperidol administration. Neither was there any observable difference between "treated" (i.e. those animals being nursed by haloperidol-treated mothers) and "untreated" litters in mortality and body weight, nor could any behavioral difference be observed when the young were kept in the nest with their mother. However, when they were placed on a surface outside the cage and started to move, a considerable difference could be observed between the "treated" and "untreated" young animals. At 8 days of age the halo-peridol-treated animals displayed considerable gait problems whereas the "untreated" animals were already moving in a way rather similar to that of adult animals with sym-metrical movements of their hind limbs. The "treated" animals, on the other hand, displayed

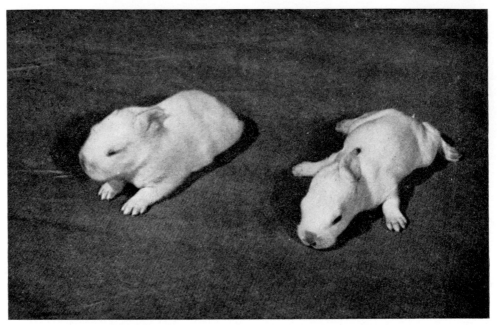

Fig. 2. Ten-day-old rabbits nursed by mothers. Right: offspring of mother treated with halo-peridol (1 mg/kg/day in 500–600 ml drinking water from days 1 to 7 after parturition). Left: offspring of untreated mother. Note inability of the young "treated" rabbit to raise its head and to elevate itself from a smooth surface.

a marked inability to elevate themselves above the smooth surface, and they moved either by crawling with an amphibious swimming motion or, when able to elevate themselves, with uncoordinated step-for-step movements without trying to jump. They also demon-strated a certain inability of head-raising, and such attempts were combined with tremor of the head. When the animals were placed on a smooth surface, the inability to elevate themselves was almost complete and the general impression was that of a muscular weakness in the proximal part of the extremities (Fig. 2).

During the period between 8 and 14 days of age, the "treated" young animals improved a little in their way of moving in that they could now elevate themselves normally on a rough surface. On a smooth surface the 14-day-old "treated" animals still demonstrated the similar impairments as described above, but they were less pronounced. The most typical abnormal sign observed in these animals was a failure of coordination of the hind-limb which appeared to be the result of weakness in the flexor muscles of the hip joint. They also moved more slowly and appeared to show less exploratory behavior than "untreated" animals of the same age. The 4-week-old "treated" animals behaved very similarly to the control animals. However, the same signs of muscular dysfunction in the hindlimbs as described above, whilst less pronounced, could still be observed.

It seems quite plausible that the behavioral changes observed in the "treated" young could be related to a specific effect of haloperidol elicited by a continuous blockade of DA receptors in the brain during a period when "dopaminergic" synapses are under maturation. Such developmental abnormalities could occur if stimulation of postsynaptic dopamine receptors is of importance for the functional development either of various postsynaptic neural pathways or of important feedback control systems. It should also be mentioned that haloperidol given as a single huge parenteral dose in an acute situation to previously untreated animals did not elicit the same effects as observed in the present study. The behavioral results observed following chronic administration of haloperidol cannot therefore be explained as a direct accumulative effect of the drug. Since the symptoms observed seemed to disappear with age, they may be reversible or the further maturation of other neural pathways may partly mask the changes caused by haloperidol. These behavioral changes induced by haloperidol have been more extensively studied in rats utilizing more specific behavioral tests (Engel *et al.*, this symposium).

Behavioral changes were noted when haloperidol was administered during the "vulnerable" period of development of DA receptors, but in a previous (unpublished) study, no behavioral effect could be noted in the offspring when haloperidol was administered prenatally to the mothers during different gestational periods. This effect was not unexpected, since, as was discussed above, no response to haloperidol (change in HVA) could be detected in foetal rabbits until the twenty-ninth day of gestation. These observations could perhaps explain the extremely inconclusive data obtained by many investigators studying behavioral responses in young animals whose mothers were treated with tranquilizers prenatally (Hoffeld and Webster, 1965; Werboff and Kesner, 1963; Jewett and Norton, 1966). Thus a critical period for drugs interacting with DA receptors may have been defined.

INDUCTION OF MOTOR ACTIVITY IN NEONATAL AND YOUNG RATS IN RESPONSE TO L-DOPA AND NA OR DA RECEPTOR-STIMULATING AGENTS

When L-DOPA (L-3,4-dihydroxyphenylalanine) is administered to adult experimental animals, a syndrome characterized by marked autonomic signs as well as signs of central stimulation is elicited. Extensive studies have been carried out to analyze the central actions of L-DOPA, and it is generally accepted that both NA and DA produced in the brain from L-DOPA are involved in the induced responses.

The central responses elicited by L-DOPA are variable but appear to have a dose-dependent relationship (Strömberg, 1970) with lower doses having a depressing effect and higher doses an excitatory effect upon locomotion. When L-DOPA is given, NA and DA are formed at many locations in the central nervous system and the amount of the two catecholamines synthesized from L-DOPA in the different brain regions is proportional to the L-DOPA decarboxylase activity and endogenous monoamine content (Bertler and Rosengren, 1959). The complexity of the adult nervous system makes it difficult to separate the various components of the L-DOPA-induced behavioral response. However, the study of the developing animals was considered a useful approach to separating into individual components the total behavioral response elicited by L-DOPA. In a previous study, the presence of neurons in the brain capable of synthesizing, retaining, and metabolizing NA and DA from L-DOPA was demonstrated following the peripheral administration of tritiated L-DOPA (Kellogg and Lundborg, 1972a).

In the present study, various pharmacological agents have been utilized to assist in separating the components of the L-DOPA-induced response in developing rats (Kellogg and Lundborg, 1972b). As in the rabbit, the rat is a nonprecocial animal with the various regions of the brain developing at different times postnatally, thus facilitating the study of centrally elicited behavioral responses.

Young rats of the Sprague–Dawley strain were studied at 1, 4, 7, 14, and 21 days post-natal age.

BEHAVIORAL OBSERVATIONS

The behavior induced in the young animals by various pharmacological manipulations was carefully observed and recorded. In all experiments the animals were independently observed and the induced activity graded by two individuals. Animals from each group were analyzed on at least two different days, with a minimum of five animals included in each group. All animals were observed from the time of injection for a period of 1–2 h. The following drugs were utilized and will be considered in the present review:

(1) L-DOPA (100 mg/kg). Pilot studies were performed in which doses of L-DOPA in the range of 50–200 mg/kg were analyzed and the dose of 100 mg/kg selected for analysis at all ages.

(2) Clonidine (2 mg/kg). Clonidine is reported to stimulate central NA receptors (Andén et al., 1970b) and was utilized for that purpose.

(3) Apomorphine (1 mg/kg) is a compound with a stimulating effect on central DA receptors (Andén et al., 1967a; Roos, 1969).

(4) Haloperidol (20 mg/kg) is a butyrophenone derivative that has been shown to block both central DA and, when given in high doses, NA receptors (Andén et al., 1970a).

Only the behavioral changes induced by the various drugs will be considered in the present review. The L-DOPA-induced behavior in the young rats could be separated into two major characteristics—crawling and head-raising. These two characteristics were graded as marked, moderate, slight, depressed, or no change from untreated animals or from the first drug when more than one drug was utilized. There was little, if any, variation between the grades given by the two observers. In cases where differences were noted, the grade has been enclosed in parentheses in Table 1.

TABLE 1. BEHAVIORAL OBSERVATIONS

	Head-raising					Crawling				
Age in days:	1	4	7	14	21	1	4	7	14	21
Treatment										
Saline	0	0	0	0	0	0	0	0	0	0
L-DOPA (100 mg/kg)	+++	+++	+++	++	+	+++	+++	+++	++	−
Clonidine (2 mg/kg)	0	+	+	−	−	++	++	++	++	−
Apomorphine (1 mg/kg)	(+)	(++)	(++)	+		0	(+)	(+)	−	−
Haloperidol (20 mg/kg) + L-DOPA (100 mg/kg)	0	0	0	0	0	0	0	0	0	0

The overt behavior was observed in rats at different postnatal ages following the subcutaneous injection of various drugs. Responses were graded as: +++ marked, ++ moderate, + slight, and − depressed. 0 indicates no changes from untreated animals or in the case of two drug treatments, no change from the first drug. The response to haloperidol alone is not listed in the table, but at all ages this drug induced a state of tranquilization. All observations were graded by two observers, and a minimum of five animals were included in each group. Parentheses around grade indicate an irregular but noticeable response.

1. L-DOPA (100 mg/kg)

This drug induced intense crawling at 1, 4, and 7 days of age and the motor activity elicited was a function of the motor ability at a particular age. At 1 day the animals crawled with an amphibious, swimming motion, at 4 days they displayed more limb extension and could elevate themselves above the crawling surface, and at 7 days the animals crawled with vigorous, strong movements and were able to readily right themselves from a back-lying position. L-DOPA also induced strong head-raising ability at these ages to the extent that they would lift their heads over a small obstacle placed in their crawling path.

At 14 days L-DOPA increased motor activity, but the induced running was sporadic with intermittent periods in which the animal appeared stuporous. They displayed an "arch-back" posture with extremely abducted hindlegs. Some stereotyped behavior such as licking the cage walls was noted at this age in accord with the developmental progress. At 21 days any hyperactivity observed was short-lasting, and often the animals appeared depressed.

2. CLONIDINE (2 mg/kg)

In the younger age groups (1, 4, and 7 days) clonidine stimulated the same type of crawling as seen following L-DOPA; however, the clonidine-induced running was slower and less frantic than after L-DOPA, and there was a noticeable decrease in head-raising in animals at these ages treated with clonidine as compared to those receiving L-DOPA. At 14 days, clonidine induced sporadic running and postural changes similar to the pattern induced by L-DOPA; however, the animals appeared less stable, tending to fall over quite frequently. Clonidine treatment also produced decreased head-raising for animals at this age as compared to the control animals. The appearance of animals at 21 days given clonidine was primarily that of a depressed state.

3. APOMORPHINE (1 mg/kg)

A definite response to apomorphine in the youngest animals was difficult to grade because the response varied from day to day. However, at 1 day of age a slight behavioral response in the form of a head-tremor was observed following apomorphine injection. At 4 and 7 days of age, apomorphine stimulated slight forward-crawling, but it was not a continuous response as was that observed after L-DOPA. Very little crawling or running was noted, however. At 21 days, apomorphine elicited definite stereotypic behavior such as digging and grooming.

4. HALOPERIDOL PLUS OTHER AGENTS

Twenty mg/kg of haloperidol inhibited the response to L-DOPA and clonidine in animals at all ages.

The information thus obtained indicates that the L-DOPA-induced behavior was elicited by NA and/or DA produced in the brain from the administered L-DOPA. Similar behavioral patterns were elicited at the respective ages by known NA and DA receptor-stimulating agents such as clonidine and apomorphine respectively. Haloperidol, a monoamine receptor-blocking agent, blocked L-DOPA and clonidine-induced responses at all ages when given in a high dose. Because haloperidol is a much more potent inhibitor of DA receptors than NA receptors (Andén et al., 1970a), the high doses were necessary to effectively inhibit the NA receptors. However, it should also be noted that at the dose administered, the animals were heavily tranquilized. To further support NA and/or DA involvement in L-DOPA-induced hyperactivity, the increase in the concentration of NA and DA measured in the brain following L-DOPA administration correlated well with the duration of the induced hyperactivity (Kellogg and Lundborg, 1972b).

The data thus obtained in the behavioral study suggest the possibility of an earlier development of sensitive and functional NA receptors than DA receptors because of an earlier repeatable response to clonidine than to apomorphine. The delay in response to apomorphine could be related to the slow development of DA concentration in the neo-striatum (e.g. Connor and Neff, 1970; Agrawal and Himwich, 1970; Loizou, 1972) since this CA is concentrated primarily in the neostriatum (Bertler and Rosengren, 1959) in the nerve terminals of ascending fibers (Andén et al., 1966). In somewhat of a contradiction to the lack of pronounced stereotypic behavior in response to apomorphine until 21 days of age in our study, others have reported D-amphetamine-induced gnawing ("gumming") in rats at 1 day of age (McGeer et al., 1971). Although such an observation suggests functional DA receptors in the neostriatum at that age, the possibility that the response was induced by an alternate neuronal pathway cannot be excluded. D-amphetamine has been demonstrated to release both NA and DA from nerve terminals.

From the observations of Loizou (1972), a functioning DA system would seem to occur prior to the NA systems because of the earlier appearance of DA terminals in the telencephalon and diencephalon at a time when there was a noted sparseness of NA terminals. However, density of the CA terminals at the different ages cannot be precisely correlated to the age-specific L-DOPA-induced behavioral responses because other neurotransmitters, e.g. acetylcholine, may be considered to influence the final behavioral expression. Evidence from studies on the effect of scopolamine on amphetamine-induced hyperactivity has suggested that a functional acetylcholine system matures at a later time in rats than an adrenergic system (Campbell et al., 1969; Fibiger et al., 1970).

Thus the behavioral study indicated that in rats as in rabbits, development of DA receptors seems to occur during the first week or two of postnatal life. The question then arises whether or not this represents a "vulnerable" period in the rat for proper development of the DA receptors. To test this, data has been gathered on rats given small doses of L-DOPA (10, 20, or 30 mg/kg) for the first 7 days after birth (de Wyngaert and Kellogg, in preparation). Behavioral observations were made at 8, 10, 14, 20, and 25 days of age. Animals were observed for their spontaneous locomotor activity, geotaxic response, and hyperactivity following a test dose of L-DOPA (100 mg/kg). Marked motor deficits were noted primarily in response to the test dose of L-DOPA, and these deficits were pronounced up to 14 days of age. By 21 days there were very little observable differences between treated and control animals. As blocking DA receptors in rabbits appeared to impair normal motor development, so it appears can overstimulation of DA and/or NA receptors during a related period in the rat.

DISAPPEARANCE OF CATECHOLAMINES FROM THE RAT BRAIN AFTER SYNTHESIS INHIBITION

In addition to analyzing the development of the postsynaptic receptors sensitive to the CA, we also wanted to analyze the onset of functional DA- and NA-containing neurons. The method selected was to follow the disappearance of the monoamines after treatment

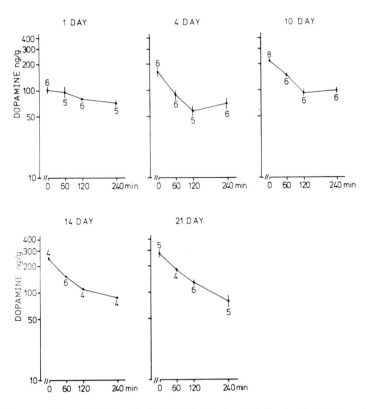

FIG. 3. Concentration of DA (ng/g) $\pm$ SEM in the brain following inhibition of tyrosine hydroxylase with H 44/68, 250 mg/kg. 0 value represents saline-treated control animals. Numbers represent number of groups determined.

with an inhibitor of tyrosine hydroxylase (Kellogg and Lundborg, 1973). This enzyme is considered to be rate-limiting in the production of CA. Inhibition of this enzyme with a subsequent decrease in NA and DA has been demonstrated to be dependent upon the presence of nerve impulses (Andén et al., 1967). This approach was considered useful in providing information on the time of development of physiologically functional DA and NA neurons.

Young rats of the Sprague–Dawley strain were analyzed at 1, 4, 10, 14, and 21 days postnatal age. Tyrosine was inhibited using H 44/68 (α-methyl-p-tyrosine methyl ester) at a dose of 250 mg/kg. Control animals received saline. All injections were made subcutaneously and animals were killed at 0 (control), 1, 2, or 4 h after injection of the synthesis inhibitor.

Figure 3 describes the disappearance of DA from whole brain over time. For each curve (at a respective age) a regression coefficient was calculated and tested for significance of linearity. Following inhibition of tyrosine hydroxylase, there was no significant linear decrease in DA concentration with time at 1 day of age ($p > 0.05$). However, at this age there was a noted decrease in the DA concentration at the 4 h time point as compared to the control, indicating some release of DA. At all other ages DA decreased over the 4 h period with a highly significant linear component. The decrease of DA over time after treatment

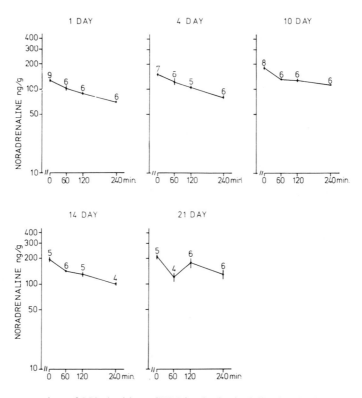

FIG. 4. Concentration of NA (ng/g) $\pm$ SEM in the brain following inhibition of tyrosine hydroxylase with H 44/68, 250 mg/kg. 0 value represents saline-treated control animals. Numbers represent number of groups determined.

with H44/68 appeared to be biphasic. Statistical analysis supported the biphasic appearance of the curves from 4 days of age.

In a few animals, at all ages, the effect of a second dose of H44/68 upon the disappearance of DA was investigated. A second dose of 250 mg/kg was administered 2 h after the initial injection and DA in the brain was determined at 4 h after the initial injection. No difference in the DA concentration was observed (data not included) at this time point between animals given one or two doses of H44/68. This observation indicates that the biphasic curve probably did not result from incomplete inhibition of tyrosine hydroxylase centrally.

Following treatment with H44/68, the NA concentration in whole brain (Fig. 4) decreased significantly over time at all ages with the exception of the 21-day-old animals. These findings provide further support to the suggestions presented above that NA-containing neurons within the brain become functionally mature at an earlier age than do DA-containing neurons. Whilst a significant decrease in NA was observed in whole brain from 1 day of age in response to inhibition of tyrosine hydroxylase, there was no significant decrease in DA noted until 4 days' postnatal age. Hence there appears to be support for the impression of a more rapid maturation of NA neurons as compared to DA neurons, not only morphologically (Loizou, 1972) and biochemically (Coyle, 1973), but also functionally.

The low rate of disappearance of DA in the 1-day-old animals and the biphasic curve of disappearance of DA thereafter could be interpreted in at least two ways—either as an inability of nerve impulses to release the transmitter substance or as an absence of impulse conduction in the DA neurons. The DA cell bodies are located exclusively in the brain stem, and processes project from this region to innervate other areas of the brain. Before the terminals develop, the DA present in proliferating axons and presumably localized in newly formed granules is probably not available for release by any impulse flow. Release of DA would increase in proportion to development of the terminal network. The increased rate of loss of DA observed after tyrosine hydroxylase inhibition with progressing age could reflect this development.

Following the other interpretation, the early DA neurons may behave similarly to postsynaptic sympathetic neurons in the periphery after presynaptic denervation. In the absence of impulse flow in the postsynaptic neuron, the transmitter release would be slow and no appreciable decrease in transmitter content would be expected in response to tyrosine hydroxylase inhibition. Perhaps both interpretations will be proven valid to a certain extent. In either case, a potential imbalance could exist in different brain regions between released transmitters if NA-containing neurons are more functional than DA-containing neurons, and this imbalance could in part account for age-specific behavioral responses, seen, e.g., in response to a large dose of L-DOPA.

The ontogeny of CA receptors and neurons in the brain has been further analyzed by examining the ability of CA receptor-stimulating agents to attenuate the decrease of NA and DA following synthesis inhibition (Kellogg and Wennerström, 1973). Young rats of the Long–Evans Hooded strain were studied at 4 and 14 days of postnatal age since the previous study suggested definite differences between the turnover rate of DA at these two ages. The brains were dissected into four regions: hemispheres, neostriatum, diencephalon, and midbrain–brain stem. NA and DA were analyzed 2 h after inhibition of tyrosine hydroxylase using H44/68 (250 mg/kg). In the experimental groups, apomorphine (1 mg/kg) or clonidine (2 mg/kg) was given 30 min before the enzyme inhibitor. These agents have been demonstrated to markedly attenuate the decrease of DA and NA respectively after synthesis inhibition.

The results were analyzed using the Mann–Whitney U test. Median values measured in the different regions are described in Table 2. A markedly significant decrease in NA following synthesis inhibition was noted at 4 days of age in the cortex and brain stem. By 14 days, the decrease of NA in the diencephalon also approached significance ($p = 0.056$). A significant decrease in DA was observed at 4 days of age in the neostriatum and diencephalon. At 14 days a significant decrease of DA was also noted in the brain stem. According to the above discussion, the brain regions demonstrating significant changes in the CA concentrations following inhibition of tyrosine hydroxylase should be considered to contain physiologically functional CA-containing neurons.

Clonidine significantly attenuated the decrease in NA at 4 days of age in the cortex ($p = 0.014$) and brain stem ($p = 0.029$), and in all regions at 14 days. Apomorphine attenuated the decrease of DA in the diencephalon and neostriatum at 4 days, but the level of significance was much lower ($p = 0.057$) than observed for NA. At 14 days of age a significant attenuation of DA was also noted in the brain stem ($p = 0.016$), but the significance in the neostriatum had dropped ($p = 0.095$).

Thus a more pronounced feedback effect was noted in response to NA receptor-stimulation than to DA receptor-stimulation at 4 days of age. In general, the magnitude of the effect increases for both NA and DA at 14 days. However, one cannot so strongly state from these results that NA receptors develop earlier than DA receptors. The mechanism of

TABLE 2

	Cortex		Neostriatum		Diencephalon		Brain stem	
	NA	DA	NA	DA	NA	DA	NA	DA
4 Days:								
Control	54	23	67	788	171	233	171	83
H 44/68	31	25	92	435	162	146	121	42
Apomorphine + H 44/68	25	15	93	618	126	162	103	37
Clonidine + H 44/68	56	27	80	591	185	146	184	50
14 Days:								
Control	70	20	64	1559	225	512	349	79
H 44/68	33	12	23	587	210	243	223	40
Apomorphine + H 44/68	26	19	22	718	175	311	198	78
Clonidine + H 44/68	100	12	66	803	272	266	331	46

Median values in ng/g of NA and DA in the brain. Groups are saline control, H 44/68 (250 mg/kg), apomorphine (1 mg/kg) given 30 min before H 44/68, and clonidine (2 mg/kg) given 30 min before H 44/68. All determinations were made 2 h after H 44/68 (or saline). The data were analyzed using the Mann–Whitney U test. See text for significance.

feedback inhibition from the receptors is not understood. It is possible that DA receptors on the effector cell can be pharmacologically stimulated and exert influence over synthesis of DA in presynaptic neurons but not be physiologically active (i.e. the effector cell is not mature). Receptor sensitivity to many agents and transmitter substances has been observed in the purkinje cells of the cerebellum prior to the appearance of any neuronal connections (Woodward *et al.*, 1971).

The mystery of the ontogeny of the CA terminals remains yet to be fully solved. However, data gathered to date from the many approaches utilized strongly indicate that understanding the ontogeny of functional terminals (release, receptor activation, feedback, etc.) will assist in elucidating mechanisms underlying such observations as ontogenic changes in the circadian rhythms of NA and serotonin in the brain (Asano, 1971) and changes in NA and DA concentrations and tyrosine hydroxylase activity in young rats following perinatal undernutrition (Shoemaker and Wurtman, 1971).

ACKNOWLEDGEMENTS

Most of the work described in this review has been sponsored by the Swedish State Medical Research Council (Nos. 14P-3266 and 14X-2464), Expressens Prenatalforskningsfond, the National Institute for Neurological Diseases and Stroke, United States Public Health Services, No. 2 FO2 NS 31010-02 and ONR Grant No. N00014-68-A-0091.

REFERENCES

AGRAWAL, H. C., and HIMWICH, W. A. (1970) Aminoacids, proteins, and monoamines of developing brain. In *Developmental Neurobiology* (W. A. Himwich, ed.), Ch. C. Thomas, Springfield, pp. 287–310.
ANDÉN, N. E., BUTCHER, S. D., CORRODI, H., FUXE, K., and UNGERSTEDT, U. (1970a) Receptor activity and turnover rate of dopamine and noradrenaline after neuroleptics. *Eur. J. Pharmac.* **11**, 303–314.
ANDÉN, N. E., CORRODI, H., FUXE, K., HÖKFELT, B., HÖKFELT, T., RYDIN, C., and SVENSSON, T. (1970b) Evidence for a central noradrenaline receptor stimulation by clonidine. *Life Sci.* **9**, 513–523.
ANDÉN, N. E., DAHLSTRÖM, A., FUXE, K., LARSSON, K., OLSON, L., and UNGERSTEDT, U. (1966) Ascending monoamine neurones to the telencephalon and diencephalon. *Acta physiol. scand.* **67**, 313–326.

ANDÉN, N. E., FUXE, K., and HÖKFELT, T. (1967b) Effect of some drugs on central monoamine nerve terminals lacking nerve impulse flow. *Eur. J. Pharmac.* **1**, 226–232.

ANDÉN, N. E., ROOS, B. E., and WERDINIUS, B. (1964) Effects of chlorpromazine, haloperidol, and reserpine on the levels of phenolic acids in rabbit corpus striatum. *Life Sci.* **3**, 149–158.

ANDÉN, N. E., RUBENSON, A., FUXE, K., and HÖFKELT, T. (1967a) Evidence for dopamine receptor stimulation by apomorphine. *J. Pharm. Pharmac.* **19**, 627–629.

ASANO, X. (1971) The maturation of the circadian rhythm of brain norepinephrine and serotonin in the rat. *Life Sci.* **10**, 883–894.

BERTLER, Å., and ROSENGREN, E. (1959) On the distribution in brain of monoamines and of enzymes responsible for their formation. *Experientia* **15**, 382.

CAMPBELL, B. A., LYTLE, L. D., and FIBIGER, H. C. (1969) Ontogeny of adrenergic arousal and cholinergic inhibition mechanisms in the rat. *Sci.* **166**, 637–638.

CONNOR, J. D., and NEFF, N. H. (1970) Dopamine concentrations in the caudate nucleus of the developing cat. *Life Sci.* **9**, 1165–1168.

COYLE, J. T. (1973) Development of the central catecholamine neurones. In *The Neurosciences*, Third Study Program (in press).

FIBIGER, H. C., LYTLE, L. D., and CAMPBELL, B. A. (1970) Cholinergic modulation of adrenergic arousal in the developing rat. *J. Comp. Physiol. Psychol.* **72**, 384–389.

HOFFELD, D. R., and WEBSTER, R. L. (1965) Effect of injection of tranquilizing drugs during pregnancy on offspring. *Nature* **204**, 1070–1072.

JEWETT, R. E., and NORTON, S. (1966) Effect of tranquilizing drugs on postnatal behavior. *Expl. Neurol.* **14**, 33–43.

KELLOGG, C., and LUNDBORG, P. (1972a) Production of (^{3}H)catecholamines in the brain following the peripheral administration of (^{3}H)DOPA during pre- and postnatal development. *Brain Res.* **36**, 333–342.

KELLOGG, C., and LUNDBORG, P. (1972b) Ontogenic variations in responses to L-DOPA and monoamine receptor-stimulating agents. *Psychopharmac.* **23**, 187–200.

KELLOGG, C., LUNDBORG, P., and ROOS, B. E. (1972) Ontogenic changes in cerebral concentrations of homovanilic acid in response to haloperidol treatment. *Brain Res.* **40**, 469–475.

KELLOGG, C., and LUNDBORG, P. (1973) Inhibition of catecholamine synthesis during ontogenic development. *Brain Res.* (in press).

KELLOGG, C., and WENNERSTRÖM, G. (1973) Ontogeny of catecholamine receptors in the brain. Society for Neuroscience, Third Annual Meeting, San Diego, Calif., November, 1973.

LUNDBORG, P. (1972) Abnormal ontogeny in young rabbits after chronic administration of haloperidol to the nursing mothers. *Brain Res.* **44**, 684–687.

LOIZOU, L. A. (1972) The postnatal ontogeny of monoamine-containing neurones in the central nervous system of the albino rat. *Brain Res.* **40**, 395–418.

McGEER, E. G., FIBIGER, H. C., and WICKSON, V. (1971) Differential development of caudate enzymes in the neonatal rat. *Brain Res.* **32**, 433–440.

ROOS, B. E. (1965) Effects of certain tranquillizers on the level of homovanilic acid in the corpus striatum. *J. Pharm. Pharmac.* **17**, 820–821.

ROOS, B. E. (1969) Decrease in homovanilic acid as evidence for dopamine receptor stimulation by apomorphine in the neostriatum of the rat. *J. Pharm. Pharmac.* **21**, 263–264.

SHOEMAKER, W. J., and WURTMAN, R. J. (1971) Perinatal undernutrition: accumulation of catecholamines in rat brain. *Science* **171**, 1017–1019.

STRÖMBERG, U. (1970) DOPA effects on motility in mice; potentiation by MK 485 and dexchlorpheniramine. *Psychopharmac.* **18**, 58–67.

WERBOFF, J., and KESNER, R. (1963) Learning deficits of offspring after administration of tranquilizing drugs to the mother. *Nature* **197**, 106–107.

WOODWARD, D. J., HOFFER, B. J., SIGGINS, G. R., and BLOOM, F. E. (1971) The ontogenic development of synaptic junctions, synaptic activation and responsiveness to neurotransmitter substances in rat cerebellar purkinje cells. *Brain Res.* **34**, 73–97.

BRAIN AND PERIPHERAL MONOAMINES: POSSIBLE ROLE IN THE ONTOGENESIS OF NORMAL AND DRUG-INDUCED RESPONSES IN THE IMMATURE MAMMAL

LOY D. LYTLE AND FRANK C. KEIL†

Department of Nutrition and Food Science, Massachusetts Institute of Technology, Cambridge, Massachusetts 02139, USA

SUMMARY

The ability of the developing, nonprecocial newborn mammal to produce mature physiological and behavioral responses may in part depend upon the functional status of monoamine-containing neurons in the brain and periphery. Alterations produced in the patterns of locomotor activity, elective food consumption, and thermoregulation produced by various drugs thought to act via monoaminergic neurons, also change as a function of the age of the organism. Monoamine-containing neurons are not fully mature at birth in neonatal animals such as the rat: they are less able to synthesize, store, inactivate, release, and respond to neurotransmitters than are corresponding neurons in adult animals; moreover, not all of their synaptic connections have been made. The significance of changes in the developing monoamine neurons are discussed in relationship to their roles in determining the course of physiological and behavioral ontogenesis.

INTRODUCTION

Brain and peripheral neurons that contain monoamine compounds as their neurotransmitters have been associated with the regulation of numerous biochemical, physiological, and behavioral functions in the adult organism. Much less is known, however, concerning the functional significance of monoaminergic neurons during the various stages of postnatal development. Whereas a considerable body of information has accumulated regarding the behavioral and neurochemical effects of various drugs in the adult organism, fewer data exist concerning the effects of these drugs on the developing animal. In previous experiments, we have compared the physiological and behavioral effects of drugs on the responses of adult and immature mammals. The results of these experiments suggest that many psychoactive compounds thought to act on brain and peripheral monoamine-

† Now at the Department of Psychology, Stanford University, Palo Alto, California, USA.

containing neurons produce differential, age-related effects on developing animals. These differential responses may reflect major developmental changes in the maturation of brain and peripheral monoaminergic neurons.

ONTOGENETIC CHANGES IN LOCOMOTOR ACTIVITY, FOOD CONSUMPTION, AND THERMOREGULATION

LOCOMOTOR ACTIVITY

Patterns of spontaneous locomotor activity develop characteristically throughout the early postnatal life of the rat (Fig. 1). For the first 10 days of age, the neonatal rat moves about relatively little in the environment; shortly thereafter, activity increases rapidly,

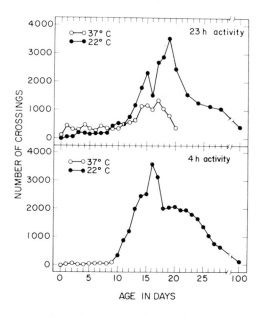

FIG. 1. Spontaneous activity of rats (as measured by stabilimeter cages) during development. The upper panel shows daily activity for groups of animals tested only once at different ages and under one of two different ambient temperature conditions. The lower panel shows the activity of a single group of animals tested for two 2 h daily periods for 28 consecutive days. (Reprinted from an article by Moorcroft et al., 1971. Copyright by the American Psychological Association, 1971.)

reaching a peak between 15 and 20 days postnatally (Moorcroft et al., 1971). This sharp rise is followed by an equally precipitous drop to near-adult activity levels by 30 days of age. The rapid increase and subsequent fall in activity presumably reflect major changes in the structure and/or functional capacity of the central and peripheral nervous systems. Prior to 10 days of age, the behavior of the rat is primarily reflexive in nature and the animal is largely unresponsive to auditory and visual stimuli. At approximately the tenth postnatal day, the sensory systems begin developing (Crowley and Hepp-Reymond, 1966; Rose, 1968; Salas et al., 1969); the maturation of these systems increases the total amount of stimuli that can impinge upon the nervous system. At the same time, the maturation of skeletal muscle and cerebellar neuronal development dramatically increases the motor and behavioral repertoire of the animal (Woodward *et al.*, 1969). The rather sharp decline in locomotor activity after the twentieth postnatal day may reflect the gradual maturation of brain and peripheral mechanisms that may serve to modulate and inhibit the overall levels of behavioral arousal. For example, damage to the frontal cortex or to the hippocampus greatly increases the level of behavioral activity following food deprivation or injections of amphetamine in adult rats (Lynch *et al.*, 1969). Removal of either of these areas in the neonatal rat, however, does not affect activity until the animals are 20–25 days of age (Moorcroft, 1971). Hence these and other neuronal systems may not become functionally involved in modulating locomotor activity until relatively late in the postnatal development of the rat.

The hamster, an animal born relatively immature, shows age-dependent changes in locomotor activity that are similar to those observed for the rat. The guinea-pig is much more developed than is the rat at birth (Dobbing and Sands, 1970; Altman, 1967). Whereas the activity of the rat and hamster peaks between the fifteenth and twentieth postnatal day and declines to adult levels by the thirtieth day of age, the locomotor activity of the newborn or juvenile guinea-pig is comparable to the activity of the adult and shows no change throughout the postnatal period (Campbell and Mabry, 1972). These data indirectly suggest that the guinea-pig may have brain and peripheral neuronal structures that are mature at birth and that are functionally equivalent to those of the adult.

ELECTIVE FOOD CONSUMPTION

The regulation of food and water intake is not fully mature until relatively late in development. The feeding and drinking patterns of the adult rat gradually emerge from reflexive components that are largely undifferentiated and nonintegrated at birth. During the pre-weaning period, the neonatal rat is greatly dependent upon the mother for the maintenance of homeostatic balance as well as for survival. Energy from milk ingested is utilized mainly for growth; regulatory processes such as thermoregulation and, to some extent, fluid balance, are controlled by the mother (Lytle *et al.*, 1971). From birth until weaning, feeding occupies a large part of the waking period, and is dependent upon the strength of the clinging, rooting, and sucking reflexes. At about the fifteenth day of age the rat is able to survive on solid food and, as weaning is instituted, the feeding pattern begins to resemble that of the adult. However, weanling rats exhibit subtle changes in the control of food and water intake that are different from those of the fully mature adult. Teitelbaum and his co-workers (Teitelbaum *et al.*, 1969; Cheng *et al.*, 1971) have used growth retardation (experimentally induced by thyroidectomy or semistarvation) as a means of slowing down the rapid developmental changes that occur in the food and water regulatory capacities of the weanling rat. With this preparation they have observed that the most retarded of these animals are completely aphagic and adipsic when offered wet palatable food or ordinary laboratory chow and water. More fully developed thyroidectomized or semistarved animals accept wet palatable food but do not eat enough to maintain weight. Still other weanling rats, even less retarded, gain weight and regulate intake on a liquid diet; however, they are still adipsic and will die if presented with dry food and water. The least retarded weanlings accept dry food and water, but drink only when they eat (*prandial drinking*); they are more *finicky* (more sensitive to food or water adulteration with quinine) than adults, and do not eat more in response to hypoglycemic challenges induced by insulin. These changes in food and water intake by the weanling rat are strikingly similar to those observed in adult rats recovering from damage to the lateral hypothalamic area (Teitelbaum and Epstein, 1962); hence, the ontogenesis of food and water intake regulation may reflect changes in the functional capacity of central and peripheral neuronal systems.

THERMOREGULATION

Neonatal rats are poikilothermic at birth (Fig. 2); body temperature becomes increasingly independent of the environmental temperature as the body size of the animal increases, insulating materials (such as hair and fat) are accumulated, and control over the cutaneous

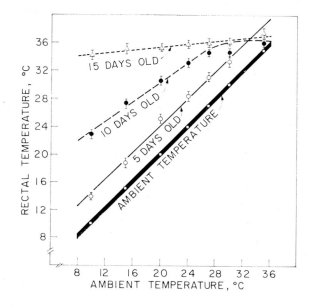

FIG. 2. The rectal temperatures of different aged animals following a 1 h period of exposure to different ambient temperature conditions (RH = 40%). Each data point represents the mean of eight animals, ± standard error. (From Lytle *et al.*, in preparation.)

circulation is acquired (Hill, 1947; Adolph, 1957; Conklin and Heggeness, 1971). Accelerated heat production following exposure to cold ambient temperatures is not present during the first 3 weeks of life; even then, it is quite unstable until long after the time of weaning (Fairfield, 1948). Heat conservation mechanisms mature gradually throughout the pre- and postnatal stages of development. These mechanisms include the thickening of the skin, eruption and growth of fur, and, early in development, attraction to the mother (Adolph, 1957). The infant rat can tolerate depressions in body temperature down approximately to 5°C, whereas in the adult the lethal limit is usually around 15°C. This early resistance to cold persists until the end of the third postnatal week (Adolph, 1957). Newborn rats lack a functional vasomotor mechanism of heat conservation and dissipation in response to changes in environmental temperature. They gradually acquire this mechanism between the first and third postnatal weeks (Poczopko, 1961). Experimentally induced changes in the growth rates of rats aged 5–20 days of age (brought on by manipulating the litter size) can alter the maturation of developmental responses to ambient temperature; core temperature

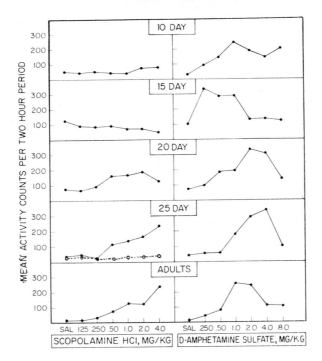

FIG. 3. The effects of the 0.9% saline vehicle (1 cc/kg) or various doses of scopolamine hydro-chloride, or D-amphetamine sulfate on the 2 h activity of rats of five different ages. Rats were habituated to the stabilimeter activity cages for 30 min prior to injection. The effect of methyl scopolamine is shown by the dotted line in the 25-day panel. All points are the means of 10–16 animals per group. The activity cages were housed in temperature-controlled cubicles main-tained at 29°C for the 10-, 15-, 20-, and 25-day-old rats and at 22°C for the 100-day-old animals. (Reprinted from Campbell et al., 1969. Copyright by the American Association for the Advancement of Science, 1969.)

decreases more slowly in large animals than in small animals following exposure to a cold ambient environment. Temperature regulation is nearly complete in large animals by the twentieth day of age, but remains immature in smaller-sized animals (Heggeness, 1962).

Many behavioral and physiological indices of maturation, thought to be mediated in adults at least in part by the activity of monoamine-containing neurons, suggest that the functional status of the immaturely born mammal is incomplete. Mature adult responses are attained only after a relatively long period of development.

ONTOGENETIC, DRUG-INDUCED CHANGES IN LOCOMOTOR ACTIVITY, FOOD CONSUMPTION, AND THERMOREGULATION

LOCOMOTOR ACTIVITY

Drugs, such as amphetamine, that presumably affect behavior by enhancing catechol-aminergic neurotransmission (Glowinski and Axelrod, 1965), increase locomotor activity very early in the postnatal development of the rat (Campbell et al., 1969); other drugs, such as scopolamine and pilocarpine, that primarily affect acetylcholinergic neurotransmission (Giarman and Pepeu, 1964; Zetler, 1968), have no effect on the activity of the developing rat until approximately the twentieth postnatal day (Fibiger et al., 1970; see Fig. 3). These psychopharmacological observations suggest that different systems in the brain that mediate behavioral arousal and behavioral inhibition become functional at different stages during development. Hence, catecholamine-containing neurons that mediate arousal may develop earlier in the rat than do acetylcholine-containing neurons that modulate these overall levels of activity. The increased levels of spontaneous locomotor activity that emerge between the fifteenth to the twentieth postnatal day in the rat may be due to the increased functional capacity of brain catecholamine-containing neurons: either a-methyl-p-tyrosine or reserpine can prevent the normal increases in activity observed at these ages; the depressive effects of these drugs can be reversed with systemic injections of L-DOPA (Campbell and Mabry, 1973).

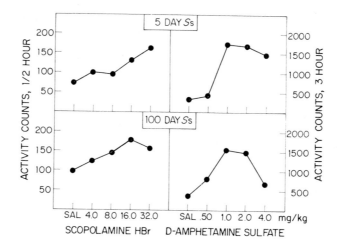

FIG. 4. The effects of saline, or various doses of scopolamine hydrobromide (left panels) or D-amphetamine sulfate (right panels) in 5-day-old and 100-day-old guinea-pigs. Animals were habituated for 30 min prior to injection; activity was measured for 30 min following the injection of scopolamine and for 3 h following the injection of amphetamine.

The differential, age-dependent responses of the rat to drugs that affect acetylcholinergic neurotransmission may reflect the immature nature of these amine-containing neurons. The newborn, more fully developed guinea-pig does not progress through a stage of hyper-activity followed by hypoactivity (Campbell and Mabry, 1972) and also responds to the activity-inducing effects of scopolamine or amphetamine in a manner very similar to that of the adult guinea-pig (Fig. 4). These data suggest that whereas acetylcholinergic-inhibitory mechanisms may not be fully mature in the neonatal rat, these systems may have attained full functional maturity in the newborn guinea-pig.

FOOD CONSUMPTION

Even though the arousal effects of amphetamine are present quite early in the development of the rat, the anorexic or appetite-reducing effects of the drug are not clearly evident until the fifteenth to the twentieth postnatal day (Lytle et al., 1971; see Fig. 5). Hence, amphetamine-induced changes in activity and appetite may be mediated via different neuroanatomical and/or neurochemical systems in the brain. Since injections of insulin do not increase feeding behavior in satiated newborn animals (as they do in the adult) until after the twenty-fifth day of age (Teitelbaum *et al.*, 1969; Lytle *et al.*, 1971), many of the brain and peripheral neurons that mediate food and water regulation in the adult may not be functionally mature in the neonatal rat.

Lesions of the lateral hypothalamic areas of the brains of adult rats produce decreases in food and water intake that eventually result in death unless appropriate therapeutic measures are instituted (Anand and Brobeck, 1951; Teitelbaum and Epstein, 1962). Electrolytic lesions of the area destroy traversing neurons that contain norepinephrine, dopamine, or serotonin (Ungerstedt, 1971a); one monoamine pathway cannot be selectively damaged with electrolytic lesions without concomitant destruction of the other pathways. Lesions in the lateral hypothalamic area radically alter the content of norepinephrine, dopamine,

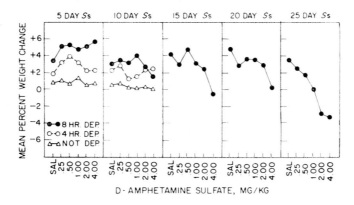

FIG. 5. The effects of various doses of D-amphetamine sulfate or the 0.9% saline vehicle on food intake, as measured by weight change, in the developing rat. Subjects were placed with a mammectomized foster mother for an 8 h period of food and water deprivation. At the end of this period, the animals were weighed, injected, and then returned to the normal dam for a 1 h test period of *ad libitum* feeding. Animals were reweighed at the end of the hour. Additional groups were tested at 5 and 10 days of age with *ad libitum* or 4 h periods of deprivation to control for the possibility ceiling effects induced by the severity of the 8 h deprivation condition. (Reprinted from Lytle *et al.*, 1971. Copyright by the American Psychological Association, 1971.)

and serotonin in more rostrally located brain structures (Heller and Moore, 1968). Ungerstedt (1971b) has speculated that the damage to the dopamine-containing neurons of the nigro-striatal pathway alone may be sufficient to reproduce the aphagia and adipsia classically associated with the lateral hypothalamic syndrome. In developing animals, the gradual maturation of monoamine-containing neurons is associated temporally with the behavioral changes that occur in the regulation of food and water consumption. Newborn (Lytle *et al.*, 1972) or 7-day-old (Breese and Traylor, 1972) rats injected with intracisternal doses of 6-hydroxydopamine, a drug that destroys catecholamine-containing neurons, or 5,7-dihydroxytryptamine (Lytle *et al.*, in preparation), a drug that destroys serotonin-containing neurons, show dose-related, severe retardations in growth. The depressions in growth rates are associated with long-lasting depletions in the levels of brain norepinephrine and dopamine following the injection of 6-hydroxydopamine, and in brain serotonin following the injection of 5,7-dihydroxytryptamine. Attempts to reverse the growth retardation with injections of growth hormone (Breese and Traylor, 1972) or stomach intubations of high caloric diets (Lytle *et al.*, unpublished observations) have been unsuccessful. No

studies have yet explored the other developmental physiological and behavioral consequences of the destruction of monoamine-containing neurons by these agents.

THERMOREGULATION

Whereas the newborn rat is poikilothermic and is unable to regulate temperature until
relatively late in the postnatal period, amphetamine-induced alterations in the thermoregulatory capacity of the rat are present from the time of birth. Amphetamine-injected
intraperitoneally or intracisternally to developing rats produces *hyper*thermia in all animals
following exposure to high ambient temperature conditions (37°C); the effects of the drug
on the body temperatures of young rats exposed to a 22°C ambient temperature are more
complex (Figs. 6 and 7). At 5 days of age the highest intraperitoneal or intracisternal doses
of the drug decrease body temperature. However, the failure to observe a dose-related effect
on rectal temperature and the lack of any other associated changes in body temperatures in
the 10-day-old animals following amphetamine at this ambient temperature condition
obscure the significance of the effect. By 15 days of age the rat is able to regulate body
temperature within small limits and the hypothermic effects of amphetamine, characteristically observed following its administration to adult rats, become evident. If the body
temperature of the developing rat is measured following amphetamine at *thermoneutral*
ambient conditions (i.e. at the minimum ambient temperature at which rectal temperature
changes less than 1°C over a 1 h time period), no hypothermia can be detected until 15 days
of age or older (Lytle *et al.*, in preparation). Whereas amphetamine-induced hyperthermia
is present in animals that apparently lack the mature physiologic mechanisms necessary for
thermoregulation, the ontogenesis of amphetamine-induced hypothermia in cold environments parallels the onset of homeothermia.

The hypothalamus (especially the anterior hypothalamic–preoptic area) is essential for
the normal regulation of temperature in adult mammals (Hammel, 1968) and may be a
possible site of action of temperature-altering drugs (Feldberg, 1969). In addition, dopaminergic neurons projecting to the olfactory tubercles may also be involved in thermoregulatory
changes following amphetamine administration to rats in cold environments. Lesions of
these projections do not alter amphetamine-induced hyperthermia but do abolish the drug-
induced hypothermia; the hypothermia is also abolished by dopamine-receptor blocking
agents (Yehuda and Wurtman, 1972a, b). Hence, the lack of response of the newborn rat
to amphetamine administered in the cold or at the thermoneutral environment may indicate
that a dopaminergic neuronal system mediating amphetamine hypothermia is immature
until approximately the fifteenth day of age.

Thus the normal ontogenetic changes that occur in the patterns of locomotor activity,
elective food consumption, and thermoregulation do not always parallel the development
of drug-induced alterations in these responses. The neonatal rat markedly increases the
basal level of spontaneous locomotor activity between the fifteenth and twentieth postnatal
days; some drugs (scopolamine and pilocarpine) have no effect on activity until this time;
other drugs (such as amphetamine) induce large increases in activity at birth or shortly
thereafter. In contrast, elective food consumption by preweanling rats is manifest from
birth although the nature of this regulatory response changes rapidly with age; at approximately the fifteenth day of age these animals develop both the capacity to begin surviving on
solid food as well as to have appetite suppressed by amphetamine. Neonatal rats are
poikilothermic at birth; however, by day 20 they have attained the ability to maintain body

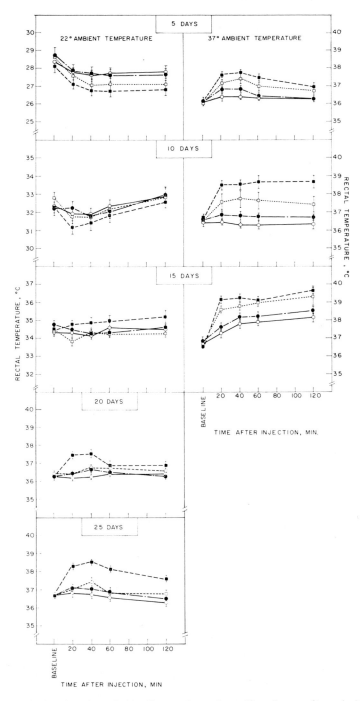

FIG. 6. The effects of various doses of D-amphetamine sulfate (intraperitoneal; 0.9% saline control: ○———○; 1.0 mg/kg: ●—·—●; 3.0 mg/kg: □·········□; or 9.0 mg/kg: ■————■) on the rectal temperatures of developing rats. Animals were adapted to one of two ambient temperatures (37°C in the right-hand panels and 22°C in the left-hand panels) for 1 h prior to injection. Baseline measurements were determined at the end of the hour. All 20- and 25-day-old animals died within 1 h following amphetamine injection under the 37°C temperature condition. (From Lytle *et al.*, in preparation.)

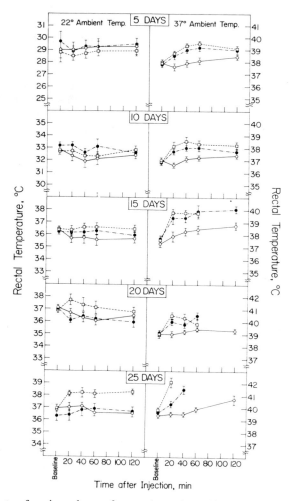

FIG. 7. The effects of various doses of D-amphetamine sulfate (intracisternal; 0.9% saline control: ○———○; 50 μg: ●—·—●: or 200 μg: □··············□). All injection volumes were 20 μl; no anesthesia was used for the injections. Adaptation periods and baseline measurements were the same as described in Fig. 6. (From Lytle *et al.*, in preparation.)

temperature over a fairly wide range of ambient temperature conditions. Whereas amphetamine-induced hyperthermia is present shortly after birth, the hypothermic effects of the drug do not become clearly evident until the fifteenth postnatal day.

In adults, many drugs simultaneously produce an array of physiological, behavioral, and neurochemical effects; it is oftentimes difficult to separate or isolate one effect of a drug from the others. For example, amphetamine anorexia could result as an indirect consequence of psychomotor stimulation at lower doses of the drug (Carlton, 1963) or from the disturbed state that reflects itself in stereotypic behavior following higher doses. The developing animal may provide a suitable experimental preparation for separating the multiple effects of drugs. Hence we have shown that rats younger than 15 days of age become hyperactive following amphetamine administration even though the drug produces no effects on food intake. If changes in response to various drugs reflect the differential maturation of neuronal systems upon which a psychoactive compound acts, then the developing animal may provide a unique opportunity for separating the relative contributions of individual monoaminergic systems to various response outputs before and after drug administration.

BRAIN AND PERIPHERAL MONOAMINE NEURONS: THEIR POSSIBLE ROLE IN ONTOGENESIS

The normal developmental maturation of various physiological and behavioral responses, as well as developmental changes that occur in response to certain drugs, may reflect the relative functional maturity of central and/or peripheral monoaminergic neurotransmitter-containing systems. Brain and peripheral monoaminergic neurons have been shown to play a critical role in mediating changes in the levels of locomotor activity, food consumption, and thermoregulation in the adult organism. Similarly, the actions of many psychotropic drugs on these responses have been attributed to their effects on monoamine-containing neurons. These neurons are not fully mature at birth in nonprecocial mammals; hence, their functional status may provide limiting factors for the ontogenesis of normal and drug-induced changes in the response capacity of the developing organism. The maturational changes in monoamine-containing neurons that might account for these age-related changes include several possibilities: (1) the total number of neurons in a population that mediates a behavioral or physiological response may attain critical levels only after a certain time following birth; (2) a sufficient number of synaptic connections necessary for a response to occur may accumulate with increasing age; (3) presynaptically, the capacity of monoamine-containing neurons to synthesize, concentrate, store, release, or catabolize sufficient neurotransmitter may increase with age; (4) the sensitivity of postsynaptic receptors for the monoamines may change with ontogenesis, as may the effectiveness of enzymatic and nonenzymatic mechanisms for inactivating the monoamines; and (5) in the case of differential developmental responses to drugs, age-related changes may occur in the distribution, metabolism, and/or neurochemical effects of the drugs.

NEURONAL PROLIFERATION

Altman and his co-workers (Altman, 1967; Altman et al., 1970) have described different rates of growth for neuronal elements that comprise a large proportion of cells in the mammalian central nervous system. Three cell types have been differentiated: *macroneurons*, *microneurons*, and *neuroglia*. The macroneurons are cells with long axons that form the major connective links in the central and peripheral nervous systems. These neurons arise early during prenatal development, with little or no neurogenesis occurring after birth. The microneurons, short-axoned interneurons with regional or local afferent and efferent connections, apparently modulate the interaction among the afferent, efferent, and interregional macroneurons. Whereas the macroneurons are localized in specific regions of the central and peripheral nervous systems by birth, the microneurons originate and differentiate during the preweanling period. The cellular proliferation of the microneurons remains high after birth around the forebrain ventricles, certain subpial zones, and in white and gray matter in various brain regions. Finally, neuroglia cells increase considerably during the early phases of postnatal development, and continue increasing at lower rates well into adulthood. These cells provide supporting elements for myelination of axons and for linking nerve cells with blood capillaries.

Although it seems likely that the macroneurons may contain monoamines as neuro-transmitters, specific neurotransmitter compounds localized in specific populations of macroneurons and microneurons have only recently begun to be identified. It is possible that the relatively late neurogenesis of microneuronal elements in the brain, spinal cord, and periphery may serve to increase the physiological and behavioral repertoire of the developing organism. For example, the maturation of the microneurons of the cerebellum (the basket cells and stellate cells of the molecular layer and the granule cells of the internal granular layer) is highly correlated with the temporal onset of motor coordination in a number of species (Altman, 1967).

INCREASED SYNAPTIC CONNECTIONS

Large increases in the number of synaptic junctions occur in rat cortex between the third and fourth postnatal weeks (Aghajanian and Bloom, 1967). These increases are apparently the result of increased size of the perikarya, the sprouting and growth of axons, increases in dendritic arborization, and increases in the number of axonal terminations (Eayrs and Goodhead, 1959). The increases in synaptic connections are highly correlated with regional changes in the maturation of brain monoamine-containing neurons. Histochemical fluorescence micrographs show that norepinephrine and dopamine-containing neural cell bodies and axons (without terminals) are detectable in the brain of the rat fetus (Loizou, 1972). At birth, brain dopamine-containing neurons are morphologically more developed than are norepinephrine-containing neurons, and these even more so than serotonin-containing neurons. Norepinephrine-containing cell bodies are present in the caudal half of the brain while only a sparse distribution of terminals can be seen in the rostral half of the cerebrum (Loizou, 1972). There follows a gradual increase in the fluorescence of cell bodies containing norepinephrine throughout the brain, with the adult pattern being attained by the fourth to fifth postnatal week in eleven brain areas. Dopamine-containing terminals are present mainly in the telencephalon, and these show large increases in density from birth to the fourth postnatal week (Loizou, 1972). Similar regional correlations between the levels of catecholamines and the activities of their biosynthetic enzymes have been reported (Porcher and Heller, 1972).

The caudal-rostral sequence of development of monoamine-containing neurons may be an important determinant of the functional capacity of various brain neuronal systems to control and modulate physiological and behavioral responses in the immature mammal. The relevance of this developmental model for the ontogenesis of normal and drug-induced changes in behavioral activity has been described (Campbell et al., 1969; Moorcroft, 1971).

ONTOGENETIC, PRESYNAPTIC CHANGES IN MONOAMINERGIC NEURONS

Recent histochemical observations demonstrate that the fluorescence intensities of post-ganglionic sympathetic neurons (presumably reflecting the contents of catecholamines) increase most rapidly in rats during the first postnatal week, whereas the fluorescence intensity of each axon terminal decreases (Champlain et al., 1970). The postnatal increases in fluorescence intensity observed within most innervated tissues or brain regions apparently result from quantitative increases in the number of monoaminergic nerve terminals. Post-natal changes in various biochemical indices of monoamine synthesis, uptake, and storage correlate well with these histochemical observations. Monoamine concentrations are low in the brain and periphery at birth (Karki *et al.*, 1962; Bennett and Giarman, 1965; Agrawal *et al.*, 1968; Loizou and Salt, 1970; Loizou, 1971; Breese and Traylor, 1972), and the capacity of tissues to take up and store catecholamines appears to be less than that of the adult (Glowinski *et al.*, 1964). The continuous increase with age in the ability of organs to accumulate radioactively labeled norepinephrine (i.e. injected intravenously or into the CSF) may reflect the growth of additional nerve terminals (Iversen *et al.*, 1967; Sachs *et al.*, 1970). In brain, monoamine concentrations continue to increase for 4–10 weeks after birth; postnatal increases in the activities of enzymes that catalyze the synthesis and metabolism of monoamine neurotransmitters correlate well with monoamine concentrations and neuronal densities within peripheral tissues and brain regions (Coyle and Axelrod, 1971, 1972a, b; Lamprecht and Coyle, 1972; Porcher and Heller, 1972). The biochemical functional maturation of the presynaptic monoaminergic neurons (as indicated by the capacity to synthesize, concentrate, store, release, or catabolize sufficient transmitter) apparently increases with age. Differential, developmental regional changes may affect the capacity of drugs such as amphetamine to alter the physiological and behavioral responses of the neonate.

ONTOGENETIC CHANGES IN RECEPTOR SENSITIVITY AND ENZYMATIC INACTIVATION MECHANISMS

Recent lines of evidence suggest that some of the receptors for brain monoamines may be associated with adenyl cyclase, the enzyme that catalyzes the formation of cyclic AMP from ATP. The activity of adenyl cyclase is high in the brains of adult rats (Sutherland *et al.*, 1962), can be altered by catecholaminergic stimulation (Klainer *et al.*, 1962; Greengard *et al.*, 1968), and some of the effects of exogenously administered norepinephrine in brain are mimicked by the application of cyclic AMP (Siggins *et al.*, 1969). The level of brain cyclic AMP in the developing rat begins to increase during the first postnatal week, and roughly parallels the developmental time course for the increases in other brain monoaminergic neurotransmitters with maximum levels being reached by 30 days of age (Schmidt *et al.*, 1970). However, the sensitivity of brain cyclic AMP to norepinephrine is absent in the newborn rat and only becomes evident after the third postnatal day. In contrast, norepinephrine stimulates the formation of cyclic AMP in the brain of newborn guinea-pigs. The increasing sensitivity of cyclic AMP to norepinephrine in the neonatal rat brain may indicate an increase in the levels of brain adenyl cyclase, an increase in the number or sensitivity of adrenergic receptors, or an increase in the concentration of monoamines that contact with these receptors (Schmidt *et al.*, 1970).

Developmental increases in the activity of the enzyme monoamine oxidase are dependent on *de nova* protein synthesis; its postnatal maturation can be prevented by the protein synthesis inhibitor cycloheximide (Black *et al.*, 1972). The activity of monoamine oxidase increases steadily from birth to reach adult levels by day twelve, with an overall fourfold increase during development (Black *et al.*, 1972). The rat fetus and neonate are also deficient in catechol-*O*-methyl transferase activity; the enzyme is present in concentrations only about 20% of that observed in the adult (Glowinski *et al.*, 1964). It is interesting to speculate that increased locomotor activity following injections of scopolamine to rats older than 20 days of age may reflect changes in the sensitivity of cholinergic receptors. Future research utilizing specific noradrenergic (phenoxybenzamine, phentolamine), dopaminergic (pimozide or haloperidol) or serotoninergic (methysergide) blocking agents may provide some indication of the changing sensitivity of monoamine receptors and their role in determining the physiological and behavioral responses of the developing organism.

DEVELOPMENTAL CHANGES IN DRUG ACTION

One or more of several alternative mechanisms could account for the differential responses of developing animals following drug treatment. These maturational changes may include (a) differential drug metabolism with age; (b) altered drug distribution; or (c) differential neurochemical effects of a drug on the uptake, synthesis, storage, inactivation and/or release of neurotransmitters.

The liver microsomal enzymes of the newborn animal are immature and have a limited ability to metabolize foreign compounds; hence, it is possible that various drugs are differentially metabolized in young animals when compared to adults. For example, in the adult rat, aromatic hydroxylation is the major degradative pathway for amphetamine and this is apparently accomplished by hepatic microsomal p-hydroxylating enzymes (Axelrod, 1954). The two major metabolites of amphetamine formed in the adult rat are p-hydroxy-amphetamine and p-hydroxynorephedrine (Goldstein and Anagnoste, 1965). It has been suggested that the long-term reduction in brain amines following large doses of amphet-amine may be due to the formation of p-hydroxynorephedrine and its uptake into catechol-amine-containing neurons (Costa and Groppetti, 1970). It has been shown that the liver microsomes of newborn animals do not readily metabolize amphetamine; hence, the drug endures longer in newborn animals than in adults (Groppetti and Costa, 1969). Either the increased half-life of amphetamine or changes in the amount of its major metabolites with age could alter the neurochemical, physiological, or behavioral responses of the developing organism.

A second possible age-related difference in the metabolism of amphetamine may involve the rate of β-hydroxylation. The enzyme dopamine-β-hydroxylase apparently catalyzes the hydroxylation of several amphetamine derivatives $in\ vitro$ and $in\ vivo$ (Goldstein and Contrera, 1962; Creveling $et\ al.$, 1962). Since the levels of activity of dopamine-β-hydroxyl-ase are low at birth and gradually increase with development (Coyle and Axelrod, 1972), the levels of norephedrine and p-hydroxynorephedrine may be low following the injection of amphetamine in neonatal animals.

If the uptake and distribution of amphetamine or its metabolites are in some way related to the extent of catecholamine innervation in various regions of the brain and periphery, then it might be expected that the differential distribution of the drug may change with age, depending upon the relative functional status of specific catecholamine-containing neurons. Similarly, the actions of this compound may affect different populations of monoamine neurons that mediate specific physiological and behavior responses in the developing animal. These alternatives are currently under investigation in our laboratory.

ACKNOWLEDGEMENTS

Part of this research was conducted while L.D.L. was a NIH postdoctoral fellow (5 FO2 MH40476-02) in the Laboratory of Neuroendocrine Regulation, Department of Nutrition and Food Science, MIT, Cambridge, Massachusetts. The authors gratefully acknowledge the excellent technical assistance of Kenneth Cottman, David Becher, and Robert Steininger and the editorial assistance of Barbara Simon and Kathy Doyle.

REFERENCES

ADOLPH, E. F. (1957) Ontogeny of physiological regulations in the rat. *Qt. Rev. Biol.* **32**, 89–137.

AGHAJANIAN, G. K., and BLOOM, F. E. (1967) The formation of synaptic junctions in developing rat brain: a quantitative electron microscopic study. *Brain Res.* **6**, 716–727.

AGRAWAL, H. C., GLISSON, S. N., and HIMWICH, W. A. (1968) Developmental changes in monoamines of mouse brain. *Int. J. Neuropharmac.* **7**, 97–101.

ALTMAN, J. (1967) Postnatal growth and differentiation of the mammalian brain, with implications for a morphological theory of memory. In *The Neurosciences—A Study Program* (G. C. Quarton, T. Melnechuk, and F. O. Schmitt, eds.), Rockefeller University Press, New York, pp. 723–743.

ALTMAN, J., DAS, G., and SUDARSHAN, K. (1970) The influence of nutrition on neural and behavioral development: I, Critical review of some data on the growth of the body and the brain following dietary deprivation during gestation and lactation. *Develop. Psychobiol.* **3**, 281–301.

ANAND, B. K., and BROBECK, J. R. (1951) Localization of a "feeding center" in the hypothalamus of the rat. *Proc. Soc. Exp. Biol. Med.* **77**, 323–324.

AXELROD, J. (1954) Studies on sympathomimetic amines: II, The biotransformation and physiological disposition of D-amphetamine, D-p-hydroxyamphetamine and D-methamphetamine. *J. Pharmac. Exp. Ther.* **110**, 315–326.

BENNETT, D. S., and GIARMAN, N. J. (1965) Schedule of appearance of 5-hydroxytryptamine (serotonin) and associated enzymes in the developing rat brain. *J. Neurochem.* **12**, 911–916.

BLACK, I. B., HENDRY, I. A., and IVERSEN, L. L. (1972) Effects of surgical decentralization and nerve growth factor on the maturation of adrenergic neurons in a mouse sympathetic ganglion. *J. Neurochem.* **19**, 1367–1377.

BREFSE, G. R., and TRAYLOR, T. D. (1972) Developmental characteristics of brain catecholamines and tyrosine hydroxylase in the rat: effects of 6-hydroxydopamine. *Br. J. Pharmac.* **44**, 210–222.

CAMPBELL, B. A., and MABRY, P. B. (1972) Ontogeny of behavioral arousal: a comparative study. *J. Comp. Physiol. Psychol.* **81**, 371–379.

CAMPBELL, B. A., and MABRY, P. B. (1973) The role of catecholamines in ontogenesis. *Psychopharmacologia* (in press).

CAMPBELL, B. A., LYTLE, L. D., and FIBIGER, H. C. (1969) Ontogeny of adrenergic arousal and cholinergic inhibitory mechanisms in the rat. *Science* **166**, 637–638.

CARLTON, P. L. (1963) Cholinergic mechanisms in the control of behavior by the brain. *Psychol. Rev.* **70**, 19–39.

CHAMPLAIN, J., MALMFORS, T., OLSON, L. and SACHS, CH. (1970) Ontogenesis of peripheral adrenergic neurons in the rat: pre- and postnatal observations. *Acta physiol. scand.* **80**, 276–288.

CHENG, M. F., ROZIN, P., and TEITELBAUM, P. (1971) Starvation retards development of food and water regulations. *J. Comp. Physiol. Psychol.* **75**, 206–218.

CONKLIN, P., and HEGGENESS, F. W. (1971) Maturation of temperature homeostasis in the rat. *Am. J. Psychol.* **220**, 333–336.

COSTA, E., and GROPPETTI, A. (1970) Biosynthesis and storage of catecholamines in tissues of rats injected with various doses of D-amphetamine. In *Amphetamines and Related Compounds* (E. Costa and S. Garattini, eds.), Raven Press, New York, pp. 231–255.

COYLE, J. T., and AXELROD, J. (1971) Development of the uptake and storage of L-[³H] norepinephrine in the rat brain. *J. Neurochem.* **18**, 2061–2075.

COYLE, J. T., and AXELROD, J. (1972a) Tyrosine hydroxylase in rat brain: developmental characteristics. *J. Neurochem.* **19**, 1117–1123.

COYLE, J. T., and AXELROD, J. (1972b) Dopamine-beta-hydroxylase in the rat brain: developmental characteristics. *J. Neurochem.* **19**, 449–459.

CREVELING, C. R., DALY, J. W., WITKOP, B., and UDENFRIEND, S. (1962) Substrates and inhibitors of dopamine-β-oxidase. *Biochim. biophys. Acta* **64**, 125–126.

CROWLEY, D. E., and HEPP-REYMOND, M. C. (1966) Development of cochlear function in the ear of the infant rat. *J. Comp. Physiol. Psychol.* **62**, 427–432.

DOBBING, J., and SANDS, J. (1970) Growth and development of the brain and spinal chord of the guinea pig. *Brain Res.* **17**, 115–123.

EAYRS, J. T., and GOODHEAD, B. (1959) Postnatal development of the cerebral cortex in the rat. *J. Anat.* **93**, 385–402.

FAIRFIELD, J. (1948) Effects of cold on infant rats: body temperatures, oxygen consumption, electrocardiograms. *Am. J. Physiol.* **155**, 355–365.

FELDBERG, W. (1969) The role of monoamines in the hypothalamus for temperature regulation. *J. Neurovisc. Rel.*, Suppl. 9, 362–379.

FIBIGER, H. C., LYTLE, L. D., and CAMPBELL, B. A. (1970) Cholinergic modulation of adrenergic arousal in the developing rat. *J. Comp. Physiol. Psychol.* **72**, 384–389.

GIARMAN, N. J., and PEPEU, G. (1964) The influence of central acting cholinolytic drugs on brain acetyl-choline levels. *Br. J. Pharmac. Chemother.* **23**, 23–30.

GLOWINSKI, J., and AXELROD, J. (1965) Effect of drugs on the uptake, release and metabolism of ³H nor-epinephrine in the rat brain. *J. Pharmac. Exp. Ther.* **149**, 43–49.

GLOWINSKI, J., AXELROD, J., KOPIN, I. J., and WURTMAN, R. J. (1964) Physiological disposition of ³H norepinephrine in the developing rat. *J. Pharmac. Exp. Ther.* **146**, 48–53.

GOLDSTEIN, M., and ANAGNOSTE, B. (1965) The conversion *in vivo* of D-amphetamine to (+)-*p*-hydroxy-norephedrine. *Biochim. biophys. Acta* **107**, 166.

GOLDSTEIN, M., and CONTRERA, J. F. (1962) The substrate specificity of phenyl amine-β-hydroxylase. *J. Biol. Chem.* **237**, 1898–1901.

GROPPETTI, A., and COSTA, E. (1969) Factors affecting the rate of disappearance of amphetamine in rats. *Int. J. Neuropharmac.* **8**, 209–215.

GREENGARD, P., ROBISON, G. A., and SUTHERLAND, E. W. (1968) Unpublished observations.

HAMMEL, H. T. (1968) Regulation of the internal body temperature. *A. Rev. Physiol.* **30**, 641–710.

HEGGENESS, F. W. (1962) Nutritional status and physiological development of the preweanling rat. *Am. J. Physiol.* **203**, 545–549.

HELLER, A., and MOORE, R. (1968) Control of brain serotonin and norepinephrine by special neural systems. *Adv. Pharmac.* **6**, 191–206.

HILL, R. M. (1947) The control of body temperature in white rats. *Am. J. Physiol.* **203**, 650–656.

IVERSEN, L. L., CHAMPLAIN, J., GLOWINSKI, J., and AXELROD, J. (1967) Uptake, storage and metabolism of norepinephrine in tissues of the developing rat. *J. Pharmac. Exptl. Ther.* **157**, 509–516.

KARKI, N., KUNTZMAN, R., and BROADIE, B. B. (1962) Storage, synthesis and metabolism in the developing brain. *J. Neurochem.* **9**, 53–58.

KLAINER, L. M., CHI, Y. M., FREIDBERG, S. L., RALL, T. W., and SUTHERLAND, E. W. (1962) Adenyl cyclase: IV, The effects of neurohormones on the formation of adenosine 3'5'-phosphate by preparations from brain and other tissues. *J. Biol. Chem.* **237**, 1239–1243.

LAMPRECHT, F., and COYLE, J. T. (1972) DOPA decarboxylase in the developing rat brain. *Brain Res.* **41**, 503–506.

LOIZOU, L. A. (1971) Effect of inhibition of catecholamine synthesis on central catecholamine-containing neurones in the developing albino rat. *Br. J. Pharmac.* **41**, 41–48.

LOIZOU, L. A. (1972) The postnatal ontogeny of monoamine-containing neurons in the central nervous system of the albino rat. *Brain Res.* **40**, 395–418.

LOIZOU, L. A., and SALT, P. (1970) Regional changes in monoamines of the rat brain during postnatal development. *Brain Res.* **20**, 467–470.

LYNCH, G. S., BALLANTINE, P., and CAMPBELL, B. A. (1969) Potentiation of behavioral arousal after cortical damage and subsequent recovery. *Expl. Neurol.* **23**, 195–206.

LYTLE, L. D., MOORCROFT, W. H., and CAMPBELL, B. A. (1971) Ontogeny of amphetamine anorexia and insulin hyperphagia in the rat. *J. Comp. Physiol. Psychol.* **77**, 388–393.

LYTLE, L. D., SHOEMAKER, W., COTTMAN, K., and WURTMAN, R. J. (1972) Long term effects of postnatal 6-hydroxy-dopamine treatment on tissue catecholamine levels. *J. Pharmac. Exp. Ther.* **183**, 56–64.

MOORCROFT, W. H. (1971) Ontogeny of forebrain inhibition of behavioral arousal in the rat. *Brain Res.* **35**, 513–522.

MOORCROFT, W. H., LYTLE, L. D., and CAMPBELL, B. A. (1971) Ontogeny of starvation-induced behavioral arousal in the rat. *J. Comp. Physiol. Psychol.* **75**, 59–67.

POCZOPKO, P. A. (1961) A contribution to the studies of energy metabolism: I, Development of mechanisms of body temperature regulation in rats. *J. Cell Comp. Physiol.* **57**, 175–184.

PORCHER, W., and HELLER, A. (1972) Regional development of catecholamine biosynthesis in the rat brain. *J. Neurochem.* **19**, 1917–1930.

ROSE, G. H. (1968) The development of visually evoked electrocortical responses in the rat. *Devl. Psychobiol.* **1**, 35–40.

SACHS, CH., CHAMPLAIN, J., MALMFORS, T., and OLSON, L. (1970) The postnatal development of noradrenaline uptake in noradrenergic nerves of different tissues from the rat. *Eur. J. Pharmac.* **9**, 67–79.

SALAS, M., GUZMAN-FLORES, C., and SCHAPIRO, S. (1969) An ontogenetic study of olfactory bulb electrical activity in the rat. *Physiol. Behav.* **4**, 699–703.

SCHMIDT, M. J., PALMER, E. C., DETTBARN, W. D. and ROBISON, G. A. (1970) Cyclic AMP and adenyl cyclase in the developing rat brain. *Devl. Psychobiol.* **3**, 53–67.

SIGGINS, G. R., HOFFER, B. J., and BLOOM, F. E. (1969) Cyclic adenosine monophosphate: possible mediator for norepinephrine effects on cerebellar Purkinje cells. *Science* **165**, 1018–1020.

SUTHERLAND, E. W., RALL, T. W., and MENON, T. (1962) Adenyl cyclase: I, Distribution, preparation and properties. *J. Biol. Chem.* **237**, 1220–1227.

TEITELBAUM, P., and EPSTEIN, A. N. (1962) Recovery of feeding and drinking after lateral hypothalamic lesions. *Psychol. Rev.* **69**, 74–90.

TEITELBAUM, P., CHENG, M., and ROZIN, P. (1969) Development of feeding parallels its recovery after hypothalamic damage. *J. Comp. Physiol. Psychol.* **67**, 430–441.

UNGERSTEDT, U. (1971a) Stereotaxic mapping of the monoamine pathways in the rat brain. *Acta physiol. scand.*, Suppl. 367, 1–48.

UNGERSTEDT, U. (1971b) Adipsia and aphagia after 6-hydroxy-dopamine induced degeneration of the nigro striatal dopamine system. *Acta physiol. scand.*, Suppl. 367, 95–122.

WOODWARD, P. J., HOFFER, B. J., and LAPHAM, L. W. (1969) Postnatal development of electrical and enzyme activity in Purkinje cells. *Expl. Neurol.* **23**, 120–139.

YEHUDA, S., and WURTMAN, R. J. (1972a) The effects of D-amphetamine and related compounds on colonic temperature of rats kept at various ambient temperatures. *Life Sci.* **18**, 851–859.

YEHUDA, S., and WURTMAN, R. J. (1972b) Release of brain dopamine as the probable mechanism for the hypothermic effects of d-amphetamine. *Nature* **240**, 477–478.

ZETLER, G. (1968) Cataleptic state and hypothermia in mice, caused by central cholinergic stimulation and antagonized by anticholinergic and anti-depressant drugs. *Int. J. Neuropharmac.* **7**, 325–335.

ENHANCED ACCUMULATIONS OF CYCLIC AMP IN BRAIN SLICES ELICITED BY NOREPINEPHRINE AFTER INTRAVENTRICULAR PRETREATMENT OF RATS WITH 6-HYDROXYDOPAMINE

M. Huang† and J. W. Daly

National Institute of Arthritis, Metabolism and Digestive Diseases,
National Institute of Health, Bethesda, Maryland 20014, *USA*

2,4,5-Trihydroxyphenethylamine (6-hydroxydopamine) and certain related compounds cause a selective degeneration of noradrenergic terminals in both peripheral organs and the central nervous system (see Malmfors and Thoenen, 1971; Tranzer and Thoenen, 1973; and references therein). Concomitant and subsequent to this "chemical sympathectomy," of the innervated organ or cell to catecholamines may develop. With heart, nictitating membrane, and blood vessels, supersensitivity to norepinephrine in 6-hydroxydopamine-treated animals appears due primarily to lack of presynaptic uptake mechanisms; i.e., the maximal response is unchanged while the threshold response to norepinephrine is shifted to lower levels (Finch and Leach, 1970); Nadeau *et al.*, 1971; Hauesler *et al.*, 1968). In the central nervous system both the type of response and threshold for the stereotypical response of rats to apomorphine, a dopaminergic agonist, are altered in animals pretreated with intraventricular 6-hydroxydopamine (Schoenfeld and Uretsky, 1972). The inhibitory effect of norepinephrine on firing of cerebellar Purkinje cells is potentiated in 6-hydroxydopamine-treated animals, while the spontaneous rate of discharge at such neurons is increased (Hoffer *et al.*, 1971). Norepinephrine appears to inhibit Purkinje cell firing by mechanisms that involve the formation and action of cyclic AMP (Siggins *et al.*, 1971). It was, therefore, of interest as to whether 6-hydroxydopamine pretreatment of animals would potentiate the responses of the cyclic AMP-generating system in brain slices during incubation with norepinephrine. In rat cerebral cortical slices norepinephrine appears to elicit enhanced accumulation of cyclic AMP via interaction with both classical α- and β-adrenergic receptors (Perkins and Moore, 1973; Schultz and Daly, 1973). Adenosine and depolarizing agents such as veratridine also stimulate formation of cyclic AMP in this

† Fellow in the Visiting Program of the United States Public Health Service.

593

tissue. An adenosine–norepinephrine combination has greater than additive stimulatory effect on cyclic AMP accumulation. The accumulation of cyclic AMP in rat cerebral slices elicited by these agents was now examined in preparations from Sprague–Dawley rats that had received an intraventricular injection of either 6-hydroxydopamine or 2,3,5-trihydroxyphenethylamine, 4–20 days before sacrifice (Huang et al., 1973). Accumulation of cyclic AMP was ascertained with the prelabeling technique of Shimizu et al. (1969). Typical results are presented in Fig. 1. Responses to isoproterenol, norepinephrine, and an adenosine–norepinephrine combination were significantly enhanced in slices from 6-hydroxydopamine-treated animals, while responses to adenosine and veratridine were virtually unchanged.

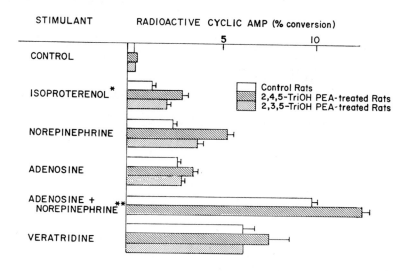

FIG. 1. Accumulation of radioactive cyclic AMP in rat cerebral cortical slices labeled during a prior incubation with radioactive adenine. Sprague–Dawley rats received an intraventricular injection of 6-hydroxydopamine (2,4,5-TriOH PEA, 250 μg free base) or 2,3,5-trihydroxyphenethylamine (2,3,5-TriOH PEA, 125 μg) 7–10 days before sacrifice and preparation of slices. The slices were labeled with 4 μM [^{14}C]-adenine for 40 min, washed, and after 10 min of post incubation, the test substances (0.1 mM, except for veratridine which was 0.08 mM) were added. The percentage of total intracellular radioactive adenine nucleotides present as radioactive cyclic AMP was assayed after a further 8–15 min incubation. *$p < 0.01$. **$p < 0.05$. (Huang et al., 1973.)

Intraventricular injection of 5,6-dihydroxytryptamine (100 μg free base) or 5,7-dihydroxytryptamine (100 μg) had no significant effect on responses of the cyclic AMP-generating system to the various stimulatory agents. No responses to dopamine or serotonin were seen in any of these experiments with rat cortical slices (Huang et al., 1973). Both α- and β-adrenergic receptor-mediated accumulations of cyclic AMP appear to be potentiated in rats pretreated with 6-hydroxydopamine (Huang et al., 1973; Table 1). Supramaximal concentrations of norepinephrine and isoproterenol were employed in these studies in order to avoid effects due to the impaired uptake of catecholamines in the slices from 6-hydroxydopamine-treated animals. Kalisker and Perkins (1973) have also investigated the response of the cyclic AMP-generating system of rat cortical slices after prior intraventricular injection of 6-hydroxydopamine, and in addition to increases in total accumulation in cyclic AMP elicited by norepinephrine or isoproterenol they report a classical super-

TABLE 1. α- AND β-ADRENERGIC RECEPTOR-MEDIATED ACCUMULATION OF RADIOACTIVE CYCLIC AMP IN RAT CEREBRAL CORTICAL SLICES

Effect of prior treatment with 6-hydroxydopamine. For experimental protocol see legend Fig. 1. (Huang *et al.*, 1973)

Agonists and antagonists (0.1 mM)	% Conversion of intracellular radioactive nucleotides to cyclic AMP	
	Control	6-Hydroxydopamine
None	0.33 ± 0.02	0.36 ± 0.10
Norepinephrine	2.8 ± 0.3	4.3 ± 0.5
Norepinephrine/phentolamine	1.8 ± 0.1	2.5 ± 0.4
Norepinephrine/dichloroisoproterenol	0.9 ± 0.1	1.4 ± 0.4
Isoproterenol	1.5 ± 0.1	2.0 ± 0.2
Isoproterenol/propranolol	0.4	0.6

sensitivity to low dosages of norepinephrine which is apparently due to the lack of pre-synaptic uptake of the amine in slices from 6-hydroxydopamine-treated animals. Weiss and Strada (1972) report a more marked increase in the response of the cylic AMP-generating system to 5 μM norepinephrine than to 50 μM amine in slices of rat cerebrum prepared 4 weeks after intraventricular administration of 6-hydroxydopamine. Palmer (1972) reports significant enhancement of the norepinephrine-elicited accumulation of cyclic AMP in slices of cerebrum, hypothalamus, and brain stem only at 10 μM and not at 1 μM norepinephrine. Slices were prepared 7 days after intraventricular administration of 6-hydroxy-dopamine (Palmer, 1972). It should be mentioned that Weiss (1969) has demonstrated that the response of adenyl cyclase to norepinephrine in rat pineal glands was enhanced after chronic denervation.

The mechanism whereby destruction of presynaptic noradrenergic terminals can cause an enhanced response of the cyclic AMP-generating system to norepinephrine in postsynaptic sites is as yet unknown. Such changes might be due to lack of neurotransmitter or other neurotrophic factors which results in (i) further synthesis or "unmasking" of α- and β-adrenergic receptor–adenylate cyclase complexes, (ii) alteration of phosphodiesterase activity, (iii) changes in availability of ATP as substrate for adenylate cyclases, or (iv) increases in levels of protein kinases with sites for sequestration of cyclic AMP. The hypothesis (i) of increases in both α- and β-adrenergic receptor–adenylate cyclase complexes is at the moment most attractive in view of the fact that enhanced accumulations following 6-hydroxydopamine pretreatment of animals are seen only in slices incubated with catecholamines. Further studies on these phenomena are in progress.

REFERENCES

FINCH, L., and LEACH, G. D. H. (1970) A comparison of the effects of 6-hydroxydopamine immuno-sympathectomy and reserpine on the cardiovascular reactivity in the rat. *J. Pharm. Pharmac.* **22,** 354–360.

HAUESLER, G., THOENEN, H., and HAEFELY, W. (1968) Chemische Sympathektomie der Katze mit 6-Hydroxydopamin: Veranderungen von Sympathiscusreizeffekten und Noradrenalineempfindlichkeit. *Helv. physiol. pharmac. Acta* **26,** CR 223–CR-225.

HOFFER, B. J., SIGGINS, G. R., WOODWARD, D. J., and BLOOM, F. E. (1971) Spontaneous discharge of Purkinje neurons after destruction of catecholamine-containing afferents by 6-hydroxydopamine. *Brain Res.* **30,** 425–430.

HUANG, M., HO, A. K. S., and DALY, J. W. (1973) Accumulation of cyclic adenosine 3',5'-monophosphate in rat cerebral cortical slices: stimulatory effect of α- and β-adrenergic agents after pretreatments with 6-hydroxydopamine, 2,3,5-trihydroxyphenethylamine and dihydroxytryptamines. *Molec. Pharmac.* **9**, 711–717.

KALISKER, A., and PERKINS, J. P. (1973) Effects of intraventricular 6-hydroxydopamine on the catecholamine-sensitive adenyl cyclase system of rat cerebral cortex. *Fed. Proc.* **32**, 680 Abs.

MALMFORS, T., and THOENEN, H. (eds.) (1971) *6-Hydroxydopamine and Catecholamine Neurons*, North-Holland, Amsterdam.

NADEAU, R. A., DE CHAMPLAIN, J., and TREMBLAY, G. M. (1971) Supersensitivity of the isolated rat heart after chemical sympathectomy with 6-hydroxydopamine. *Can. J. Physiol. Pharmac.* **49**, 36–44.

PALMER, G. C. (1972) Increased cyclic AMP response to norepinephrine in the rat brain following 6-hydroxydopamine. *Neuropharmacology* **11**, 145–149.

PERKINS, J. P., and MOORE, M. M. (1973) Characterization of the adrenergic receptors mediating a rise in adenosine 3',5'-monophosphate in rat cerebral cortex. *J. Pharmac. Exp. Ther.* **185**, 371–378.

SCHOENFELD, R., and URETSKY, N. (1972) Altered response to apomorphine in 6-hydroxydopamine-treated rats. *Eur. J. Pharmac.* **19**, 115–118.

SCHULTZ, J., and DALY, J. W. (1973) Accumulation of cyclic adenosine 3',5'-monophosphate in cerebral cortical slices from rat and mouse: stimulatory effect of α- and β-adrenergic agents and adenosine. *J. Neurochem.* **21**, 1319–1326.

SHIMIZU, H., DALY, J. W., and CREVELING, C. R. (1969) A radioisotopic method for measuring the formation of adenosine 3',5'-cyclic monophosphate in incubated slices of brain. *J. Neurochem.* **16**, 1609–1619.

SIGGINS, G. R., BATTENBERG, E. F., HOFFER, B. J., BLOOM, F. E., and STEINER, A. L. (1971) Noradrenergic stimulation of cyclic adenosine monophosphate in rat Purkinje neurons: an immunocytochemical study. *Science* **173**, 585–588.

TRANZER, J. P., and THOENEN, H. (1973) Selective destruction of adrenergic nerve terminals by chemical analogues of 6-hydroxydopamine. *Experientia* **29**, 314–316.

WEISS, B. (1969) The effects of environmental lighting and chronic denervation on the activation of adenyl cyclase of rat pineal gland by norepinephrine and sodium fluoride. *J. Pharmac. Exp. Ther.* **168**, 146–147.

WEISS, B., and STRADA, S. J. (1972) Neuroendocrine control of the cyclic AMP system of brain and pineal gland. *Adv. Cyclic Nucleotide Res.* **1**, 357–374.

ENHANCED SENSITIVITY TO THE NORADRENALINE RECEPTOR STIMULATING AGENT, CLONIDINE, FOLLOWING DEGENERATION OF NORADRENALINE PATHWAYS: STUDIES ON ARTERIAL PRESSURE, HEART RATE, AND RESPIRATION

PER BOLME, KJELL FUXE, LARS-GÖRAN NYGREN, LARS OLSON, AND CHARLOTTE SACHS

Department of Histology, Karolinska Institutet, Stockholm, Sweden

INTRODUCTION

The aim of the present study was to investigate if degeneration of central noradrenaline (NA) neurons could lead to an increased sensitivity of the NA receptors to known agonists. Evidence has previously been presented that removal of the dopamine (DA) input into the neostriatum will result in an increased sensitivity of the DA receptors to DA receptor stimulating agents (Ungerstedt, 1971). Such a supersensitivity phenomenon could occur also in central NA receptors following degeneration of the NA nerve terminals. In fact some recent reports clearly suggest that this may occur and involve changes in adenylcyclase. Thus it has been found that the accumulation of cyclic AMP in brain slices following exposure to NA or α- and β-adrenergic agents was significantly higher in brains from rats pretreated with 6-hydroxydopamine (6-OH-DA) intraventricularly (Huang and Daly, this symposium), which produces degeneration of central NA neurons (Uretsky and Iversen, 1970). All these findings constitute indirect evidence that a supersensitivity development in NA receptors takes place after denervation.

We have tested the action of the antihypertensive drug clonidine on arterial pressure, heart rate, and respiration rate in anaesthetized rats. Clonidine produces hypotension and bradycardia (Kobinger and Walland, 1967) and a decreased respiration rate (Bolme and Fuxe, 1973). Clonidine is believed to exert its action by stimulating central NA receptors (Andén *et al.*, 1970; Bolme and Fuxe, 1971; Schmitt *et al.*, 1971).

The exact localization of the effect of clonidine within the brain is not known, but the nucleus tractus solitarii and the nucleus motorius n. vagi have been suggested as important relay stations for autonomic impulses, and they are also densely innervated by catechol-amine (CA) nerve terminals (Fuxe, 1965). Direct activation of NA receptors in the sym-pathetic lateral column could certainly be another site of exerting action on blood pressure and heart rate (see review by Bolme *et al.*, 1972).

METHODOLOGY

The experiments were performed on male Sprague–Dawley rats, anaesthetized with halothane. Arterial pressure was measured via a catheter in the carotid artery by a Statham pressure transducer. Heart rate was determined by counting the blood pressure pulses from the chart of the Grass Polygraph on which the recordings were made. Respiration rate was measured by direct counting. Clonidine was administered into a jugular vein. The rats were pretreated in the following ways in different sets of experiments.

(a) One group of rats were given 6-OH-DA neonatally 100 mg/kg s.c. daily on the first three days of life. Controls were given saline. These rats were tested at 4–6 months of age. (b) A second group of rats were given, by a stereotaxical technique, 8 μg of 6-OH-DA (in 4 μl saline-ascorbic acid solution) into the dorsal coeruleo-cortical NA bundle lying ventro-lateral of griseum centralis in the tegmentum. The effects of clonidine were tested and compared with those in saline controls 2 weeks after the administration of 6-OH-DA or saline respectively. (c) In a third group of rats, 6-OH-DA (4 μg) in (2 μl) saline ascorbic acid solution, was administered bilaterally into the centrum of the spinal cord at the C1 level. Controls only given the solvent were prepared at the same time and in the same way. These rats were tested 2–3 weeks after the procedure. The completeness of the denervations was tested by fluorescence histochemical examinations (Falck *et al.*, 1962; Fuxe *et al.*, 1970).

RESULTS

A. DENERVATION OF ASCENDING AND DESCENDING NA NEURONS
   (Bolme *et al.*, unpublished results)

Systemic injections of 6-OH-DA to newborn rats led i.a. to a marked reduction of NA nerve terminals in the cortex cerebri and in the spinal cord, whereas the pons-medulla region became highly innervated by NA terminals. This has been demonstrated both histochemically, biochemically and by uptake of ^{3}H-amines (Sachs and Jonsson, 1972; Clark *et al.*, 1972; Singh and de Champlain, 1972; Jonsson *et al.*, 1974). The result of the present study is illustrated in Table 1. The resting values of arterial pressure, heart rate, and respiration rate were in the same order of magnitude in the treated animals and in the controls. The effect of clonidine on arterial pressure and heart rate did not differ between the groups, but there was a potentiation of the respiratory rate lowering effect in the 6-OH-DA-treated group. This finding was interpreted as due to a supersensitivity development of the NA receptors in areas lacking NA terminals, e.g. the cerebral cortex and spinal cord.

B. DENERVATION OF ASCENDING NA NEURONS (Bolme and Fuxe,
   unpublished results)

6-OH-DA was injected into the dorsal NA bundle. After 2 weeks there was an almost complete denervation of the NA projections to the limbic cortex and neocortex (see

TABLE 1. CLONIDINE 10 μg/kg I.V. EFFECTS ON ARTERIAL PRESSURE, HEART RATE, AND RESPIRATION RATE IN RATS TREATED AT BIRTH WITH 6-OH-DA (Bolme et al., unpublished)

	Resting values Mean ± SEM (n = 6)	% Decrease from resting values Mean ± SEM (n = 6)					
		5'	10'	15'	30'	45'	60'
Arterial pressure (mm Hg):							
Control	117.4 ± 3.1	19.8 ± 3.2	22.9 ± 2.7	21.7 ± 2.9	11.4 ± 4.5	7.7 ± 2.2	3.6 ± 2.1
6-OH-DA	110.1 ± 3.2	17.7 ± 2.0	17.2 ± 2.3	14.0 ± 2.8	7.4 ± 2.3	1.8 ± 2.8	+0.9 ± 2.4
Heart rate (beats/5s):							
Control	32.5 ± 1.3	18.3 ± 2.9	15.5 ± 2.4	10.9 ± 2.0	13.0 ± 3.0	8.1 ± 2.1	4.0 ± 3.0
6-OH-DA	34.9 ± 1.2	23.1 ± 1.4	18.1 ± 3.6	16.9 ± 4.8	12.4 ± 4.0	7.0 ± 3.4	8.2 ± 1.7
Respiration rate (breaths/30s):							
Control	39.8 ± 1.8	15.7 ± 6.5	17.1 ± 5.8	7.3 ± 6.2	+1.2 ± 5.6	+3.4 ± 4.2	+4.7 ± 5.3
6-OH-DA	39.2 ± 1.4	30.5 ± 5.4*	27.0 ± 6.1*	19.5 ± 7.2*	+3.3 ± 3.6	+2.5 ± 4.1	+2.0 ± 3.1

* Significantly different $p < 0.05$.

Lidbrink, this symposium). Clonidine was given to these rats and the effects were compared with controls. In Table 2 these results are summarized. There was no significant difference in the resting levels of arterial pressure, heart rate or respiration rate between the treated rats and the controls. There was, furthermore, no significant difference in the blood pressure lowering effect of clonidine between the groups. However, the heart rate and respiration rate lowering effects of clonidine were clearly potentiated in the group treated with 6-OH-DA. This was again interpreted as due to a supersensitivity development in the NA receptors lacking NA boutons.

C. DENERVATION OF DESCENDING NA NEURONS
(Bolme *et al.*, unpublished results)

Due to technical difficulties the sympathetic lateral column was insufficiently denervated in six out of the eight experiments in this group. However, in the ventral and dorsal horns, there was a marked reduction of NA terminals as tested histochemically in the group given 6-OH-DA. When clonidine was tested the only significant difference between treated and control rats was a potentiation of the respiration rate lowering effect at 5 and 10 min after administration. The two rats in which the NA terminals in the sympathetic lateral column were greatly reduced had a lower heart rate and arterial pressure than their matched controls, but there was no evident potentiation of the effects of clonidine on heart rate and arterial pressure in these rats. Of course, these experiments must be further developed in order to understand the role of the spinal NA receptors in autonomic control.

DISCUSSION

In the present experiments indications have been obtained that a supersensitivity develops in central NA receptors following denervation. With the present lesions it seems as if those NA terminals modulating *respiration* are mainly affected, since mainly the respiration rate lowering effect is potentiated by clonidine. Denervation by dorsal NA bundle lesion was evidently more efficient in this respect than denervation caused by neonatal administration of 6-OH-DA systemically. The heart rate lowering effect of clonidine was potentiated in the dorsal NA bundle denervated rats, but no such effect was noticed on the arterial pressure. These findings indicate that the heart rate lowering and the blood pressure decreasing effect of clonidine are not necessarily coupled. Taken together the present results suggest that respiration and heart rate can be modulated by NA nerve terminals in the limbic and neocortex, since mainly the cortical NA nerve terminals were affected by the present lesions.

In the present experiments no potentiation of the blood pressure lowering effect of clonidine was observed. This finding points indirectly to a main effect of clonidine on arterial pressure at the pons-medulla oblongata level, since the NA terminals in these areas were not degenerated. These results are in good agreement with recent studies on effects of L-DOPA on arterial pressure in rats with transections in the lower brain stem (Henning *et al.*, 1972; Schmitt *et al.*, 1973). However, an effect at the hypothalamic level cannot be ruled out, since both following systemic 6-OH-DA treatment neonatally and after dorsal NA bundle lesion by 6-OH-DA locally, hypothalamic NA terminals are to a large extent unaffected.

After lesioning the descending NA tracts to the spinal cord with local 6-OH-DA injections, clonidine caused an increased reduction of respiration rate. The mechanism underlying this effect can be the development of supersensitivity in NA receptors in the ventral horn, from which fibres to the respiratory muscles emanate.

TABLE 2. Clonidine 10 µg/kg i.v. Effects on Arterial Pressure, Heart Rate, and Respiration Rate in Rats 2 Weeks after giving 6-OH-DA in the Dorsal NA Bundle (Bolme and Fuxe, unpublished)

	Resting values Mean ± SEM (n = 6)	% Decrease from resting values Mean ± SEM (n = 6)					
		5'	10'	15'	30'	45'	60'
Arterial pressure (mm Hg):							
Control	95.2 ± 3.7	14.0 ± 1.8	13.8 ± 2.0	15.5 ± 2.3	12.4 ± 3.0	11.0 ± 4.3	10.4 ± 2.9
6-OH-DA	89.7 ± 4.0	21.3 ± 4.7	16.2 ± 2.2	13.0 ± 1.5	8.5 ± 3.4	13.5 ± 4.6	8.2 ± 5.0
Heart rate (beats/5s):							
Control	32.7 ± 1.1	7.5 ± 1.2	5.2 ± 1.1	5.7 ± 1.9	5.0 ± 2.1	5.4 ± 2.9	5.2 ± 1.5
6-OH-DA	33.0 ± 1.0	16.8 ± 3.2*	18.5 ± 2.6**	15.7 ± 2.1*	10.0 ± 4.3	11.2 ± 4.1	12.0 ± 3.3*
Respiration rate (breaths/30s):							
Control	50.0 ± 1.7	13.8 ± 2.4	10.5 ± 2.0	7.0 ± 2.1	+1.2 ± 3.2	+8.2 ± 2.6	+10.4 ± 2.6
6-OH-DA	49.2 ± 3.0	22.8 ± 2.5	21.3 ± 2.8*	19.2 ± 3.4*	11.7 ± 1.6**	9.5 ± 2.6**	1.7 ± 2.8*

* Significantly different $p < 0.05$.
** Significantly different $p < 0.01$.

Finally, it was interesting to note that systemic 6-OH-DA treatment of rats neonatally (Sachs and Jonsson, 1972; Jonsson *et al.*, 1973) which leads to an increased accumulation of NA in terminals of the pons-medulla region, did not lead to any difference in resting values or in the response of arterial pressure to clonidine. This finding suggests that it is not the absolute level of the transmitter but rather the frequency of amine released that is a factor of importance for the receptor sensitivity. It may be pointed out that the adrenergic innervation of blood vessels is intact in these animals treated with 6-OH-DA at birth (Finch *et al.*, 1973).

ACKNOWLEDGEMENTS

This work has been supported by Grants 04X-4246, 04X-715, 04X-3185 and 04X-3881 from the Swedish Medical Research Council. For excellent technical assistance we thank Miss Beth Hagman.

REFERENCES

ANDÉN, N.-E., CORRODI, H., FUXE, K., HÖKFELT, B., HÖKFELT, T., RYDIN, C., and SVENSSON, T. (1970) Evidence for a central noradrenaline receptor stimulation by clonidine. *Life Sci.* **9**, 513.

BOLME, P., and FUXE, K. (1971) Pharmacological studies on the hypotensive effects of clonidine. *Eur. J. Pharmac.* **13**, 168.

BOLME, P., and FUXE, K. (1973) Pharmacological studies on a possible role of central noradrenaline neurons in respiratory control. *J. Pharm. Pharmacol.* **25**, 351.

BOLME, P., FUXE, K., and LIDBRINK, P. (1972) On the function of central catecholamine neurons—their ro!e in cardiovascular and arousal mechanisms. *Res. Communs. Chem. Pathol. Pharmac.* **4**, 657.

CLARK, D. W., LAVERTY, R., and PHETAN, E. L. (1972) Long-lasting peripheral and central effects of 6-hydroxydopamine in rats. *Br. J. Pharmac.* **44**, 233.

FALCK, B., HILLARP, N.-Å., THIEME, G., and TORP, A. (1962) Fluorescence of catecholamines and related compounds condensed with formaldehyde. *J. Histochem. Cytochem.* **10**, 348.

FINCH, L., HAEUSLER, G., and THOENEN, H. (1973) A comparison of the effects of chemical sympathectomy by 6-hydroxydopamine in newborn and adult rats. *Br. J. Pharmac.* **47**, 249.

FUXE, K. (1965) Evidence for the existence of monoamine neurons in the central nervous system: IV, The distribution of monoamine nerve terminals in the central nervous system. *Acta physiol. scand.* **64**, Suppl. 247, 39.

FUXE, K., HÖKFELT, T., JONSSON, G., and UNGERSTEDT, U. (1970) Fluorescence microscopy in neuroanatomy. In *Contemporary Research in Neuroanatomy* (S. Ebbesen and W. Nauta, eds.), Springer, New York.

HENNING, M., RUBENSON, A., and TROLIN, G. (1972) On the localisation of the hypotensive effect of L-dopa. *J. Pharm. Pharmacol.* **24**, 447–451.

JONSSON, G., PYCOCK, CH., FUXE, K., and SACHS, CH. (1974) Changes in the development of central noradrenaline neurons following neonatal administration of 6-hydroxydopamine. *J. Neurochem.* **22** (in press).

KOBINGER, W., and WALLAND, A. (1967) Investigations into the mechanisms of the hypotensive effect of 2-(2,6-dichlorophenylamino)-2-imidazoline HCl. *Eur. J. Pharmac.* **2**, 155.

SACHS, CH., and JONSSON, G. (1972) Degeneration of central noradrenaline neurons after 6-hydroxydopamine in newborn animals. *Res. Communs. Chem. Pathol. Pharmac.* **4**, 203.

SCHMITT, H., SCHMITT, H., and FENARD, S. (1971) Evidence for an α-sympathomimetic component in the inhibitory effects of Catapresan on vasomotor centres: antagonism by piperoxane. *Eur. J. Pharmac.* **14**, 98.

SCHMITT, H., SCHMITT, H., and FENARD, S. (1973) Localization of the site of the central sympatho-inhibitory action of L-DOPA in dogs and cats. *Eur. J. Pharmac.* **22**, 212.

SINGH, B., and DE CHAMPLAIN, J. (1972) Altered ontogenesis of central noradrenergic neurons following neonatal treatment with 6-hydroxydopamine. *Brain Res.* **48**, 432.

UNGERSTEDT, U. (1971) Postsynaptic supersensitivity after 6-hydroxydopamine-induced degeneration of the nigro-striatal dopamine system. *Acta physiol. scand.*, Suppl. 367, 69.

URETSKY, N. J., and IVERSEN, L. L. (1970) Effects of 6-hydroxydopamine on catecholamine-containing neurons in the rat brain. *J. Neurochem.* **17**, 269.

LEARNING DEFICITS IN OFFSPRING
OF THE NURSING MOTHERS GIVEN PENFLURIDOL

J. Engel, S. Ahlenius, R. Brown, and P. Lundborg

Department of Pharmacology, University of Göteborg, Göteborg, Sweden

It has been shown that the monoamine neurons develop mechanisms for synthesis and storage of the monoamines at a very early stage during ontogeny (Olson and Seiger, 1972; Coyle, 1973). However, as has been shown in numerous studies, the brain levels of serotonin, noradrenaline (NA), and dopamine (DA) increase progressively with age and do not reach adult levels until several weeks after birth or, as in the case of dopamine, not until adult life (Kato, 1960; Nachmias, 1960; Karki *et al.*, 1962; Smith *et al.*, 1962; Bennet and Giarman, 1965; Agrawal *et al.*, 1966, 1968; Loizou and Salt, 1970; Kellogg and Lundborg, 1972). This progressive increase in the brain monoamine levels of the developing rat is in all probability a consequence of the postnatal centrifugal outgrowth of axons and terminals from the cell bodies (see Loizou, 1972). Furthermore, there seems to be a differential time of functional development between noradrenaline and dopamine neurons. Recently, Kellogg and Lundborg (1972, 1973) investigated the gross behavioral response of neonatal and young rats to noradrenaline and dopamine receptor stimulating agents, clonidine and apomorphine respectively. Results from these experiments indicate that the DA systems gradually develop their functions postnatally, whereas the NA systems are more mature at birth. Further support for this idea was found from experiments analyzing the disappearance of NA and DA after inhibition of the tyrosine hydroxylase (Kellogg and Lundborg, 1973). Taken together these observations indicate that the early postnatal period in rats could be considered as the vulnerable period for the functional maturation of the central DA nervous system.

In the present experiment we have administered the neuroleptic drug, penfluridol, to the nursing mothers and examined the result of this drug on the offspring 4 weeks after birth by measuring the acquisition of a conditioned avoidance response.

The acquisition of a conditioned avoidance response was measured by means of a two-way shuttle-box. The rats were trained to avoid an electric shock (unconditioned stimulus, UCS) in the box, with the sound of a house buzzer as warning stimulus (conditioned stimulus, CS).

In each trial the CS was presented for maximally 10 s followed by the CS plus the UCS for a maximum of another 10 s. A *conditioned avoidance response* (CAR) is defined as a crossing through the opening within 10 s after the CS has been presented. An escape is a cross within 10 s after the shock (UCS) had been delivered. Prior to the first training session the rats were allowed to adapt to the shuttle-box for 30 min. Training sessions lasted for 20 min and consisted of twenty trials.

The Sprague–Dawley mothers of five different litters were randomly assigned to one of the following two treatments. The nursing mothers in two of the litters were given penfluridol, 1 mg/kg orally at days 1, 3, and 5 after delivery. The nursing mothers of the three other litters received 5.5% glucose orally at corresponding time intervals.

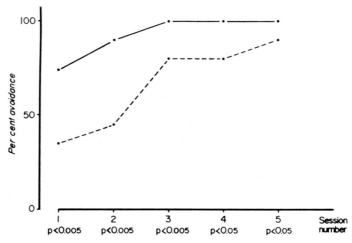

FIG. 1. Nursing rat mothers were given penfluridol (1.0 mg/kg p.o.), or 5% glucose (5 ml/kg), at days 1, 3, and 5 after delivery. The offspring was trained to a CAR 4 weeks after birth, in five consecutive daily sessions. Shown percent CAR values are medians of 11 "penfluridol"-treated and 15 "glucose"-treated infants. Statistical comparisons were performed by means of the Mann–Whitney U-test. (– – – –) penfluridol group. (———) glucose group.

At the age of 28 days the male littermates were taken out from their homecages and given five daily consecutive acquisition sessions.

As shown in Fig. 1, the infants of mothers given glucose started with 75% CAR and reached 100% CAR from the third training session. The infants of mothers given penfluridol showed an initial avoidance responding of only 35%, and after the fifth session they had reached the level of 90% avoidance responding. During every session a significant difference appeared between control and treated animals. As assessed by gross observation there was no difference between "penfluridol-treated" and "glucose-treated" animals.

There was no difference in the weight at the start of training 4 weeks after birth between the "penfluridol-treated" and the "glucose-treated" rats ($p < 0.05$). However, the "penfluridol-treated" animals were found to be more heavy than controls at the age of 8 weeks after birth ($p < 0.001$) (Table 1).

The importance of undisturbed catecholamine neurotransmission for the maintenance of conditioned avoidance behavior in adult rats and mice have been implicated in several investigations during the last decade (for rev. see Engel, 1972). In the present experiment we have found that treatment with the catecholamine receptor blocking agent penfluridol, which seems to have a preferential effect on DA receptors (Janssen *et al.*, 1970) during early

TABLE 1. BODY WEIGHT (g) AT DIFFERENT AGES IN OFFSPRING OF NURSING MOTHERS GIVEN PENFLURIDOL OR GLUCOSE

Age (weeks)	Treatment		
	Glucose	Penfluridol	Difference
4	77.8 ± 12.63 (31)	73.9 ± 20.51 (53)	$p > 0.05$
8	227.8 ± 22.65 (24)	256.1 ± 23.31 (30)	$p < 0.001$

Penfluridol, 1.0 mg/kg p.o., or 5.5% glucose (5 ml/kg p.o.) was given to the mothers at days 1, 3, and 5 after delivery. Shown are the means ± SD. Statistical comparison was performed by means of the Student's t-test.

postnatal life interfered with the acquisition of a conditioned avoidance response in rats. In view of the considerations given in the introduction this effect of penfluridol may be due to an impaired development of central catecholamine mechanisms which are involved in the acquisition of avoidance behavior.

ACKNOWLEDGEMENTS

R. B. was supported by a postdoctoral fellowship from the Swedish Medical Research Council, J. E. from the Swedish Board for Technical Development.

This research was also sponsored by the Swedish Medical Research Council (project No. 4247), the Medical Faculty, University of Göteborg, Expressens Prenatalforskningsfond, and Magnus Bergwalls Stiftelse. For generous supply of penfluridol we thank Dr. P. A. J. Janssen, Janssen Pharmaceutica, Beerse. The technical assistance of Mr. Kenn Johannessen is gratefully acknowledged.

REFERENCES

AGRAWAL, H. C., GLISSON, S. N., and HIMWICH, W. A. (1966) Changes in monoamines of rat brain during postnatal ontogeny. *Biochim. biophys. Acta* **130**, 511–513.

AGRAWAL, H. C., GLISSON, S. N., and HIMWICH, W. A. (1968) Developmental changes in monoamines of mouse brain. *Int. J. Neuropharmac.* **7**, 97–101.

BENNET, D. S., and GIARMAN, N. J. (1965) Schedule of appearance of 5-hydroxytryptamine (serotonin) and associated enzymes in the developing rat brain. *J. Neurochem.* **12**, 911–918.

COYLE, J. T. (1973) Development of the central catecholamine neurons. In *The Neurosciences, Third Study Program.* (In press.)

ENGEL, J. (1972) Neurochemistry and behaviour: a correlative study with special reference to central catecholamines. Thesis, Göteborg, Erlanders Boktryckeri AB.

JANSSEN, P. A. J., NIEMEGEERS, C. J. E., SCHELLEKENS, K. H. L., LENAERTS, F. M., VERBRUGGEN, F. J., VAN NEUTEN, J. M., and SCHAPER, W. K. A. (1970) The pharmacology of penfluridol (R 16341) a new potent and orally long-acting neuroleptic drug. *Eur. J. Pharmac.* **11**, 139–154.

KARKI, N., KUNTZMAN, R., and BRODIE, B. B. (1962) Storage, synthesis and metabolism of monoamines in the developing brain. *J. Neurochem.* **9**, 53–58.

KATO, R. (1960) Serotonin content of rat brain in relation to sex and age. *J. Neurochem.* **5**, 202.

KELLOGG, C., and LUNDBORG, P. (1972) Ontogenic variations in response to L-DOPA and monoamine receptor-stimulating agents. *Psychopharmacologia* **23**, 187–200.

KELLOGG, C., and LUNDBORG, P. (1973) Inhibition of catecholamine synthesis during ontogenic development. *Brain Res.* **61**, 321–329

LOIZOU, L. A. (1972) The postnatal ontogeny of monoamine-containing neurones in the central nervous system of the albino rat. *Brain Res.* **40**, 395–418.

LOIZOU, L. A., and SALT, P. (1970) Regional changes in monoamines of the rat brain during postnatal development. *Brain Res.* **20**, 467–470.

NACHMIAS, V. T. (1960) Amine oxidase and 5-HT in developing rat brain. *J. Neurochem.* **6**, 99–104.

OLSON, L., and SEIGER, Å. (1972) Early prenatal ontogeny of central monoamine neurons in the rat: fluorescence histochemical observations. *Z. Anat. EntwGesch.* **137**, 301–316.

SMITH, S. E., STACEY, R. S., and YOUNG, I. M. (1962) 5-HT and 5-HTPD activity in the developing nervous system of rats and guinea-pigs. In *Proc. 1st Int. Pharmacol. Meeting* (B. Uvnäs, ed.), Oxford: Pergamon Press, Oxford, pp. 101–105.

EFFECTS OF PRE- AND POSTNATAL INJECTION OF 6-HYDROXYDOPAMINE ON SLEEP AND BIOGENIC AMINES OF ADULT RAT

J. L. Valatx and J. F. Pujol

Département de Médecine Expérimentale, Université Claude Bernard, Lyon

Sixty-three rats from nine litters have been studied. Of 39 rats treated with 6-OH-DA (100 mg/kg), 20 were injected *in utero* and on the first postnatal day, and 19 with only one subcutaneous injection. The last 24 rats were injected with Ringer solution.

Fetal injection has been performed at the seventeenth day of gestation under ether anesthesia of the mother. After median laparotomy, each fetus was injected in a vitelline vein collateral wth 6-OH-DA solution (5 μl) or with Ringer solution plus ascorbic acid (1 mg/ml).

After birth, animals were regularly weighed.

Thirty days after birth, animals have been implanted with cortical and muscular electrodes and continuously recorded for a 6-day period in order to study their sleep–waking cycle.

At 60 days, 32 rats (17 6-OH-DA, 15 control) were sacrificed for cerebral biogenic amines study.

Our results showed:

(1) Growth of 6-OH-DA-treated rats was faster than in the Ringer group. At 27 days of age the weight of 6-OH-DA rats was 70 g versus 53 g in control group.

(2) Waking–sleep cycle, slow wave sleep, and paradoxical sleep were not different from control group. These results are similar to those of Matsuyama *et al.* (1973).

(3) Alterations of cerebral catecholamines and indolamines have been, however, observed:

   (a) A decrease of endogenous caudate dopamine (-35%) and telediencephalic nor-adrenaline (-30%) without alteration of brainstem NA.

   (b) A large increase of endogenous tyrosine in the brainstem ($+157\%$) in agreement with the results of Petitjean *et al.* (1972), observed on cats (2).

   (c) An increase of endogenous tryptophan ($+40\%$) associated with an augmentation of 5-HIAA/5-HT ratio in the brainstem, meaning a greater utilization of 5-HT.

These results confirm that 6-OH-DA acts on catecholamine terminals (cortex, caudate nucleus) and not on perikarya (brainstem). That could explain the normal patterns of waking and paradoxical sleep in treated rats.

REFERENCES

MATSUYAMA, S., COINDET, J., and MOURET, J. (1973) 6-Hydroxydopamine intracisternale et sommeil chez le rat. *Brain Res.* **57**, 85–95.

PETITJEAN, F., LAGUZZI, R., SORDET, F., JOUVET, M., and PUJOL, J. F. (1972) Effets de l'injection intra-ventriculaire de 6-hydroxydopamine: I, Sur les monoamines cérébrales du chat. *Brain Res.* **48**, 281–293.